Life's Rewards

Life's Rewards
Linking Dopamine, Incentive Learning, Schizophrenia, and the Mind

Richard J Beninger

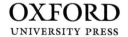
OXFORD
UNIVERSITY PRESS

OXFORD
UNIVERSITY PRESS

Great Clarendon Street, Oxford, OX2 6DP,
United Kingdom

Oxford University Press is a department of the University of Oxford.
It furthers the University's objective of excellence in research, scholarship,
and education by publishing worldwide. Oxford is a registered trade mark of
Oxford University Press in the UK and in certain other countries

Published in the United States of America by Oxford University Press
198 Madison Avenue, New York, NY 10016, United States of America

British Library Cataloguing in Publication Data
Data available

Library of Congress Control Number: 2018931003

ISBN 978-0-19-882409-1

Printed and bound by
CPI Group (UK) Ltd, Croydon, CR0 4YY

Oxford University Press makes no representation, express or implied, that the
drug dosages in this book are correct. Readers must therefore always check
the product information and clinical procedures with the most up-to-date
published product information and data sheets provided by the manufacturers
and the most recent codes of conduct and safety regulations. The authors and
the publishers do not accept responsibility or legal liability for any errors in the
text or for the misuse or misapplication of material in this work. Except where
otherwise stated, drug dosages and recommendations are for the non-pregnant
adult who is not breast-feeding

Links to third party websites are provided by Oxford in good faith and
for information only. Oxford disclaims any responsibility for the materials
contained in any third party website referenced in this work.

To Judith, Mariah, Max, and Samantha

Preface

While writing this book over the years 2012–2017, I frequently began my day with an electronic literature search beginning with the word "dopamine." I would then add terms to narrow the search to the specific topic that I was studying at the time. The term "dopamine" always came up with over 75,000 hits, immediately revealing the volume of work on this neurotransmitter and challenging the confidence of any writer who seeks to organize the information into a coherent story. It would take several volumes to achieve that goal. My aim in writing this book was a more focused effort to bring together a wide range of findings about the role of the neurotransmitter dopamine in reward-related learning so that the reader can develop a broad integrated overview of its function in day-to-day life and use that as a basis for understanding how disruptions of dopaminergic neurotransmission can lead to puzzling and sometimes paradoxical features of diseases, including schizophrenia, Parkinson's disease, attention deficit hyperactivity disorder (ADHD), and drug abuse.

To achieve this goal it is necessary first to understand the role of dopamine in reward-related or incentive learning and to place this type of learning and memory within the broader framework of multiple memory systems. I review evidence resulting from the use of a wide range of different techniques in different species, including humans, implicating increases in dopaminergic neurotransmission in the incentive learning effects of rewarding stimuli on behavior and then argue that events that lead to decreases in dopaminergic neurotransmission produce the opposite effect, inverse incentive learning. I show that cooperative social stimuli activate dopaminergic neurotransmission and serve as rewarding stimuli producing incentive learning. This background provides a basis for understanding the positive symptoms of schizophrenia, the sometimes-paradoxical symptoms of Parkinson's disease, and the symptoms and response to medication of people with ADHD. The powerful influence of conditioned incentive stimuli produced by the effects of drugs of abuse on dopaminergic neurotransmission provide a basis for better understanding drug addiction.

The book includes an overview of neuroanatomy with specific reference to the position of dopaminergic neurons in the brain. Using this neuroanatomical framework, it is possible to understand the interaction of signaling molecules activated by dopamine working in conjunction with those activated by glutamatergic inputs to the same dendritic spines that leads to synaptic changes that are the biological foundation of incentive learning. Finally, the relationship between these brain mechanisms and mental experience is considered in the last chapter.

My general approach in writing this book has been to try as much as possible to place relevant discoveries about dopamine into their historical context, emphasizing especially major scientific findings that provided the techniques and theory for further discoveries about dopamine and its role in reward-related learning. I have also emphasized the apparent conservation of dopamine function across vertebrate species and even across phyla.

This book should be accessible to senior undergraduate and graduate students with a background in neuroscience and psychology. It is relevant to students and practitioners of psychiatry and neurology. It contains a number of novel insights that should be of interest to principle investigators. For the general "educated" lay reader, portions of the book may be of interest, even if some parts prove to be too technical. All readers will find a level of integration and a common theme of neuroscience and psychology of dopamine running throughout this volume that is not available in any other book.

I am deeply indebted to many people who contributed their valuable time to this enterprise and generously provided comments and insights. Sincere thanks to David Andrew, Max Beninger, Robert Carey, Judith Davidson, Nicholas Delva, Samantha Drover, Paul Fletcher, Todor Gerdjikov, Jon Horvitz, Sheena Josselyn, Marco Leyton, Mary (Cella) Olmstead, Vern Quinsey, Robert Ranaldi, and Jeffery Rocca. Each read one chapter—Cella Olmstead read two—and provided editorial and conceptual feedback that in many cases led to major revisions, additions, or reorganization that improved the narrative and clarified the arguments. Thanks also to Carolyn Woogh, R. John MacLeod, and many others too numerous to name whose comments and discussions helped me find my way through some of the material in this book. I alone am responsible for any inaccuracies or errors that remain in the text.

Kingston artist Aida Šulcs did the artwork. Aida studied fine arts at Queen's University Kingston and graphic design at the Kootenay School of Art in Nelson, British Columbia. She began her art career in editorial illustration 45 years ago and has since worked in art education, including a residency at the Faculty of Education, Queen's University. Her exploration of human behavior through an inter-disciplinary art practice incorporates drawing, painting, photography, and performance art. Of the figures in this book she wrote:

> In imagining an oeuvre that would bring together the collected graphs and figures of this book, I decided to use a centuries' old method of intaglio printing because it exudes a human presence through the hand-drawn line, which I think is appropriate

in illustrating an act of discovery. To me the appearance of this printing process brings continuity between the history and currency of research, as well as between human agency and the scientific precision of laboratory testing.

Thank you Aida for your valuable contribution.

I thank the funding agencies that have provided support for my research for decades. In particular, I acknowledge the support of the Natural Sciences and Engineering Research Council of Canada and the Ontario Mental Health Foundation. Thank you to Tomás Palomo and the Fundatión Cerebro y Mente of Madrid, Spain; through their support of numerous international meetings, bringing together experts in neuroscience and psychiatry, they provided me with exposure to a wide range of neuroscientific topics, and to many colleagues whose ideas and insights helped me understand the role of dopamine in reward-related incentive learning.

Finally, a special thank you to my wife and fellow scientist Judith Davidson. In writing and publishing her own book, Judith showed me how it is done. Judith was always generous with her time, listening patiently to my struggles with difficult material, and, through questioning and feedback, often helped me find a solution.

Richard J. Beninger, Kingston, Ontario, September 2017

Contents

1 Introduction *1*

2 Dopamine and reward-related learning *23*
Stimulus–response learning and the law of effect *23*
Incentive learning *28*
Dopamine and incentive learning *29*
Avoidance conditioning *35*
Summary *41*

3 Dopamine and the elements of incentive learning *44*
Lever pressing for food *45*
Amphetamine-produced conditioned place preference *50*
Conditioned activity based on cocaine *54*
Conditioned avoidance responding *58*
Summary *66*

4 Multiple memory systems *68*
Multiple memory systems in humans *68*
Multiple memory systems in non-human animals *75*
Competition and cooperation among memory systems in animals *82*
Competition and cooperation among memory systems in humans *84*
Why did we evolve multiple memory systems? *87*
Summary *89*

5 Dopamine as the dependent variable *91*
Postmortem biochemistry of dopamine and its metabolites *92*
Intracerebral microdialysis *95*
Electrophysiology *99*
In vivo electrochemistry *105*
Neuroimaging *111*
Summary *121*

6 Dopamine and inverse incentive learning *123*
Novel stimuli and dopamine *124*
Intense stimuli and dopamine *126*
Aversive stimuli and dopamine *126*
The bar test *132*

Sensitization of descent latency in the bar test *132*

Conditioned increases in descent latency *137*

Habituation *139*

Understanding sensitization and conditioning of descent latency *141*

Summary *148*

7 Dopamine receptor subtypes and incentive learning *149*

Discovery of D1 and D2 receptors *149*

Discovery of D1- and D2-like receptor families *153*

Differential locomotor function of D1- and D2-like receptors *155*

Differential incentive learning function of D1- and D2-like receptors *158*

Dopamine receptor-knockout mice and incentive learning *164*

Psychopharmacology of D3 and D4 receptors *167*

Receptor heteromers that include dopamine receptors *174*

Summary *176*

8 Dopamine and social cooperation *177*

Dopamine and social cooperation in humans *177*

Dopamine and social cooperation in non-humans animals *184*

Dopamine and social cooperation in monkeys *186*

Dopamine and social cooperation in rats *186*

Dopamine and social cooperation in voles *190*

Dopamine and social cooperation in hamsters *191*

Dopamine and social cooperation in avians *192*

Dopamine and social cooperation in reptiles *196*

Dopamine and social cooperation in amphibians *198*

Dopamine and social cooperation in fish *198*

Dopamine and social cooperation in insects *200*

Summary *201*

9 Schizophrenia, Parkinson's disease, and attention deficit hyperactivity disorder *203*

Schizophrenia and dopamine *205*

Parkinson's disease and dopamine *218*

Dopamine receptor antagonist medications *226*

Dopamine agonist medications *234*

Attention deficit hyperactivity disorder and dopamine *236*

Summary *242*

10 Drug abuse and incentive learning *245*

Drugs of abuse activate dopaminergic neurotransmission *246*

Drugs of abuse produce incentive learning *248*

Role of conditioned incentive stimuli in drug abuse *251*

Mechanisms of the need state *256*

Treating drug abuse *258*

Summary *264*

11 Neuroanatomy and dopamine systems *266*

Functional anatomy of vision *267*

Functional anatomy of audition *270*

Functional anatomy of olfaction *272*

Functional anatomy of gustation *273*

Functional anatomy of somatosensation *275*

Multimodal cortical cells *277*

Functional anatomy of motor systems *279*

Anatomy of dopamine systems and the basal ganglia *285*

Summary *293*

12 Mechanisms of dopamine-mediated incentive learning *295*

The wave of phosphorylation *296*

The wave of phosphatase activity *298*

Local enhancement of dopamine signaling *302*

Effects of the dopamine signal *304*

Signaling molecules in incentive learning *308*

Short-term and long-term incentive learning *310*

Role of the indirect pathway in incentive learning *316*

Possible mechanism of inverse incentive learning *320*

Incentive stimuli and dopamine release *325*

Summary *328*

13 Dopamine and mental experience *330*

Evidence linking brain and mind *330*

Evidence linking dopamine and mental experience *335*

Do non-human animals have mental experiences? *345*

Summary *350*

References and notes *353*

Index *457*

Chapter 1

Introduction

The effects of rewarding stimuli on behavior are like the effects of the moon on the tides.[1] Whether or not the mechanisms of planetary influences are understood, the oceans' waters relentlessly rise and fall. So it is with the effects of rewarding stimuli on behavior. Whether or not the mechanisms of dopamine-mediated incentive learning are understood, the behavioral changes produced by rewarding stimuli inevitably occur. Rewarding stimuli constantly mold the organization of the behavior of organisms by altering the ability of stimuli in the environment to control responding. The effects of rewarding stimuli take place without conscious awareness. This book is about those effects and their underlying mechanisms. As you will see, the neurotransmitter dopamine is a central player, but no neurotransmitter system operates in a vacuum; in later chapters I discuss how dopamine operates within complex brain circuitry to organize the response tendencies of individuals to the various people, places, and things that they encounter in day-to-day life. In this chapter, I provide an overview of the remaining chapters so that the reader can get a general sense of the big picture before wading into the multiple details of each section. Extensive references for all of the points presented in this chapter are provided in Chapters 2–13.

In the early decades of the twentieth century, departments of psychology began to spring up at universities. At the time, the influence of Charles Darwin's (1809–1882) writings about evolution was widespread and biology was making great strides toward the modern evolutionary synthesis that would reach fruition in the 1930s and 1940s. Throughout the twentieth century, the biological bases of animal, including human, behavior, encompassing its genetic and environmental causes, underlying neurophysiology and evolutionary origins began to be understood. Research in psychology departments increasingly sought to explain behavior in terms of the influence of environmental stimuli, genetic, and epigenetic interactions with early experience, to identify brain regions, neurotransmitters, and circuits that control behavior, and to understand the possible evolutionary origins of human nature.

One line of investigation focused on the modification of behavior by its consequences. In the late nineteenth century Edward Thorndike's (1874–1949) observations of the problem-solving behavior of cats led him to propose a putative law of learning stating that responses in a particular situation that are followed by satisfying consequences tend to be repeated when that situation is encountered again. Behaviorists developed this idea but replaced Thorndike's "satisfier" with the term "reinforcer" to refer to the class of stimuli that can lead to the apparent strengthening of stimulus–response connections suggested by Thorndike. The behaviorists' quest for universal laws of learning gave rise to an extensive research enterprise involving many prominent scientists, including John B. Watson (1878–1958), Clark Hull (1884–1952), Kenneth Spence (1907–1967), Burrhus F. Skinner (1904–1990), and many others. The behaviorists' approach held wide sway in psychology during the early half of the twentieth century.

Beginning around the middle of the twentieth century a number of observations began to challenge the generality of the putative laws of learning and the influence of behaviorism began to decline. Observations of phenomena such as conditioned taste aversion, instinctive drift, and sign tracking violated behaviorists' principles of the need for temporal contiguity between stimulus and response for response strengthening by a reinforcer, and the ability of reinforcers themselves to strengthen stimulus–response connections. The observation of avoidance responses in the presence of stimuli previously paired with an aversive event, an example of behavior that was maintained in the absence of an overt reinforcer, challenged behaviorisms' goal of describing behavior based on observable variables without reference to internal states of the organism. Although the experimental analysis of behavior carried out by behaviorists provided many valuable findings that continue to have an influence in basic neuroscience research and in areas such as behavior therapy and education, their quest for universal laws of learning failed.

Incentive theory arose as an alternative framework for explaining the effects of rewarding stimuli on behavior. Incentive theorists replaced the term "reinforcer" or "reinforcing stimulus" with the more neutral term "reward" or "rewarding stimulus" in an effort to avoid some of the strong links to behaviorism suggested by "reinforcer." Although the term "incentive motivation" appears in the earlier literature, it was psychologists, including Robert Bolles (1928–1994) and Dalbir Bindra (1922–1980), who showed how the flexibility of incentive theory could provide a framework for understanding behavioral observations that appeared to fall outside of the purview of behaviorism. For example, as you will see later, incentive theory provides a framework for understanding conditioned avoidance responding. According to incentive theory, rewarding stimuli produce *incentive learning: the acquisition by neutral stimuli of an increased ability to elicit approach and other responses.* "Other responses" could include pushing, pulling, digging, biting, and so on, depending on the situation and the natural abilities of the animal.

While the effects of rewarding stimuli on behavior were being debated during the transition from behaviorism to modern incentive theory, James Olds (1922–1976) and Peter Milner discovered that direct electrical stimulation of the brain could serve as a rewarding stimulus. In the years that followed, Annica Dahlström and Kjell Fuxe discovered the dopamine pathways in the brain. It then began to emerge that brain areas that would support electrical self-stimulation showed considerable overlap with areas that contained dopaminergic neurons. Subsequently, Roy Wise and co-workers discovered that drugs that block dopamine receptors in the brain reduce the rewarding effects of food. These findings suggested that dopamine is involved in incentive learning.

Chapter 2 discusses further details of the link between dopamine and reward-related learning. It also discusses the finding that dopamine is involved in avoidance learning. Rats with reduced brain dopaminergic neurotransmission are impaired in their ability to learn to avoid mild electric shock by shuttling to the safe side of a test chamber; rats trained to perform the avoidance response before dopamine reduction continue to make avoidance responses for a time after dopamine reduction but responding gradually declines over trials. These important findings implicate dopamine and reward-related incentive learning in learning to avoid an aversive stimulus, as well as in learning to respond to an appetitive stimulus as shown by Wise and colleagues. Furthermore, they show that *once incentive learning has occurred, conditioned incentive stimuli can control responding for a time even when dopaminergic neurotransmission is greatly reduced.* This applies to incentive learning based on shock avoidance or food. Keeping this observation in mind will help to understand many of the experimental results discussed in this book.

A number of behavioral approaches are taken to the study of incentive learning. Perhaps the most defining of behaviorism is rats lever pressing for food in a Skinner box. As discussed in Chapter 3, training begins by feeding the rat from a food hopper affixed to one of the walls of the test chamber. Each food pellet delivery is signaled by the click of the feeder magazine. During this stage of training, the click and the food hopper will become conditioned incentive stimuli because they are among the stimuli encountered just prior to eating the food pellet. The release of dopamine produced by consumption of the food pellet will lead to an increase in the ability of the click and food hopper to elicit approach and other responses; *those stimuli will also acquire the ability themselves to produce dopamine release and can be used to produce further incentive conditioning about stimuli that precede them.* Once this conditioning has taken place, if the click occurs only when the rat is near the lever, the lever and lever-related stimuli will gradually become conditioned incentive stimuli with an increased ability to elicit approach and other responses. As the rat approaches and manipulates the lever, it will learn that a downward displacement produces the click and food and will then have acquired the lever-press response. As a result, in addition to the click and food hopper, the lever and lever-related stimuli will be conditioned incentive stimuli. If dopaminergic neurotransmission is blocked during the training phase, incentive learning will be impaired and the lever-press response will be acquired slowly or not at all. When an animal trained while dopamine function is intact is returned to the Skinner box it will likely approach the food hopper soon after being placed there and then approach the lever, demonstrating the conditioned incentive value of those stimuli. If dopamine function is blocked when the trained rat is returned to the Skinner box, lever-pressing responses will be observed at the beginning of the session, revealing the previous incentive learning. However, *with continued exposure to conditioned incentive stimuli while dopaminergic neurotransmission is blocked, those stimuli (the lever and lever-related stimuli in this case) will gradually lose their incentive value and lever-press responses will decline*; similarly, in this case, the click and food hopper will gradually lose their incentive value and approaches to those stimuli will also decline.

Conditioned place preference learning, often used to evaluate the possible rewarding properties of various drugs, can also be understood to involve incentive learning. In this procedure, one side of a test chamber with two distinct sides is paired with the drug in daily 30-minute sessions, for example. Equal exposure is given to the other side but no drug is given there. A place preference is demonstrated on a test day when the animals in an un-drugged state are given access to both sides and are observed to spend more time in the side previously paired with the drug. Drugs, for example, amphetamine, that augment dopaminergic neurotransmission produce a place preference; if dopamine receptor-blocking drugs are given prior to amphetamine during pairing sessions, no place preference is observed. From an incentive learning point of view, the stimuli from the side of the test chamber associated with the dopamine-augmenting drug become conditioned incentive stimuli with an increased ability to elicit approach and other responses. On the test day, even though the animals are drug free, they are observed to spend more time in the drug-paired chamber putatively because of the increased incentive value of the stimuli there. We have found that the dopamine receptor blocker haloperidol dose-dependently blocks the establishment of place preference conditioning based on amphetamine; if the lowest effective dose of haloperidol for blocking establishment of conditioning is given to amphetamine-conditioned rats for the first time on the test day, place preference is still seen. This demonstrates again that once incentive learning has occurred, conditioned incentive stimuli can control responding for a time, even when dopaminergic neurotransmission is greatly reduced.

As mentioned above, dopamine-mediated incentive learning is also involved in conditioned avoidance responding. Chapter 3 discusses the elements of avoidance learning. Results show that dopamine is not necessary for learning the association between a signal for shock, for example, a tone, and the shock itself. Neither is dopamine necessary for learning the cognitive map of the test environment, including the location of safety, nor is dopamine required for demonstrating improved efficiency of escaping from electric shock. Dopaminergic neurotransmission seems to play a critical role in incentive learning, the acquisition by safety-related stimuli of an increased ability to elicit approach and other responses. If avoidance training begins while dopaminergic neurotransmission is blocked, animals fail to learn to shuttle towards safety related stimuli during exposure to shock-associated stimuli even though they appear to be threatened by the shock-associated stimuli. If animals are first trained to make avoidance responses and then tested following treatment with a dopamine-depleting drug, they continue to make avoidance responses for a number of trials but gradually the avoidance response is lost. From an incentive learning point of view, the initial performance of the avoidance response in these trained animals occurred because safety-related stimuli had acquired an increased ability to elicit approach and other responses; when testing took place with dopaminergic neurotransmission reduced, that learning initially controlled responding but was gradually lost.

These observations reveal that there are multiple memory systems; this is the topic of Chapter 4. This idea emerged in the middle of the twentieth century in part as a result of the findings of neuropsychologist Brenda Milner working at McGill University in Montreal. In her studies of the now-famous neurological patient HM, Milner revealed evidence of learning and memory in an amnesic patient. HM's amnesia resulted from the bilateral surgical removal of the medial temporal lobes for the treatment of his severe epilepsy. HM was unable to learn new information about facts and events following the surgery, although it did cure his epilepsy. However, Milner found that he showed day-to-day improvement on a drawing task involving observing his hand reflected in a mirror while he traced between parallel lines. Even though HM was unable to remember having done the task the day before, his performance improved. This and a number of related observations from studies with HM and other neurological patients revealed learning and memory in apparently amnesic patients and led to the recognition that there are multiple memory systems.

One system for classifying memories identifies them as declarative or nondeclarative. Declarative memories are memories for facts and events, explicit information that can be recalled consciously in humans; non-declarative memories are implicit, revealed, for example, in the development of skills and habits and are not consciously recalled in humans. People with bilateral damage to their medial temporal lobes show declarative memory impairments; the hippocampus is located in the medial temporal lobe and it has become recognized as an important neural substrate of declarative memory formation. There appear to be a number of subtypes of non-declarative memory and each appears to be associated with a different brain region. For example, aversive conditioning, that is, learning the relationship between a particular environmental stimulus and threat, relies on the amygdala. Incentive learning leads to another form of non-declarative memory; it appears to rely on dopamine and dopamine-innervated brain regions, including the striatum. People with Parkinson's disease who suffer from a loss of brain dopamine show intact learning on declarative memory tasks but impaired learning on incentive learning tasks.

The use of the term "conscious" in the definition of declarative memory limits its applicability to non-human animals. Consciousness is defined by a person's ability to describe his/her mental experiences or to respond to written or spoken instructions; it is difficult to assess the possible mental experiences of non-human animals because of our limited ability to communicate with them about what they may be experiencing. However, it is possible to evaluate the effects on memory of damage to brain areas in animals that are homologous to those areas in humans that have been identified to be the possible neural substrates of declarative or non-declarative memory types. Thus, damage to the hippocampus in animals impairs their ability to learn tasks that require memory for spatial details of an environment. Just as HM was greatly impaired in learning the path from point A to point B in a new building, rats with bilateral hippocampal damage are impaired in their ability to learn the path in a maze from the start box to the goal box. This suggests that spatial learning in rats may be a form of declarative memory, even though rats cannot tell us if they are conscious of spatial arrangements. Rats with bilateral damage to dopaminergic neurons that project to the striatum, like humans with Parkinson's disease, are impaired in the acquisition of incentive learning tasks. This reveals a similar role for dopamine in the striatum in incentive learning in human and non-human animals. As already mentioned, multiple memory systems is the topic of Chapter 4.

Studies of the possible role played by various brain regions or neurotransmitter systems in the control of behavior involve observing the behavioral consequences of either activating or inactivating the region or system. Alternatively, the activity of the brain region or neurotransmitter systems can be recorded while observing behavior, allowing identification of possible correlations between the two. In the latter case, if dopaminergic systems are the target of investigation, dopamine is the dependent variable, that is, the quantity measured. Numerous studies fall into this category. Recording methods include postmortem biochemistry, intracerebral microdialysis, electrophysiology, in vivo electrochemistry, and imaging techniques, including fiber photometry, positron emission tomography, and functional magnetic resonance imaging (fMRI). Results provide compelling evidence for a role for dopamine in incentive learning.

At least two major findings have come out of recording studies of dopamine as the dependent variable. One is that primary rewarding stimuli such as food and water, or sexual stimuli lead to increased firing of dopaminergic neurons and increased concentrations of dopamine in the terminal regions of those neurons. The second is that cues that reliably predict a primary rewarding stimulus gradually acquire the ability themselves to increase firing of dopaminergic neurons and to increase the concentration of dopamine in the terminal regions of those neurons. In conjunction with the second finding, it has been observed that primary rewarding stimuli that are reliably signaled by a particular cue begin to lose their ability to activate dopaminergic neurons in parallel with the acquisition by the cues of the ability to activate dopaminergic neurons. However, it is important to note that if those cues are presented repeatedly without being followed by a primary rewarding stimulus, they lose their ability to activate dopaminergic neurons. This means that *even though reliably signaled primary rewarding stimuli no longer activate dopaminergic neurons, those primary rewarding stimuli remain critical for conditioned stimuli to retain their ability to activate dopaminergic neurons.*

Cues that reliably predict primary rewarding stimuli become conditioned incentive stimuli with an increased ability to elicit approach and other responses. Once a cue is established as a conditioned incentive stimulus, it can for a time control behavior even when dopaminergic neurotransmission is greatly reduced as already stated. This means that even though conditioned incentive stimuli acquire the ability themselves to activate dopaminergic neurotransmission, their conditioned incentive properties do not depend on that ability. What that ability does is to make it possible for conditioned incentive stimuli themselves to act as rewarding stimuli, leading to the acquisition by neutral stimuli that precede them of an increased ability to elicit approach and other responses. Incentive learning and the acquired ability of conditioned stimuli to activate dopaminergic neurons are separable aspects of reward-related learning that probably rely upon different mechanisms.

Chapter 5 reviews studies of dopamine as the dependent variable. The remarkable convergence of findings from diverse approaches to recording the responses of dopaminergic neurons to rewarding stimuli is striking. The chapter also covers imaging studies mostly done with human participants. Positron emission tomography studies provide further evidence that dopamine concentrations increase in dopamine terminal areas as a result of primary rewarding stimuli and the cues that reliably signal them. fMRI studies are included, although they do not measure dopamine as the dependent variable, but rather they measure blood oxygenation level-dependent (BOLD) responses. Results show that rewarding stimuli lead to increases in BOLD responses in dopamine terminal regions, consistent with the results of positron emission tomography studies and with numerous studies using other methodologies in non-human animals.

Dopaminergic neurons are activated by novel and intense stimuli. In the case of novel stimuli, the level of activation of dopaminergic neurons decreases rapidly from one presentation to the next if those stimuli do not signal biologically important outcomes such as food reward or safety from danger; the gradual loss of behavioral responses such as orientation and approach to novel stimuli following their repeated presentation is referred to as "habituation." In the case of intense stimuli, behavioral orienting and dopaminergic responses do not appear to habituate. However, the maximal level of dopaminergic neuron activation by intense stimuli is only about half of that seen when rewarding stimuli are presented. Electrophysiological studies show that the pattern of dopaminergic neuron activation following novel or intense stimuli is also different from that seen following rewarding stimuli: the peak response is earlier for novel or intense stimuli and activation is followed by a period of *decreased* dopaminergic neuronal firing that is not normally seen following rewarding stimuli.

Aversive stimuli such as mild electric foot shock also activate dopaminergic neurons, but they may do so because they are either novel or intense. The similar electrophysiological signature produced by aversive stimuli to that produced by novel or intense stimuli supports this suggestion. Intracerebral microdialysis studies show that aversive restraint leads to increased dopamine release in dopaminergic neuron terminal areas but that over a period of chronic restraint (e.g., two hours), the dopamine signal gradually is lost and then if restraint continues, dopamine levels begin to fall below baseline.

The effects of novel, intense, and aversive stimuli on dopaminergic neuron activity and dopamine levels in terminal areas are discussed in Chapter 6. That chapter also discusses a phenomenon termed "inverse incentive learning:" *the loss by stimuli of their ability to elicit approach and other responses*. Inverse incentive learning may take place when dopamine levels are reduced below normal; this occurs, for example, when an expected rewarding stimulus fails to arrive and has been termed "negative prediction error." Werner Schmidt (1950–2007) and colleagues at Tubingen University discovered that rats (paired group) injected with a low dose of the dopamine receptor antagonist haloperidol and placed in a rearing position with their forepaws resting on an elevated horizontal bar got down right away on the first test, but when the test was performed from day to day, a gradual increase in descent latency was observed. Control (unpaired) rats tested daily on the bar and then given haloperidol later in their home cage showed no comparable increase in descent latency. When both the paired and unpaired groups were tested with haloperidol after a number of trials, only the paired group showed increased descent latencies. Since both groups had a similar drug history prior to the time when they were both tested with haloperidol, the elevated descent latencies in the paired group cannot be attributed simply to repeated haloperidol injection. Instead, it appears that it is the pairing of dopamine receptor blockade by haloperidol and the testing environment that leads to the increased descent latencies.

My students and I have termed this phenomenon "inverse incentive learning," arguing that stimuli repeatedly paired with reduced levels of dopaminergic neurotransmission produced by, for example, haloperidol gradually lose their ability to elicit approach and other responses, manifested by increased descent latencies in the bar test. Perhaps the brief period of reduced dopamine neuron firing observed after the elevation produced by novel stimuli leads to the gradual loss by those stimuli of the ability to elicit approach and other responses that is defined as habituation. In the case of intense stimuli, the brief period of inhibition following excitation of dopaminergic neurons may prevent incentive learning to those stimuli. When aversive stimuli are encountered, the initial elevation of dopaminergic neuron firing may increase the likelihood of the animal finding safety and of incentive learning occurring to safety-related stimuli. If the animal fails to find safety in the presence of chronic aversive stimuli, the activation of dopaminergic neurons gradually subsides and then they become inhibited. This may lead to inverse incentive learning resulting in a loss of responding to stimuli associated with chronic aversion, similar to the phenomenon of learned helplessness. These ideas are discussed in Chapter 6.

Dopamine produces its effects by acting on five major receptor subtypes that are members of two families: D1-like receptors, including D1 and D5 receptors, are defined by their ability to stimulate the second messenger cyclic 3',5'-adenosine monophosphate (cAMP); D2-like receptors, including D2, D3, and D4 receptors, do not stimulate cAMP and, in fact, inhibit signaling by this second messenger. In the course of discovering the dopamine receptors, it was found that antipsychotic drugs used to treat the positive symptoms of schizophrenia act as antagonists of dopamine receptors. A strong positive correlation was found between the average clinical doses of a number of antipsychotic medications and their ability to compete with radioactively labeled dopamine for dopamine D2-like receptors. This suggested the hypothesis that dopaminergic neurotransmission was overactive in the brains of people suffering from schizophrenia. As discussed later, it also suggests the hypothesis that people with schizophrenia suffer from excessive incentive learning.

As discussed in Chapter 7, the identification and development of drugs that act with relative selectivity at D1- or D2-like receptors enabled an investigation of the possible differential role of the two dopamine receptor families in the control of behavior. Elevations of dopaminergic neurotransmission produce a stimulant effect on behavior, for example by increasing locomotion in a test box. Conversely, decreases in dopaminergic neurotransmission produce a sedating effect on behavior and decrease locomotion in a test box. Studies with relatively selective pharmacological agents revealed that blockade of either D1- or D2-like receptors led to decreased locomotion and stimulation of D1- or D2-like receptors elevated locomotion; D2-like receptor agonists generally produced greater locomotor stimulation than D1-like receptor agonists. These results implicated both dopamine receptor families in the control of locomotor activity.

Studies of the possible role of D1- and D2-like receptors in reward-related incentive learning similarly implicated both families. For example, lever pressing for food by trained animals showed a gradual decline following treatment with an antagonist of either receptor family, replicating the observations of Roy Wise and co-workers mentioned above showing that dopamine receptor blockade gradually decreases the ability of food-related incentive stimuli to elicit approach and other responses. Agonists with relative selectivity for either receptor family produced a conditioned place preference. When studies evaluated further details of the effects of dopamine receptor family-selective compounds, some differences were found. Thus, in a discrete-trial task, D2-like receptor antagonists seemed to have a greater effect than D1-like receptor antagonists on lengthening the duration of head entries into the feeder aperture, whereas D1-like receptor antagonists reduced the proportion of responses to the conditioned incentive stimulus more than D2-like receptor antagonists. In studies where a conditioned incentive stimulus was being used to control an operant lever-press response, D1-like receptor agonists impaired learning, whereas D2-like receptor agonists did not. This result putatively showed that tonic activation of D1-like receptors with an agonist masked the conditioned reward-related signal at D1-like receptors leading to impaired learning. Agonists acting selectively at D2-like receptors, however, preserved the reward-related signal at D1-like receptors allowing learning to proceed. Because stimulation of D2-like receptors also stimulates motor activity, animals treated with D2-like receptor-selective agonists not only showed learning to respond for conditioned rewarding stimuli, but also showed an enhanced effect by making more lever presses overall.

An alternative to using relatively selective pharmacological tools to target the D1- or D2-like receptor family is to use molecular biological techniques to genetically engineer mice that do not express a particular dopamine receptor type and to evaluate them in incentive learning tasks. One potential difficulty with this approach is that the nervous system compensates for alterations during development; the outcome following damage to the developing brain is often less severe than comparable damage to the developed brain. Notwithstanding this concern, studies with D1 receptor-knockout and D2 receptor-knockout mice have shown that they are impaired in a variety of incentive learning tasks.

D3 receptors seem to play a unique role in incentive learning. A number of studies using a variety of D3 receptor-selective compounds showed that D3 receptors play a more important role in the *expression* than in the *acquisition* of incentive learning. For example, in conditioned place preference based on amphetamine, a D3 receptor-selective antagonist blocks expression at a lower dose than it blocks acquisition. This can be contrasted with D1-like or D2 receptor-preferring antagonists that block acquisition at a lower dose than expression. Postmortem biochemical assays for D3 receptor protein or messenger RNA showed elevated levels in animals that were killed after removal from an environment previously paired with cocaine (a drug that enhances dopaminergic neurotransmission) versus control animals with a similar drug history but that had not been exposed to an environment paired with the drug before sacrifice. Results suggest that exposure to conditioned incentive stimuli leads to an up-regulation of D3 receptors.

Dopamine receptor subtypes form heteromers with each other and with the receptors of other neurotransmitters (e.g., N-methyl-D-aspartate glutamate receptor, adenosine 2A receptor, growth hormone secretagogue receptor 1a for the neuropeptide ghrelin) and the signaling properties of these heteromers can differ from those of either receptor in isolation. These findings have opened up a new area of investigation. A complete understanding of the role of dopamine receptor subtypes in the control of locomotor activity and learning will require the integration of new findings from studies of dopamine receptor subtype-containing heteromers.

Chapter 8 shifts from these considerations of the possible functions of individual dopamine receptor subtypes in the control of behavior to a discussion of the many links between dopamine and socially cooperative behavior. From these links it appears that for many species incentive learning may play a central role in the formation of social bonds between individuals and in the formation of groups. As mentioned above, fMRI studies do not measure dopamine directly but rather BOLD changes in various brain areas are monitored. Results show increased BOLD changes in dopamine terminal areas, including the nucleus accumbens or dorsal striatum, when participants are imaged while engaging in a cooperative social interaction with a stranger or viewing a picture of a person with whom they are romantically in love, respectively. These findings show that neuronal activity is enhanced in dopamine terminal areas when human volunteers are engaged with a socially significant other person.

In vivo microdialysis of the nucleus accumbens shows increased dopamine release in mother rats when they parent their pups and neurotoxic damage to dopaminergic neurons decreases maternal behavior. Mother rats will perform an operant response to gain access to their pups and juvenile rats show a conditioned preference for a place associated with social contact with another juvenile rat. These finding show that social interactions produce reward-related learning leading to acquisition by the cooperative interlocutor and other associated environmental stimuli of the ability to elicit approach and other responses in the future.

Prairie voles are one of the rare mammalian species that forms lifelong pair bonds. The bond is formed when a male and female engage in courtship behavior that culminates in copulation. Treatment with dopamine receptor antagonists while courting and copulation are taking place blocks the formation of the pair bond. However, treatment with a dopamine receptor agonist during courting that does not end in copulation leads to the formation of a pair bond; pair bonding does not normally occur when copulation does not take place. Adult male Syrian hamsters show a preference for a place previously associated with the scent of vaginal secretions from a female conspecific. A dopamine receptor antagonist given during pairing sessions blocks this effect and in vivo microdialysis studies show increased dopamine release in the preoptic area of the males when they encounter the female scent. These findings with prairie voles and Syrian hamsters implicate dopamine in incentive learning about social stimuli.

Male songbirds sing directed song to attract a mate and to defend their territory; dopamine may play a role in the formation of mating pairs. Measures of dopamine levels in the preoptic area of finches were higher in birds paired with an opposite-sex conspecific compared with those paired with a same-sex conspecific. An index of dopaminergic neuron activity in the ventral midbrain was positively correlated with number of directed songs and the amount of courtship behavior received from the partner during the observation periods before sacrifice. Individual species of finches show phenotypic differences in affiliation behavior; postmortem immunohistochemical experiments show larger numbers of dopamine cells in the ventral midbrain of more affiliative species.

Results reveal a possible link between dopamine and sociality, with more social species having more dopamine cells.

Members of bird species that form larger flocks have more dopamine cells than members of species that form smaller flocks. In zebrafish, shoaling behavior develops over the first several weeks post-fertilization and whole-brain levels of dopamine increase over the same period. Fish treated with a dopamine receptor blocker show less of a tendency to approach a shoaling stimulus. In untreated fish, exposure to animated images of other zebrafish leads to postmortem increases in measures of dopamine in several brain areas and the magnitude of the increase is associated with the duration of exposure. In migratory locusts, decreases in dopamine are associated with the transition from the gregarious to the solitary phase and, conversely, increases in dopamine are associated with the transition from solitary to gregarious. Perhaps in many species, dopamine may mediate incentive learning about conspecific stimuli that increases the ability of those stimuli to elicit approach and other responses that, in turn, lead to aggregation.

As already mentioned above, evidence suggests that dopaminergic neurotransmission is overactive in the brains of people who suffer from schizophrenia and the medications that are used to treat the psychotic symptoms of schizophrenia are dopamine receptor blockers. Under normal conditions, increases in dopamine associated with cooperative social interactions may lead to incentive learning about the cooperative interlocutor, that person acquiring an increased ability to elicit approach and other responses in the future; if dopaminergic neurotransmission is overactive, excessive incentive learning may occur. In unmedicated, afflicted individuals, the apparent increase in the incentive value of other people and environmental stimuli while encountered in a hyperdopaminergic state may lead to the development of delusions. Delusions may be formulated using declarative memory systems that remain relatively intact. Thus, delusions may be understood as somewhat reasonable interpretations of the world as it appears to a person with excessive incentive learning. For example, the delusion may be one of persecution by other people or by technology; alternatively, the delusion may be one of grandiosity, the sufferer apparently believing that others see her as a great person. In either case, the delusion can be understood as issuing from the attribution of incentive value to stimuli, including other people, that normally would be ignored. As discussed in Chapter 9, the observation that the content of delusions shows a strong cultural link supports this interpretation.

In Parkinson's disease, dopamine neuron numbers are substantially decreased. This hypodopaminergic state is characterized by bradykinesia, rigidity, and tremor. Although Parkinson's disease is often characterized as a motor disturbance, patients periodically show apparently intact motor capacities, such as the ability to walk or run, a phenomenon termed *kinesia paradoxa*. If patients with Parkinson's disease are conceptualized as suffering from a loss of incentive learning and perhaps excessive inverse incentive learning, symptoms of bradykinesia and the observation of *kinesia paradoxa* can be understood. From this point of view, the gradual loss of motor ability of patients with Parkinson's disease is seen as the failure of new incentive learning and the loss by conditioned incentive stimuli of their ability to elicit approach and other responses. In an unmedicated patient who has become severely bradykinetic, a conditioned incentive stimulus that has not been encountered before while in a hypodopaminergic state should retain its ability to elicit approach and other responses providing a basis for understanding *kinesia paradoxa*.

Medications used to treat Parkinson's disease include the dopamine precursor 3,4-dihydroxyphenylalanine (L-DOPA). By elevating brain levels of dopamine, L-DOPA may prolong incentive learning that normally would be lost with the death of dopamine neurons. Patients with Parkinson's disease who take too much L-DOPA may experience excessive incentive learning, leading to the formulation of delusions, a phenomenon well documented in this population. Conversely, patients with schizophrenia who are treated with doses of antipsychotic medications that interfere with normal incentive learning might be expected to begin to show symptoms of Parkinson's disease, a phenomenon well documented in this population. Results suggest that there is a continuum of synaptic concentrations of dopamine with too little on one end leading to a loss of incentive learning and possibly inverse incentive learning, and too much on the other end leading to excessive incentive learning. Normal functioning appears to require synaptic concentrations of dopamine within a range between these two extremes.

Attention deficit hyperactivity disorder (ADHD) appears to be another condition related to low dopamine. One of the most remarkable observations about ADHD is that psychomotor stimulant drugs such as methylphenidate or amphetamine have an apparent calming effect. How can low dopamine lead to the classic triad of Parkinson's symptoms in some individuals and to hyperactivity and inattention in others? The answer may lie in the age of the patients: Parkinson's disease is usually seen in the elderly, although cases in younger adults also occur; ADHD is normally seen in children or early adolescents. Young adults can also show symptoms related to inattention but usually not hyperactivity. In animal studies, depletions of dopamine in adults leads to hypokinesia like that seen in Parkinson's disease; however, similar depletions done in young animals around the time of birth have an opposite effect, leading to hyperactivity. Novel stimuli have an unconditioned ability to elicit approach and other responses. The preponderance of novel stimuli in the environments of young animals may have an energizing effect on locomotor activity that masks the loss of dopamine. However, dopamine-mediated incentive learning may serve to focus animals on particular environmental stimuli, those associated with primary rewarding stimuli. If dopamine levels are low, incentive learning may be limited and young individuals may move from stimulus to stimulus in their environment, failing to focus on particular stimuli and appearing to be impaired in their ability to stay on task. The activating effects of novelty may lessen in young adults, but if they have low dopamine, attention deficits may persist. From this point of view, dopamine-enhancing drugs will increase incentive learning and improve the ability of environment stimuli to control behavior. As discussed in Chapter 9, these considerations raise the intriguing question of whether people who suffer from ADHD are more likely to develop Parkinson's disease in later life.

Drug addiction is another disorder that involves dopamine. Drugs of abuse, including nicotine, ethanol, marijuana, amphetamine, cocaine, morphine, heroin, and numerous related drugs, rely on dopamine for their ability to produce reward-related learning. All of these agents are self-administered by animals, all produce a conditioned place preference, all produce increased concentrations of extracellular dopamine in dopamine neuron terminal areas, and dopamine receptor antagonist drugs block the reward-related learning effects of these drugs. Especially with relatively fast-acting drugs of abuse such as amphetamine, cocaine, heroin, and perhaps nicotine, environmental stimuli associated with drug taking will become conditioned incentive stimuli. In the future those stimuli will have an increased ability to control behavior by eliciting approach and other responses. In the case of slower-acting agents a gradient of incentive learning may lead gradually to the stimuli associated with drug-taking acquiring conditioned incentive value. Drugs of abuse collectively have a characteristic that sets them aside from more natural rewarding stimuli, including food, water, and possibly social cooperation. As already mentioned, stimuli that reliably signal food acquire the ability to activate dopaminergic neurons and, in parallel, the primary rewarding food stimulus loses its ability to do so. In a similar fashion, stimuli that signal a drug of abuse gradually begin to activate dopamine neurons. However, in the case of drugs of abuse, the unconditioned drug stimulus retains its ability to enhance dopaminergic neurotransmission. As a result, *repeated drug users experience two activations of dopaminergic neurotransmission, one upon exposure to the conditioned stimuli signaling the drug and another upon actually taking the drug.* This unusual double activation of dopaminergic neurons may lead to compensatory changes that contribute to aversive withdrawal symptoms. A drug-addicted person will experience a gradual amelioration of withdrawal symptoms in a detoxification treatment facility. However, spending time in the treatment facility will not expose the addict to the conditioned incentive stimuli that support drug taking. Once the detoxified addict returns to the environment where those stimuli are encountered, they may elicit approach and other responses, possibly leading to renewed drug taking. As discussed in Chapter 10, these considerations suggest that the most effective treatments for drug addiction will include not only detoxification, but also systematic exposure to drug-associated conditioned incentive stimuli in the absence of primary drug rewards.

Incentive learning is mediated by mechanisms operating within the intricate circuitry of the brain. Neuroanatomy is dizzyingly complex with different brain regions specialized for the specific abilities of various species; neuroanatomy is not yet fully worked out with new connections, circuits, and their various neurotransmitters being identified each year. In spite of this complexity, there are organizational generalities that help to recognize the common structure of the nervous system across species. One is the extraction of features by sensory/perceptual systems. Our senses of vision, audition, olfaction, taste, and somatosensation all have specialized transducers (e.g., rods and cones in the retina for vision) for converting various forms of energy from the environment into signals in the nervous system. Through a series of brain nuclei where the elements of sensory systems converge onto the next level of neurons, perceptions are gradually built up until, at the level of the cerebral cortex, assemblies of cells represent complex stimuli such as faces or the vocal communications of conspecifics. At each level, sensory inputs also connect to nuclei that contain neurons projecting either directly or indirectly to the muscles for the production of responses to those stimuli. At the earlier levels, the features that are extracted from sensory input are less complex and the responses they produce more stereotyped, for example orienting to a sound. Subsequent levels of sensory processing influence correspondingly more complex levels of motor organization. At a subsequent level, for example a stimulus that was oriented to may be recognized as a food source and motor output signals may activate responses resulting in the procurement of that food. The most complex aspects of the environment may specifically activate assemblies of cells in the cerebral cortex. Those cells project to the basal ganglia where they make contact with medium spiny output neurons of the dorsal striatum (caudate and putamen nuclei in primates) and the ventral striatum (nucleus accumbens and olfactory tubercle). Striatal outputs influence motor nuclei in the brainstem region. Those motor nuclei project to motor regions located earlier in the hierarchy of motor control and, in addition, bypass some of the earlier motor regions and project to motor nuclei closer to the muscles they control. In this way, each motor level can exert its influence on response systems while also controlling intermediate motor regions thereby avoiding conflicting messages to the muscles.

Different assemblies of cells in the cerebral cortex are activated by different stimuli, but *it must be the case that any stimulus we can discriminate activates a unique subset of cells in the brain.* As environmental stimuli change the subset of cortical cells activated by those stimuli will change and so will the subset of synapses that is activated in the striatum where cortical input neurons contact medium spiny neurons. Dopamine-containing neurons are located in the ventral mesencephalon and they project to the same medium spiny neurons that receive cortical input. Rewarding stimuli activate dopamine neurons and the increased concentration of dopamine that results modifies the strength of corticostriatal synapses that were *most recently active.* As a result, stimuli that precede rewarding stimuli acquire an increased ability to elicit approach and other responses. In the future, when those stimuli are encountered they will lead to stronger output signals from the striatum that influence brainstem motor circuitry as described in the previous paragraph.

As discussed in Chapter 11, some vertebrates, notably primates, have evolved a further level of motor control known as the corticospinal or pyramidal tract. Via these pathways, motor signals from the cerebral cortex project all the way to motor nuclei closest to the muscles. On their way to these targets, corticospinal neurons also project to other motor regions in the hierarchy, including the striatum, mesencephalon, and other brainstem motor regions, thereby avoiding conflicting messages from these regions to the motor nuclei closest to the muscles. However, the motor control exerted by the corticospinal tract is heavily influenced by the striatum. Especially in species that have developed corticospinal tracts, striatal output, instead of flowing heavily in the caudal direction to influence mesencephalic motor regions, projects more heavily in the rostral direction. Striatal output nuclei project to ventral nuclei of the thalamus and thence back to the cortex where they influence corticospinal neurons. Through this circuitry, incentive learning produced by the action of dopamine on corticostriatal synapses influences the control of behavior by the corticospinal tract.

The putative mechanism by which dopamine modifies glutamatergic corticostriatal synapses to produce incentive learning is discussed in Chapter 12. Many of the axons of cortical cells projecting to the striatum end on the spines of medium spiny neurons. Those spines also receive input from extensively branched dopaminergic neurons; estimates suggest that a single dopamine neuron may have as many as 400,000 synaptic regions. The cortical cells that are activated at any specific time by a combination of internal proprioceptive stimuli and/or external environmental stimuli will produce glutamate release at their corresponding synapses onto medium spiny neurons in the striatum. As the stimuli change, the subset of active corticospinous glutamatergic synapses will change. Glutamatergic inputs that are of sufficient strength produce a number of biochemical events in the postsynaptic dendritic spines, including increased calcium concentrations that can lead to molecular changes characterized as a wave of phosphorylation. If no rewarding stimulus is encountered in close temporal proximity to this putative wave, a subsequent putative wave of phosphatase activity quickly undoes the molecular changes produced by the wave of phosphorylation and the spine returns to its preactivated state. If, however, a rewarding stimulus is encountered and bursts of activity are produced in dopaminergic neurons, the rise in synaptic concentrations of dopamine and stimulation of D1 receptors leads to activation of cAMP, protein kinase A (PKA), and a cascade of intracellular events that arrests the wave of phosphatases, thereby prolonging the initial wave of phosphorylation in those dendritic spines that recently received an input. These intracellular events that result from a close temporal combination of a glutamate input followed by a dopamine input act synergistically to influence gene expression and the production of new proteins that may participate in producing long-term strengthening of the glutamatergic input. This strengthening is thought to contribute to the biological basis of incentive learning: stimuli that were present just prior to a rewarding stimulus will have an increased ability to elicit approach and other responses in the future because they will activate cortical neurons that have strengthened synapses onto striatal medium spiny output neurons.

There are two major subsets of medium spiny neurons in the striatum defined according to the subtype of dopamine receptor, D1 or D2, they express. The anatomical connections of the two subsets differ with D1 receptor-expressing medium spiny neurons forming the direct pathway and their D2 counterpart forming the indirect pathway. Some authors have referred to the direct pathway as the "go" pathway and the indirect pathway as the "no go" pathway. Evidence suggests that when incentive learning takes place and corticospinous synapses onto direct pathway neurons are strengthened, recently active corticospinous glutamatergic synapses onto medium spiny neurons of the indirect pathway are weakened. Far less is known about the mechanism by which corticospinous synapses onto indirect pathway medium spiny neurons are weakened, but evidence implicates endocannabinoids. When inverse incentive learning takes place, recently active corticospinous synapses of the indirect pathway may be strengthened and those onto direct pathway neurons may be weakened. Again, relevant molecular data are relatively sparse. Recall that inverse incentive learning is associated with a decrease in synaptic concentrations of dopamine. When synaptic levels of dopamine are high, dopamine acts at D2 receptors to inhibit the ability of adenosine to stimulate A2A receptors and thereby inhibits activity in the cAMP–PKA signaling pathway in D2 receptor-expressing medium spiny neurons. When dopamine neuron firing is inhibited and synaptic levels of dopamine decrease, this inhibitory effect is removed and adenosine is able to act at A2A receptors to stimulate the cAMP–PKA cascade. This effect in conjunction with the molecular events associated with recent activity at the glutamatergic input to the indirect pathway neurons may lead to strengthening of the glutamate synapses through a series of molecular events like those observed in direct pathway neurons when incentive learning occurs. At the same time, corticospinous glutamatergic synapses onto medium spiny neurons of the direct pathway may be weakened. The possible mechanism is poorly understood but may also involve endocannabinoids.

Recall from the discussion above that cues that reliably predict a primary rewarding stimulus gradually acquire the ability themselves to increase firing of dopaminergic neurons and to increase the concentration of dopamine in the terminal regions of those neurons. The mechanisms for altering the strength of corticostriatal glutamatergic synapses onto dendritic spines of medium spiny neurons as a basis for incentive learning do not account for this phenomenon. A number of findings discussed near the end of Chapter 12 suggest that synaptic modifications of inputs to dopaminergic neurons in the ventral midbrain may underlie the acquisition by stimuli that reliably signal a rewarding stimulus of the ability to activate dopamine neurons. Dopamine cells receive glutamatergic inputs from a number of brain regions, including the cortex. They also receive cholinergic inputs that are active when a rewarding stimulus is encountered. Some data suggest that activity at cholinergic inputs may modify the strength of glutamatergic afferents to dopamine cells leading to the ability of conditioned stimuli that signal a rewarding stimulus to augment dopamine release. Much remains to be done to identify the molecular mechanisms of incentive learning.

As discussed in Chapter 13, there is extensive evidence that brain activity produces mental experiences in humans and that changes in brain activity lead to changes in mental experiences. For example, Wilder Penfield (1891–1976) stimulated cortical regions in awake patients undergoing brain surgery and in some cases they reported vivid mental experiences of sounds and/or sights from their past. Psychoactive drugs, for example opiates, LSD, or cocaine, affect various neurotransmitters and produce sometimes-spectacular changes in mental experience. Positron emission tomography studies show that cocaine-produced verbal reports of "high" or "rush" are highly correlated with dopamine receptor occupancy in the striatum. Similar studies with food show that ratings of "pleasantness" of the food are correlated with dopamine receptor occupancy in the striatum. Diseases that involve pathological changes in dopaminergic neurotransmission also lead to changes in mental experience. People with schizophrenia who are thought to suffer from increased dopaminergic neurotransmission report that stimuli become more "interesting" or are difficult to ignore. People with Parkinson's disease who suffer from a loss of dopaminergic neurons lose interest in environmental stimuli and may report a loss of feelings such as "happiness" or "sadness." The dopamine receptor-blocking medications used to treat schizophrenia produce a loss of interest and creativity and the medications used to treat Parkinson's disease that replace lost dopamine produce reports of increased interest. These and many related findings show the strong relationship between the brain and mental experience in humans.

Reports of mental experiences rely on language-based communication in humans. In the absence of these communication capacities, can we access possible mental experiences in other animals? Generally, the answer is "no." Rats can be trained to discriminate the stimulus effects of a particular dose of a particular drug, for example cocaine, from the absence of the drug or from other doses of the same drug or from other drugs. Although there is good evidence that these pharmacological compounds affect the brain, we have no way of knowing whether this discrimination is based on mental experiences of the drugs. In studies of non-human animals, behavioral neuroscientists should avoid the use of language that implies mental states that are not accessible to reliable measurement. Thus, terms such as "incentive learning" or "reward-related learning" are preferable to "pleasure" or "wanting." A disciplined use of non-mentalistic vocabulary will reduce the confusion of reliable behavioral phenomenon and their corresponding brain mechanisms from possible mental experiences associated with them.

Summary

This chapter provides a brief overview of the contents of this book. The central theme is dopamine and the form of learning it produces, termed "reward-related learning" or "incentive learning." *Incentive learning is the acquisition by neutral stimuli of an increased ability to elicit approach and other responses.* "Other responses" could include pushing, pulling, digging, biting, and so on depending on the situation and the natural abilities of the animal. The brain has multiple memory systems broadly defined as "declarative" and "non-declarative" and incentive learning produces only one form of non-declarative memory. Rewarding stimuli produce incentive learning by activating dopaminergic neurons and changing non-dopaminergic synapses so that *once incentive learning is established it is only gradually lost when the rewarding stimulus is no longer available, when dopamine receptors are blocked or when dopamine is depleted.* Conditioned incentive stimuli acquire the ability to activate dopaminergic neurons and to themselves produce incentive learning about stimuli that precede them. Once conditioned incentive stimuli acquire this ability, the primary rewarding stimuli they signal no longer activate dopaminergic neurons (unless those primary rewarding stimuli are drugs of abuse). When expected rewarding stimuli fail to occur, dopamine neuron activity is inhibited, a phenomenon termed, "negative prediction error." Decreases in dopaminergic neurotransmission may produce *inverse incentive learning, the loss by stimuli of their ability to elicit approach and other responses.*

Rewarding stimuli include food, water, sex, and other cooperative social interactions. Thus, social cooperators acquire an increased ability to elicit approach and other responses in the future. People who suffer from schizophrenia have hyperactive dopaminergic neurotransmission possibly leading to excessive incentive learning. Other people, for example, who are not cooperators and normally would not be incentive stimuli may inappropriately acquire incentive value in schizophrenia sufferers. Delusions may rely on relatively intact declarative memory to construct a somewhat reasonable interpretation of the world as it appears with excessive incentive learning. Parkinson's disease, associated with a loss of dopaminergic neurons, may be characterized by a gradual loss of incentive learning and possibly by increased inverse incentive learning. People with this disorder will lose their ability to respond to stimuli but may retain the ability to respond to previously established incentive stimuli not encountered while in a state of hypodopaminergia; this may explain the phenomenon of *kinesia paradoxa.* Drugs of abuse activate dopaminergic neurotransmission leading to incentive learning about stimuli associated with drug taking. Unlike the case with other primary incentive stimuli, drugs of abuse retain their ability to activate dopaminergic neurons even when they are signaled by conditioned incentive stimuli. As a result, *repeated drug users experience two activations of dopaminergic neurotransmission, one upon exposure to the conditioned stimuli signaling the drug and another upon actually taking the drug.* This may lead to compensatory changes that contribute to withdrawal symptoms. Even after withdrawal symptoms have been alleviated by a period of treatment in a detoxification center, conditioned incentive stimuli in environments previously associated with drug taking will retain their ability to elicit approach and other responses until they are repeatedly experienced in the absence of primary drug rewarding stimuli.

Incentive learning may occur by the action of dopamine at dendritic spines of medium spiny neurons of the striatum that have recently had an active glutamatergic input. Medium spiny neurons provide striatal output that strongly influences responses. A major input to medium spiny neurons comes from the cerebral cortex where assemblies of neurons are activated by environmental and proprioceptive stimuli. As the environmental stimuli and on-going behavioral responses of the organism change, so does the active subset of corticospinous glutamatergic afferents onto medium spiny neurons. Activity at glutamatergic synapses initiates a putative wave of phosphorylation in the postsynaptic dendritic spine that normally is followed by a putative wave of phosphatase activity that quickly returns the spine to a pre-excited state. If a rewarding stimulus occurs and dopaminergic neurons increase their firing rate, stimulation of dopamine D1 receptors, acting through cAMP and PKA, initiates a cascade of signaling events that arrests the putative wave of phosphatase activity thereby prolonging the wave of phosphorylation begun by the glutamate input; through synergistic interactions glutamate and dopamine inputs lead to transcription and translation events that contribute to strengthening of the glutamatergic synapse. This strengthening is thought to be an important part of the mechanism of incentive learning. Incentive learning may also involve weakening of corticostriatal synapses onto D2 receptor-expressing medium spiny neurons.

Activity in dopaminergic neurons in humans appears to affect mental experience. Increased activity produced by cocaine leads to reports of "high" or feeling a "rush" and natural rewarding stimuli such as food lead to reports of "pleasant." There is a strong correlation between the intensity of these mental experiences and the level of dopamine receptor occupancy measured by positron emission tomography. It is difficult to access the possible mental experiences of non-human animals and therefore the language of behavioral neuroscience should avoid terms that conflate mental experience and behavioral observation. Terms such as "incentive learning" or "reward-related learning" are preferable to the terms "pleasure" or "wanting."

Chapter 2

Dopamine and reward-related learning

Dopamine is involved in reward but what does such a statement actually mean? Reward can refer to an event like the presentation of food to a food-restricted rat. Reward can be an amount of money indicated in a display on a computer screen, perhaps being viewed by someone who is lying in a brain-scanning machine. Reward might be a treat given to a child who has performed well on a task, or, as you will see in Chapter 8, reward can be a cooperative social interaction. So what does it mean to say that dopamine is involved in reward?

Stimulus–response learning and the law of effect

Long before anyone had any idea about a link between reward and dopamine, there was a lot of interest in reward. In psychology, rewards were stimuli that could be used to modify behavior. Psychologists found that by controlling access to rewarding stimuli, they could systematically shape the behavior of animals, including people. To those familiar with training animals, none of this work of psychologists came as any surprise; they used rewarding stimuli routinely and to good effect to train their dogs, for example. If you think about training your dog to heel using doggie yummies as the rewarding stimulus, what would it mean to say that dopamine is involved in reward?

When people say that dopamine is involved in reward, what they really mean is that dopamine is involved in reward-related learning. Reward-related learning has been studied for over a century. The radical behaviorists of the first half of the twentieth century had a lock on reward-related learning, but they did not call it that. Instead of the term, "reward," they used the term, "reinforcer," referring to a stimulus that strengthens (reinforces) stimulus–response connections. The presentation of a reinforcer was termed "reinforcement." Decades of research, especially with rats, but also with other species, including pigeons and monkeys, produced a highly systematized set of putative *laws of learning*. For example, habit strength, the speed at which an organism will perform a particular response in a particular situation (e.g., a rat running down a runway alley) for a particular rewarding stimulus (e.g., food), was a function of a number of variables including the drive state of the animal (quantified as the period of time since it last ate) and the number of times in the past that the animal had been reinforced for performing the response in the test environment.[1] Behaviorists thought the laws of learning might have the same natural law status as the laws of physics, but it did not turn out that way.

I began my career in 1969 as a psychology student studying the effects of reinforcement on behavior while the behaviorists were still influential but cracks were beginning to show in their paradigm. It would be wrong, however, to throw out all the scientific findings from the period of behaviorism. These scientists provided us with a wealth of data about how adjusting the contingencies of reinforcement could systematically modify behavior. One of the first studies I carried out while working with Professor Stephen Kendall (1936–2015) at the University of Western Ontario (now Western University) was on behavioral contrast. This is the phenomenon whereby the value of a rewarding stimulus changes when the value of other rewarding stimuli presented in the same context changes. We trained rats on a multiple schedule of reinforcement in daily one-hour sessions. According to this schedule, in alternating two-minute periods, one signaled by an illuminated light and the other by darkness, rats could press a lever for a reinforcer that was presented on average every 30 seconds; in one component the reinforcer was milk (0.1 mL) presented in a tiny dipper and in the other it was a small (45 mg) pellet of food that dropped automatically through a tube into a cup. The rats learned to lever press reliably according to this multiple schedule of reinforcement and, although individual rats differed in how frequently they pressed the lever, the behavior of all rats became stable from day to day and highly predictable. Then we changed one of the components of the multiple schedule so that lever presses during that component no longer produced food. As you might expect, responding gradually decreased in that component. What was amazing to me as a young scientist was that responding in the other, alternating, component systematically increased. Even though the rats were getting the same amount of food that they always got in that component, they pressed more when it was alternated with a component where a rewarding stimulus was no longer given.[2] This is a reliable behavioral phenomenon known as behavioral contrast and it has been studied extensively.[3] What was novel about our study was that we observed behavioral contrast with two different reinforcers. The study of behavioral contrast provides insight into the effects of context on the valuation of rewarding stimuli.[4] For example, if a person gets income from two jobs and then loses one of them, the income from the remaining job will increase in value perhaps because it is now compared with no other income instead of some other income. I included a description of this study here as an example of the type of experiments that were being carried out by behaviorists in their heyday. Before moving on to why the radical be-haviorist paradigm crumbled, it is important to acknowledge that we learned a lot from the work of the behaviorists and that their behavioral methods are the backbone of contemporary behavioral and neuroscience studies of reward-related learning and of many behavioral clinical interventions used by clinical psychologists.[5]

The behaviorist dream of a set of laws of learning began to unravel in the middle of the twentieth century. There were a number of observations of animal behavior that failed to conform to the putative laws of learning. One finding was conditioned taste aversion. It was found that if a rat ate a novel-tasting food and then became ill, even hours later, it subsequently showed an aversion to that food. If, instead, the rat ate its usual food but associated with novel noise and flashing lights and became ill hours later, no aversion was subsequently shown to the food when it was again associated with the noise and light cues. There were at least two things about this observation that violated the so-called laws of learning. One was the timing of events. The laws of learning had shown a systematic relationship between delay of reinforcement and the strength of learning. For example, if a dog was presented with a food reinforcer that was preceded several seconds earlier by a brief light stimulus, the strength of the learning, measured in amount of salivation to the brief light stimulus, was much weaker than if the brief stimulus had preceded the food by only half a second. The observation that rats learned a strong taste aversion to a novel taste when that taste preceded the outcome of eating the food, the illness, by min-utes or hours undermined the apparent lawful timing relationship for learning the association between stimuli and outcomes. The other observation that gave behaviorism trouble was the finding that an aversion was learned to a taste when the illness followed the taste by several hours but no similar aversion was learned to the novel noise and flashing lights when they preceded illness by minutes or hours. The laws of learning were thought to be universal, applying to any stimuli that were presented according to the same temporal parameters. The finding that learning took place with a taste stimulus but not with a visual–auditory one was problematic.[6] I recall sitting in a graduate seminar in the early 1970s when these new findings were discussed and being struck by the utter dismay in the face of one of my behaviorist professors as he pondered the impli-cations of these new findings.

Another nail in the coffin of the behaviorists' universal laws of learning was findings from efforts to train animals for entertainment. Keller Breland (1915–1965) and Marian Breland (1920–2001), former students of B.F. Skinner (1904–1990), worked privately on a farm in Minnesota where they trained a variety of animals for circus acts and other commercial enterprises. The Brelands soon began to realize the limitations of the formal descriptions of animal learning that they had been taught as graduate students. They published their observations in a paper with the title "The Misbehavior of Organisms," parodying the title of Skinner's influential 1938 book, *The Behavior of Organisms*. In one example, raccoons were trained to put wooden coins into a box for food reward. At first this worked well and made for an entertaining act. However, gradually from one repetition to another of the act, the behavior broke down as the raccoons spent more and more time manipulating the coins, rubbing them against the box as if the coins themselves were food objects rather than depositing them into the box. Pigs were similarly trained to put large coins into a piggy bank and they too initially performed well but gradually began to spend more time with the coins, manipulating and rooting them as if they were food objects. Both of these examples of instinctive drift violated the putative laws of learning. Food reinforcement continued to be presented for performance of the conditioned behaviors by the raccoons and pigs, yet they failed to continue to reliably perform the conditioned response. Their behaviors toward the coins actually reduced the amount of food reward that they received.[7]

One more example of the many observations that began to emerge in the middle of the twentieth century and challenged the hold of behaviorism was pigeons key pecking for food or water. When a pigeon pecked the key for food, its beak was wide open as it is when the pigeon eats food; when a pigeon pecked for water, its beak was only slightly open as it is when the pigeon drinks. Apparently, the pigeons *ate* the key when key pecks were reinforced with food and *drank* the key when key pecks were reinforced with water. The putative laws of learning stipulated that reinforcers strengthened stimulus–response connections. They had no provisions for the response associated with the reinforcer working retroactively to alter the topography of the conditioned response.[8]

These and many related observations presaged the end of behaviorism's intellectual hegemony over the study of animal behavior,[9] especially in North America. While behaviorism had dominated the study of animal behavior in North America during the early decades of the twentieth century, European animal behaviorists were focusing their studies on the behavior of animals in their natural environment.[10] Ethologists such as Nikolaas Tinbergen (1907–1988) and Konrad Lorenz (1903–1989), recipients of the Nobel Prize in Physiology or Medicine in 1973, provided explanations for many of the observations that undermined behaviorism. The case of conditioned taste aversion began to make sense when it was realized that rats are unable to vomit. When a rat encounters a new food it typically will show caution, only eating a small amount. If the rat does not become ill in the coming hours, it will subsequently eat larger quantities of the food. If it becomes ill, it will show an aversion as already described. By considering the physiology of the rat and its natural history, it follows that it has evolved mechanisms that allow it to detect safe and dangerous foods. Rats in their natural environment do not normally encounter toxic foods associated with sounds and lights and so they have not evolved mechanisms for learning associations between sound and light stimuli and illness.[11]

The behavior of Breland and Breland's animals toward the wooden coins and the topography of the pigeons' key-pecks for food or water reveal mechanisms of learning that were not anticipated by behaviorism but that reflect how animals behave towards food- or water-related stimuli in their natural environment. Raccoons in the wild obtain food by manipulation and wash food before they eat it, and pigs obtain food by rooting. Pigeons obtain food by pecking with their beak wide open and water by drinking with their beak slightly open. If a stimulus is repeatedly paired with food, as was the case with the coins in the circus act or the food and water in the pigeon experiment, that stimulus *acquires* some of the response-eliciting properties of the rewarding stimulus itself. Thus, the raccoons and pigs began to treat the coins as food, manipulating and rooting them, respectively, and the pigeons began to *eat* and *drink* the keys that preceded the respective presentation of food and water. Understanding the way that animals find and eat food in their natural environments provided a way to understand the apparent violations of the laws of learning.

During the same period of the twentieth century when ethological perspectives were modifying or replacing behaviorists' notions about the putative laws of learning, behavioral psychologists were making other observations that also challenged some of the ideas of behaviorism. Behaviorism was founded on Edward Thorndike's (1874–1949)[1] *law of effect* stating that when a response in a particular situation was followed by a satisfier (i.e., reinforcer), the strength of the connection between the stimuli associated with the response and the response was strengthened. Thus, rewarding or reinforcing stimuli strengthen or reinforce stimulus–response connections. A problem began to emerge with this rather rigid formulation when researchers found that once animals learned a response for food, for example, they could substitute other responses. One of the classic experiments involved training rats to run a maze for food. The rats learned the maze well and soon were making few errors between the start point and the goal box that contained food. The maze was then partially immersed in water so that the rats had to swim to get the food. The rats made few errors, even on the first swim. Parallel experiments began by training the rats to swim first and then switching them to running and produced the same results. If the effects of food reinforcement were to strengthen stimulus–response connections and if the response was *running* the maze, then how could it be that the rats could use a different response, *swimming*, requiring different movements and different sequences of muscle contractions to get the food? Apparently, animals did not learn strict stimulus–response connections.[12]

Incentive learning

Findings like this and the findings of apparent violations of the putative laws of learning led researchers to reconsider stimulus–response connectionist notions of learning in favor of explanations based on incentive learning.[13] Because the term "reinforce" was strongly linked to stimulus–response thinking, the incentive-learning theorists used instead the term "reward." In both cases, the terms referred to the presentation of food to a food-restricted animal or similar events that entail an animal getting something that satisfies its biological needs. The rejection of behaviorism was partly indicated by the shift away from the use of the term "reinforcer" and towards the use of the term "reward;" you will see the term "reward" much more frequently in the contemporary animal learning literature. In incentive learning theory, rewarding stimuli produce *incentive learning, the acquisition by neutral stimuli of an increased ability to elicit approach and other* responses.[14] "Other responses" could include pushing, pulling, digging, biting, and so on, depending on the situation and the natural abilities of the animal. This formulation accommodated both the observation of transfer of the response-eliciting properties of rewarding stimuli to the stimuli that signaled them and the response flexibility that animals showed in learning to attain rewarding stimuli.

Incentive learning notions posited that stimuli associated with rewarding stimuli themselves acquire the ability to activate responding. In the case of the circus animals putting coins into a piggy bank in order to receive food reward, the coins, being regularly associated with food reward, gradually acquired the ability to elicit approach and other responses; in the case of raccoons and pigs, *other responses* included the species-typical responses that normally were directed toward the food itself. For the pigeons, the key that was pecked to get food was repeatedly associated with food and acquired food-like properties. Like food itself, it elicited pecking and, like food, it elicited a particular topography of pecking. In the maze the cues associated with the correct alleys were repeatedly associated with food and acquired the ability, like food itself, to attract the animal. The cues closest to primary rewarding stimuli would acquire the strongest ability to elicit approach and other responses. Once this learning had taken place, the animals were capable of using a range of response alternatives to get to the food, as was shown in the rapid transfer from running to swimming when the situation demanded it. In all of the situations, stimuli associated with rewarding stimuli acquired incentive value, an increased ability to elicit approach and other responses. They became conditioned incentive stimuli.

Dopamine and incentive learning

We know that dopamine is involved in reward-related learning from the results of many, many studies.[15] Some of the earliest investigations involved brain stimulation reward. In the 1950s, before the dopaminergic systems in the brain had been discovered and before the possible role of dopamine in reward-related learning was on anyone's radar, James Olds (1922–1976) and Peter Milner at McGill University in Montreal discovered that reward-related learning could be produced by direct stimulation of the brain. They had implanted an electrode into the brain of a rat and had placed the animal in a small arena where they periodically stimulated its brain to investigate the behavioral effects of the stimulation. They noticed that the rat kept returning to the area of the arena where it received the brain stimulation. Being observant and creative scientists, they decided to set up a circuit with a switch in it that the rats could operate, by pressing a small lever, to close the circuit and stimulate their own brains. They found that the rat pressed the lever vigorously to get the stimulation. When the stimulator was turned off so that switch closures no longer provided brain stimulation, the rat stopped lever pressing.[16] This was recognized as a scientific breakthrough at the time because it suggested that parts of the brain contained centers for reward (nowadays, the idea of centers has been replaced with the notion of circuits). News of the discovery was reported on the front page of the *Montreal Gazette* on March 12, 1954, under the headline, "McGill opens vast new research field with brain 'pleasure area' discovery."[17] In subsequent years, Olds and Milner and many others mapped the regions of the brain that supported responding for brain stimulation reward and the phenomenon was widely studied.[18]

There was an exciting convergence of the findings from mapping studies of the brain regions that supported brain stimulation reward and the subsequent discovery of monoaminergic (e.g., histaminergic, dopaminergic, norepinephrinergic, serotonergic, etc.) neurotransmitter systems in the brain. As discussed in Chapter 11, in 1964, with the development of new techniques for visualizing specific molecules in the brain, Annica Dahlström and Kjell Fuxe, working at the Karolinska Institute in Stockholm, Sweden, discovered that there were dopamine-containing neurons in the brain with cell bodies in the ventral midbrain and axonal projections to a number of forebrain regions.[19] Researchers began to notice the overlap between the location of dopaminergic neurons and axons and brain sites that supported brain stimulation reward.[20] Many studies investigated the hypothesis that dopamine neurons were mediating reward-related learning.[15]

One of the central challenges faced by behavioral scientists who are interested in investigating the possibility that a particular brain region mediates aspects of behavior, for example spatial learning, memory, reward-related learning, aversively motivated learning, and so on, is sorting out possible effects on the function of interest from non-specific changes in motor capacity, perception, or motivation. Often behavioral scientists have to design experimental proced-ures that pit various explanations against one another in order to unequivo-cally implicate a particular brain region in a particular function. This challenge was front and center in behavioral studies of dopamine function because it was realized early on that changes in dopamine neurotransmission produced cor-responding changes in locomotor activity. Drugs or other interventions that increased dopaminergic neurotransmission generally increased locomotor activity and those that decreased dopaminergic neurotransmission decreased locomotor activity.

If an animal was trained to press a lever for brain stimulation reward and then treated with a dopamine receptor-blocking drug that would reduce dopamin-ergic neurotransmission, lever-pressing rates were often seen to decline. The decline was not only consistent with a reduction in reward-related learning, but it was also consistent with a general motor slowing. Thus, such an observa-tion on its own would not provide knockdown evidence that dopamine was in-volved in reward-related learning. In 1979, Peter Zarevics and Paulette Settler, working at the laboratories of Smith Kline and French in Philadelphia, came up with an ingenious solution to this problem. They trained rats to lever press for brain stimulation reward in a situation where there were two levers. Pressing one lever provided the rewarding brain stimulation, but each press also resulted in a small reduction in the intensity of the stimulation. As the animal continued to press the lever and get brain stimulation reward, the intensity decreased apace. When the intensity reached a level where it was no longer rewarding, the rat could press the other lever to reset the intensity to the starting level. The rat could then resume pressing on the lever that produced the brain stimulation re-ward and again receive high-intensity reward that again decreased in intensity with each press.

The authors examined the effects of drugs that affect dopaminergic neuro-transmission. They found that treatment with the dopamine receptor antag-onist pimozide caused the rats to press the reset lever sooner. The rats pressed the lever producing brain stimulation reward in the usual manner, but at a higher intensity the stimulation apparently was no longer rewarding and the reset lever was pressed. The authors also found a dose-dependent effect, observing that with a higher dose of pimozide the rats opted to press the reset lever even sooner, suggesting that an even higher minimum intensity was needed for the stimulation to maintain reward-related learning. The beauty of this experimental design was that the results could not easily be attributed to a drug-related general motoric inhibition. The drug did not stop the rats from lever pressing for brain stimulation reward but instead lessened the magnitude of reward so that lower intensities that maintained responding when the animal was not treated with pimozide no longer maintained responding when the animal was treated with the drug. By definition, these intensities were no longer rewarding. Further strengthening their case, the authors showed that rats treated with amphetamine, a drug that increases dopaminergic neurotransmission, pressed the lever that produced brain stimulation at lower intensities than those that were self-administered when the animal was not drugged. The rat would then press the reset lever and begin again on the descending staircase of rewarding intensities. Results provide good evidence for a role for dopamine in reward-related learning.[21]

In the same year, Keith Franklin and S.N. McCoy, researchers at McGill University in Montreal, took a different approach to the question of whether dopamine receptor-blocking drugs were reducing the rewarding effects of brain stimulation or simply producing motor inhibition that led to less lever pressing. They trained rats to press a lever for brain stimulation reward made available according to a schedule consisting of two alternating six-minute components. During the first component, brain stimulation reward was available intermittently for three minutes and this was followed by a three-minute period during which no explicit rewarding stimulus was available. Then a flashing light came on and remained on for six minutes; the light signaled the renewed availability of brain stimulation reward, again intermittently for three minutes and then not at all for the next three minutes. The offset of the flashing light at the end of six minutes signaled the switch back to the first component of the schedule. They then treated the rats with the dopamine receptor antagonist pimozide and put them back into the lever-pressing situation with the flashing light turned off. The rats could lever press for brain stimulation as usual only the stimulation remained available beyond the usual three minutes used in training. The rats were observed to show a gradual decline in lever pressing for the brain stimulation reward. At this point it could be argued that the drug had diminished the reward-related response-maintaining effects of the stimulation, but it equally could be argued that the drug had produced a motor impairment that was responsible for the decline in responding.

The ingenious part of this experiment was to present the flashing-light stimulus that had been used in training to signal the renewed availability of rewarding brain stimulation at a time when responding in the first component had declined to zero for two consecutive minutes. The authors found that the rats resumed vigorous responding and again showed a gradual decline. If responding had originally declined because the drug had caused the motor capacity of rats to be impaired, they would not have been expected to resume responding when the flashing-light signal came on. If, however, the drug decreased the reward-related response-maintaining effects of the stimulation, then the arrival of the usual cue for renewed stimulation would result in a resumption of responding, as was seen. Before concluding that this experiment provided unequivocal evidence for a role for dopamine in reward-related learning, one additional control experiment was needed. What if just presenting a stimulus, any stimulus, to a rat that had been treated with a dopamine receptor antagonist and ceased responding resulted in a resumption of responding? Perhaps stimuli have activating effects that are independent of their previous signal properties. The authors included a control group that tested for this possibility. The control group had been similarly trained to lever press for food and the flashing-light stimulus was presented periodically, but its presentation was random, that is, it was not associated with the renewed availability of brain stimulation reward. When these rats were treated with pimozide, they showed the gradual decline in responding for brain stimulation reward like that observed in the group already described where the light signaled renewed availability of the rewarding stimulus. When the flashing-light stimulus was turned on, responding did not resume in this additional control group. Simply presenting a stimulus was not sufficient to produce a resumption of responding.[22] My colleague Nelson Freedman and I, working at Queen's University in Kingston, replicated this finding using different responses in each component.[23] Taken together, these data provide strong evidence for a role for dopamine in reward-related learning produced by electrical stimulation of the brain.

Dopamine was implicated in reward-related learning produced by natural stimuli too. In what has become a classic study in behavioral neuroscience, Roy Wise, Joan Spindler, Harriet de Wit, and Gary Gerber, working at Concorida University in Montreal in 1978, found that animals trained to lever press for food gradually decreased responding when treated with the dopamine receptor-blocking drug pimozide. The decrease resembled that seen when the food was removed, a pattern often referred to as *extinction*. The authors had trained rats to lever press in daily 45-minute sessions for food reward and observed stable responding from day to day. They then treated the rats with pimozide prior to the next three test days. They observed that the rats initially lever pressed at the same rate that was seen prior to drug treatment but responding gradually declined over the course of the session. The next day the rats again responded but rates declined further and this pattern continued on the third day, with rates continuing to decline. They tested two doses of pimozide and observed a larger decline in responding with the higher dose, showing that the effect was dose-dependent. Remarkably, the rats continued to receive food for responding and they continued to eat the food. In spite of this, response rates showed a decline similar to that seen in extinction.[24]

As is always the case with behavioral experiments, control groups are needed to examine alternative explanations of the data. One possible explanation for the results of Wise et al. is that there was residual drug from the first dose that added to the effects of the next dose on the next day, making the effective day-to-day dose larger; according to this view, with the larger dose resulting from the cumulative effect, a greater inhibition of responding was seen from day to day. To test this possibility, the authors included a control group that received three home-cage injections of pimozide, one on each of the three days preceding the first test day with pimozide. If the observed day-to-day decline in responding resulted from the drug accumulating in the system, responding on the first test day for this group should have been lower than the first test day for the experimental group. Results revealed that this group responded at the same level as the experimental group on the first day of testing. This finding argued against the possibility that the gradual decline in responding resulted from the drug building up over days.

The results of Roy Wise and his co-workers were important because they suggested that blocking dopamine receptors produced a brain state that was similar to that resulting from the discontinuation of presenting a rewarding stimulus for a particular response. The animals treated with the dopamine receptor blocker retained the ability to respond. They retained their motivation to eat as evidenced by the observation that they ate the food. However, the food did not have its usual effect on responding. Normally, when food presentation to a food-restricted animal follows a particular response in a particular situation, incentive learning occurs resulting in an increased ability of those stimuli associated with the response to elicit approach and other responses (see Chapter 3). If the dopamine system is blocked, even though a lever-press response occurs in the test environment and is followed immediately with the presentation of a food pellet, that pellet fails to have the effect of a rewarding stimulus—it fails to produce incentive learning. Thus, the ability of the lever and lever-related stimuli to elicit approach and other responses is gradually lost and responding is observed to decline from day to day.

The paper of Wise et al. contained the statement "A history of testing with normal reward and pimozide was the apparent *equivalent* to drug-free testing without reward" (p. 263, italics added). The claim for equivalence between pimozide plus reward, on the one hand, and non-reward, on the other, was unfortunate because it was easily shown to be inaccurate and it deflected attention away from the really important finding that treatment with pimozide produced behavioral changes that resembled the effects of discontinuing the presentation of a rewarding stimulus in several aspects. For example, responding declined gradually over time in both cases. However, animals treated with pimozide and continuing to receive food (that they ate) are different from animals in the non-reward condition that do not receive food—the difference is that they are spending some time eating. Response rate was the behavioral measure and food was given for each response. Response rates would not be expected to be equivalent if one group of animals is eating and the other is not. Therefore, feeding time in the pimozide-treated rats confounded apparent equivalence. However, the *pattern* of responding, showing a gradual decline over time, was similar for both groups and supported a role for dopamine in reward-related learning.[24].

The title of the publication by Wise and his co-workers was, "Neuroleptic-induced 'anhedonia' in rats: pimozide blocks reward quality of food." This was a provocative title that led to many publications by other investigators who took issue with Wise's conclusions.[25] The discussion of dopamine can cover a number of levels of explanation. At the behavioral level, it is possible to describe what animals do or do not do when dopamine function is manipulated, for example with the use of drugs like pimozide. The experimental results from the behavioral studies discussed in this chapter are an example. At the physiological level, electrophysiologial and biomolecular changes associated with manipulations of dopaminergic neurotransmission can be described, as they are in Chapters 5 and 12, respectively. I argue in Chapter 12 that theoretical concepts like incentive learning that are used to describe what is happening at the behavioral level can also be reduced to a biomolecular level of explanation that provides an understanding in terms of synaptic change produced by dopamine.

Discussions of dopamine can be at the level of neuropsychiatric disorders where the symptomatology and responses to treatment are related to changes in dopamine function (see Chapters 7 and 9). Sometimes the symptoms are discussed in behavioral terms, for example level of motor activity, that make comparisons to the results of animal studies possible. Sometimes the symptoms are discussed in phenomenological terms, reflecting mental changes associated with changes in dopamine function. It was this latter realm that Wise et al. touched on in their title when they used the term "anhedonia." In their paper's closing comments they suggested that dopamine receptor blockade by pimozide takes away "pleasure," "euphoria," or "goodness" (p. 263).[24]. These terms refer to mental experiences that are described by people. They are inferred in animals by observing their behavior. Thus, another level of discussion of dopamine function is the relationship between brain dopamine neurotransmission and mental experience. This is the topic of Chapter 13. Much confusion about dopamine has arisen because of the careless intermixing of these levels of explanation.

Avoidance conditioning

I turn now to a discussion of the role of dopamine in aversive conditioning. Aversive stimuli cause pain and tissue damage. In the natural environment, aversive stimuli might include temperature extremes, hostile conspecifics, predators, and, depending on the species, painful stimuli such as sharp rocks underfoot, barbs on vegetation, or the bark of certain trees. For small prey animals such as rats, mice, and voles, being in the open where they are subject to possible aerial predation is aversive. In the laboratory, the delivery of mild electric shock through a metal grid floor in part of a test chamber serves as a non-natural aversive stimulus that can be easily quantified and instrumented. Animals learn to avoid aversive stimuli and dopamine is involved in this avoidance learning.

Although there are many ways to evaluate aversively motivated learning,[26] a typical avoidance-learning situation in studies using rats as subjects involves the use of a shuttle box consisting of two chambers connected by an opening in a common wall (for further details of the apparatus see Chapter 3). In the one-way version of this task, there are, for example, ten discrete trials per session and one session per day. Each trial begins by placing the rat into one of the two chambers, always the same one. This chamber is outfitted with an electrifiable grid floor that can be used to deliver mild electric shock to the rat through its feet, which are in contact with the floor.[27] The shock is programmed to come on after a specific time, for example ten seconds. The shock might be signaled by, for example, a tone or light that comes on at some point after the rat is placed into the shock side of the shuttle box.[28] Once the shock comes on, the rat begins to seek safety from the shock by rapidly trying alternate locations within the shock side of the shuttle box and by running through the opening into the other, safe, chamber. Movement into the safe chamber achieves the goal of escaping the aversive stimulus and is therefore rewarding. After a delay, for example 30 seconds, the rat is again picked up and placed into the shock side of the shuttle box and the warning stimulus, if there is one, is turned on. After ten seconds, the shock is again presented and the rat can again escape it by shuttling to the safe side. After only a few trials, the rat is observed to make the shuttle response shortly after being placed into the shock side and during the warning stimulus if one is used, *before* the shock comes on. The rat has now learned to make avoidance responses instead of escape responses.

Efforts to understand what is learned in avoidance learning led to the development of two-factor theory, attributed to Orval Hobart Mowrer (1907–1982), who spent most of his career working at the University of Illinois in Urbana. According to this framework, there are at least two separate elements (factors) of learning in avoidance learning. One is learning the association between the signal for shock (e.g., the stimuli associated with the shock side or a warning stimulus if one is used) and the shock itself, and the other is the reward-related learning produced by offset of the aversive stimulus when the shuttle response is made. The former element is often described as classical conditioning, originally discovered by Ivan Pavlov (1849–1936), working at the Institute of Experimental Medicine in St. Petersburg, Russia. Pavlov received the Nobel Prize in Physiology or Medicine in 1904, although the prize was for his work on the physiology of digestion rather than his equally important work on classical conditioning. Classical conditioning is often referred to as "Pavlovian conditioning" in recognition of Pavlov's pioneering work. Classical conditioning occurs in avoidance learning when the signals for the shock themselves acquires aversive properties by association with shock. In Pavlov's terms, the shock is the unconditioned stimulus and the discomfort that it produces as a result of activation of pain pathways and the sympathetic nervous system, for example increased heart rate and threat (see Chapter 13), is the unconditioned response. The signals for the shock, as a result of pairings with the shock on initial trials when an avoidance response is not made, acquire the aversive properties of the shock so that they now produce discomfort, for example increased heart rate, threat, like that produced by the shock itself. The signals for the shock are termed a "conditioned stimulus" and the responses it produces are termed "conditioned responses." Thus, the signals for shock have now become aversive just like the shock itself. As a result of classical conditioning, offset of the signals for shock is rewarding because their offset terminates the discomfort in the same manner that the offset of shock itself serves as a rewarding stimulus.[29]

The second element of Mowrer's two-factor theory is termed "operant conditioning" because it involves responding for reinforcement (I am using here the behaviorists' terminology in wide use at the time). However, the reinforcement in this case was not the onset of a stimulus that satisfies a biological need but the offset of a stimulus that produces pain or discomfort, termed "negative reinforcement." Negative reinforcement refers to the effects of a stimulus that reinforces behavior by its offset in contrast to positive reinforcement that refers to the effects of a stimulus that reinforces behavior by its onset. In Mowrer's time, the radical behaviorist paradigm was still dominant and he described the operant conditioning element of two-factor theory in those terms. Thus, the negative reinforcement produced by making the avoidance response strengthened the stimulus–response connection between the signal for shock and the shuttle response, increasing the frequency of the shuttle response when the animal is exposed to the classically conditioned shock-associated stimuli. Two-factor theory posed some problems for behaviorists, as discussed in the next paragraph, and the rigidity of the stimulus–response framework eventually yielded to incentive learning interpretations of avoidance learning.

One of the problems that behaviorists had with avoidance learning was the apparent persistence of behavior in the absence of any explicit reinforcing stimulus. In the typical one-way avoidance task described earlier, a rat would receive a few shocks in the first session and then begin to shuttle to safety during the signals for shock, avoiding further shocks. Often, shuttle responding was observed to persist for days, even though the rats received no further shocks. Two-factor theory provided a clear means to understand what was going on, but for the behaviorists, who eschewed explanations based on unobservable internal states, the suggestion that stimuli associated with shock produced a state of threat that was reduced, and therefore reinforced, by the shuttle response was difficult to swallow. Various attempts were made to explain avoidance responding without recourse to internal states, but they were unable to stand up to empirical testing.[30] It is a credit to Mowrer that his two-factor theory endured the scrutiny of the behaviorists; in fact, it has proven to be one of the more influential explanations of behavior that came out of the behaviorist era.

The influence of two-factor theory can be found in present-day clinical psychology in the understanding and treatment of anxiety disorders and phobias. Anxiety and phobias are states of discomfort often associated with increased heart rate and other physiological signs of activation of the sympathetic nervous system and feelings of fear. Just as rats will make a response—such as shuttling—to the other side of the test apparatus to escape conditioned aversive stimuli, humans will learn to perform responses that succeed at removing them from the presence of anxiety provoking stimuli. Someone who has a fear of open places, that is, agoraphobia, for example, will be able to mitigate their feelings of anxiety and fear by avoiding open places, perhaps by staying at home. The agoraphobia may have come about through the prior experience of strong discomfort while in an open space and the discomfort was escaped by moving indoors. Subsequent movement into open spaces may again bring about feelings of discomfort and again they are lessened—negatively reinforced—by avoiding the open places. Once this conditioning has taken place, just as was the case for avoidance learning in rats, the response of escaping particular conditioned aversive stimuli is rewarded even though the primary aversive stimulus is no longer encountered. It is easy to see how such behaviors might persist for a long time even though the primary aversive stimulus is seldom encountered.

Psychologists use applied behavioral analysis to treat anxiety and phobias.[31] The goal is to weaken the aversive conditioning so that the ability of aversive stimuli to provoke feelings of anxiety and fear is mitigated. Once that is achieved, avoiding those stimuli will no longer be negatively reinforcing and the avoidant behavior will decline. To do this, psychologists often use a technique termed systematic desensitization. Once the main anxiety provoking stimuli are identified, open places in the earlier example, then other, related stimuli can be identified so that a hierarchy of anxiety-provoking stimuli can be constructed. An example might be as follows, although the hierarchy for any individual will be idiosyncratic and the first step listed (mental images) might actually involve several steps: mental images of being out of doors, standing at the doorway, walking out to the street from the front of a house, going to a neighbor's house, walking around the block, driving to a mall parking lot, driving to the mall parking lot and getting out of the car, going into the mall for a brief period, going into the mall for longer periods. Once the hierarchy is constructed, the psychotherapist will begin with the first item on the list. The therapist will instruct the patient in relaxation and when the patient is in a relaxed state will ask her to construct explicit mental images of going out of doors. Once the patient can remain relaxed and comfortable while forming mental images of going out of doors, the psychologist will move to the next item on the list, standing at the doorway. Again the patient will be instructed to relax and then she will be asked to stand at the door. This will continue until the patient can remain comfortable while standing at the doorway. The therapist moves up the hierarchy to stimuli more and more proximal to the primary anxiety provoking stimulus until the patient finds herself in the presence of that stimulus and in a relaxed state. Now there is no longer any reward for escaping from those stimuli and the ability of those stimuli to control responding is extinguished.

Another problem that avoidance learning posed for behaviorists who adhered to rigid stimulus-response learning theories was the response flexibility that was observed for avoidance responding. This response-flexibility problem was discussed earlier with reference to the apparent ease of transfer of a running to a swimming response for food. In a similar manner, Mowrer commented that rats that had learned to perform a running response to avoid could readily substitute other responses such as jumping onto a platform to achieve the same end.[29]. Stimulus–response theories did not provide for this response flexibility. However, as discussed for appetitive conditioning, incentive learning theories provide a framework that can accommodate response flexibility. In the case of avoidance learning, the rewarding stimulus is the offset of discomfort produced by the conditioned aversive stimulus. Rewarding stimuli produce incentive learning, increasing the ability of safety related stimuli to elicit approach and other responses. Thus, the stimuli from the safe side of the shuttle box acquire an ability to elicit approach leading to avoidance responses. As discussed in the following and in the next chapter, there is considerable evidence that dopamine mediates the effects of reward in avoidance learning in a similar manner to its role in mediating the effects of reward in appetitive learning.

Aversive conditioning provided other observations that contributed to the downfall of the behaviorists' quest for universal laws of learning. Robert Bolles (1928–1994), who worked at the University of Washington in Seattle for much of his career, wrote an influential paper with the title "Species-typical defense reactions and avoidance learning" that contributed importantly.[32] He discussed findings showing that animals learned avoidance responses most readily when those responses matched species-typical responses, for example running away or jumping for a rodent, flying away for a bird, and that avoidance responses were learned poorly or not at all when they were not species-typical, for example lever pressing for a rat. The laws of learning held that a reinforcer could condition any response if that reinforcer was made contingent upon the response. The fact that different responses were differentially conditioned by the same reinforcer and the same arrangement of contingencies, some responses apparently not learned at all, flew in the face of the putative lawfulness of learning.

Bolles' emphasis on the importance of considering species-typical defense reactions in studies of avoidance learning provides a basis for understanding the difficulty some rats have in learning two-way avoidance. In this paradigm, training begins like that for one-way avoidance described earlier. However, after the animal receives the first shock and eventually finds its way to safety on the other side of the shuttle box, it is not picked up by the experimenter and replaced into the first side of the shuttle box to begin the next trial. Instead, it is left in the "safe" side and after an inter-trial interval, for example 30 seconds, a warning stimulus, for example a tone, comes on and now the correct response is to shuttle back to the original side to escape the shock or avoid the impending shock. In a recent study carried out by my former doctoral student, Stuart Fogel, working in the laboratory of his co-supervisor and my colleague Carlyle Smith at Trent University in Peterborough, Ontario, we used two-way avoidance training in rats, in part because we were interested in possible differences in the electrophysiological architecture associated with sleep in learners and non-learners. Rats were trained for 50 trials a day for two days and only about half of them learned the task in that period of time.[33] Most or all rats would have learned *one*-way avoidance responding in many fewer trials. The reason rats find the two-way version of avoidance learning difficult may be because it requires them to go against their natural tendency to avoid places previously associated with harm and danger.

You might wonder why some rats actually do learn two-way avoidance. One possibility is that different rats learn about different features of the task. As I discussed earlier,[28] in one-way avoidance rats do not need a signal, for example a tone, to learn the task because contextual cues provide a reliable signal of impending shock. In two-way avoidance, attention to the tone cue and the reward provided by its offset may lead to successful learning, but attention to the contextual cues may impair learning because threat reduction may not occur when the animal shuttles back to a place where it previously received shock. There is evidence from studies with pigeons that, when multiple cues are provided for making a response, different birds attend to different cues. George Stanley Reynolds (1936–1987), another student of B.F. Skinner, working at the University of California in San Diego, trained pigeons on a discrimination task with two pecking keys, circular plastic disks that could be pressed for grain reward. In each trial, one of the keys was red and the other green; additionally, the red key had a triangle drawn on it and the green key had a circle drawn on it. The two birds in the experiment learned the discrimination to a high degree, selecting the appropriate key, red with triangle, and receiving grain reward. Then Reynolds did some probe trials with just color (red or green) or geometric shape (triangle or circle) on the keys. Results revealed that for one of the birds, color was controlling responding and, for the other, geometric shape was controlling responding.[34] These results showed that when different stimuli occurred together, some animals used one stimulus and some used the other to control their responding. If the same phenomenon occurred in rats trying to learn two-way avoidance, those for which the warning cue controlled responding might learn the task; those for which contextual cues controlled responding might not learn the task. This may provide an explanation for why some rats learn two-way avoidance and some do not.

Even before Roy Wise and his co-workers identified the important role for dopamine in the rewarding effects of food in 1978, it was well known that dopamine played a role in avoidance learning. Barrett Cooper, George Breese, Lester Grant, and James Howard, working at the University of North Carolina in Chapel Hill in 1973, were the fist to show that depletion of brain dopamine led to deficits in conditioned avoidance responding in rats. Using the neurotoxin 6-hydroxydopamine, they were able to selectively damage dopaminergic neurons in the ventral midbrain (I discuss the anatomy of dopamine systems in Chapter 11). They observed that if a sufficient number of these dopaminergic neurons were destroyed, leading to a critical level of dopamine depletion in dopamine neuron terminal areas, rats failed to acquire avoidance responses.

If rats were trained first to perform the avoidance response and then had their dopamine systems depleted, they initially made avoidance responses but gradually lost the ability to perform the responses over trials. In both acquisition experiments and those carried out in trained animals, the rats continued to make *escape* responses when the shock was presented.[35] Results implicated dopamine in aversive learning where the rewarding stimulus for responding was offset of conditioned aversive stimuli.

Many years before Cooper et al. explicitly implicated dopamine in avoidance learning, it was reported that the drug chlorpromazine blocked avoidance responding.[36] As I discuss in more detail in Chapter 9, chlorpromazine was discovered in the 1950s to be an effective treatment for schizophrenia. Simone Courvoisier, working in 1956 in the pharmaceutical division of Rhône Poulanc, a company in France, reported that chlorpromazine blocked avoidance but not escape responses in rats. In these studies, rats were trained to climb a rope to avoid electrical foot shock and readily learned to do so. Rats treated with chlorpromazine failed to avoid the shock during a warning stimulus but still leapt onto and grasped the rope when shock occurred.[37] Although this observation provided evidence for the role of dopamine in avoidance learning, it was not known at the time because the effects of chlorpromazine on dopaminergic neurotransmission were not yet known.

The link between chlorpromazine and dopamine was first made in 1963 by Nobel laureate Arvid Carlsson and his co-worker Margit Lindqvist working at the University of Göteborg in Sweden. They found that chlorpromazine elevated levels of a metabolite of dopamine in the brain of mice and reasoned correctly that this resulted from the action of chlorpromazine on dopamine receptors.[38] Combining this information with the finding of Cooper et al. strongly suggested that the effects of chlorpromazine on avoidance learning resulted from its ability to block dopamine receptors.

Summary

This chapter has discussed the term "reward" and placed it into its historical context. The intellectual dominance of behaviorism in the early part of the twentieth century led to the use of the term "reinforcer" instead of "reward" to refer to biologically important stimuli (e.g., food presentation) that lead to modifications of behavior by increasing the frequency of responses that precede those stimuli. The intellectual influence of behaviorism began to decline in the middle of the twentieth century as descriptions of behavioral phenomena that appeared to violate the putative laws of learning accumulated. Among others, these included: conditioned taste aversion learning, the misbehavior of animals described by Breland and Breland, the apparent flexibility of responses used to attain rewarding stimuli once learning had taken place, and the observation of species-specific defense reactions. Incentive theory along with an ethological perspective that emphasized animals' specific behavioral adaptations for survival in their natural environment provided an alternative to the rigid stimulus–response learning framework of behaviorism. Because behaviorism had used the term "reinforcer" and it had come to connote the behaviorist perspective, the term "reward" came into broader use. Rewarding stimuli produce *incentive learning, the acquisition of neutral stimuli of an increased ability to elicit approach and other responses.*

During the years of transition from behaviorism to incentive learning perspectives on the effects of rewarding stimuli on behavior, the neurotransmitter dopamine began to emerge as a critical link in the neural circuitry underlying these effects. The relatively newly discovered phenomenon of brain stimulation reward was shown to depend on dopamine and subsequently the reward-related learning effects of food were shown to depend on dopamine. The importance of the latter discovery was somewhat obscured by the unfortunate use of the term "anhedonia" to describe the effects of dopamine receptor blockade on food-rewarded responding. It eventually emerged that the ability of reward-related stimuli to elicit approach and other responses from a trained animal was gradually lost when those stimuli were encountered while dopaminergic neurotransmission was blocked; this gradual loss took place even though lever pressing-contingent food presentations continued to be made.

Behaviorism struggled with avoidance learning. For an explanatory framework that shunned the use of any explanation that relied on unobservable events, the persistent responding of animals to *avoid* aversive stimuli such as mild electric shock presented a challenge. What was the reinforcer? Two-factor theory provided an answer. The first factor was learning the association between a conditioned stimulus (e.g., tone, contextual cues) and an aversive unconditioned stimulus, that is, mild electric shock; the pairing of these stimuli led to acquisition by the conditioned stimulus of aversive properties like those of the unconditioned stimulus. Initially, *escape* responding led to offset of the unconditioned aversive stimulus, termed "negative reinforcement." Eventually, *avoidance* responses similarly led to negative reinforcement by producing offset of the conditioned aversive stimulus. From an incentive learning point of view, the presentation of rewarding stimuli—offset of unconditioned or conditioned aversive stimuli—would lead to an increase in the ability of previously neutral stimuli to elicit approach and other responses. Thus, safety-related stimuli would become conditioned incentive stimuli. Around the time that dopamine was implicated in the ability of food reward to control responding, dopamine was also implicated in avoidance learning. Results suggest that in untrained animals, tested while in a dopamine-depleted state, conditioned incentive stimuli fail to acquire the ability to elicit approach and other responses and in trained animals similarly tested, conditioned incentive stimuli gradually lose their ability to elicit approach and other responses (e.g., avoidance responses). Note that *trained animals subsequently tested while dopaminergic neurotransmission is reduced initially retain the ability to respond but lose that ability with repeated testing while in a low dopamine neurotransmission state*; this observation is central to understanding the role of dopamine in reward-related incentive learning and reappears many times throughout the book. In the next chapter I provide further details of the elements of incentive conditioning.

Chapter 3

Dopamine and the elements of incentive learning

Incentive learning is the acquisition by neutral stimuli of an increased ability to elicit approach and other responses. "Other responses" could include pushing, pulling, digging, biting, and so on, depending on the situation and the natural abilities of the animal. Rewarding stimuli produce incentive learning. We all know that rewarding stimuli can be used to modify behavior and probably all have experience training an animal to perform a trick by using food rewards. If you have a cat or dog that is regularly fed with food taken from a can or plastic bag, you probably have noticed that the sound of opening the can or rustling the bag can cause the animal to come bounding to the kitchen from somewhere else in the house. Even if the can you were opening or the bag you were rustling was not a can or bag of pet food, the pet came. What has happened in this situation?

The simple answer to that question is that the pet has learned to associate the sound of opening the can or bag with food. However, this explanation provides no information about the neural mechanisms underlying this learning. Neither does it acknowledge that there may be dissociable elements of the learning that are mediated by different parts of the brain. Research has shown that in a situation like the one described here, where an animal learns to approach cues signaling food, at least two things are learned: (i) animals learn associations between stimuli; and (ii) they undergo incentive learning mediated by brain dopamine systems.

Incentive learning theory provides a descriptive framework for what is going on when reward-related learning takes place and learning theory in general describes the elements of multiple forms of learning. Incentive learning theory does not provide the mechanism for how the learning actually takes place in terms of neuronal connections in the brain. Since dopamine has been shown to play a critical role in incentive learning, it follows that dopamine probably modulates neuronal connections that are the basis of the learning. In Chapters 11 and 12, I discuss the brain nuclei and neuronal pathways that have been implicated in incentive learning and how dopamine is thought to influence their synaptic strengths. Before that, it is important to recognize the elements that are involved in reward-related learning. That is the topic of this chapter.

Lever pressing for food

Let's start with a rat learning to press a lever for food, a *sine qua non* of behaviorism. The rat will be hungry because it will not have been fed for some hours before the test session. What does the animal learn in this situation? The testing apparatus is a clear plastic chamber, 20 cm in each dimension, frequently referred to as a "Skinner box," named after B.F. Skinner, an influential behaviorist in the twentieth century. The chamber is housed in a larger, opaque, ventilated cubicle that reduces the rat's exposure to light and sounds in the room. The front wall of the chamber is the door through which the rat can be placed into it. On one side a small lever, 2.0 cm wide and 0.5 cm thick protrudes 2.0 cm into the chamber at a height of 3.0 cm. On the other side on the floor against the wall is a semicircular food cup 2.5 cm in diameter and 1.0 cm deep with a hole in the wall just above it. Outside of the chamber is a food dispenser (food magazine), a devise like a gumball machine with a disk with holes around the edge; the disk is situated in the bottom of a plastic cylinder. In each hole is a 45-mg food pellet. There is an opening in the bottom of the plastic cylinder so that when the disk rotates a pellet drops through the hole. Below the hole a plastic tube runs down to the hole above the feeder cup in the chamber. Electrical circuits are arranged so that when the rat presses the lever it closes a switch, sending an electrical pulse to the stepping motor that operates rotation of the disk in the food disperser and a pellet appears in the food cup. Thus, the rat can learn to press the lever to get food.

If a rat is placed into the chamber with no food in the food cup and the electrical circuit for operating the food dispenser by pressing the lever disabled, what will the rat do? Since the chamber is novel, the first thing the rat might do is freeze. This is a natural response to novelty for rats. Being prey animals in their natural environment, they have evolved to be cautious in unfamiliar situations where there may be a predator lurking. As the chamber is located in an outer cubicle, the rat will not be out in the open and will soon begin to explore the environment. During exploration the rat will sniff, make vibrissae (whisker) contact with, and touch and manipulate with its forepaws the walls, floor, corners, lever, and food cup. The rat will form a *cognitive map* of the chamber environment. The term "cognitive map" was used by Edward C. Tolman (1886–1959), a psychologist who worked at the University of California, Berkeley, and who challenged the radical behaviorists' focus on observable events.[1] A cognitive map can be understood as a set of relationships or associations among stimuli (Chapter 4). If the rat is left in the chamber for an hour and its movement is recorded, the movement will be seen to diminish over time. If the rat is removed from the chamber after an hour and then returned the next day, it again will explore, exploration will diminish over time, and the total amount of exploration will likely be less than the previous day. The diminution of exploration both within and across days reflects a form of learning termed "habituation;" this is a different form of learning from incentive learning, but the two may be related, as discussed in Chapter 6. If the rat is returned to the chamber for an hour each day and the environment remains unchanged, it may lie down there and may sleep.

Prior to beginning to train the lever press response itself, let's now introduce food into the situation by placing a couple of food pellets into the food cup before putting the rat into the chamber. When the now-habituated rat is placed into the chamber it will initially check it out to see that nothing has changed and in so doing will find the food and, if it is familiar food, will probably immediately eat the food. The food will have a general activating effect on the rat (as a result of the release of dopamine, as you will see in Chapter 5) and it will begin to vigorously explore the chamber, returning often to the food cup to see if there is any more food. If no more food arrives, activity will diminish like on previous days. If instead a food pellet is delivered periodically by activating the feeder (that makes a click), say once a minute on average but with a variable time between pellets, the rat will readily eat each pellet when it arrives and in between deliveries will vigorously explore the chamber, especially the food cup area, *as if it is trying to figure out how to control food delivery*. I cannot know if the rat is trying to figure something out; I can only observe its behavior. Behaviorally, the rat is sniffing, biting, gnawing, licking, clawing, pushing, pulling, climbing onto, and doing whatever else it can to the food cup. It sure looks like the rat is trying to figure out how to control food delivery.

This is incentive learning in action. Eating the food activated dopamine neurons in the brain of the rat (see Chapter 5) and they produced incentive learning, increasing the ability of neutral stimuli to elicit approach and other responses. The affected stimuli are those associated with the food. In this example, the stimuli associated with food are the click of the pellet dispenser, the food cup, and the region of the chamber around the food cup. Those stimuli acquire the ability to elicit approach and other responses and this learning is manifested by the animal's barrage of behavior towards the food cup and surrounding area. This phase in lever-press training is often referred to as magazine training. Overall, the animal will be much more active in the chamber after having been fed there compared to its previous days there when the chamber was familiar but not associated with food. Not only will the rat direct more responding towards the food cup, but it will also direct more responses towards the other areas of the chamber, including the corners, opposite walls, floor, and lever. There is some incentive learning about all of the cues in the chamber because the chamber now is associated with food; in addition, there is a gradient of incentive learning in the chamber with the focus being on the stimuli most temporally and spatially proximal to the food, that is, the click of the pellet dispenser and the food cup.

Now the fun part begins. We are going to *shape* the lever press response of the rat. Skinner may have first used the term "shape" in 1951 to refer to the process of training a particular response.[2] The circuit in the test box will now be reconnected so that the lever can activate the feeder. In addition, we, the experimenter, will connect a hand-held switch to the feeder so that we can manually operate the feeder by pressing a button. A couple of food pellets will be dropped into the feeder cup and the rat will be placed into the chamber. The rat will eat the food pellets and begin its routine of directing species-typical responses at the food cup: biting, sniffing, and scratching, for example. It may sniff one of the corners of the wall behind the food cup. Soon, it will turn towards the opposite wall, the location of the lever. At this point, we press the button and deliver a food pellet. The pellet dispenser clicks and the rat whips around and snatches the food pellet from the feeder. Again the rat will direct responses at the food cup and related stimuli, but its likelihood of turning towards the opposite wall will increase and as soon as it does so, we deliver another pellet. The pattern repeats itself, but the turn towards the other wall comes sooner. We wait. The rat pauses as if waiting to hear the wonderful click but nothing happens. A flurry of responses towards the food cup is followed by a more vigorous response directed towards the opposite wall and this time the rat almost touches the lever. "Click." A dash to the food cup and back to the opposite wall. It usually does not take very many approximations before the rat is directing a variety of responses towards the lever, for example licking, biting, pushing, pulling, and so on, and in so doing, displaces the lever to operate the pellet dispenser and deliver a food pellet. It quickly learns that a downward displacement is the effective action. The lever press response has been shaped.

What has happened here? One important aspect of this learning that is discussed at some length in Chapter 5 is that stimuli that are reliably associated with a rewarding stimulus themselves acquire the ability to release dopamine and produce incentive learning. This learning is dissociable from incentive learning involving the click of the pellet dispenser becoming a conditioned incentive stimulus, acquiring an increased ability to elicit approach and other responses (see Figure 3.1).

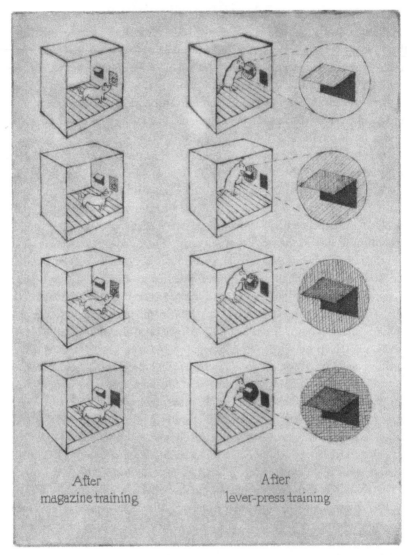

After magazine training

After lever-press training

Figure 3.1 *Incentive learning underlying lever pressing for food*: Magazine training (left-hand column) involves periodic presentations of a food pellet into the recess in the right-hand wall of the chamber. For the rat, the recess gradually (top to bottom) acquires incentive value—an increased ability to elicit approach and other responses—with repeated food presentations; the gradual darkening of the recess is a heuristic device used to show how incentive learning strengthens with repeated presentations of food into the recess. Lever-press response learning (middle column) involves gradual (top to bottom) acquisition by the lever and lever-related stimuli (images enlarged in right-hand column) of incentive value.

When I first began working with rats, I used the response-shaping procedure described to train my animals to lever press for food. Over the years, however, I learned that for most animals it was not necessary to manually shape the lever-press response. If food was periodically delivered to the food cup in the chamber and the lever circuit to operate the feeder was engaged, most rats learned to press the lever for food on their own. Apparently the activating effects of the food were vigorous enough to produce a sufficient volume and variety of responses from the rat that displacement of the lever to produce the click of the pellet dispenser and a food pellet took place, and the incentive learning mechanism looked after the rest. One of the tricks-of-the-trade often used by animal behaviorists to accelerate lever-press response learning is to put a bit of powdered food pellet onto the lever after magazine training has taken place.[3] A rat that has just eaten a pellet from the food cup and is vigorously responding towards the features (stimuli) of the chamber will quickly find the food powder on top of the lever. This will elicit sniffing, reaching, scratching, and related responses towards the top of the lever that quickly serve to depress the lever and operate the switch to produce the click of the pellet dispenser. It can save the experimenter a lot of time!

B.F. Skinner's last book was entitled, *Upon Further Reflection*.[4] In it, Skinner talks about the effects of reinforcement on behavior in terms of selectionism by analogy to natural selection. Charles Darwin (1809–1882) first described the elements of natural selection. These included two things: (i) an at-the-time-unknown mechanism of variation; and (ii) a mechanism of selection that acted on that variation.[5] We now know that the variation is produced through genetic mechanisms of mutation, combination, and crossing over;[6] those variations that confer a fitness advantage, defined by the number of offspring left by that individual, are selected. In the case of learning produced by reinforcement, Skinner argued that the mechanism of variation is the behavioral repertoire of the individual; basically, the individual tries to act on her environment in a variety of ways until she finds something that apparently works to produce another reinforcement (cf, the description of lever-press learning in the previous paragraph). According to Skinner, reinforcement then selects that response by strengthening it, making that response more likely to recur when the same situation is encountered in the future. According to the incentive-learning framework being elaborated in this book, the effect of reward presentation is not so much to select a particular response, but to strengthen the response-eliciting properties of the stimuli associated with the reward. However, the response also has a stimulus aspect (proprioception, efference copy) that can become incorporated into the stimulus complex controlling responding as discussed in Chapters 11 and 12. At this point, it is useful to think of behavioral variation by analogy to genetic variation, and to think of rewarding stimuli operating on behavioral variation by selecting, through incentive learning, those stimuli that are reliably associated with the rewarding stimulus by analogy to natural selection operating on genetic variation.

Before continuing the discussion of the elements of reward-related learning, I want to mention *creativity* in the context of the present ideas. Without an understanding of the two essential elements of Darwin's theory of evolution, genetic variation and natural selection, it is difficult to understand the variety of species on Earth and many alternate explanations have been suggested such as those provided by some religious doctrines. Perhaps one of the most difficult aspects of evolutionary theory to accept is that there is no purposeful creative process behind it; genetic mutations follow physical laws but are essentially random in terms of possible functional consequences. Occasionally, a variation comes along that confers a fitness advantage and that mutation endures in the gene pool. Richard Dawkins, evolutionary biologist from Oxford, UK, addressed this issue in his illuminating book *The Blind Watchmaker*.[7] Continuing on the analogy proposed by Skinner for the effects of reinforcement on behavior, it follows that apparent creativity manifested behaviorally can be understood as variation in action. Organisms emit a variety of actions towards stimuli associated with rewarding outcomes and those actions and associated stimuli that lead to a successful (rewarding) outcome get an enhanced ability to elicit responses in the future and thereby come to control responding. In the end the behavior of the animal may appear to be creative, but it can be understood as resulting from the selectionist effects of incentive learning operating on environmental and response-related stimuli. Although the present section is focused on understanding several animal-learning paradigms from the point of view of incentive learning, this framework has implications extending well beyond these paradigms to more complex human behavior that is often deemed to be creative. Just as apparent creativity in nature can be understood with reference to the elements of natural selection, apparent human creativity may be best understood with reference to the elements of reward-related incentive learning.

Amphetamine-produced conditioned place preference

One of the lines of evidence implicating dopamine in reward-related learning comes from studies of conditioned place preference. In these studies, rats show a preference for a particular place by spending more time there when given a choice, after the place has been paired with a drug that enhances dopamine neurotransmission. Generally, drugs that are abused by people (e.g., amphetamine, cocaine, alcohol, nicotine, heroin, etc.) produce a conditioned place preference in animals and there is good evidence that this learning depends on dopamine (see Chapter 10). In this section I use amphetamine-produced conditioned place preference to describe incentive learning in this situation.

The testing apparatus consists of two chambers, approximately 35 cm^2, connected by a short tunnel, 8.0 cm^2. The two chambers are arranged linearly with the tunnel between them, centered at floor level on a wall of each chamber. Guillotine doors can be inserted to block access to the tunnel from either chamber. The two chambers are made distinctive from each other by varying the floor and walls. The floor in one chamber is stainless steel rods spaced 1 cm apart and the floor in the other is wire mesh that forms 1-cm squares. The walls in one of the chamber are urethane-sealed natural wood and in the other they are vertical alternating black-and-white stripes 1 cm wide. The walls are covered with clear plastic. In my lab, I have four of these apparatus and each has a different configuration of wall and floor stimuli; thus, in two apparatus, the wire mesh floors are on the right and, in two, on the left. In two, the striped walls are on the right and, in two, on the left, but not the same two as for the floors so that one apparatus has black and white stripes on the left paired with a wire-mesh floor and the other has clear plastic-covered natural wooden walls paired with the wire mesh floor on the left. Each apparatus has a hinged top with holes in it for ventilation, is dimly and indirectly illuminated by a 7.5-watt incandescent bulb placed between the chambers, and is situated inside a larger, opaque, ventilated cubicle that mutes outside noise and blocks most outside light.

The conditioned place preference apparatus is outfitted with six infrared emitters and detectors (sensors) that make it possible to monitor the location of the rat and provide an index of level of activity in each chamber. Each chamber is outfitted with two emitters and sensors at a height of 5 cm that trisect the chamber along the long axis; similarly, the tunnel is trisected by a pair of emitters and sensors at a height of 3 cm.

Rats are tested one at a time in each apparatus at about the same time each day. One version of the protocol begins by placing the rat into one side of the apparatus with the tunnel open. Half of the rats in a group will regularly begin on one side and half on the other, with the start side remaining constant for any particular animal. The first three sessions over the first three days are preconditioning sessions that simply measure the time the rat spends on each side and in the tunnel; each session is 15 minutes in duration. You might have wondered about the choice of wall and floor patterns; they were chosen because previous work has shown that they are about equally attractive or unattractive to rats so that they spend about an equal amount of time in each side.[8] Over the three preconditioning days the typical rat will spend about 420 seconds in each side and about 60 seconds in the tunnel for a total of 900 seconds or 15 minutes.

The next eight days are conditioning days during which the tunnel is blocked. During daily 30-minute sessions, one side is paired with the dopamine-activating drug amphetamine (2.0 mg/kg injected immediately before placing the rat into the chamber) and the other side is paired with saline, the vehicle used to dissolve amphetamine. Thus, prior to sessions 1, 3, 5, and 7, amphetamine is injected and the animal is placed on one side and prior to sessions 2, 4, 6, and 8, saline is injected and the animal is placed on the other side. Some rats are conditioned in the right-hand chamber and some in the left, and each configuration of wall and floor patterns is associated with drug for some rats and with saline for others. All of this counterbalancing assures that any possible influence of a particular side (left or right) or pattern of wall or floor stimuli is randomized across animals within each group. During conditioning sessions, activity can be quantified by the number of beam breaks.

The final day is the test day and the tunnel is open as it was during preconditioning. No drug in injected prior to the 15-minute test. Results reveal that the animals spend significantly more time in the side of the apparatus where they had amphetamine. Whereas initially they spent about 420 seconds in the side that was to be paired with amphetamine, now they spend more than 500 seconds there and proportionally less time in the other side. They show a preference for the amphetamine-paired side that is referred to as a conditioned place preference.

Amphetamine reverses the dopamine transporter, a molecule in the membrane of the presynaptic cell that normally removes dopamine from the synapse. As a result of the action of amphetamine, the level of synaptic dopamine increases because more is released and the releasing cell reuptakes less. The higher concentrations of synaptic dopamine putatively produce incentive learning, increasing the ability of neutral stimuli to elicit approach and other responses. The stimuli that are encountered in association with amphetamine are those of the side of the apparatus that was paired with amphetamine, *viz.*, the particular wall pattern and floor type, as well as the place in space, that is, the right or left side of the apparatus, depending on the rat. When the rat is placed in the apparatus with the tunnel open on the test day, the stimuli from the drug-paired side will attract the animal more than the stimuli from the saline-paired side resulting in the animal spending more time there, manifested as the conditioned place preference (see Figure 3.2).

If dopamine is critical for the ability of amphetamine to produce incentive learning in the conditioned place preference experiment, it should be possible to block the place preference effect by blocking dopamine receptors

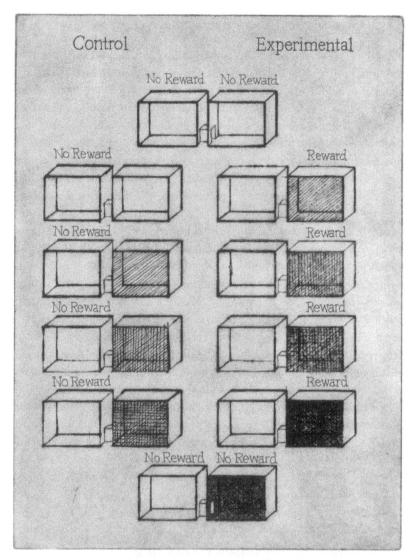

Figure 3.2 *Incentive learning underlying the establishment of a conditioned place preference*: During three 15-minute pre-exposure sessions, rats are placed into an apparatus consisting of two distinct chambers connected by a tunnel (top image) and the amount of time spent in each chamber is measured. During eight conditioning sessions, with the tunnel blocked, rats experience four 30-minute exposures (days 1, 3, 5, and 7, top to bottom) to the left (no reward) chamber following an injection of saline and four 30-minute exposures (days 2, 4, 6, and 8, top to bottom) to the right (reward) chamber after being injected with a dopamine agonist such as amphetamine. During amphetamine sessions, the stimuli of the right-hand chamber gradually become incentive stimuli indicated by progressive darkening (top to bottom). On the test day (bottom image), rats are *not* injected and again have access to both chambers. Conditioned place preference is revealed as increased time spent in the chamber previously associated with amphetamine reflecting the increased incentive value of those stimuli, i.e., their increased ability to elicit approach and other responses.

before injecting amphetamine on conditioning days. This is exactly what has been found using a number of different dopamine receptor-blocking drugs.[9] It should be possible to produce a conditioned place preference with other drugs, for example cocaine, that augment dopamine neurotransmission and to block their effect with dopamine receptor-blocking drugs, and it is.[10] In fact, the rewarding properties of a number of drugs, for example nicotine, alcohol, and Δ^9-tetrahydrocannabinol (the active ingredient of marijuana), that are not primarily dopamine receptor agonists have been shown to be mediated by dopamine (see Chapter 10),[11] further strengthening the claim that dopamine is critical for incentive learning.

There is a difference in the specificity of the incentive learning in the lever-press situation compared with the conditioned-place-preference situation that should be noted. In the lever-press situation there is a gradient of incentive learning with the strongest incentive stimuli being those associated with the food cup, then those associated with the lever, and, finally, the rest of the stimuli of the test chamber, all of which will have some incentive strength because they are part of a place where the animal has received food. In the conditioned place preference situation, however, there is no obvious comparable gradient within the side of the apparatus associated with amphetamine. The strength of incentive learning associated with the stimuli of the floor or walls, the corners, and the entrance area to the tunnel should all have about the same incentive value. None has been specifically associated with increased synaptic dopamine produced by amphetamine.[12] This difference in the specificity of incentive learning associated with lever pressing for food versus incentive learning in conditioned place preference will be important when considering the effects of various dopaminergic agents, including dopamine receptor subtype-specific agonists, on responding in Chapter 7.

Conditioned activity based on cocaine

Cocaine and amphetamine are similar but not identical in their action at synapses. Where amphetamine reverses the transporter, increasing dopamine release and blocking the reuptake of dopamine already in the synapse, cocaine only blocks the transporter thereby blocking reuptake. The result is that the concentration of synaptic dopamine increases with both drugs, but perhaps amphetamine compared to cocaine more clearly amplifies the ongoing signals in dopamine neurons. I discuss some results in Chapter 7 that inform this consideration. When discussing conditioned activity it would be equally possible to base the discussion on amphetamine or cocaine or other related agents, for example methylphenidate; I have chosen to use cocaine here.

Conditioned activity refers to the phenomenon of increased locomotor activity in the presence of stimuli previously associated with a drug that increases dopamine neurotransmission and itself produces increases in locomotor activity. The instrumentation for this task is the simplest of the three discussed so far; all that is needed is a chamber and the capacity to assess locomotor activity. We use clear plastic chambers, 41 × 50 × 37 cm high outfitted with two tiers of infrared emitters and detectors. Each chamber (we have six of them) is located in an outer, ventilated cubicle that provides some insulation from sounds and light in the room. There is a clear plastic window in the front of the cubicle and it is illuminated inside with a 2.5-watt incandescent bulb, allowing the experimenter to view a rat inside the chamber. The tiers of infrared emitters and detectors are at a height of 5 and 15 cm, respectively. The beams are located at 10-cm intervals along the walls of the chamber creating a 4 × 3 grid at each tier. A count is made each time a rat passes through a beam. The lower tier of beams generally produces counts as a result of the rat moving about the chamber and the upper tier produces counts when the rat rears or jumps. Counts are collected by a small, dedicated computer and subsequently downloaded to a general-purpose computer for analyses.[13]

The conditioned place preference procedure discussed in the previous section relied on a within-animal comparison of time spent in the drug-paired side before and after conditioning. The conditioned activity procedure relies on a between-group comparison of independent groups that undergo slightly different training. One version of the protocol consists of three phases: three 60-minute preconditioning sessions, five 60-minute conditioning sessions, and one 60-minute test session. To begin with, each rat from two groups is pre-exposed to an activity chamber for 60 minutes a day for three days. For the next five days, each group is injected just prior to a 60-minute session in an activity chamber. Each rat in the paired group is injected with cocaine (10 mg/kg) and each rat in the unpaired group is injected with the saline vehicle used to dissolve cocaine. Some time after the test session, say one hour, the animals from the unpaired group receive cocaine (10 mg/kg) in their home cage and the animals from the paired group receive saline in their home cage. Thus, after five conditioning days, all animals have had five one-hour exposures to the activity chambers, each following an injection, and all animals have had five injections of cocaine and five injections of saline. The critical difference between the two groups is that the paired group had the cocaine in the activity chamber and the unpaired group had it in their home cage. Assessment of the activity counts during the five conditioning sessions will show greater activity in the paired group revealing the unconditioned locomotor-stimulating ability of this compound.

On the test day, rats in both groups are injected with saline and given one 60-minute session. Conditioned activity based on cocaine is observed as significantly more activity counts in the group that had cocaine paired with the test environment than in the group that had saline paired with the test environment. By including home-cage injections in the experimental procedure it is not possible to attribute the conditioned activity effect to simply having received cocaine on the five previous days, as this was the case for both groups. What was critical for producing the conditioned activity effect was the *pairing* of the drug with the test environment.

From an incentive learning point of view, the features of the activity boxes that were experienced while the animal was under the influence of cocaine and therefore with enhanced dopamine neurotransmission became conditioned incentive stimuli, acquiring an increased ability to elicit approach and other responses. This conditioning was manifested as increased activity counts. The group that received cocaine in their home cage did not experience the pairing of the stimuli of the activity chamber with increased dopamine neurotransmission and did not show conditioned activity (see Figure 3.3).

For the unpaired group, it might be expected that stimuli in the home cage that are associated with cocaine will become conditioned incentive stimuli by the same mechanism that leads to incentive learning in the paired group. However, those same stimuli would also be associated with no cocaine for many hours after the effects of the cocaine wore off. During this time any conditioning effect would be expected to be lost because repeated exposure to conditioned incentive stimuli in the absence of the unconditioned incentive stimulus upon which they are based (e.g., food, amphetamine, cocaine, etc.) leads to a loss of incentive conditioning, a phenomenon termed "extinction."[14] In fact, extinction can also be observed in the rats of the paired group if they are tested in the activity chambers on several occasions following an injection of saline. If both groups are tested several times following an injection of saline, the initial difference between the paired and unpaired group will gradually diminish over sessions, revealing extinction of the conditioned incentive properties of the cocaine-paired stimuli.[15]

As might be anticipated, if a dopamine receptor-blocking drug is given before cocaine injections during conditioning days, the locomotor-enhancing effect of cocaine is lost and so is the conditioned activity effect.[16] Cocaine only produces conditioned activity if its dopamine neurotransmission-enhancing effects are intact during conditioning sessions. Other drugs that enhance dopamine neurotransmission, for example amphetamine, produce conditioned activity and it too is blocked by treatment with dopamine receptor-blocking drugs prior to conditioning sessions.[17]

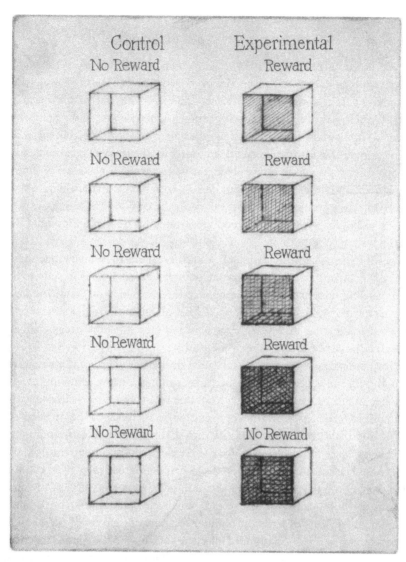

Figure 3.3 *Incentive learning underlying the establishment of conditioned activity*: Two independent groups of rats are tested. The control group receives four (left-hand column, top to bottom, first four images, "no reward") 60-minute exposures to a chamber outfitted with detectors that record amount of motor activity. One hour following each of these sessions, rats in the control group are injected with the dopamine agonist cocaine in their home cage. The experimental group receives four (right-hand column, top to bottom, first four images, "reward") 60-minute exposures to the same chamber, but this group is injected with cocaine prior to each exposure; one hour following each of these sessions, rats in the experimental group are injected with saline in their home cage. During cocaine sessions, the stimuli of the chamber gradually become incentive stimuli indicated by progressive darkening (top to bottom). On the test day (bottom image in each column), rats are *not* injected and again have access to the chamber. Greater activity is observed in the experimental group, even though both groups have the same history of cocaine treatments. This reveals incentive learning to the stimuli associated with dopamine activation, i.e., those stimuli have acquired an increased ability to elicit approach and other responses.

Sensitization is a phenomenon related to conditioned activity. Sensitization is observed as an increasing response to the same dose of the same drug when it is given from session to session, for example, with one session per day. Sensitization has been reported with cocaine, amphetamine, and a number of related compounds.[18] A sensitization experiment can be carried out using the same experimental design as described earlier for the study of conditioned activity. During the conditioning phase, the paired group is observed to show a larger response to each subsequent dose of cocaine. On the test day, instead of giving each group saline, as was done in the conditioned activity experiment, each group is tested with cocaine at the same 10 mg/kg dose that was given during conditioning sessions (sometimes lower doses are given to both groups on the sensitization test day). Results reveal that the paired group shows a greater response to cocaine than the unpaired group. This is in spite of the similar drug history of the two groups. In these experiments, sensitization is not simply the result of giving repeated doses of the same drug; sensitization is greater in the group that is tested for sensitization in the presence of environmental stimuli previously paired with the drug.

The observation of greater sensitization in the paired group can be understood from the point of view of incentive learning. During conditioning, the pairing of the test environment with cocaine results in incentive learning, the stimuli from the test environment acquiring an increased ability to elicit approach and other responses. This incentive learning adds to the unconditioned stimulant effects of the drug to produce the elevated response to the drug observed as sensitization. On the test day, when both groups are given cocaine, the paired group experiences the unconditioned stimulant effect of the drug plus the response-activating effects of the environmental stimuli; the unpaired group experiences only the unconditioned stimulant effects of the cocaine. The addition of the unconditioned effects of cocaine and the learned incentive properties of the environmental stimuli where the drug was experienced in the past results in greater locomotor activity in the paired group compared with the unpaired group that experiences only the unconditioned effects of cocaine.[19]

Conditioned avoidance responding

As discussed briefly at the end of the previous chapter, for many years, the conditioned avoidance responding procedure was used by the pharmaceutical industry to screen drugs that may be useful in the treatment of psychosis. Drugs that blocked conditioned avoidance responding without blocking escape responding were identified as good candidates. In this section, I review this procedure, the effects of dopamine receptor-blocking drugs, and what they tell us about the elements of incentive learning. Considerable insight into incentive learning can be gained from a study of conditioned avoidance responding.

A number of different apparatuses have been used in the study of conditioned avoidance responding, even a rope dangling above the floor that can be climbed to escape mild foot shock or avoid impending mild foot shock (see Chapter 2). A more typical apparatus is a rectangular chamber, for example $25 \times 78 \times 33$ cm high. The chamber is divided along its long axis into two equal compartments by a partition that has an opening, for example 13 cm², in the middle at floor level. In the one-way avoidance version of the procedure, the rat is placed into one side, a tone is turned on and after ten seconds the rat receives mild electric foot shock; this is termed the "shock side." The foot shock can be escaped by passing through the opening in the partition to the other side, termed the "safe side." The two sides are spatially distinct insofar as they remain in the same position relative to one another and normally the entire apparatus remains in the same place in a testing room so that room cues such as light fixtures remain constant; the experimenter stands beside the apparatus to manually move the animal between compartments and she always stands in the same place so that cues related to the experimenter also remain relatively constant. The two compartments may have distinct features such as wall pattern or floor texture, but even if they are quite similar, their relative spatial location remains different.

A typical testing protocol might include ten trials per day with a 30-second inter-trial interval. Each trial will begin by placing the rat into the shock side of the apparatus and turning on the tone. After ten seconds, mild electric foot shock comes on. (The foot shock is not like the intense electrical shock that some of us may have experienced by inadvertently coming into contact with a live wire in our home. It is much less intense. If the experimenter touches the electrified grid with her hand, she experiences mild cramping feelings in her fingers.[20]) The rats find the shock uncomfortable and try to escape it. They may jump, move into the corners of the box, and go through the partition. When they have entered the safe side the tone turns off and they escape the shock. When 30 seconds have elapsed since the end of the trial, the rat is picked up by the experimenter and placed back into the shock side and the tone is again turned on, beginning another ten-second pre-shock period followed by shock. After an average of about five trials, rats begin to make the shuttle response to the safe side during the tone stimulus prior to the onset of foot shock; rather than making an *escape* response during the shock, the rat has made an *avoidance* response during the pre-shock stimulus, termed a "conditioned avoidance response." For the remaining trials on the first day and for almost all of the trials on subsequent days, rats are observed to make avoidance responses and they seldom experience the shock again.

If an animal is treated with a dopamine receptor-blocking drug before conditioned avoidance response training begins, it fails to acquire the avoidance response.[21] From trial to trial the rat sits in the shock side through the entire ten seconds of the signal and then receives foot shock at the end of the signal. When the shock comes on, the rat moves about the chamber and eventually makes the escape response to the safe side. It would appear that the rat has failed to learn that the tone signals shock. However, I will show you that that is not the case. The dopamine receptor blocker-treated rat learns a number of things in the conditioned avoidance situation but it does not undergo incentive learning.

One thing the dopamine receptor blocker-treated rat learns is the location of safety. I discovered this in one of those rare and wonderful moments in a scientist's career when he begins to organize his data from individual animals into group averages and variances and an unexpected picture emerges. I was calculating the average latency, for each of the ten trials of the first test session, to make the shuttle response from the shock side to the safe side starting from the beginning of the trial when the rat is placed into the shock side and the tone is turned on. There were three groups: a control group that was injected with drug vehicle (but no drug) prior to the session and two drug groups that had been treated with two different doses (0.5 and 1.0 mg/kg) of the dopamine receptor-blocking drug pimozide prior to the session. The data revealed an impressive learning curve for the control group. This group took an average of about eight seconds to make the *escape* response on the first trial. Over the first five trials, the latency to make the *escape* response got shorter and shorter until by the fifth trial it reached about two seconds, close to the time when the shock comes on. Over the next five trials, average latencies continued to decline as the rats became more and more efficient at *avoiding* the foot shock by scrambling to safety prior to its onset. This learning curve revealed normal avoidance learning over ten trials (Figure 3.4).[21]

When I calculated the points for the corresponding curves for the two drug groups, I made an important discovery. Over the first five trials, the two drug groups showed the same decrease in latencies as the control group, beginning with an *escape* latency of about 9–10 seconds on trial one and showing progressively shorter *escape* latencies over the next four trials. The drug groups then diverged from the control group, failing to progress to shorter and shorter latencies. Apparently, during the period when the shock was on and an escape response was required, the drug groups learned from trial to trial how to more effectively get to the safe side. They must have learned that there was a safe side and where it was. In spite of this learning, they showed significant deficits in learning to make *avoidance* responses during the tone before the shock came on.[21]

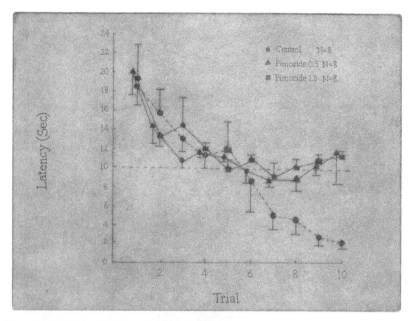

Figure 3.4 *Effects of a dopamine receptor antagonist on conditioned avoidance learning*: Mean (± standard error of the mean) avoidance latencies (seconds) over ten training trials in a control group and two groups treated with the dopamine receptor-blocking drug pimozide (0.5, 1.0 mg/kg). The conditioned stimulus (tone) comes on at time 0 and remains on for ten seconds (indicated by the broken horizontal line), then mild electric foot shock is presented. The performance of all groups improves over the first six trials; the control group continues to improve over the next four trials, but the pimozide-treated groups show no further improvement. Analysis of variance yielded a significant group × trial interaction.

Adapted from RJ Beninger, ST Mason, AG Phillips, and HC Fibiger, The use of conditioned suppression to evaluate the nature of neuroleptic-induced avoidance deficits, *Journal of Pharmacology and Experimental Therapeutics*, 213 (3), pp. 623–627, Figure 3 (top panel) © The American Society for Pharmacology and Experimental Therapeutics, 1980. With permission from ASPET.

What does this observation tell us? To answer that question, it is important first to identify the elements of learning in this situation. Recall that incentive learning is the acquisition by neutral stimuli of an increased ability to elicit approach and other responses. In the conditioned avoidance-learning situation, incentive learning occurs when the stimuli associated with the safe side of the chamber acquire the ability to elicit approach responses (Figure 3.5). Presumably, during the initial stages of avoidance learning, dopamine neurons are activated by the offset of foot shock that takes place when the rat physically moves itself from the shock side to the safe side (I said, "presumably" here because this point is not yet resolved as discussed further in Chapter 6). The

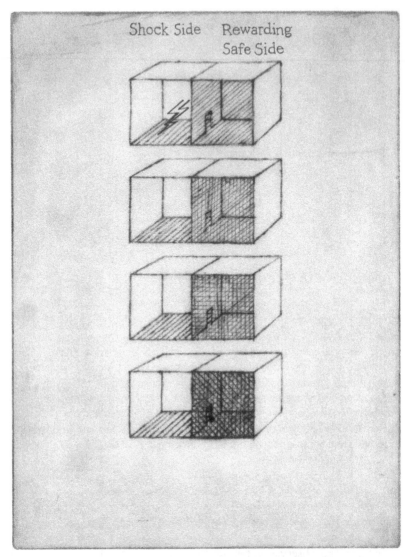

Figure 3.5 *Incentive learning underlying conditioned avoidance responding*: During each conditioning day, rats are placed into the left (shock side) of an apparatus consisting of two chambers separated by a wall outfitted with an opening allowing access to both chambers. A tone is sounded and at the end of ten seconds, mild electric foot shock is presented on the shock side only. Over several trials (top to bottom) rats quickly learn to shuttle to the rewarding safe side during the tone stimulus, thereby avoiding aversive mild electric foot shock. The gradual darkening of the rewarding safe side is a heuristic device used to show how incentive learning strengthens with repeated presentations of safety. Presumably (see text), exposure to safety-related stimuli activates dopaminergic neurons that produce incentive learning, increasing the ability of those stimuli to elicit approach and other responses.

putative increased release of dopamine associated with the safety-related stimuli leads to those stimuli acquiring the ability subsequently to elicit avoidance responding. Animals undergoing initial training while treated with a dopamine receptor-blocking drug fail to show incentive learning and avoidance responses are seldom seen. However, from the latency data discussed earlier, it is clear that the animals have learned something, *viz.*, the location of safety, because they show a learning curve during the period of foot shock, becoming progressively more efficient at making the escape response.

When a rat is treated with a dopamine receptor blocker and tested a second day, it generally fails to avoid but always escapes in the first second or two of mild foot shock, showing clear evidence that it has retained the learning of the place of safety from the first day. There is other evidence of learning in this situation. Our anecdotal observations of the dopamine receptor blocker-treated rats in the conditioned avoidance task suggested that they were threatened during the tone presentation. Recall that the tone is on for ten seconds before the shock comes on. The rats would crouch, their fur would stick up somewhat, sort of like a Halloween cat only not that extreme (a phenomenon termed "piloerection"), they would sometimes urinate or defecate, and occasionally vocalize. The rats sure seemed to know something bad was imminent. To empirically test the hypothesis that the rats have learned that the tone signals shock, one possibility would be to engage some observers, armed with a rating scale of response intensity, for example crouching posture (mild (score 1), moderate (score 2), severe (score 3)); piloerection (mild (score 1), moderate (score 2) severe (score 3)), and so on. The observers could be kept blind to the treatment condition of the animals, obviating any possibility of observer bias in their scoring, that is, if the observer knew a rat had been treated with a dopamine receptor-blocking drug and if he knew the hypothesis was that such a rat will show increased scores on the rating scales, such knowledge might influence the ratings, biasing them towards the hypothesis. An alternative would be to use a more formal, automated method to evaluate the hypothesis; that is what we did.

We used a procedure known as conditioned suppression to test the hypothesis that the rats, treated with a dopamine receptor-blocking drug and failing to learn to avoid foot shock, have learned that the tone signals shock. Many previous studies had shown that if a rat that is pressing a lever for intermittent food reward is presented with a conditioned stimulus previously paired with an aversive stimulus such as foot shock, the rat's lever-pressing rate declines during the period of stimulus presentation. This phenomenon is termed "conditioned suppression." It is nicely quantifiable. If the conditioned stimulus is presented for, say, 60 seconds, the experimenter takes the number of lever presses made by the rat during the period of the conditioned stimulus and divides it by the number of lever presses made during the 60-second period preceding the conditioned stimulus plus the number of lever presses during the conditioned stimulus to produce a suppression ratio. This ratio has a value of 0.5 if no suppression occurs and approaches a value of 0 with greater suppression.

We trained rats to lever press for intermittently presented food and after eight days with a 40-minute session each day their responding was quite stable. The rats were then assigned to groups that underwent conditioned avoidance response training: one group was pretreated with drug vehicle, the second with a low dose of a dopamine receptor-blocking drug, and the third group with a high dose of a dopamine receptor-blocking drug. A fourth group remained in their home cage during these sessions and never received conditioned avoidance response training. Suppression ratio results are show in Figure 3.6. The first thing to note is that the group that never received avoidance training had a suppression ratio of about 0.45, showing little suppression to the tone when it was presented while rats in that group were lever pressing for food. The next thing to note is the suppression ratio of the group treated with drug vehicle during conditioned avoidance training. This group had learned to avoid the foot shock by running to safety during the tone, indicating that the tone had acquired aversive properties and those are reflected in the suppression ratio of about 0.23, significantly lower than that seen in the group that never received shock. The third thing to note is the suppression ratios of the groups that were treated with a dopamine receptor blocker during avoidance training; ratios were, respectively, about 0.11 and 0.19 for the groups that had received 0.5 and 1.0 mg/kg of pimozide during avoidance training. Although these groups showed little avoidance learning, they clearly learned the association between the tone and the aversive foot shock.[21]. These suppression ratio results are consistent with our anecdotal observations that the rats looked threatened during the tone. Clearly, they learned the tone-shock association, yet they failed to avoid the shock.

Together these results present a complex situation. Rats that fail to show avoidance learning learn the location of safety and they learn the tone-shock association. Before considering the implications of this constellation of results, I want to deal with one specific interpretation and try to convince you that it is a nonstarter. In the previous chapter I introduced the idea that the effects of dopamine receptor blocking drugs might be interpreted as primarily motoric, that is, interfering with the ability to initiate or carry out motor responses. In the conditioned avoidance situation, it might be argued that the dopamine receptor-blocking drug is impairing the ability to initiate motor responses and that this accounts for the failure of avoidance responses to occur. This argument

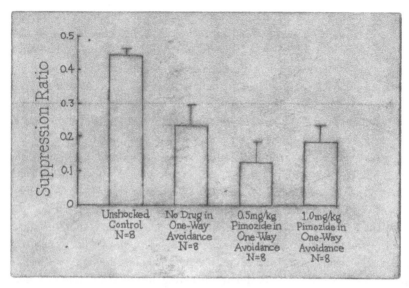

Figure 3.6 *Mean (± standard error of the mean) lever-press response suppression ratios to a 60-second tone stimulus in four groups of rats*: Values of 0.5 indicate no suppression and lower values indicate greater suppression. None of the groups received any drug injection before this test. The bar to the left is for a group that had no previous exposure to the tone or mild electric foot shock. The three remaining bars are for groups that were previously trained in one-way avoidance with no drug or following injection of the dopamine receptor-blocking drug pimozide (0.5, 1.0 mg/kg). The two groups previously treated with pimozide failed to learn to avoid mild electric foot shock by running to safety during the tone. However, their suppression ratios indicate that, like the no-drug control group that had received avoidance training and learned to make the avoidance response, they learned that the tone signaled shock.

Adapted from RJ Beninger, ST Mason, AG Phillips, and HC Fibiger, The use of conditioned suppression to evaluate the nature of neuroleptic-induced avoidance deficits, *Journal of Pharmacology and Experimental Therapeutics*, 213 (3), pp. 623–627, Figure 3 (top panel) © The American Society for Pharmacology and Experimental Therapeutics, 1980. With permission from ASPET.

may seem more compelling in the face of the observations that the location of safety and the tone-shock association are clearly learned. Perhaps, for the sake of argument, the drug impairs the ability to initiate motor responses, but the onset of the foot shock, by providing intense sensory input, overcomes that impairment and a rapid escape response is seen. The trouble with this argument is that rats that are first trained in the conditioned avoidance response task and then tested while treated with a dopamine receptor-blocking drug are observed to perform the avoidance response like rats that have not received drug.[22] This observation clearly flies in the face of the suggestion that treatment with a dopamine receptor-blocking drug simply produces a motor impairment. Something more complex is going on and it involves incentive learning.

Remember that incentive learning is the acquisition by neutral stimuli of an increased ability to elicit approach and other responses. In the conditioned avoidance response task, dopamine putatively mediates incentive learning so that safety-related stimuli acquire the ability to elicit an approach response and avoidance responses emerge. If training in the task while drug-free occurs first and then testing following treatment with a dopamine receptor-blocking drug takes place, the incentive learning has already occurred so the drug no longer blocks avoidance responses. Avoidance responses will gradually decline with repeated testing while treated with a dopamine receptor-blocking drug, but the initial resistance to the effects of the drug shows that treatment with the drug does not simply impair motor performance. The account presented here provides a more complete and accurate statement of what is occurring when rats treated with a dopamine receptor antagonist are tested in the conditioned avoidance task than simply attributing the failure to avoid to a motor impairment.

Before continuing with a discussion of the role of dopamine in incentive learning, it is important to expand on the theme of multiple memory systems. By about the middle of the twentieth century it was becoming clear that there was more than one memory system and that is was possible to dissociate memory systems by observations of neurological patients with damage to specific brain areas. That is the topic of the next chapter.

Summary

In lever pressing for food tasks, the first step is to feed the animal in the Skinner box by periodically presenting food pellets. The animal learns that the click of the feeder apparatus signals food. Food activates dopaminergic neurons and the click and food cup become conditioned incentive stimuli, acquiring the ability to elicit approach and other responses. Conditioned incentive stimuli acquire the ability to activate dopaminergic neurons; those stimuli can themselves act as rewarding stimuli so that the animal will begin to direct approach and other responses towards stimuli that are encountered just prior to hearing the click. With the use of response shaping techniques, the experimenter can arrange that the click occurs when the animal is near the lever, then when it is touching the lever, and, finally, only when it is pressing the lever. The lever and lever-related stimuli, being the stimuli encountered just prior to the click and delivery of food, become conditioned incentive stimuli with an increased ability to elicit approach and other responses. In the future, when the trained rat is returned to the Skinner box, it will likely first check the food magazine because that stimulus has become a conditioned incentive stimulus, and it will likely then go over and press the lever because it is also a conditioned incentive stimulus. Incentive learning has produced a gradient of attractiveness of stimuli in the test environment.

In place preference conditioning, one side of a two-chambered test apparatus is paired with a drug such as amphetamine that enhances dopaminergic neuro-transmission. The stimuli from that side of the test apparatus become conditioned incentive stimuli with an increased ability to elicit approach and other responses. When the rat is subsequently exposed to the whole apparatus, it is observed to spend more time in the presence of the stimuli previously paired with amphetamine, revealing the incentive learning that took place during pairing sessions.

In conditioned activity experiments, comparisons are made between a group that has had the test apparatus paired with a dopamine enhancing drug such as cocaine and one that has the same history of cocaine injections but where the injections were not paired with the test apparatus. Results reveal that the paired group shows greater activity than the unpaired group. This can be understood as revealing incentive learning in the paired group, stimuli from the test apparatus having acquired an increased ability to elicit approach and other responses manifested as increased activity.

In conditioned avoidance responding, animals learn to shuttle to the safe side of a test apparatus when a warning stimulus portending mild electric foot shock is presented. The warning stimulus will be a conditioned aversive stimulus as a result of its association with aversive foot shock and its offset will be rewarding (negative reinforcement) and putatively activates dopaminergic neurons. As a result, safety-related stimuli encountered just prior to a rewarding stimulus become conditioned incentive stimuli with an increased ability to elicit approach and other responses. If naïve animals begin training while treated with a dopa-mine receptor blocker, they learn the association between the warning stimulus and mild electric foot shock and they learn the location of safety. However, safety-related stimuli fail to become conditioned incentive stimuli with an increased ability to elicit approach responses and avoidance responses fail to develop. If previously trained animals are tested while treated with a dopamine receptor blocker, they are observed to continue to make avoidance responses but responding gradually declines over trials, presumably because the previous incentive learning is gradually being lost.

Chapter 4

Multiple memory systems

Concepts of memory have changed over the years and there is now general agreement that there are multiple forms of memory. In the following I will discuss declarative and non-declarative memory, providing definitions and a discussion of how the two are related. Non-declarative memory itself has many subtypes. What most people think of as memory is probably what psychologists and neuroscientists now refer to as declarative memory. The content of declarative memory is facts and events. For example, the recollections of the first school you attended—the building, its location, the teachers, your classmates—are an example of declarative memory. Defining characteristics of this type of memory are that it is explicit and the information is recalled consciously.[1]

Multiple memory systems in humans

Declarative memory appears to depend on the integrity of specific brain regions: the medial temporal lobes, including the hippocampus, and medial diencephalic nuclei. The medial temporal lobe was linked to memory by the finding that people with amnesia had damage to this area. The most famous example is the patient Henry Molaison (1926–2008).[2] Until the time of his death the scientific community knew him simply as HM. HM suffered from severe epilepsy that was refractory to medication; his seizures were so frequent and so intense that something had to be done. In 1953 at the age of 27 HM was referred to William Scoville (1906–1984), a neurosurgeon at the Hartford Hospital. Scoville had had some success in treating severely epileptic patients by removing the portion of the brain that was triggering the seizures. In the case of HM, he found that the medial temporal lobes, one on each side of the brain, were the trigger zones for his epileptic seizures, and Scoville surgically removed them. The good news is that the operation was successful in treating HM's seizures; the bad news is that the operation affected HM's memory.[3]

HM had severe anterograde amnesia subsequent to his operation. "Anterograde" means "forward in time." Apparently, HM could not remember anything new. A more modern statement of HM's symptoms would be that he could not learn new declarative memories. He retained memories from before the operation, although there was some relatively mild retrograde amnesia, too.

Thus, HM could remember his name, his family, and talk about his time serving in the US navy. He could provide details of his schooling and his early life as a boy in Hartford Connecticut. However, he could not remember having gone to the hospital for his surgery; this is an example of the relatively mild retrograde amnesia that accompanied the operation. If HM met someone new and had a conversation with her about the topics just mentioned and then saw her the next day, he would have no memory of ever having seen that person or the topic they had discussed. If he walked a new route in the city or inside a large building and then returned the next day, he would have no recall of having been there before.

It turned out that HM did not forget everything new, however. This was discovered by the insightful neuropsychologist Brenda Milner, working at the Montreal Neurological Institute, associated with McGill University. Shortly after HM's operation, she made the startling discovery that HM, and patients like him with temporal lobe amnesia, characterized by an apparent inability to remember any new recent information, showed evidence of learning on some tasks. For example, they improved from day to day in their ability to trace between parallel lines while seeing their hand reflected in a mirror in spite of remaining severely impaired in their ability to remember having done the task from day to day.[4] This pioneering work ushered in the concept of multiple memory systems that is now widely accepted.

Another researcher found that HM improved over days on a sensorimotor task known as the pursuit rotor. HM was charged with trying to keep a metal stylus on a spot of light that rotated in a circle on a flat surface. Nowadays such a task would be implemented with a computer. The task requires coordination of motor movements of the arm with the visual input from the spot of light. Normal (i.e., non-amnesic) participants show improvement in this task from day to day if they spend about three minutes on the task each day. HM similarly improved from day to day. This was even more remarkable because he did not remember the experimenter from day to day, in this case neuropsychologist Suzanne Corkin (1937–2016), who was a student of Brenda Milner. Each day she would introduce herself again and go through the usual formalities of meeting someone new. Then she would explain to HM that she was going to ask him to perform some tests. HM was an agreeable sort and would always politely acquiesce. Then Corkin would show him the pursuit rotor apparatus and ask him if he knew what it was or if he had seen it before. His answer would always be "no." She would explain what was required to perform the task and then HM would begin the trial. It was here that the evidence of learning revealed itself. HM would perform at a higher level of proficiency than he had shown the previous day. This pattern continued from day to day until performance reached an asymptotic level.[5] Clearly, HM's memory was severely impaired yet he learned on the mirror-drawing and pursuit-rotor tasks.

What the mirror-drawing and pursuit-rotor tasks have in common is that they rely on feedback that can be viewed as a rewarding stimulus. In both tasks the participant is motivated to perform well. In the mirror-drawing task, successfully remaining between the lines is rewarded by avoidance of the aversive outcome of crossing a line, recorded as an error. The fewer the line crossings, the fewer the errors and the better the performance. In the pursuit-rotor task, successfully remaining on the target increases the time-on-target score, reflecting proficiency at the task. These tasks are sometimes referred to as motor learning or habit learning tasks. However, if feedback is viewed as providing a rewarding stimulus, they can also be seen as incentive learning tasks. In the mirror-drawing task, the area between the parallel lines putatively acquires an increased ability to control responding; in the pursuit-rotor task, the illuminated disk putatively acquires an increased ability to control responding.

One system of classifying different types of memory specifies two large categories: declarative and non-declarative.[1] The content of declarative memory is facts and events, it is explicit, and this information is recalled consciously. As already mentioned, declarative memory appears to depend on the integrity of the medial temporal lobes, including the hippocampus, and medial diencephalic nuclei. By contrast, the content of non-declarative memory includes a collection of abilities such as skills and habits, simple forms of conditioning and priming. Priming refers to the enhanced likelihood of using a word that has recently been heard or read, for example in a list. Amnesic patients generally show normal priming effects, even though they are severely impaired in recalling the list of words they have just heard or read.[6] Non-declarative memory is implicit and *it is not recalled consciously* but is manifested as improved performance of the tasks where it is used. Different brain regions have been implicated in different forms of non-declarative memory. Thus, classical conditioning relies upon the cerebellum or amygdala, priming and perceptual learning upon the neocortex, and the learning of skills and habits upon the striatum. These relationships are summarized in Figure 4.1.

Dopamine and incentive learning did not appear in the original classification system, although reference was made to habit learning and its reliance on the striatum (an area of the brain that receives input from dopaminergic neurons; see Chapter 11). The term "habit learning" is frequently used to describe learning in tasks like mirror drawing and rotary pursuit. However, as discussed above, those tasks can be seen as reward-related learning tasks, with feedback providing the rewarding stimulus. As discussed in Chapters 2 and 3, in animal studies lever press responding is an incentive learning task that depends on

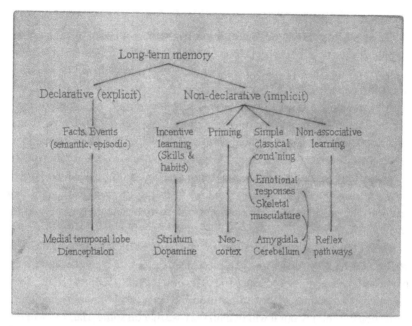

Figure 4.1 *Multiple memory systems and the brain regions where they are thought to be located*: Non-declarative incentive learning, skills, and habits appear to depend on dopamine. cond'ning: conditioning.

Adapted and modified from Gazzaniga, Michael S., ed., *The Cognitive Neurosciences*, figure 53.10, p. 834, © 1994 Massachusetts Institute of Technology, by permission of The MIT Press.

dopamine; lever press learning is also referred to as a form of habit learning. These considerations suggest that habit learning and incentive learning refer to the same thing. I will use the term "incentive learning" in this book.

In recent years, researchers have developed a number of tasks that require incentive learning and appear to rely on striatal dopamine. One of the things that distinguishes these tasks from declarative memory tasks is that their solution cannot be found in a single trial or even in a small number of trials. Feedback (e.g., the participant being told he is "correct" or "incorrect") is provided on every trial and being told he is correct is a rewarding stimulus. However, the best choice is not followed with feedback that he is correct on every occasion that he chooses it. For a simple example, suppose there are two choices, A and B. The participant's task is to get as many choices correct as possible. In this example, suppose further that choice A is rewarded with the feedback "correct" on 67% of the trials that it is chosen; on the other 33% of trials that choice A is made, the feedback is, "incorrect." For the alternative B, rewarding feedback, "correct" will occur on 33% of the occasions it is chosen and the feedback "incorrect" on 67%

of the trials on which it is chosen. This is a probabilistic selection task with the choice of A being correct on 67% of the trials and the choice of B being correct on 33% of the trials. Because the outcome of each trial is probabilistic, there is no way to know on a particular trial whether choice A or B will be rewarded with the feedback "correct". However, over many trials, choice A will be the best choice to maximize reward. Once the rule "always choose A" is learned, this task can be done using declarative memory of the rule without paying particular attention to the feedback provided on each trial. Before the rule is learned and especially on early trials, it is almost impossible to declare what is going on.

A large number of different sequences of events can take place for a participant learning the two-choice task described in the previous paragraph. For example, the participant might choose A on the first trial and be told he is incorrect. He might then choose B on the next trial and be told he is incorrect. The next choice of A might be rewarded with "correct" but then the next choice of B might be rewarded with "correct." At this point four choices have been made and there is no way to know the best choice. With additional trials, it will gradually emerge that the rewarding feedback "correct" occurs more frequently with choice A than B, but it will remain the case that on some trials (33% in this case) choice A will be followed by the feedback "incorrect" and on some trials (again 33% in this case) choice B will be rewarded with the feedback "correct." It should be easy to see that learning of this probabilistic selection task will be gradual and that it may take some time before a declarative rule such as 'always choose A' emerges. (In fact, many people will continue to "play the odds" and choose B some of the time, leading to less-than-maximal performance.)

Probabilistic classification learning tasks that are more complicated than the example provided have been developed for studies with humans.[7] The weather-prediction task is a probabilistic classification task that involves prediction of one of two outcomes—rain or shine—on each trial, given the particular cues provided on that trial. In one version of the task, there are four cues (rectangles with geometric symbols inside them) and up to three appear on each trial (i.e., on some trials there is just one cue, on some trials there are two cues, and on some, three). Each cue is probabilistically associated with either outcome but participants are not told this. For example, the four cues may predict rain with probabilities of 75%, 57%, 43% and 25%; the same four cues would predict shine with probabilities of 25%, 43%, 57%, and 75%, respectively. On trials where just the 75% rain cue appears, the choice "rain" will be followed by rewarding feedback, "correct" 75% of the time, but 25% of the time that choice will receive the feedback "incorrect." As you might imagine, it is very difficult to figure out what is going on in the early stages of learning this task. In spite of this challenge, normal control participants gradually learn this task based on the feedback they receive, improving their prediction of rain or shine over five blocks of ten trials. A group of amnesic patients with medial temporal lobe or medial diencephalic damage also showed learning and did not differ significantly from the controls. The ability of these amnesic patients to recall details of the task (e.g., the geometric symbols used in the cues) was significantly impaired, confirming that they suffered from a loss of declarative memory. This result from amnesic patients provides another example of learning in amnesia and of the dissociation of declarative and non-declarative memory. Importantly, a group of participants with Parkinson's disease, known to suffer from a loss of striatal dopamine,[8] failed to learn the probabilistic classification task in spite of showing intact declarative memory for details of the task.[9] These results show a double dissociation that implicates medial temporal cortical regions and the medial diencephalon in declarative but not non-declarative memory, and striatal dopamine in non-declarative but not declarative memory. My former doctoral student, James Perretta, neurologist Giovana Pari of Queen's University in Kingston, and I replicated this finding in participants with advanced Parkinson's disease and showed further that a group of participants with early Parkinson's disease with milder symptoms was less impaired.[10] Together, these results indicate that people with impaired striatal dopamine function have impaired incentive learning and that incentive learning is non-declarative.

In the probabilistic classification task reward is provided as positive feedback on some trials indicating that the weather prediction is correct. Rewarding stimuli activate the dopamine system (Chapter 5) and increase the incentive value of the stimuli associated with the rewarding outcome. In the weather-prediction task, those stimuli that are associated with a higher probability of rain (those that are correct 75% or 57% of the time in the earlier example) will become stronger incentive stimuli for controlling the "rain" response than those that are associated with a lower probability of rain (the 43% and 25% correct stimuli in the example) because the high probability stimuli will, on average, be followed by more positive feedback reward. In the same way, those stimuli that are associated with a higher probability of shine will become stronger incentive stimuli for controlling the "shine" response. Positive feedback putatively activates dopamine neurons (see Chapter 5) and produces incentive learning, increasing the ability of previously neutral stimuli to elicit approach and other responses. In this case, the responses are the weather predictions—rain or shine—associated with the appropriate higher-probability stimuli.

In patients with Parkinson's disease with reduced striatal dopamine, incentive learning will be impaired. My former doctoral student Danielle Charbonneau, now at the Royal Military College in Kingston, neurologist Richard Riopelle, now at McGill University, and I verified this prediction in a study testing patients with Parkinson's disease, arthritic patients with a level of disability comparable to that of the patients with Parkinson's disease, and normal controls on a point-loss avoidance task and on a declarative learning paired-associates task.[11] The point-loss avoidance task is an incentive learning task that is the human equivalent of the conditioned avoidance task for rats described in Chapters 2 and 3. In point-loss avoidance, participants begin with a number of points that are exchangeable for money and are required to avoid point loss by pressing a button during a signal that is a warning stimulus for impending point loss. We found no group differences in learning the declarative memory paired-associates task but the Parkinson's group was significantly impaired in learning the point-loss avoidance task compared with the other two groups. This finding, like that from the probabilistic classification task, showed the dissociation of declarative and non-declarative memory in patients with Parkinson's disease, with deficits specific to non-declarative memory in this group. The observation that the arthritic group, although impaired in activities of daily living at a similar level to the Parkinson's group, was not impaired on the point-loss avoidance task rules out level of disability as an explanation for the deficit in the Parkinson's group. The probabilistic classification and point-loss avoidance tasks are incentive learning task, relying on a form of non-declarative memory, and are sensitive to reductions in striatal dopamine.

The Iowa gambling task is another task that relies on non-declarative memory, in general,[12] and incentive learning, in particular. This task involves choosing cards from four decks that have different payoffs and penalties; choices from two decks lead to eventually making money over trials and choices from the other two lead to eventually losing money over trials. As was the case with the weather-prediction task, multiple trials are needed to learn which are the best decks. Importantly, normal controls shift to choosing from the good decks before they are aware (conscious) of the differential payoffs, suggesting that learning in this task is non-declarative. One difference between the probabilistic classification task and the Iowa gambling task is that the latter provides cumulative feedback in the form of net dollars earned or lost over trials. In functional imaging studies Iowa gambling task learning activated the medial frontal gyrus,[13] and learning of the task was impaired by damage to the ventromedial prefrontal cortex,[12,14] although the subregion(s) of the prefrontal cortex that are critical for Iowa gambling task learning remain the topic of debate.[12,14,15] The Iowa gambling task is another example of an incentive learning task with behavior being (non-consciously) shaped by rewarding stimuli; however, the cumulative aspect of the Iowa gambling task and the additional penalty contingencies may require the use of planning. This may explain why the prefrontal cortex seems to play an important role in mediating this task. In the scheme of multiple memory systems shown in Figure 4.1, the Iowa gambling task might define another subtype of non-declarative memory (incentive learning with planning?) and the involvement of another brain region, the medial prefrontal cortex.

In summary, within the multiple memory systems model, two broad categories of memory—declarative and non-declarative—have been defined and a number of subtypes of non-declarative memory have been described. Incentive learning or habit learning is one subtype of non-declarative memory. Striatal dopamine plays a critical role in incentive learning evaluated with probabilistic classification learning tasks and studies of the Iowa gambling task suggest further that the medial prefrontal cortex may be involved in incentive learning in some tasks. Whether medial prefrontal cortical dopamine (see Chapter 11) contributes to the putative role of this structure in incentive learning remains an open question.

Multiple memory systems in non-human animals

One of the problems with the definition of declarative memory is that it is conscious. People are aware of their declarative memories and can talk about them. Since animals cannot talk or directly tell us what they are aware of, it does not seem possible to assess declarative memories in animals. This makes the classification of memory systems into declarative and non-declarative based on whether learning is conscious or non-conscious of limited use for classifying animal memories. One alternative is to seek behavioral definitions of different memory types that do not require language to be observed.

Declarative memories are often classified as semantic or episodic (see Figure 4.1). University of Toronto cognitive psychologist Endel Tulving suggested that episodic memory "receives and stores information about temporally dated episodes or events, and temporal-spatial relations among these events" (p. 385).[16] This has become known as the *what–when–where* of events and some researchers have shown that animals have memories of this type. University of Cambridge psychologists Nicola Clayton and Anthony Dickinson showed episodic-like memory in scrub jays (*Aphelocoma coerulescens*) by observing their cache-retrieval behavior. They found that scrub jays visited less-preferred peanut cache sites after a long delay, but they visited more-preferred wax-moth larvae cache sites after a short delay. Wax-moth larvae decay quite rapidly and are no longer desirable after a long delay. Results show that the scrub jays appeared to have memory of what they had cached, where they had cached it, and when they had cached it, demonstrating episodic-like memory.[17]

Stephanie Babb and Jonathon Crystal, working at the time at University of Georgia in Athens, subsequently observed evidence of episodic memory in rats. They trained rats to find food in four arms of an eight-arm radial maze with one of the arms (randomly chosen each day) containing preferred chocolate food pellets. After a short delay the rats received access to all arms of the maze and the four previously un-baited arms were now baited. On other days similar access was given after a long delay but this time the former chocolate-pellet arm was again baited. Rats made more visits to the chocolate-pellet arm after long delays than after short delays. When chocolate taste was devalued using a taste-aversion procedure, rats made fewer visits to the chocolate-pellet arm on long-delay trials. Results showed that the rats had memory of what was in the chocolate-pellet arm (normal or devalued chocolate food), when it was available (after a long delay, not after a short delay), and where it was (the randomly selected chocolate-pellet arm each day).[18] These data, like those of Clayton and Dickinson suggest that animals have episodic-like declarative memories.

The declarative–non-declarative classification system also includes brain regions that are associated with the different types of memory. In animal studies, it is possible to assess memory in a variety of tasks and to see if learning and memory for these different tasks relies on different brain areas. If it does, animal memories would similarly be shown to be of multiple types, each associated with a different region of the brain. In the following, I discuss studies that relate different types of memory to different brain regions in animals.

Robert McDonald, now at the University of Lethbridge in Alberta, and Norman White, working at McGill University in Montreal, carried out a brilliant memory experiment that supported the hypothesis of multiple memory systems in animals.[19] It involved training rats on an eight-arm radial maze in three different types of tasks. The radial maze is like a spoked wheel with a central hub and arms radiating from it; often there are eight arms, each being about one meter long. The arms are flat runways that a rat can travel along to retrieve a morsel of food that has been placed by the experimenter into a small cup at the end of the arm. By training all three types of tasks on the same apparatus, the experimenters minimized possible differential demands on sensory/perceptual or motor systems that might arise if the tasks were instrumented in different apparatus. A description of each of the three tasks follows.

One of the tasks was a spatial task in which all of the arms were baited, each with a small piece of food. A food-restricted animal will be motivated to find and eat the food as quickly as possible. If it learns the spatial location of the arms of the radial maze within the test room, it will be able to retrieve the baits quickly and make few errors; by remembering where it has been, the rat can avoid entering previously baited arms from which it has already retrieved the food. Spatial learning requires learning about relationships among stimuli in the test environment. McDonald and White had various stimuli arranged in the test room where the maze was located, for example a storage box, poster, door to a closet, black cardboard circle attached to one of the walls, and so on. Importantly, the maze remained in the same location and orientation throughout the experiment. As discussed in the previous chapter, Edward Tolman (1886–1959) suggested that this type of learning involves forming a cognitive map of the test environment. If the rat can form an effective cognitive map, it will be better able to identify the locations in space, that is, arms of the radial maze, where it has already retrieved the food and thus make fewer re-entry errors as it goes about collecting all eight of the food baits. This radial maze task requires intact spatial memory abilities.

The second task was a cue task, carried out on the same radial maze that was used for the spatial task. In this case, six of the arms were blocked and only two arms were used. For each rat, the same two arms were used throughout the experiment, but different pairs of arms were used for each rat; the two arms were randomly selected except that they were not adjacent. A black curtain surrounded the maze to remove the room cues that were available in the spatial memory task and the room was dimly lit to further reduce the influence of spatial cues. A small light illuminated one of the arms and the other one was dark. Over a period of eight days, each rat was placed on the maze once each day, on half the days into the illuminated arm and on half the days into the darkened arm. On these days, access to the central hub was blocked so that the rats were confined to a single arm. Each rat was fed in one of the two arms; half of the rats were fed in the light arm and half were fed in the dark arm. The critical test was carried out on the next day by placing the rat into the central hub with both arms open. If the rat had learned that the light cue (for half of the animals) or the dark cue (for the other half) signaled the location of food, it should spend more time in the presence of that cue. This form of learning is referred to as conditioned cue preference. It can be seen to rely more heavily on learning about a specific cue than on learning the relationships among multiple spatial cues as was required in the first task.

The third task required learning about a cue, but the cue was not simply paired with food but signaled where the rat had to go to get food. The third task also had a spatial learning component insofar as the rats had to remember places where they had found food on any particular test day. However, unlike the first two tasks, the third task had a strong response component. The black curtain again surrounded the maze, eliminating room cues, and the room was dimly lit. Each day, four of the eight maze arms were illuminated, each arm by a dim light. The illuminated arms were randomly selected except that no more than two of the four of them could be adjacent. A different set of four arms was selected each day. The rat could collect a maximum of eight food pellets, two from each of the four illuminated arms. On the first visit to an illuminated arm, one pellet was available. After the rat returned to the central hub of the maze, a second pellet was delivered to the food cup at the end of the arm just visited. The rat continued to run the maze until it retrieved all eight pellets or ten minutes elapsed. For the rats to learn this task, they needed to learn that the dim light cue is associated with food as in the second task, but perhaps more importantly, they needed to remember their responses to specific arms. As each arm was baited twice and only twice, the rats needed to remember which arms they had visited once and which arms they had visited twice. Because the curtain surrounded the maze and the room lights were dimmed, spatial cues were minimized. Instead, the rats had to rely more on recalling their response patterns to remember which arms they had already visited once or twice. Thus, the third task had a stronger stimulus–response learning component than the other two.

Using these three tasks, McDonald and White found a triple dissociation. They studied three different brain areas and found that each appeared to be uniquely responsible for successful performance of one of the three tasks. The brain areas were the hippocampus, lateral amygdala, and dorsal striatum. They found that lesions of the fornix (the major output pathway of the hippocampus), but not the lateral amygdala or dorsal striatum, impaired performance of the spatial memory task. Lesions of the lateral amygdala, but not lesions of the fornix or dorsal striatum, impaired performance of the conditioned cue preference task. Lesions of the dorsal striatum, but not lesions of the fornix or lateral amygdala, impaired memory of the stimulus–response learning task (Figure 4.2). These results showed that different brain regions mediate different types of memory. Non-human animals, like rats, have multiple memory systems.

How does incentive learning come into the tasks used by McDonald and White? As each of the three tasks used food reward to train the animals, it would follow that each involved incentive learning. Although the effects of dopamine receptor antagonist on the learning and maintenance of these tasks were not tested by McDonald and White, others have evaluated the effect of dopamine receptor antagonists in similar tasks. For example, radial maze-trained animals retrieved food from the ends of four of the arms on a radial maze and were then injected with the dopamine receptor antagonist haloperidol shortly afterward. Upon retest several hours later, these animals were impaired in their ability to remember the arms from which they had retrieved the food.[20] These results implicate incentive learning in the spatial memory task. As discussed by

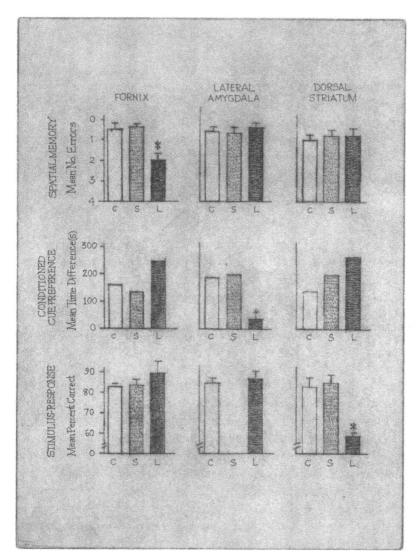

Figure 4.2 *Triple dissociation of the effects of brain lesions on learning and memory of rats in different tasks*: Lesions of the fornix, but not the lateral amygdala or dorsal striatum, impair learning (mean number of errors ± standard error of the mean on day 10 of testing for fornix and dorsal striatum groups and day 7 of testing for lateral amygdala groups) of a spatial memory task; note that the vertical axis is inverted so that higher bars indicate fewer errors. Lesions of the lateral amygdala, but not the fornix or dorsal striatum, impair learning (mean time difference (seconds) in the two arms) of a conditioned cue preference. Lesions of the dorsal striatum but not the fornix or lateral amygdala impair stimulus–response learning (mean percent correct ± standard error of the mean on trial block 11 of testing). C: control; L: lesion; S: sham. *Significantly different ($p < 0.05$) from C and S in pairwise comparisons following a significant group effect in analysis of variance; †only the lateral amygdala lesion group *failed* to show a significant difference in mean time spent in the two arms.

Derived with permission from data presented in McDonald RJ, White NM (1993) A triple dissociation of memory systems: hippocampus, amygdala and dorsal striatum. *Behavioral Neuroscience* 107: 3–22, published by the American Psychological Association.

McDonald and White, the conditioned cue preference task could also be called a conditioned reward task, the cue acquiring rewarding (incentive) properties as a result of pairing with food. Working with my postdoctoral supervisor, Anthony Phillips at the University of British Columbia in the late 1970s, we showed that treating animals with the dopamine receptor antagonist pimozide during the pairing of a tone with food blocked the subsequent ability of the tone to act as a conditioned reward.[21] These results strongly implicate dopamine-mediated incentive learning in the cue preference task. The third task was a somewhat unusual version of the radial maze task, with the same four of the eight arms being baited twice in each session. I do not know of any studies evaluating the effect of dopamine receptor blocking drugs in this particular version of the radial maze task. However, as dopamine receptor antagonists impair redial maze performance by blocking the effects of food reward on behavior, it is reasonable to assume that these drugs would also impair the stimulus–response version of the task.

If each of the tasks used by McDonald and White involves incentive learning, how can the results be understood to provide evidence of multiple memory systems? The answer to this question relates to the type of information that is processed in the brain areas where the lesions were placed in the study of McDonald and White. The hippocampus is well known to play an important role in learning the relationships among stimuli, allowing the formation of cognitive maps.[22] As is discussed in more detail in Chapter 11, one of the projection areas of the hippocampus is the nucleus accumbens, a ventral region of the striatum that is a major target of dopaminergic neurons from the ventral midbrain. It is thought that dopamine produces incentive learning by acting on neuronal projections to the striatum to alter their synaptic strength (see Chapter 12), thereby altering their ability to elicit approach and other responses in the future. The lateral amygdala processes (non-spatial) stimuli and is involved in assessing their possible threat to the animal; the lateral amygdala via the basal nucleus of the amygdala also projects to the nucleus accumbens,[23] where dopaminergic neurons can modify the synaptic effectiveness of these projections leading to incentive learning. The third area that was studied by McDonald and White was not an input area to the striatum but a region of the striatum itself, the dorsal striatum. Among the input regions of the dorsal striatum are motor regions of the frontal cortex that carry information about an animal's own responses.[24] Dopamine may act in dorsal striatal regions to alter the strength of certain responses themselves as those responses have frequently been followed by food reward and activation of dopaminergic neurons (see Chapter 12). As already mentioned earlier in this chapter, this type of dopamine-mediated learning is sometimes referred to as habit learning.

These considerations make it possible to understand the differential results of McDonald and White, even though the three tasks that they employed all involved incentive learning. Thus, the fornix lesions damaged projection neurons from the hippocampus, the brain region specialized in processing information about spatial relationships. In fornix-lesion animals, intact spatial information was no longer projecting into the ventral striatal region where dopaminergic signals produced by rewarding stimuli (see Chapter 5) putatively modulate the strength of synaptic terminals carrying this information (Chapter 12). In the case of animals with damage to the lateral amygdala, neurons normally activated by (non-spatial) sensory cues that project via the basal nucleus to the ventral striatum were damaged. As a result, the dopamine signal produced by a rewarding stimulus was unable to modify the ability of reward-associated stimuli to elicit approach and other responses. In the case of the animals with lesions of the dorsal striatum, the lesions were not placed in the cortical areas projecting to the dorsal striatum that carry information about the responses being made by the animal but in the projection region itself. The lesion would impair the ability of activity in dopaminergic neurons produced by encountering food reward to strengthen the synaptic terminals of neurons that activate motor responses of the animal.[25]

Under normal circumstances in an intact animal, inputs to the dorsal and ventral striatum would be arriving from the frontal cortex, and from the hippocampus and basolateral amygdala, respectively, when an animal is performing any one of the three tasks employed by McDonald and White. McDonald and White ingeniously manipulated the relative importance of these different inputs for maximizing food reward in each of the tasks, tipping the balance towards one input and away from the others. They were then able to show that damage to a specific region, that is, the fornix, lateral amygdala, or dorsal striatum, selectively affected only one of the tasks. Even though all of their tasks relied on incentive learning, they were able to clearly show that there are multiple memory systems in the brains of animals.

In a paper on the evolution of multiple memory systems that I further discuss later in this chapter, David Sherry and Daniel Schacter, working at the time at the University of Toronto in Canada, commented that multiple memory systems implies different memory mechanisms, not simply different content.[26] Clearly, the hippocampus, amygdala and dorsal striatum process different content. All of this information is carried by neurons that project to the striatum, some to the ventral region and some to the dorsal regions; then the synapses of these neurons are modulated by dopamine putatively via a similar mechanism in all regions of the striatum (see Chapter 12). This raises the question: are these really multiple memory systems? On the basis of this evidence alone, perhaps not. However, there is abundant evidence for synaptic plasticity underlying the formation of memory in each of the regions that projects to the striatum, some of it discussed in Chapter 12, that makes a strong case for different molecules being involved in memory storage in these brain regions,[27] supporting different mechanisms of memory in different regions.

Competition and cooperation among memory systems in animals

Different memory systems appear to compete for the control of behavior. An example of this phenomenon can be seen in the data of McDonald and White. On the spatial learning task, as already discussed, lesions of the hippocampal output pathway, the fornix, impaired learning and memory (Figure 4.2); the group that received lateral amygdala lesions, however, showed a non-significant trend towards *improved* performance on the spatial leaning task (this is most apparent in the earlier trials; only the last trial is shown in Figure 4.2). On the stimulus–response learning task, animals with lesions of the dorsal striatum were impaired (Figure 4.2), but animals with lesions of the fornix showed sig-nificantly *better* performance (as in the case of spatial learning, this can be seen best on earlier trials; only the last trial is shown in Figure 4.2 where the better performance of the fornix lesion group can also be seen). These results support the idea that different memory systems normally compete for the control of be-havior. In a spatial learning task that relies heavily on the hippocampus, learning is actually augmented by reducing the influence of the lateral amygdala. In a stimulus–response task that relies heavily on the dorsal striatum, learning is improved by reducing the influence of the hippocampus. As is discussed in the following section, similar observations suggest that different memory systems compete for the control of behavior in humans.

Another way that multiple memory systems can be inferred from findings from animal research is through the observation of stimulus–stimulus asso-ciative learning in animals that have dopamine neurotransmission blocked. As discussed in Chapter 3, animals tested for conditioned avoidance learning while treated with a dopamine receptor blocker failed to learn to make avoid-ance responses but learned the association between the tone and shock, and they learned the location of safety. This observation was used to support the role for dopamine in incentive learning. However, it equally supports the existence of multiple memory systems, that is, some that rely on dopamine, *viz.*, incentive learning, and some that do not rely on dopamine.

The possible differential role for dopamine in various types of learning was also suggested by the results of a study by Sven Ahlenius (1944–2001) and colleagues working at the University of Göteborg, Sweden.[28] These researchers were employing a behavioral procedure in animals to study a phenomenon termed "latent learning."[29] The phenomenon was named by behaviorists in the early twentieth century and refers to the observation that animals apparently learn about an environment they have visited, even though they do not find any explicit rewarding stimuli there. This was discovered during a time when some behaviorists were arguing that rewarding stimuli were necessary for learning (see Chapter 3). These studies involved pre-exposing rats to a maze without any food reward in the maze and then subsequently training the rats to traverse that maze to find food at the end. Hugh Carlton Blodgett (1896–1972), in a paper published in 1929,[30] and his PhD supervisor, Edward Tolman, working with Charles H. Honzik (1897–1968), in a paper published in 1930,[29] all working at the University of California in Berkley, found that rats that had been pre-exposed to the maze learned to find the food faster when the maze was subsequently baited with food, that is, they made fewer errors than non-pre-exposed rats on their first trials with food reward. From these observations it was implied that the rats must have learned something about the maze when they were pre-exposed to it, even in the absence of food reward; because that learning was not apparent until the rats were subsequently trained to run the maze for food, it was termed latent learning.

Mice that were treated with the dopamine receptor blocking drug haloperidol or its vehicle were pre-exposed by Ahlenius et al. to a maze for 30 minutes. They included a non-drug, non-pre-exposed control group. The next day, mice in each group were given ten trials with food reward located in the end area of the maze. Ahlenius et al. found that the groups that had been pre-exposed to the maze learned faster (i.e., made fewer errors by entering the wrong arms) than the non-pre-exposed group; this effect was observed in the vehicle- and haloperidol-treated pre-exposed groups. This result showed that treatment with a dopamine receptor-blocking drug had not blocked latent learning. One of the effects of being treated with a higher dose of haloperidol is a reduction in locomotor activity. The authors measured the amount of exploration (total number of arm entries) during the pre-exposure session and found that the haloperidol-treated mice explored less, showing the expected motor slowing. This clearly revealed that the drug was having an effect during the pre-exposure session. In spite of this reduction in the amount of exploration during pre-exposure, the haloperidol group showed latent learning like that observed in the vehicle group and reported previously by other researchers. Subsequently, Kenji Ichihara and co-workers at Meijo University in Nagoya, Japan, similarly found that treatment of mice with the dopamine receptor blocker pimozide during pre-exposure to a water-finding apparatus failed to block the latent learning effect.[31] Results suggest that there was learning when dopaminergic neurotransmission was reduced by haloperidol or pimozide. From the point of view of the theme of this chapter, these results suggest that there may be more than one memory system. One is dopamine-dependent and involves incentive learning, and the other is relatively independent of dopamine and involves learning stimulus-stimulus associations such as those needed to form cognitive or spatial maps.[32]

Competition and cooperation among memory systems in humans

Russell Poldrack, working at the Harvard Medical School in Cambridge, Massachusetts, and his collaborators there and at Rutgers University in Newark, New Jersey, were among the first to show good evidence for competition between memory systems in the human brain.[33] They used functional magnetic resonance imaging (fMRI) to look at blood oxygenation level-dependent (BOLD) differences in brain regions of people who were performing the weather-prediction task described earlier or a version of the task that used paired-associate learning, known to rely on declarative memory. They observed activation of a number of brain regions when participants were performing the standard feedback-based version of the weather-prediction task, including a region of dorsal striatum known as the caudate nucleus. They also observed deactivation of a number of brain regions when participants were performing the same task, including the medial temporal lobe region that contains the hippocampus. In a further study, they compared activations in these two regions in participants who were performing the feedback-based version of the weather-prediction task to those who were performing the paired-associate version and found greater activity in the caudate versus the medial temporal lobe for the feedback-based task and greater activity in the medial temporal lobe versus the caudate nucleus for the paired-associate version.

Poldrack and his co-workers also looked at how the BOLD responses in the medial temporal lobe and dorsal striatum changed over the course of learning the standard weather-prediction task. At the beginning of learning, the medial temporal lobe showed the strongest response but that rapidly changed as activity of the dorsal striatum increased and that of the medial temporal lobes decreased. Further analyses showed that activity in the two areas was negatively correlated. Results suggested that there may be competition between memory systems in the human brain. Possible mechanisms mediating this correlation continue to be the topic of intense research.[34]

When people are learning the standard weather-prediction task, they have to learn the set of stimuli that make up the task and the general arrangement of those stimuli in space; they also have to learn the rules of the task provided by verbal instructions from the experimenter or presented on a computer screen. This learning is relatively rapid and is of the declarative type, putatively relying on the medial temporal lobe, including the hippocampus, located there. However, as discussed above, identifying the probability associated with each stimulus cannot be easily learned using declarative memory because multiple exposures to the stimuli are required to identify these probabilities. That learning appears to be mediated by the dorsal striatum and to rely on dopamine-mediated incentive learning, as discussed earlier in this chapter. As learning progresses in the task, the medial temporal lobe is initially active as the declarative knowledge of the task is rapidly acquired and then its activity quickly declines once that information is learned. The dorsal striatum is initially relatively inactive as little incentive learning has taken place, but as incentive learning progresses, gradually building up the ability of high probability stimuli to elicit the appropriate "rain" or "shine" responses, more and more activation of the dorsal striatum is seen.

Recall that McDonald and White found that performance mediated by one memory system was enhanced by damage to another memory system (Figure 4.2). For example, rats with damage to the hippocampal output tract, the fornix, had impaired learning and memory of a spatial task but *enhanced* learning and memory of a task with a strong stimulus–response component. Similar results have been found in studies with human neurological patients. Aleksandra Klimkowicz-Mrowiec and colleagues working at Jagiellonian University in Kraców, Poland, evaluated explicit (declarative) memory and implicit (nondeclarative) memory in patients with Alzheimer's disease. [35] Alzheimer's disease is functionally characterized by a loss of explicit memory with the extent of the memory loss increasing with the level of severity of the disease.[36] These researchers tested implicit memory in patients with Alzheimer's disease using the weather-prediction task and found that patients with moderate explicit memory impairments actually performed *better* on the task than those with mild explicit memory impairments. The explicit memory impairments of Alzheimer's disease are associated with dysfunction of the medial temporal lobe, including the hippocampus; as already discussed, performance of the weather-prediction task relies on the dorsal striatum. The results of Klimkowicz-Mrowiec et al. therefore show that damage to one of these systems, possibly the medial temporal lobe and hippocampus in Alzheimer's disease, leads to enhanced learning and memory mediated by the other. These results show evidence in humans of competition between memory systems like that observed by McDonald and White in rats.

In a related study, Nicol Voermans, working at the University of Nijmegen in The Netherlands, along with colleagues there and at the Karolinska Institute in Stockholm, Sweden, and the University of Bonn in Germany, compared BOLD activity in the hippocampus and the striatal region, the caudate nucleus, in humans performing a route recognition task.[37] Navigational memory is thought to be produced by both the hippocampus and caudate nucleus working in parallel, the hippocampus representing relationships among stimuli to make a cognitive map and the caudate gradually building up the correct route through incentive learning produced by positive feedback for correct choices. Voermans et al. studied patients in the early stages of Huntington's disease, characterized by a gradual loss of neurons in the caudate.[38] They were interested in the relative level of activation of the hippocampus and caudate during a route recognition task and found that as the contribution of the caudate diminished with disease progression, the level of activity in the hippocampus during performance of the task increased. The authors preferred to view these results as evidence for cooperation instead of competition between memory systems, the hippocampus compensating for the loss of caudate function in the route recognition task. Whether the interaction of memory systems is viewed as cooperative or competitive (and this may depend on the nature of the task), it appears that the activity of one system often increases when the activity of another system decreases.

A fMRI study has reported an apparent reciprocal interaction between the hippocampus and amygdala in memory. Mark Richardson, Bryan Strange, and Raymond Dolan, working at the Institute of Neurology, Queen Square, London, UK, evaluated verbal learning in people with variable degrees of hippocampal or amygdala pathology.[39] Some of the words to be learned were relatively neutral (e.g., carrot, group) and some were emotionally aversive (e.g., massacre, morgue). They found that hippocampal pathology predicted memory performance for both types of words as would be expected from the role of the hippocampus in declarative memory. The extent of amygdala pathology, however, predicted memory performance for emotional words more than for neutral words; the amygdala has been strongly implicated in the processing of emotional stimuli,[23] so this finding was not unexpected. They also found correlations between hippocampal and amygdala activity. Encoding-related hippocampal activity for successfully remembered emotional words was correlated with the extent of amygdala damage; that is, the greater the amygdala damage, the stronger the role of the hippocampus in memory. Encoding-related amygdala activity for successfully remembered emotional items was correlated with the extent of hippocampal damage; this is the converse, that is, the greater the hippocampal damage, the stronger the role of the amygdala in memory.

Reminiscent of the interdependence between the hippocampus and amygdala suggested in the data of McDonald and White, the results of Richardson et al. reveal a reciprocal dependence of amygdala and hippocampus during the encoding of emotional memories.

In summary, Klimkowicz-Mrowiec et al. showed that in Alzheimer's disease where the function of the hippocampus may be diminishing with disease progression, dorsal striatal activity increased during learning of the weather-prediction task, and Voermans et al. showed that in Huntington's disease where the function of the caudate (part of the dorsal striatum) is diminishing with disease progression, hippocampal activity increases during learning of a navigational task. Richardson et al. showed that the involvement of the hippocampus and amygdala in the learning of emotional stimuli was reciprocally related. All of these studies reveal competition and cooperation among multiple memory systems in humans.

Why did we evolve multiple memory systems?

David Sherry and Daniel Schacter took up this question[26]. They argue that learning abilities in animals are adaptive specializations for the solving of specific environmental problems. Some forms of learning, although being exquisitely tuned to the solution of one set of problems, may be functionally incompatible with the solution of another set. As a result, a different adaptive specialization takes place for the new set of problems. This leads to multiple memory systems. They used song learning and seed caching in food-storing birds as examples of functionally incompatible adaptive specializations of memory.

Male oscines use songs during the breeding season, but seldom during the non-breeding period, to attract mates and to defend their breeding territory. Song learning in a number of songbirds, for example, black-capped chickadees, requires exposure to conspecific song (not just any birdsong) during an early critical period, even though the song is not sung until months later when the bird is mature. Seed caching is used by black-capped chickadees to store food throughout an area in multiple sites that are then visited to retrieve the food, sometimes many days later. Several hundred cache sites may be used in a day and once the food is retrieved from a site it is not reused. Sherry and Schacter argue that the functional demands of song memory and memory for cache sites are very different—so different, in fact, that separate systems are needed to solve each problem. For example, song learning is restricted to a subset of songs heard by the young bird, *viz.*, conspecific song, during a critical period, but memory for cache sites would be suboptimal if some of the sites were not learned. Song learning is restricted to a critical period but similarly restricting food cache learning would limit the usefulness of this behavior as a strategy for maintaining a constant food supply. Once bird songs are learned, they are relatively resistant to modification; food cache learning, however, is most functional if the memory of the cache site can be modified by information about whether or not the cached food has been removed from the site. With this example, Sherry and Schacter argue that the song memory system is poorly adapted to the demands of successful use of food caching and that evolutionary pressure therefore favored the development of a different memory system for food caching. As a result of similar functional incompatibilities, animals, including our species, may have multiple memory systems.

Sherry and Schacter went on to consider how song learning and food caching memory systems might relate to memory types postulated in humans and other primates. They suggested that song learning is comparable to habit or incentive learning and food caching is comparable to declarative memory. Recall that non-declarative memory systems like the one for incentive learning acquire information gradually over multiple trials and they preserve invariance. Such a system would be well suited to song learning. Declarative memory systems acquire information more quickly and the information often contains specific details about individual episodes. This sort of system would be well suited to remembering the sites where food has been hidden. In a similar manner to the anatomical distinctions outlined above between declarative and non-declarative memory systems in mammals, the latter focusing on incentive learning, there is now plenty of evidence for similar anatomical distinctions for food caching and song learning memory systems in oscines. The hippocampal region of the oscine avian brain mediates food caching and regions analogous to the striatum mediate song learning.[40] As is discussed further in Chapter 8, dopamine has been strongly implicated in song learning in songbirds.

Would multiple memory systems work in parallel or serially? At the end of the day, the information stored in memory is in the service of behavior that operates on the environment to better position the individual for controlling those things that she needs for survival. There is only one set of muscles so there must be a mechanism for allowing different memory systems to access control of that musculature. Such a mechanism could involve competition or cooperation or both. As discussed earlier in this chapter with reference to the work of McDonald and White, the different memory systems that they identified all involve incentive learning. In the case of the hippocampal and amygdala systems, both structures send strong projections to the ventral striatum. The third memory system studied was the dorsal striatum that receives strong projections from the frontal cortex. At the level of the striatum, incentive learning mediated by dopamine may select for strengthening those projections that are most strongly associated with rewarding outcomes. I discuss a mechanism for this dopamine-mediated learning in Chapter 12. According to this view, different (forebrain) memory systems project in parallel to the striatum where the outcomes and their effect on dopamine neuron firing determine which memory system eventually gets the strongest ability to control behavior.

Summary

The observation by Brenda Milner and others that the amnesic patient HM and similar patients could learn some tasks, including mirror drawing and pursuit rotor, even though they had no apparent knowledge of having done the task on previous occasions, contributed importantly to the emergence of the concept of multiple memory systems. According to one theoretical framework, memories are classified as declarative or non-declarative. Declarative memories are explicit memories for facts or events (episodes) that are experienced consciously by humans. Non-declarative memories are memories for, among other things, skills and habits and are non-conscious in humans. Skill and habit learning may involve incentive learning.

Different brain regions appear to be associated with different types of memory. The declarative memory deficits of HM were associated with bilateral damage to the medial temporal lobe, a brain region that contains the hippocampus, linking the hippocampus and surrounding temporal lobe tissue to declarative memory. People with Parkinson's disease, characterized by a loss of dopaminergic neurons and their projections to one of their terminal regions, the striatum, show impairments in some non-declarative memory tasks, including incentive-learning tasks identifying striatal dopamine as a possible neural component of incentive memories; patients with Parkinson's disease showed no deficit on declarative memory tasks such as paired-associates learning. These results demonstrate a double dissociation: hippocampal damage leads to impaired declarative memory but intact non-declarative memory; Parkinson's disease leads to impaired non-declarative (including incentive) memory but intact declarative memory.

In non-humans, the distinction between declarative and non-declarative memories based on whether or not they are conscious is difficult to apply because non-human animals generally lack the language skills needed to communicate about their possible mental experiences. Non-human animals such as rats, however, have homologous brain structures to those found in humans, making it possible to evaluate the possibility that different brain regions may play a critical role in different types of memory. Using this approach, McDonald and White in a highly influential paper showed a triple dissociation of brain regions and memory types: lesions of the fornix (the major output pathway of the hippocampus), but not the lateral amygdala or dorsal striatum, impaired performance of a spatial memory task; lesions of the lateral amygdala, but not lesions of the fornix or dorsal striatum, impaired performance of a conditioned cue preference task; lesions of the dorsal striatum, but not lesions of the fornix or lateral amygdala, impaired memory of a stimulus–response learning task. Although all three were incentive learning tasks, results were consistent with findings from humans. Lesions of the fornix impaired the ability of spatial information from the hippocampus to influence responding; lesions of the amygdala impaired the ability of cue information to influence responding; lesions of the dorsal striatum, an important terminal region of midbrain dopaminergic neurons, impaired stimulus-response learning.

Studies in humans and other animals reveal not only that there are multiple memory systems, but also that they interact, possibly inhibiting one another in their effort to control responding. McDonald and White found that the group that received lateral amygdala lesions was impaired on the cue task but showed a non-significant trend towards improved performance on the spatial leaning task and the group that received fornix lesions was impaired on the spatial learning task but improved on the habit (incentive) task. In evidence from humans, hippocampus damage was associated with improvement on an incentive learning task and striatal damage in patients with Huntington's disease was associated with increased involvement of the hippocampus in a route recognition task. Findings suggest that multiple memory systems may compete with one another in their control of behavior.

Chapter 5

Dopamine as the dependent variable

All of the varied and wonderful technologies that can now be used in the service of psychological and neuroscience research can generally be grouped into three broad categories: stimulation, lesion, and record. When studying a system, a researcher can learn about its function by seeing what happens when the system is turned on (e.g., by chemical stimulation) or turned off (e.g., by placement of a lesion), or she can see what the system is doing under normal circumstances (i.e., by recording).[1] Up until now much of the research related to studying the dopamine systems of the brain that I have discussed has involved variations on the former two approaches, although some neuroimaging studies are discussed in Chapter 4; they would fit into the "record" classification. This chapter focuses on studies in the "record" classification.

Evidence for activity in dopamine neurons can be recorded in a number of ways. Some of the earliest work involved postmortem assessment of levels of dopamine and dopamine metabolites in various brain areas after the animal was exposed to a rewarding stimulus such as food compared with control animals that had not received food. A system for extracting brain fluid using a push–pull perfusion technique was also used early on to examine possible changes in dopamine release associated with feeding. In vivo microdialysis and in vivo electrochemical studies monitor the level of extracellular dopamine and/or its metabolites in various brain areas in awake, behaving animals. Extensive electrophysiological work has assessed the activity of putatively dopaminergic neurons in animals that are undergoing reward-related learning. Positron emission tomography (PET) has been used to assess the displacement of a dopamine receptor ligand by dopamine released by rewarding stimuli. Functional magnetic resonance imaging studies (fMRI) cannot image dopamine but can identify blood oxygenation level-dependent (BOLD) changes in brain regions that contain dopamine cell bodies or receive strong dopamine inputs in people who are performing cognitive tasks that have a reward component. Studies in these various categories are discussed in this chapter.

Postmortem biochemistry of dopamine and its metabolites

Some of the earliest recording studies to address the question of dopamine's involvement in food reward were postmortem studies of the level of dopamine and its metabolites in dopamine-innervated brain regions following the presentation of food to mildly food-restricted rats. In one of the first studies, published in 1971, Pierre Bobillier and Jean-Roch Mouret, working at the School of Medicine in Lyon, France, measured dopamine in the anterior part of the brain (including the midbrain and forebrain) every two hours over a day in independent groups.[2] In the control condition, the rats had unrestricted access to food and water, and in the experimental condition they were fed only during the 12-hour light period, running from 7:00 a.m. to 7:00 p.m. Results for both groups revealed a circadian rhythmicity of dopamine levels, with levels rising from the first half to the second half of the dark period, the time of day when rats are most active; levels then dropped during the light period when rats are least active and often asleep. Overall, the concentration of dopamine in brain tissue was slightly higher in the experimental (partially food-restricted) rats and they showed a drop in dopamine concentrations from the end of the dark period to the beginning of the light period when food was taken away. The control group did not show this drop. This study does not really tell us a lot about the effects of feeding on dopamine, but I have included it here for two reasons. First, it was one of the first to manipulate food availability while measuring dopamine concentrations; and, second, results suggested that such manipulations influence dopamine concentrations.

One of the earliest reports of changes in dopamine concentrations in specific brain areas appeared in 1980. By this time, most researchers were using radio-immunoassay techniques for the detection of biological molecules. Rosalyn Yalow (1921–2011) and Solomon Aaron Berson (1918–1972), working at the Bronx Veterans Administration Hospital in New York, developed the radio-immunoassay in the 1950s.[3] Rosalyn Yalow received the Nobel Prize in Medicine in 1977 for this discovery. This technique employed antibodies artificially made radioactive using methodologies discovered in the 1930s that also contributed to the development of PET, discussed at more length later in this chapter.

Thomas Heffner and John Hartman, along with Lewis Seiden (1934–2007), working in Seiden's laboratory at the University of Chicago, radio-immunologically measured dopamine and the dopamine metabolite 3,4-dihydroxyphenylacetic acid (DOPAC) in a number of brain areas following feeding in food-restricted rats.[4] By calculating the ratio of DOPAC to dopamine, they could estimate the relative rate of dopamine neuronal activity; the more often dopamine neurons fire, the more dopamine they will release and the greater the level of the metabolite. Thus, higher DOPAC:dopamine ratios indicate greater dopamine neuron activity. Their study included free-fed control rats and experimental rats that had been food restricted for 20 hours, then fed for four hours each day during a prior of two weeks. On the test day, one group of food-restricted rats was sacrificed at the end of the 24-hour food-restriction period and the remaining food-restricted rats were sacrificed one hour after the beginning of feeding. Rats from the control group were sacrificed at the same times. They used a radioenzymatic assay to measure the amounts of DOPAC and dopamine in brain tissue from a number of regions. They found higher DOPAC:dopamine ratios in the nucleus accumbens, amygdala, and hypothalamus of the animals that had fed for one hour prior to sacrifice than in the unfed food-restricted group and the control group. The observation of a difference between unfed food-restricted versus fed food-restricted rats ruled out food restriction alone as a condition leading to increased dopamine release and strongly suggested that it was feeding that led to increased dopamine release. The three areas that showed increased dopamine release associated with feeding receive input from dopamine neurons, the projection to the nucleus accumbens being especially strong. Other regions that also receive a strong dopamine input, including the striatum (caudate putamen) and frontal cortex, showed no significant change in DOPAC:dopamine rations following feeding. Results were among the first to provide strong evidence that dopamine neurons projecting to specific brain regions increase their activity in association with food reward.

A subsequent study focused on two dopamine terminal regions, the nucleus accumbens and striatum (caudate nucleus), in food-restricted control rats and rats that had fed for one hour after a 20-hour period of food restriction. James Blackburn, Anthony Phillips, Alexander Jakubovic, and Hans Fibiger carried out this study in 1986 at the University of British Columbia in Vancouver, Canada, where Phillips and Fibiger had established one of the world-leading laboratories investigating brain neurotransmitters involved in reward-related learning. Their rats fed on food pellets or a liquid diet. In addition to looking at DOPAC:dopamine ratios, they measured another dopamine metabolite, homovanillic acid (HVA) and calculated HVA:dopamine ratios. They found that only the liquid diet led to increases in DOPAC:dopamine ratios in the nucleus accumbens and striatum like those reported by Heffner et al. for the nucleus accumbens. Both the liquid diet and the food pellets diet led to increases in HVA:dopamine ratios in both regions. The authors suggested that different results for the two metabolites may reflect different foods (pellets vs. liquid)[5] or different timing for the two metabolic pathways, as previously suggested by others.[6] Results supported those of Heffner et al., implicating dopamine in food reward.

Kenny Simansky, Kathy Bourbonais, and Gerald Smith, working in Smith's laboratory at Cornell University Medical College in New York, expanded on the original work done in Seiden's lab to further implicate hypothalamic dopamine in food reward.[7] In their study, like that of Heffner et al., they maintained rats on a 20-hour food-restriction schedule with food available for four hours per day. In addition to the groups included by Heffner et al., they added a third food-restricted group that was not fed at the usual time on the test day but was exposed to many of the cues normally signaling the availability of food and was then sacrificed one hour later. Their results revealed increased DOPAC:dopamine ratios in the hypothalamus of the food-restricted group that had fed for one hour versus the food-restricted group that was sacrificed before the beginning of the feeding period, replicating the result of Heffner et al. Their novel finding was that the food-restricted group that was exposed to feeding-related cues but not provided with food similarly showed increased DOPAC:dopamine ratios in the hypothalamus. These were among the first data to show that *stimuli that reliably signal the availability of food can activate dopaminergic neurons*. The data were consistent with findings published by Stanley Schiff, working at the Albert Einstein College of Medicine in New York, who showed in 1982 that stimuli that reliably signal drugs of abuse known to activate dopaminergic neurotransmission, for example amphetamine, produce increases in the dopamine metabolite HVA in striatal regions.[8] From an incentive learning point of view, these results suggest that conditioned incentive stimuli themselves should be able to act as rewarding stimuli, augmenting the ability of stimuli that signal the conditioned incentive stimuli to increase approach and other responses. This is suggested in the description of lever-press learning in Chapter 3, where magazine cues produce incentive learning of the lever-related stimuli leading to the acquisition of lever-press responding.

A further study from the laboratories of Tony Phillips and Chris Fibiger in Vancouver used postmortem biochemical techniques to show that stimuli predictive of food reward acquired the ability to produce dopamine release in the nucleus accumbens.[9] They presented rats with a stimulus that reliably predicted food and with a stimulus that was never followed by food. After a number of days of pairings, they analyzed dopamine, DOPAC, and HVA in the nucleus accumbens and striatum of control rats that had been exposed to the non-food-paired stimulus prior to sacrifice and rats that had been exposed to the food-paired stimulus prior to sacrifice. Results showed higher DOPAC:dopamine ratios and a trend towards higher HVA:dopamine ratios in the nucleus accumbens for rats that had been exposed to the food-paired stimulus. These results supported those of Simansky et al. and Schiff showing that stimuli that reliably predict food or drug reward, like food or drug reward itself, have the ability to activate dopamine neurons.

Sexual stimuli such as access to a receptive female by a male or access to a sexually active male by a female act as rewarding stimuli, that is, rats will learn to perform an operant response to attain such access.[10] A sexually inexperienced female rat will show a preference for a place that previously contained bedding used by a sexually active male.[11] Postmortem biochemistry studies provided evidence that dopamine neurons were activated by rewarding sexual stimuli. Manuel Mas and colleagues, working at the University of La Laguna in Tenerife in the Canary Islands in 1987, showed increased dopamine and DOPAC in the preoptic area of male rats that were given access to a receptive female versus male rats given access to another male.[12] In the same year, the late Sven Ahlenius (1944–2001), at Astra Alab AB in Södertälje, and colleagues, including future Nobelist Arvid Carlsson, from the University of Göteborg, Sweden, found that male rats engaged in sexual activity compared to male rats running in a treadmill showed increased levels of DOPAC in the nucleus accumbens.[13] In a subsequent experiment, Ahlenius and co-workers showed that exposure to a receptive female for 20 minutes without sexual contact versus exposure to the empty cage without the female present was sufficient to produce increases in DOPAC in the nucleus accumbens, dorsolateral striatum, and medial prefrontal cortex.[14] Increases in dopaminergic neurotransmission produced by a sexually receptive female may produce incentive learning, increasing the ability of environmental stimuli associated with the female to elicit approach and other responses in the future.

By comparison to electrophysiological and in vivo neurochemical techniques, the postmortem biochemical techniques discussed in this section have relatively poor temporal and spatial resolution. Nevertheless, these studies are noteworthy because they blazed the trail for subsequent studies using more precise methodologies.

Intracerebral microdialysis

Although postmortem studies provided valuable information about the relationships between behavior and neurotransmitter levels in various brain regions, neuroscientists searched for ways to measure neurotransmitters in an ongoing manner in awake, behaving animals. One attempt involved placing a small cup on the cortex that could be used to collect extracellular fluid that could then be drawn off and assayed for neurotransmitter levels.[15] My colleague and long-time collaborator Khem Jhamandas at Queen's University in

Kingston, Canada, used the cortical cup technique in our first joint research project to measure concentrations of the neurotransmitter acetylcholine in rats that had been fed choline-deficient or choline-enriched diets.[16] This technique proved useful for measuring cortical levels of neurotransmitters and their metabolites but did not allow for measurements from specific brain nuclei located deeper in the brain.

Neurotransmitter release from structures below the cortex was measured using the push–pull cannulae technique that involved the use of two concentric tubes, one for "pushing" fluid into the targeted brain area and the other for "pulling" fluid from that area; the extracted fluid could be assayed for the substance of interest.[17] Robert D. Myers (1931–2011), working at the time at Purdue University in West Lafayette, Indiana, developed this technique for use in the neurosciences.[18] Along with one of his students, Myers used the push–pull technique to show increased dopamine concentrations in 30-minute fluid samples taken from a number of diencephalic sites while rats were eating, drinking, or lever pressing for food.[19] These results provided some of the earliest evidence suggesting that rewarding stimuli may lead to activation of dopamine neurons.

The push–pull technique was quickly replaced with intracerebral microdialysis. It was first introduced by Laszlo Bito and colleagues working at the University of Louisville in Kentucky in 1966,[20] refined by José Manuel Rodriguez Delgado (1915–2011, well known for his studies of electrical stimulation of the brain) et al., working at Yale University in 1972,[21] and then made more efficient by Urban Ungerstedt and Christopher Pycock at the Karolinska Institute in Stockholm, Sweden, in 1974.[22] Intracerebral microdialysis involves placing a dialysis membrane over the tip of a push–pull cannula assembly similar to that developed by Myers. Small molecules diffuse across the membrane down their concentration gradient. The membrane protects the brain from large molecules such as bacteria and from the turbulence produced by injection of the perfusate; the low flow rate of perfusion also reduces depletion of the analyte. Intracerebral microdialysis is now extensively used to analyze brain dopamine and other neurotransmitters in awake, behaving animals.[23]

Researchers at Emory University in Atlanta, Georgia, in 1987 were the first to report the use of intracerebral microdialysis to measure changes in extracellular dopamine associated with feeding. Working in the laboratories of Joseph Justice and Daryl Neill, William Church reported increased dopamine release in the "central" striatum of rats shortly after they began to receive and eat food pellets delivered by a feeder on a fixed time one-minute schedule over a 15-minute period; dopamine remained elevated for another 15 minutes after food delivery and feeding ceased.[24] Results were in good agreement with postmortem neurochemical findings reported earlier and ushered in the era of automated monitoring of extracellular dopamine in behavioral studies of reward-related learning.

Many subsequent studies reported supportive findings. Feeding-associated increases in extracellular dopamine and its metabolites were found in the nucleus accumbens core and shell,[25] medial prefrontal cortex,[26] and ventral tegmental area,[27] but not the caudate nucleus,[25] of rats that were food restricted prior to testing; the dynamics of changes in the subregions of the nucleus accumbens differed across acquisition sessions. Water-restricted rats drinking sucrose that was prevented from reaching the stomach by a gastric fistula showed concentration-dependent increases in nucleus accumbens dopamine.[28] This study showed that it was the orosensory stimulation produced by sucrose and not postingestive consequences that led to nucleus accumbens dopamine release.

Some studies were carried out with non-food-restricted rats eating highly palatable sweet or fatty foods and results suggested that the level of food restriction affects the brain region of the dopamine response following feeding. Work carried out in the productive laboratory of Gaetano Di Chiara and colleagues at the University of Cagliari in Italy showed that non-food-restricted rats fed a novel fatty and salty food had increases in extracellular dopamine in the medial prefrontal cortex and nucleus accumbens core and shell.[29] The shell response habituated quickly, but the extracellular increases in dopamine in the medial prefrontal cortex and nucleus accumbens core continued to be seen with repeated presentations of the rewarding stimuli; this region-specific effect showed that all dopamine terminal areas do not respond in a uniform manner to rewarding stimuli.

Di Chiara and colleagues showed that conditioned stimuli that reliably signal sweet or fatty and salty foods produce increased dopamine release in the medial prefrontal cortex and the nucleus accumbens core but not the nucleus accumbens shell of non-food-restricted rats.[30] Conditioned stimuli increased extracellular dopamine in the nucleus accumbens shell of food-restricted rats.[31] Repeated presentation of the conditioned stimulus in the absence of the primary food reward led to a gradual loss of the medial prefrontal cortical dopamine response.[29]. The release of dopamine by conditioned stimuli makes it possible for those stimuli to operate like rewards, producing incentive learning by increasing the ability of stimuli that precede them to elicit approach and other responses in the future.

Rewarding stimuli other than food produce increases in extracellular dopamine in several brain areas. Brain stimulation reward is discussed in Chapter 2; lateral hypothalamic brain stimulation reward produces increased levels of extracellular dopamine and its metabolites in the nucleus accumbens shell and the ventral tegmental area, the origin of dopamine neurons projecting to the nucleus accumbens.[32] As discussed in Chapter 10, animals will learn to self-administer rewarding drugs that are abused by humans. Roy Wise, my former doctoral student Robert Ranaldi, and others, working in the laboratory of Roy Wise at the time at Concordia University in Montreal, showed that rats self-administering amphetamine or cocaine maintain increased levels of dopamine in the nucleus accumbens by responding at regular intervals during a session.[33] Conditioned stimuli associated with drug rewards also increase extracellular dopamine levels in the nucleus accumbens core and shell, amygdala, and pre-frontal cortex.[34]

Intracerebral microdialysis studies have shown that sexual behavior increases extracellular dopamine in a number of brain areas. In one of the earliest studies, James Pfaus, now at Concordia University in Montreal, and colleagues, working in the laboratories of Tony Phillips and Chris Fibiger at the University of British Columbia in Vancouver in 1990, reported that sexually experienced male rats, when placed into a mating chamber previously associated with access to a sexu-ally receptive female, showed increased dopamine concentrations in the nu-cleus accumbens; this result showed that conditioned stimuli associated with sexual reward increased extracellular dopamine. When a sexually receptive fe-male was placed into the chamber with the male and copulation took place, a further increase in nucleus accumbens dopamine and an increase in striatal dopamine was observed in the male.[35] Thus, sexual reward activated dopamine. Many related studies showed increases in dopamine and its metabolites in the medial preoptic area, medial basal hypothalamus, paraventricular nucleus of the hypothalamus, dorsal striatum, and/or nucleus accumbens of male rats[36] (and male Japanese quail[37]) and female rats[38] (and female Syrian hamsters[39] and prairie and meadow voles[40]) engaged in sexual activity. Increases in dopamine and its metabolites in the nucleus accumbens were also observed during ex-posure to stimuli that signaled to male rats or Japanese quail access to a sexually active conspecific female,[41] or to female rats access to a sexually active male.[42]

The studies reviewed in this section provide strong evidence that rewarding stimuli produce increases in the release of dopamine from dopaminergic neurons, as assessed using intracerebral microdialysis. Conditioned stimuli that signal primary rewarding stimuli, such as food or a sexual partner, acquire the ability to produce increases in extracellular dopamine and they lose this ability when the conditioned stimulus is presented repeatedly in the absence of the pri-mary reward. Exposure to primary rewards results in the release of dopamine leading to incentive learning, the stimuli that precede primary reward acquiring an increased ability to produce approach and other responses. These conditioned incentive stimuli also acquire the ability to activate dopamine neurons and to produce further incentive learning about the stimuli that precede them. As discussed in the next section, a wealth of electrophysiological evidence converges with intracerebral microdialysis evidence supporting this view.

Electrophysiology

Recording of the electrical activity of cells has its origins in the nineteenth century and became possible when it was discovered that current flow in a wire loop could produce the movement of a magnetic needle.[43] The Italian neurophysiologist Carlo Matteuchi (1811–1868) was the first in 1838 to record electrical currents in animal tissues, in this case muscle.[44] In Germany, professors Alexander von Humboldt (1769–1859) and Johannes Müller (1801–1858) brought Matteucci's discovery to the attention of Emil du Bois-Reymond (1818–1896), a promising young physiologist, as a possible thesis topic. Du Bois-Reymond, working at the University of Berlin, went on to develop sophisticated electrical recording devices and became the first person to record the action potential of neurons in the frog.[45] Du Bois-Reymond is often referred to as the founder of modern electrophysiology.

Du Bois-Reymond's student, Julius Bernstein (1839–1917), assisted by findings issuing from rapid developments in the physical and biological sciences at the turn of the century, in particular that osmotic processes can give rise to electric currents, went on to develop the idea that neurons were enclosed in a membrane that had an electrical potential across it.[46] Nobel laureate Edgar Adrian (1989–1977) further developed electrophysiological recording techniques and was the first to record the electrical activity of a single muscle fiber and nerve cell.[47] After the Second World War, Alan Hodgkin (1914–1998) and Andrew Huxley (1917–2012) carried out Nobel Prize-winning electrophysiological studies at Cambridge and Plymouth in the UK, using intracellular electrodes to identify the ionic mechanisms underlying excitation and inhibition in neurons.[48] Around the same time, another Nobel laureate, John Eccles (1903–1997), working with colleagues in Dunedin, New Zealand, and, independently, J. Walter Woodbury and Harry Patton (1918–2002), working in Seattle, Washington, performed the first intracellular recordings from neurons in the central nervous system using glass ultra-microelectrodes.[49] These findings provided the technical armamentarium that made possible exploration of the electrical activity of dopamine neurons, first in anesthetized animals and then in behaving animals.

One of the first tasks was to electrophysiologically characterize dopamine neurons so that a researcher could be fairly certain that he was recording from one. The first reports of recording from dopaminergic neurons in anesthetized rats came from Benjamin Bunney, George Ajhajanian, and colleagues in 1973 working in New Haven, Connecticut.[50] They recorded from single units in the ventral midbrain and distinguished dopaminergic from non-dopaminergic neurons on the basis of a number of electrophysiological characteristics and their responses in the presence of drugs that affect dopaminergic neurotransmission. For example, dopaminergic neurons were found to have a broader action potential, slower conduction velocity, lower firing rate, and to show characteristic burst firing. These became widely used criteria in subsequent studies by numerous researchers to identify dopaminergic neurons.[51]

Joseph Miller, Manjit Sanghera, and Dwight German, working at the University of Texas Health Science Center in Dallas in 1981 were the first to use these criteria to identify putative dopaminergic neurons in awake, behaving rats.[52] They presented the rats with two different conditioning tasks; in one, the onset of a light signaled the availability of food for pressing a lever and in the other a conditioned stimulus (tone or light) was presented for 2.5 seconds and food was presented during the last 0.5 seconds. They found a number of putative dopamine cells that showed an increase in firing rate when food was presented in either task and in the second task, some putative dopamine cells fired during the conditioned stimulus prior to the presentation of food. Results corroborated those from postmortem biochemical and in vivo microdialysis studies, suggesting that dopamine neurons are activated by food reward.

One of the most influential electrophysiologists studying dopaminergic neurons in awake, behaving animals is Wolfram Schultz, who worked for many years at the University of Fribourg in Switzerland. Schultz and his co-workers studied *Macaca fascicularis* monkeys. They were able to record from single putative dopaminergic neurons while the monkey was awake and learning and performing a food-rewarded task. They inferred that the recorded neurons were dopamine neurons by their response profile, as described above. When they slowly moved a microelecrode through a brain region rich in dopamine cells, their electrode would eventually pass close enough to a neuron that they could record the activity of that individual neuron. They would distinguish neuronal fiber discharges from somatodendritic discharges on the basis of very short duration of impulses. Dopaminergic neurons were characterized as having low-frequency impulses and polyphasic waveforms of relatively long duration. Using these criteria, the researchers could be reasonably confident that they were recording from a dopamine neuron.

Schultz and his co-workers observed that dopamine neurons showed a low and fairly regular response rate when the animal was quiet and little was happening around it.[53] This was referred to as the *tonic* level of activity of the neuron. They then presented the monkeys with a stimulus, the opening of a small guillotine-type door on a panel in front of the monkey. They observed that dopamine neurons responded to this stimulus by showing a small burst of activity, referred to as *phasic* dopamine neuron activity, on the first couple of presentations, but then the response faded away and with continued repeated presentations of the door-opening stimulus, no change in the firing of dopaminergic neurons was seen. This showed that dopamine neurons can be activated by novel stimuli, but as the stimulus becomes more familiar and is not associated with any rewarding outcomes, the stimulus rapidly loses its ability to activate dopamine neurons. I return to this aspect of dopamine neuron firing in Chapter 6.

The researchers then investigated what happened when the animal was given food in the small box behind the door. They periodically presented a small portion of apple (e.g., one gram), a treat for the monkey, behind the door. Thus, the door-opening stimulus now became a signal for periodic food presentations. Schultz and his colleagues observed that the food led to a burst of activity in the dopamine neurons, that is, they fired in a phasic manner. The burst was a rapid series of action potentials superimposed on the tonic level of activity of the neuron. This was similar to the preliminary findings of Miller and colleagues in their study with rats, discussed above, and to previous findings reported by Schultz with monkeys.[54] Schultz and co-workers showed further that the phasic activity of dopamine neurons was not related to saccadic eye movements or to limb movements. Thus, dopamine neurons were observed to have a background, ongoing low level of tonic activity and a periodic phasic burst of activity when a rewarding food stimulus was presented. From an incentive learning point of view, the phasic burst of dopamine activity associated with food will produce incentive learning, increasing the ability of stimuli associated with food to elicit approach and other responses.

Schultz and co-workers made another important discovery.[53] At first, during the phase of the experiment when food was periodically presented behind the door, the dopamine neurons did not change their firing rate when the door was opened but showed phasic activity when food was present. Gradually, over approximately the first 100 trials of pairings of the door-opening stimulus with the food, they found that the dopamine neurons began to fire during the door-opening stimulus, that is, the door-opening stimulus led to phasic activity. They observed further that the magnitude of the dopamine neuron response on trials when the door-opening stimulus revealed food was greater than on trials when the door-opening stimulus revealed an empty box. During this period, the door-opening stimulus was becoming a conditioned incentive stimulus, gradually acquiring an increased ability to elicit approach and other responses, as Schultz and co-workers showed subsequently using a light stimulus.

Schultz and co-workers carried out a second experiment to further evaluate the electrophysiological responses of putative dopamine neurons during learning of a lever-press response for food, in this case a drop (0.2 mL) of diluted apple juice delivered to a spout close to the monkey's mouth.[53] The monkeys were required to keep their hand on a resting key for a trial to take place; after a variable delay of 6–10 seconds, a yellow light on a panel in front of the monkeys signaled that they could press the lever (located on the panel in front of them) for food. Before lever-press training began, presentations of the yellow light, like presentation of the novel door-opening stimulus in the previous experiment, had little effect on the activity of dopamine neurons, except for a small number of neurons that responded during the first few stimulus presentations but then showed no further responding. Once the light stimulus began to signal food, the monkeys acquired the lever-press response, rapidly moving their arm from the resting key to the lever when the light stimulus was presented. In this case, the light stimulus was becoming a conditioned incentive stimulus, acquiring the ability to elicit lever-press responses. The researchers observed that dopamine neurons began to develop a significant phasic response to the presentation of the light, similar to the responses seen to the door-opening stimulus when it began to signal food in the previous experiment, and larger than the response to the light stimulus alone, observed prior to conditioning.

The lever-pressing experiment involved extensive conditioning, perhaps as many as 40,000 trials in all! In the earlier stages of training (the first 5,000–10,000 trials), the phasic response of dopamine neurons to the yellow stimulus light increased over trials and then continued to be observed on every trial. During the same phase, the response of dopamine neurons to the presentation of food began to lessen, as if the dopamine response was being transferred gradually from the primary food reward (apple juice) to a stimulus (the yellow light) that reliably predicted it. The response of dopamine neurons to the light stimulus during the second 10,000 trials remained present but showed some diminution. Schultz and co-workers found that during the first 10,000 trials, 58% of recorded dopamine neurons showed phasic activity to the yellow light, during the next 10,000 trials the corresponding number was 46%, and during the final 20,000 trials it was 34%. The magnitude of response was also observed to decrease over this period. It is perhaps most surprising that a substantial dopaminergic response to a reliable signal for food was still present after tens of thousands of trials.

Before continuing with further details of findings from electrophysiological studies of putative dopamine neurons in behaving animals learning
and performing operant tasks for food reward, a short review. The behavioral pharmacology studies discussed in Chapter 2 show that dopamine is important for incentive learning, the acquisition by previously neutral stimuli of
an increased ability to elicit approach and other responses. The electrophysiological studies discussed earlier, in agreement with the postmortem biochemical and intracerebral microdialysis studies reviewed in the previous sections,
provide direct evidence that putative dopamine neurons are activated by rewarding stimuli as would be expected if signaling by dopamine neurons is critical for reward-related learning. The postmortem biochemical, intracerebral
microdialysis and electrophysiological studies show further that dopamine
neurons begin to be activated by conditioned incentive stimuli that reliably
signal primary rewards. *It is important to recognize that this dopamine response
to conditioned incentive stimuli is not* necessary *for the ability of those stimuli to
elicit responding.* Recall the finding of Roy Wise and colleagues that rats well
trained to lever press for food continued to respond for food, even when dopamine receptors were blocked by pimozide.[55] This responding while treated
with a dopamine receptor antagonist was transient, showing a gradual decline
within and across sessions, revealing that conditioned incentive stimuli lose
their ability to control responding when repeatedly presented in the absence of
primary rewarding stimuli. However, the initially high level of responding seen
in pimozide-treated rats reveals the ability of conditioned incentive stimuli to
control responding, even when dopamine receptors are blocked. The dopamine
neuron activation by conditioned incentive stimuli, although not required for
the ability of those stimuli to (transiently) control responding, allows those
stimuli to act themselves as rewarding stimuli, imbuing stimuli that reliably
precede them with incentive qualities.[56]

I return now to further findings from electrophysiological studies.
Astoundingly, electrophysiological recordings of the activity of putative dopamine neurons located in the substantia nigra of *humans* were reported while
the participants learned a probabilistic card-choice task for financial reward
like those described in Chapter 4.[57] This study, carried out by researchers at the
University of Pennsylvania in Philadelphia, was performed during the implant-
ation of deep brain stimulation electrodes into the subthalamic nucleus of patients with Parkinson's disease. In agreement with the results of Schultz and his
colleagues, increased firing was observed following choices that led to financial
reward. The authors concluded: "Our findings should serve as a point of validation for animal models of reward learning" (p. 1499).

Researchers at the University of Otago in New Zealand, working in the laboratories of Jeffrey Wickens and Bryan Hyland,[58] examined the responses of putative dopamine neurons in trained, water-restricted rats that continued to receive a stimulus (tone or click) that had previously been paired with reward (water in this case) but when water reward was no longer presented, that is, during extinction. They found that the activity of putative dopamine neurons decreased over extinction trials. Similar to the findings of Schultz and colleagues, the New Zealand researchers had found that putative dopamine neurons that originally responded to the presentation of rewarding stimuli gradually lost that response when the rewarding stimulus was predicted reliably by a cue and, instead, dopamine neurons were activated by the cue.[59] The observations following removal of primary reward, that is, from extinction, showed that, even though only the cue and not water reward activated dopamine neurons in well-trained rats, removal of the primary rewarding (water) stimulus led to a loss of the ability of conditioned incentive stimuli to activate dopamine neurons. This shows that *the primary rewarding stimulus was critically important in maintaining the incentive value of conditioned cues, even though the primary rewarding stimulus was no longer activating dopamine neurons when it followed the cues.*

Schultz and his co-workers proposed that dopamine neurons encode reward prediction errors.[60] When an unexpected rewarding stimulus appears, dopamine neurons are activated. If the rewarding stimulus is reliably signaled by a previously neutral stimulus, for example a light, the light stimulus begins to activate dopamine neurons and, in parallel, the predictable rewarding stimulus gradually loses its ability to do so. Because the light stimulus occurs unpredictably, it activates the dopamine neurons. In his 1998 paper, Schultz suggested that positive reward prediction error is the signal that produces incentive learning.[60]. Schultz's research team made another discovery that supported the prediction error framework. They found that in a well-trained animal where the stimulus signaling food was observed to fire dopamine neurons, if the predicted food failed to materialize, the dopamine neurons at that point became silent, showing a transient *decrease* in activity.[61] The possible function of this transient decrease is discussed in some detail in Chapter 6.

The concept of prediction error proved to be useful for researchers working in the area of computational neuroscience. This area involves developing computer programs in which the processing is carried out using algorithms that reflect characteristics of neurons and brain organization. Programs that modeled the activity of dopamine neurons at different phases of learning were able to learn in a similar manner to animals performing operant tasks for rewarding stimuli.[62] Computational neuroscience is a large research field in it own right that will not be covered further in this book; Schultz's reward prediction error framework has proven to be of great value for this field. In spite of these successes, the debate continues about the relevance of the prediction error framework for understanding the function of dopamine in the incentive learning framework.[63]

To summarize this section on electrophysiology, putative dopamine neurons were identified using a number of established criteria. Recording from these neurons in awake, behaving rats or monkeys showed that the putative dopamine neurons were activated by primary rewarding stimuli such as food and water. After many trials of repeated presentations of a cue that reliably signaled the primary reward, dopamine neurons began to be activated by the cue and not by the primary reward itself. If primary reward was then withheld, the dopamine activation associated with the cue gradually diminished with repeated presentations of the cue. In addition, dopamine neurons were observed to become silent, showing a decrease in activity at the time of the expected rewarding stimulus that failed to materialize. The meaning of this aspect of dopamine neuron function is discussed in Chapter 6. The observations from electrophysiological studies support a role for dopamine in reward-related incentive learning.

In vivo electrochemistry

The 1959 Nobel Prize in Chemistry went to the Czech Jaroslav Heyrovsky (1890–1967) who worked at Charles University and the Czechoslovak Academy of Sciences in Prague. Heyrovsky received the honor for his discovery and development of polarographic methods of chemical analysis. He found that application of an appropriate potential to a specialized electrode could produce a chemical change in organic molecules that gave rise to a current that could be used to quantify the molecule; different molecules had different polarographic signatures, making it possible to use this technique to identify and quantify specific molecules at the electrode tip.[64] Heyrovsky's work laid the foundation for amperometric (fixed potential) and voltammetric (varying potential) in vivo electrochemical techniques.[65]

Ralph Adams (1924–2002) and co-workers at the University of Kansas published the first report of the use of in vivo electrochemistry in brain tissue in 1973,[66] and paved the way for many scientists in subsequent decades to examine possible changes in brain dopamine associated with reward-related learning. The idea of Adams and co-workers was to use in vivo electrochemical techniques to measure the concentration of specific neurotransmitters in specific brain regions. They implanted carbon paste electrodes into the caudate nucleus (a dopamine terminal area) of rats and, using cyclic voltammetry, were able to measure an oxidation current. Although they hoped to detect dopamine and norepinephrine directly, they were not able to discriminate these substances from ascorbic acid that has a similar oxidation current. Adams and co-workers viewed their results as "modest and quantitatively uncertain ... " (p. 209). However, later workers, using modified electrodes and a number of criterion observations, were able to improve the resolution and to discriminate dopamine from other molecular species also detected by the electrode. Adams's pioneering work paved the way for these developments.

A major advance in in vivo electrochemistry was the subsequent development of the carbon-fiber electrode by François Gonon and colleagues from the Université Claude Bernard in Lyon, France.[67] Using this electrode in anesthetized rats, they were able to better discriminate dopamine and its metabolites from ascorbic acid in the caudate nucleus. This finding set the stage for workers from the University of Pittsburg to carry out some of the first in vivo electrochemical studies using caudate electrodes in awake, behaving rats exposed to various environmental stimuli, including food reward. Richard Keller, Edward Stricker, and Michael Zigmond recorded responses every four minutes following exposure to the stimuli. They found that food-restricted rats, when given food, showed a gradual increase in the electrochemical signal that peaked some minutes after feeding ceased and gradually declined. Non-food-restricted rats similarly exposed to chow showed no electrochemical response. Based on the ability of pharmacological compounds known to interfere with dopaminergic neurotransmission to blunt the electrochemical responses observed in their rats, they argued that the bulk of the signal was linked to dopamine release.[68] This was among the first studies using in vivo electrochemistry in behaving rats to suggest that food reward led to increased release of dopamine.

Many reports of evidence of increased dopamine release measured with in vivo electrochemistry followed. As discussed in more detail in Chapter 11, the cell bodies of most dopaminergic neurons are found in the ventral midbrain, but dopamine neurons project to a number of brain areas. In vivo electrochemists placed their electrodes in many of these different dopamine terminal areas and results generally showed evidence consistent with increased dopamine following rewarding stimuli such as food. Some researchers putatively measured the dopamine metabolites DOPAC or HVA as evidence of changes in dopamine release and results showed that food or stimuli that reliably signal food reward led to evidence of dopamine release, in agreement with the electrophysiological studies of Wolfram Schultz and others reviewed earlier. In one study, when a food-restricted rat ate food, putatively increased levels of the dopamine metabolite DOPAC, recorded every two minutes, were observed in the prefrontal cortex; exposure just to the odor of food, a stimulus that reliably predicts food, also increased the signal.[69] Researchers at the Institute of Psychiatry in London found that rats lever pressing for food showed evidence of increased levels of HVA in the caudate nucleus and the nucleus accumbens,[70,71] both measured every 12 minutes. These results suggest that food reward may lead to increased dopamine release in the nucleus accumbens, caudate nucleus, and prefrontal cortex terminal areas.

Nicole Richardson, working with Alain Gratton at his laboratory at McGill University in Montreal, was able to sample putative dopamine responses in the nucleus accumbens or medial prefrontal cortex every two seconds,[72] a substantial temporal improvement over the previous studies looking at dopamine metabolites. They recorded over several sessions of lever pressing for condensed milk reward presented in a dipper to rats for 30 seconds. They found that putative dopamine levels initially rose during the 30 seconds of drinking; over days, the magnitude of the signal associated with drinking milk reward decreased and, instead, the response began to appear during the signal for milk reward. This finding was in good agreement with Schultz's electrophysiological results already discussed. An interesting finding from these experiments was that putative dopamine levels in the nucleus accumbens began to rise as soon as the rat was placed into the operant testing apparatus. The initial period in the apparatus was associated with the odor of the milk reward being poured into the reservoir located outside the chamber just on the other side of one of the chamber walls. The observation of an increase in putative dopamine release to food-related cues is consistent with the electrophysiological results reported for dopaminergic neurons recorded in monkeys by Schultz and others, but the dopamine selectivity of the in vivo chronoamperometric methodology of Richardson and Gratton has been questioned.[73]

By the beginning of the twenty-first century, as a result of the pioneering work of Mark Wightman and others at the University of North Carolina in Chapel Hill, fast-scan cyclic voltammetry was developed and could be used to reliably measure changes in extracellular dopamine concentrations at the sub-second level. This provided temporal resolution that approached that of electrophysiology and could detect changes in dopamine resulting from vesicular release.[74] The laboratories of Mark Wightman and Regina Carelli at the University of North Carolina at Chapel Hill subsequently produced a series of sophisticated studies characterizing changes in dopamine during reward-related learning. In untrained rats, the presentation of food produced an increase in dopamine in the dopamine terminal region, nucleus accumbens core.[75] In previously trained rats, they showed rapid (latency of approximately 200 ms) increases in dopamine in the nucleus accumbens core and shell regions during the presentation of a cue that signaled food or that signaled the opportunity to lever press for food.[75-77] They found that dopamine increases associated with food itself disappeared in the core region, in agreement with the electrophysiological studies of dopamine neurons by Schultz and others, but persisted in the shell region.[76]. In more recent studies, Richardson and Gratton similarly found that nucleus accumbens core dopamine release increased during cues that predicted food reward,[78] and workers in the laboratory of Miguel Nicolelis at Duke University in Durham, North Carolina, similarly found that food reward (intravenous glucose) increased dopamine release in the nucleus accumbens shell.[79] Results reveal possible regional differences in the dynamics of dopamine release associated with rewarding stimuli.

Researchers have examined changes in extracellular dopamine in several brain regions. Taizo Nakazato from Juntendo University in Tokyo found increased dopamine release in the ventral region of the striatum of trained rats when they heard a tone and then lever pressed for food; the response was relatively stable for over five months of testing and recording.[80] In agreement with previous studies, a former postdoctoral fellow of Dr. Carelli, Mitchell Roitman, and colleagues at the University of Illinois in Chicago found that untrained rats showed increased dopamine release in the nucleus accumbens core when food was presented. In trained rats, the presentation of food or conditioned stimuli associated with food increased dopamine release in the nucleus accumbens core and the dorsomedial striatum but not the dorsolateral striatum, both dopamine terminal regions. These results further emphasized regional differences in the dynamics of dopamine release associated with rewarding stimuli.[81]

Japanese researcher Shigeru Kitazawa of Juntendo University in Tokyo and colleagues, using fast-scan cyclic voltammetry or amperometry, showed increases in extracellular dopamine associated with food reward in species other than the rat. They found that food led to an increase in dopamine release in the dorsal striatum of the mouse.[82] In studies with Japanese macaque monkeys, they observed increased putative dopamine release in the dorsal striatum (caudate nucleus) following the presentation of a juice reward or a cue that preceded the juice.[83] Chinese researchers using amperometric recording recently reported that a food stimulus increased dopamine release in dopamine-neuron terminal areas of the larval zebrafish (*Danio rerio*),[84] further extending voltammetric finding from rats, mice, and monkeys to fish.

Ann Graybiel from the Massachusetts Institute of Technology in Cambridge, Massachusetts, and co-workers recently used fast-scan cyclic voltammetry to track the concentration of extracellular dopamine in the ventromedial and dorsolateral regions of the striatum of trained rats running mazes for food reward. They found that dopamine concentrations increased from the start box to the goal box of the mazes. The increases were not significantly correlated with running speed or trial length.[85] The results of this sophisticated study clearly show that conditioned incentive stimuli associated with food reward acquire the ability to activate dopamine neurons; elevated dopamine may produce incentive learning by increasing the ability of stimuli associated with it to elicit approach and other responses. In a manner reminiscent of fractional anticipatory goal responses posited by Clark Hull (1884–1952) and Kenneth Spence (1907–1967)[86] over 60 years ago, a chain of conditioned incentive stimuli is set up backward in time from the primary food reward with the more proximal stimuli being stronger incentive stimuli than the more distal ones. This may result in the dopamine increases or "ramps" described by Graybiel and co-workers.

In vivo voltammetry studies have shown increases in extracellular dopamine produced by rewarding stimuli other than food and the conditioned stimuli that signal them. The rewarding drug cocaine produced increases in extracellular dopamine in the nucleus accumbens.[87] Stimuli that reliably signaled intravenous cocaine infusions rapidly acquired the ability to produce dopamine release from the nucleus accumbens core.[88] (Dopamine and drug reward is covered in Chapter 10.) Brain stimulation reward and some of the evidence that its effects were mediated by dopamine are discussed in Chapter 2; perhaps not surprisingly, electrochemical studies showed that brain stimulation reward increased extracellular dopamine concentrations in dopamine terminal areas of the rat, including the nucleus accumbens and caudate.[89,90] Stimuli that reliably signaled brain stimulation reward increased dopamine concentration in the nucleus accumbens shell of rats.[91] The opportunity to engage in sexual intercourse is a rewarding stimulus and male rats engaged in active sexual behavior showed increased levels of extracellular dopamine in the nucleus accumbens.[92] Male rats exposed to olfactory cues associated with sexual reward—bedding that had been used by sexually receptive females—showed rapid increases in nucleus accumbens dopamine concentrations; exposure to bedding used by non-sexually receptive females produced much less of a change.[93]

A recent study co-published by researchers from the Universities of Michigan and Washington challenged the idea that dopamine neurons code prediction error,[94] as was suggested by the results of electrophysiological studies discussed earlier. Rats were exposed to pairings of a signal, an eight-second extension of an illuminated bar from one of the walls of a chamber, with presentation of food into a food cup. The rats were observed to learn about the signal, but some of them approached and contacted the illuminated bar when it was extended and the others learned to approach and contact the feeder cup when the illuminated bar signal was presented. Recordings of dopaminergic voltammetric signals in the core of the nucleus accumbens showed that dopamine levels increased when the food reward was presented. As trials progressed, dopamine levels also increased when the illuminated bar signal was presented, replicating Schultz's findings from electrophysiological studies. Apparently, the illuminated bar had become an effective predictive stimulus for food for all of the rats, but some of them responded to this signal by approaching the bar and others by approaching the food cup. The authors found that those rats that responded to the illuminated bar signal by approaching it also showed a shift towards higher dopamine responses to the signal than to food itself. This replicated the findings of Schultz and his co-workers that they used to formulate their hypothesis that dopamine neurons code for prediction error; since the food was predicted by the illuminated bar signal, dopamine neurons fired strongly to the signal but weakly or not at all to the food itself. However, Flagel et al. also found that for the rats that responded to the signal by approaching the feeder, the strength of the dopamine response to the signal and to the food itself remained about the same; in this case, extension of the illuminated bar clearly was acting as a signal predicting food because the rats approached the feeder when the illuminated bar appeared. The elevated firing of dopamine neurons to the reliably predicted presentation of food contradicted the hypothesis that dopamine neurons code for prediction error. Although these findings bring into question the prediction error hypothesis, a much more important aspect of these and the other experiments discussed here is that signals for food acquire the ability to elicit approach or other responses. In the present example, the illuminated bar elicits approach responses to the bar in some rats and to the food cup in others, but it elicits approach response in all rats. These are examples of dopamine-mediated incentive learning.

The studies discussed in this section show that when in vivo electrochemistry is used to measure dopamine concentrations in several brain areas, a number of different rewarding stimuli, including food, drugs of abuse, brain stimulation reward, and sexual reward, are seen to produce increases. These dopamine increases would be expected to produce incentive learning, increasing the ability of stimuli that signal these rewarding stimuli to elicit approach and other responses in the future. As was observed in electrophysiological experiments discussed in the previous section, conditioned incentive stimuli associated with primary rewards themselves acquire the ability to produce increases in dopamine release and to produce incentive learning of stimuli that precede them. This chain of conditioned incentives was seen most clearly in the ingenious study of Ann Graybiel and colleagues.

These in vivo electrochemical findings and the postmortem biochemical, intracerebral microdialysis and electrophysiological results discussed in this chapter reveal clearly that rewarding stimuli activate dopamine neurons. They also reveal that stimuli that signal rewarding stimuli themselves acquire the ability to activate dopamine neurons. If rewarding stimuli are termed "primary incentive stimuli," these stimuli can be termed "conditioned incentive stimuli." Because conditioned incentive stimuli have the ability themselves to activate dopamine neurons they might be expected to be able to produce incentive learning. Indeed, they can. One of the defining characteristics of a conditioned reward or conditioned reinforcer in the twentieth century was its demonstrated ability to control responding.[95] If a rat would press a lever for a stimulus, for example a click that previously was reliably paired with food, that stimulus was a conditioned reward. Psychologist B. Richard Bugelski (1913–1995), for example, showed this in 1938 while working at Yale University.[96] If repeated testing of the ability of a previously food-paired stimulus to control responding was carried out, it was found that gradually the conditioned rewarding properties of the stimulus were lost. This implies that stimuli that signal rewarding stimuli and acquire the ability to produce dopamine release lose that ability with repeated presentation in the absence of the primary incentive stimulus.

Neuroimaging

History of neuroimaging

The path to modern neuroimaging, specifically PET and fMRI, begins at least in the late nineteenth century and stretches throughout the twentieth and into the current century. It is studded with Nobel Prizes and stunning interdisciplinarity.

Perhaps the most appropriate starting point is with Wilhelm Conrad Roentgen's (1845–1923) discovery of X-rays in 1895 that was distinguished with the first ever Nobel Prize in Physics awarded in 1901. X-ray techniques developed subsequently and were applied in medicine beginning in the early twentieth century.[97] In the late 1960s, Godfrey Hounsfield (1919–2004), an electrical engineer working at EMI Group Limited in the UK, paralleling the pioneering work on tomography carried out by David E. Kuhl at the University of Pennsylvania,[98] developed the idea of using X-rays to image a slice (tomogram) through the human brain. Hounsfield was experienced in the early development of computers and his idea was to use them to create an image produced from digital data acquired from multiple X-rays taken from different points around a plane passing through the head. This led to the development of X-ray computed tomography (CT). Unbeknownst to Hounsfield, physicist Allan Cormack (1924–1998), working at the University of Cape Town in South Africa, independently developed the theoretical bases of CT scanning and published them in two papers in the *Journal of Applied Physics* in 1963 and 1964. The two of them were honored with the 1979 Nobel Prize in Physiology or

Medicine for their discovery and development of computer-assisted tomography. In his Nobel Prize banquet speech, Cormack commented on the irony of a physicist and an engineer winning the Prize in Physiology or Medicine.[99] Different disciplines are merely convenient ways for librarians to classify books.

Along with a number of earlier discoveries and developments in the twentieth century, this set the stage for the invention of PET. In the 1930s, wife-and-husband team Irène Joliot-Curie (1897–1956) and Frédéric Joliot-Curie (1900–1958), working in France, discovered that exposing some nuclides to alpha particles from the radioactive element polonium led to the nuclides becoming radioactive themselves. For this discovery they received the Nobel Prize in Chemistry in 1935.[100] Ernest O. Lawrence (1901–1958), working at the University of California in Berkley, subsequently developed the cyclotron, a device that provided a source of accelerated positive ions that could be used to make artificially radioactive nuclides like those discovered by the Joliot-Curies. This discovery received the 1939 Nobel Prize in Physics. Some of the radionuclides that were developed were useful in biology, including those based on oxygen (^{15}O), carbon (^{11}C), nitrogen (^{13}N), and fluorine (^{18}F), and some were used in studies with humans; for example, ^{11}C-labeled carbon monoxide was used to study the activity of carbon monoxide in humans.[101] These studies were done without any apparent thought of eventually applying these compounds to tomographic imaging of the human brain and body.

In parallel with the invention of new radioactive compounds, the idea that regional blood flow in the brain could be used as an index of regional brain activity was developing. The work of the Italian physiologist Angelo Mosso (1846–1910) in the late nineteenth century showed that blood flow to different brain areas varied with emotional and cognitive state.[102] In the middle of the twentieth century, Seymour S. Kety (1915–2000), working at the University of Pennsylvania in Philadelphia and at the National Institute of Mental Health in Maryland, developed quantitative methods for measuring whole-brain blood flow and, in animal studies with colleagues, including Louis Sokoloff (1921–2015), used radiolabeled glucose and autoradiography to identify regional metabolism in the brain.[103] Kety's work led David Ingvar and Jarl Risberg, working at the University of Lund in Sweden, to use radioactive gas injected into the carotid artery of humans to measure regional blood flow changes associated with mental activity. They placed scintillation counters that detected gamma particles from the radioactive tracer around the head of the experimental participant and were able to detect differences in cortical blood flow to various cortical regions when participants engaged in different cognitive activities.[104] I remember reading a *Scientific American* article by Niels Lassen, David Ingvar, and Erik Skinhøj in 1978 about this work,[105] and being fascinated by the possibilities of actually measuring regional brain activity associated with mental experience. This topic is discussed in more detail in Chapter 13.

Michel Ter-Pogossian (1925–1996), a physicist working at Washington University in St. Louis, Missouri, where one of the first cyclotrons had been built, recognized the potential of radioisotopes discovered by the Joliot-Curies for use in medicine. The work of Nobel laureate Allan Cormack showed the advantages of imaging the products of annihilation events resulting from the emission of positrons by disintegrating radioisotopes. Emitted positrons collide with electrons leading to their annihilation and the emission of two photons that travel in orthogonal directions. By detecting these two photons simultaneously using a ring of detectors located around the head, it was possible to localize the origin of the annihilation event by using calculations similar to those used by Hounsfield and Cormack in computer-assisted tomography.[99] Kety's principles made possible the measurement of regional blood flow and localized functional activity in PET.[102],[106] Ter-Pogossian's associates at Washington University, including Michael Phelps and Edward Hoffman (1942–2004), were among the first to develop a positron imaging tomographic instrument for the three-dimensional imaging of the human brain that became commercially available in 1976.[107],[108]

In yet another parallel set of developments, physicists Felix Bloch (1905–1983) at Stanford and Edward Purcell (1912–1997) at Harvard independently discovered nuclear magnetic resonance in the 1940s for which they received the Nobel Prize in Physics in 1952. Nuclear magnetic resonance is the property of some molecules, when placed into a magnetic field, to absorb and re-emit certain frequencies of electromagnetic radiation. The Swiss chemist Richard Ernst, working in Palo Alto, California, expanded on the work of Bloch and Purcell to develop nuclear magnetic resonance spectroscopy, using concepts of phase and frequency coding with Fourier transformation. His work greatly increased the speed of acquisition of images; he received the Nobel Prize in Chemistry in 1991 for this work. Paul Lauterbur (1929–2007), a chemist working at State University of New York at Stony Brook, applied the idea of introducing magnetic gradients to determine the origin of radio waves emitted from nuclei. British physicist Peter Mansfield, working at Nottingham University, developed the mathematical analyses needed to construct images from magnetic resonance signals and he developed a system known as echo-planar imaging for rapid image acquisition. Lauterbur and Mansfield shared the 2003 Nobel Prize in Physiology or Medicine for the development of magnetic resonance imaging (MRI).[99].

Much of MRI is based on hydrogen nuclei (protons) of water. These nuclei resonate at frequencies in the radiofrequency range when exposed to those frequencies and the exact resonant frequency is determined by the strength of the magnetic field. The use of Lauterbur's technique of magnetic gradients changes the resonance frequencies of hydrogen nuclei. The MRI machine has emitters for generating the radiofrequencies and the scanner detects the emitted frequencies allowing localization of the proton.[97]. The 1954 Nobel laureate chemist Linus Pauling (1901–1994) and his colleague Charles Coryall (1912–1971), working in California, found that oxygenated and deoxygenated hemoglobin had different magnetic properties. Japanese researcher Seiji Ogawa, working at AT & T Bell Laboratories in Murray Hill, New Jersey, drew on this finding to create a contrast that could be used to infer blood flow to different brain regions; blood flow was higher in regions where the relative concentration of oxygenated hemoglobin was higher. By imaging people while they were engaged in various cognitive tasks, it was possible to use the BOLD contrast to identify the brain regions that were active during that task.[107]. One of the first published studies using this technique of fMRI appeared in 1991; it showed increased blood flow to the visual cortex during the processing of visual information.[109]

Positron emission tomography

Studies have provided evidence that food reward increases dopamine release in the human brain. Researchers from McGill University in Montreal and their collaborators from Northwestern University in Chicago used the dopamine receptor antagonist raclopride labeled with the radionuclide ^{11}C. Each participant was imaged twice. On one occasion, they measured [^{11}C]raclopride binding in their participants in the morning after an overnight fast of about 16 hours. On the other occasion, they had the participants eat a meal of their favorite food (varying from sushi to fried chicken) for 15 minutes after fasting for a similar period and they then imaged them immediately after the meal. If eating the meal increased brain dopamine release, the dopamine would occupy dopamine receptors and compete with [^{11}C]raclopride for those sites. The prediction was that [^{11}C]raclopride binding would *decrease* after the food reward, and that is what they found. As expected, [^{11}C]raclopride binding was highest in the dopamine terminal region known as the striatum where there is a high concentration of dopamine receptors. After the meal, the level of [^{11}C]raclopride binding in the dorsal striatum was lower, supporting the hypothesis that dopamine released by the food reward competed with [^{11}C]raclopride for dopamine receptor sites, thereby reducing [^{11}C]raclopride binding in this region. These were perhaps the first results to show that food reward increased dopamine release in humans.[110] The authors also found a strong positive relationship between the participants' ratings of pleasantness of the meal and their changes in

[^{11}C]raclopride binding, linking changes in brain function to changes in mental experience; this relationship is the topic of Chapter 13.

A similar approach was taken by researchers working at Hammersmith Hospital and at the Imperial College of Medicine in London, UK. Matthias J. Koepp and colleagues assessed [^{11}C]raclopride binding in two sessions on two separate days, one when the participants viewed a blank screen and another when they played a video game for monetary reward. The video game involved moving a virtual tank through a virtual battlefield using a mouse held by the right hand while the participant lay on his back in the scanner with his head immobilized by a molded head rest; the goal was to destroy enemy tanks while trying to collect flags that allowed the player to move to the next level of the game. Participants were financially compensated in proportion to the level they achieved in the game. The researchers found that [^{11}C]raclopride binding decreased in the dorsal and ventral striatum when the participants were playing the video game. This result suggested that dopamine was released when the participants played the video game and the dopamine competed with the [^{11}C]raclopride for dopamine receptor binding sites, reducing [^{11}C]raclopride binding. They found further that the magnitude of the reduction of [^{11}C]raclopride binding was positively correlated with the performance level achieved in the game; this finding suggested that more dopamine was released when a higher level of performance, and therefore greater financial reward, was achieved.[111]

One concern with the pioneering PET study of Koepp et al. of [^{11}C] raclopride displacement by endogenous dopamine during performance of a task for monetary reward was that the control condition compared with playing the video game was simply inactivity, the participants lying passively in the scanner. Was the observed increase in dopamine release a result of playing the video game for monetary reward or did it reflect the motor activity of moving the mouse, the sensory activity of watching the images on the screen, or perhaps the cognitive activity of anticipating the next move? A subsequent study addressed this question by comparing [^{11}C]raclopride binding in participants successfully performing a number comparison task for monetary reward to that of the same participants performing the same task but failing to achieve a level of performance that produced monetary reward. The researchers did this by adjusting the minimum reaction time required to achieve financial reward. Results confirmed that ventral striatal [^{11}C] raclopride binding decreased (reflecting increased dopamine release) when participants were performing the task for monetary reward.[112] A number of subsequent studies confirmed this finding.[113],[114]

The results of one study are noteworthy because of their implications for the concepts of prediction error and incentive learning. David Zald from

Vanderbilt University and co-workers carried out PET imaging of people carrying out a monetary reward task. In one condition, monetary reward was presented on a *fixed* ratio schedule so that every fourth response was rewarded; in the other condition monetary reward was presented on a *variable* ratio schedule so that, on average, every fourth response was rewarded but financial reward was unpredictable on any given trial. The variable reward schedule would produce more reward prediction errors. They found greater decreases in [^{11}C]raclopride binding (indicating increased dopamine release) in several regions of the striatum in the fixed ratio condition compared with the variable ratio condition.[114]. Because monetary reward was more predictable in the fixed ratio condition, there would have been many conditioned incentive stimuli, for example trial number, that predicted the rewarding stimulus; these conditioned stimuli would not have been present in the variable ratio condition. The observation of greater dopamine release during fixed ratio responding compared with variable ratio responding is consistent with the role of dopamine in incentive learning.

Amphetamine is an abused drug that reverses the dopamine transporter in dopamine synapses thereby increasing dopamine synaptic concentrations and postsynaptic effects. As expected from knowledge of its mechanism of action, researchers at the Montreal Neurological Institute and McGill University in Montreal, Canada, observed that amphetamine decreased [^{11}C]raclopride binding in the dorsal and ventral striatum. They carried out three scanning sessions with amphetamine separated by at least 48 hours and then a fourth session at least two weeks later where the participants thought they were receiving amphetamine but actually received no drug. Decreased [^{11}C]raclopride binding was observed in the ventral striatum during this fourth session, showing that stimuli that had come to signal amphetamine reward, that is, conditioned incentive stimuli, themselves acquired the ability to activate dopamine neurons,[115] as was seen in animal studies reviewed above.

Money is a conditioned incentive stimulus. Money itself has little or no value for the survival of an individual. Perhaps paper money could be burned to generate heat but otherwise it is of little intrinsic value. The value of money arises from the things for which it can be exchanged. Money can be exchanged for primary rewards such as food, drink, sex, and protection from heat or cold or other threats, all things that we need in order to survive and reproduce. The observation that monetary reward leads to increased dopamine release in the striatum is consistent with postmortem biochemical, intracerebral microdialysis, electrophysiological, and in vivo voltammetric results reviewed earlier, showing that stimuli that signal primary rewards themselves can produce activation of dopamine neurons and thereby produce incentive learning. The conditioned nature of monetary stimuli can be appreciated in a number of ways. For example, young children who have not yet learned about the exchange value of money treat money with the same passing interest that they treat most other novel objects. In countries where the currency has changed, for example in a number of European countries where the national currencies were replaced with the Euro in the late twentieth century, the rewarding quality of devalued currencies quickly decreased as their exchange value was lost. I recall from my first international travels the slightly uneasy sense of purchasing the local currency that was unfamiliar to me. Only after exchanging it for primary rewards did it quickly acquire incentive value. After many years of international travel, I am now familiar with many currencies and no longer have this experience. Even when I travel to a new country and encounter a new currency for the first time, that currency quickly acquires incentive value by generalization to my past experiences.

Functional magnetic resonance imaging

Studies generally compare the BOLD response during a control condition that does not involve an explicit rewarding stimulus to an experimental condition that does. If the BOLD response is greater in some brain areas during the experimental condition involving a rewarding stimulus, results suggest more neuronal activity in those areas. *This methodology does not explicitly measure dopamine* and therefore cannot be used alone to make a strong link between rewarding stimuli and dopamine. However, a number of approaches have been taken that strongly suggest a relationship between BOLD responses in some brain areas and dopamine neuron activity. These include comparisons of fMRI and PET imaging, sometimes in the same participants doing the same tasks, and comparisons of functional magnetic resonance images taken during performance of a cognitive task that involves a rewarding stimulus to images taken following administration of a drug such as amphetamine that is known to increase brain dopaminergic neurotransmission. I will discuss these approaches in the context of reviewing fMRI studies of BOLD responses to rewarding stimuli.

The earliest fMRI studies of primary reward involved using liquid to introduce a taste directly into the mouth through a tube while the participant lay in the scanner. These studies, carried out by researchers in the UK at Oxford and Nottingham Universities, sometimes in collaboration with researchers from other institutions, focused on the cerebral cortex and identified a region of the medial orbital frontal cortex that was activated by glucose.[116] They subsequently showed that the odor of food (in this case banana), a conditioned stimulus based on the taste of the food, also activated the orbitofrontal cortex.

The rating of pleasantness of the odor and the level of activation decreased after the food was eaten.[117] At about the same time, researchers at Emory University in Atlanta, Georgia, and Baylor College in Houston, Texas, were among the first to report that fruit juice or water rewards led to activation of the orbital frontal cortex and the nucleus accumbens,[118] both known to receive dopaminergic projections from the midbrain.

John O'Doherty and colleagues from the Institute of Neurology in London, UK, pre-trained participants with pairings of a visual stimulus and glucose squirted into the mouth prior to scanning the participants during the presentation of these stimuli. They found that the visual conditioned stimulus led to activations in the ventral mesencephalic region containing dopamine cell bodies and in dopaminoceptive brain areas, including the nucleus accumbens, right dorsal striatum (putamen), the posterior dorsal amygdala, and the orbital frontal cortex.[119] The US team from Emory and Baylor similarly found the nucleus accumbens response to a conditioned visual stimulus that signaled juice and found further that un-signaled juice activated the nucleus accumbens, implicating this structure in food reward.[120] Corroborative findings were reported in a number of subsequent papers.[121] Researchers at Princeton University in New Jersey imaged the ventral striatum and ventral tegmental area of the midbrain, the origin of the dopamine neurons that project to the ventral striatum, while participants were performing a task for juice or water reward and found a BOLD response in both areas. Their further observation of a significant positive correlation between the two signals led the authors to conclude that the signals reflected dopaminergic neuron activation.[122] Results support many related findings implicating dopamine in reward-related learning.

Korean researchers from Chonnan National University in Kwangju carried out fMRI in men and women who watched a two- or four-minute erotic film and compared the BOLD responses to those seen when the participants viewed a non-erotic documentary film. They found differential activation in a number of regions, including the caudate nucleus, a dopamine terminal region.[123] Using a similar approach with male and female participants, groups from Stanford University in California, and from the University of Montreal and McGill University in Montreal, Canada, found that sexually arousing stimuli activated, among other regions, the medial prefrontal cortex, caudate, putamen, and ventral striatum.[124] These results are consistent with those from studies using food as the primary rewarding stimulus in providing indirect evidence for an involvement of dopamine in the effects of rewarding stimuli.

Attractive faces may have primary rewarding properties; people will perform operant responses to gain access to images of attractive faces.[125] Participants viewing attractive faces while lying in a fMRI scanner showed increased BOLD activity in the orbital frontal cortex and nucleus acccumbens,[126] especially if the stimuli provided eye contact.[127] Visual stimuli paired with attractive faces became conditioned incentive stimuli, eliciting increased pleasantness ratings after pairing and elicited increased BOLD responses in the ventral striatum.[128] These results are consistent with those reviewed above and include attractive faces among primary incentive stimuli such as food as stimuli that can activate brain reward circuitry and produce incentive learning. The role of dopamine in the rewarding effects of social stimuli is discussed further in Chapter 8.

As further discussed in the following paragraphs, beginning in or around the year 2000, numerous studies used fMRI to evaluate BOLD changes produced by monetary rewards. Before the first of these studies appeared and around the time of appearance of PET studies using [^{11}C]raclopride to assess endogenous levels of occupation of dopamine receptors by dopamine, some PET studies using radiolabeled water, $H_2{}^{15}O$, reported changes in regional cerebral blood flow produced by monetary rewards. One of the first was carried out in 1997 in Switzerland at the Paul Scherrer Institute in Villigen, north-west of Zurich, and was co-authored by electrophysiologist Wolfram Schultz, who had done much of the pioneering work identifying the electrical activity of dopaminergic neurons associated with reward presentation, as discussed earlier in this chapter. This study compared regional cerebral blood flow during monetary reward (an amount indicated on the computer monitor that was paid to the participant at the end of the experiment), given during performance of a visual discrimination task, to the regional cerebral blood flow seen when the feedback was simply receiving the message "ok" on the computer monitor. Results revealed increased blood flow in the dorsolateral and orbitofrontal cortex during monetary reward.[129] A related study carried out by researchers in Cambridge and Nottingham, UK, similarly identified regions of orbitofrontal cortex that were involved in processing reward-related information.[130] These studies implicated cortical regions that receive dopamine input in reward-related learning.

A flood of fMRI studies reported BOLD changes associated with the receipt of monetary reward. Like the original PET study of Koepp et al..[111], using [^{11}C] raclopride displacement to identify increased dopamine release in the dorsal and ventral striatum associated with monetary reward, fMRI studies identified BOLD changes in regions of the dorsal and ventral striatum, including the nucleus accumbens, as well as the amygdala, ventral midbrain, and orbital frontal cortex in association with monetary rewards or cues that signal monetary rewards;[131] these results are consistent with activation of dopamine neurons by monetary reward or cues repeatedly associated with monetary reward. Some studies showed that the magnitude of the BOLD response in the nucleus accumbens, dorsal striatum or orbital frontal cortex correlated positively with the magnitude of monetary reward.[132]

Within some published papers, both PET and fMRI have been carried out on the same individuals doing similar or related tasks to allow a comparison of the regions of [11C]raclopride displacement and the regions showing a BOLD change. The observation of overlap would provide evidence that the BOLD response reflects changes in dopamine neuron activity. US researchers from the University of Michigan in Ann Arbor and the University of Maryland in Baltimore took this approach. They showed that a cue for a painful challenge accompanied by the expectation of receipt of an analgesic led to decreased [11C]raclopride displacement in the nucleus accumbens, showing that the cue elicited increases in dopamine neuron activity. They also showed, like many others, that a cue that signaled monetary reward led to increased BOLD activity in the nucleus accumbens. The strength of the fMRI response was correlated positively with [11C]raclopride displacement in the nucleus accumbens, providing evidence that the BOLD response is related to the level of dopamine neuron activity. An interesting feature of this work was that the authors were studying the placebo response. A placebo response resulting from anticipation of analgesia can be understood as an expectation of a rewarding effect (pain reduction); part of the mechanism of the placebo effect appears to be dopamine release in the nucleus accumbens.[133] Others have similarly observed good correlations between dopamine-related signals detected using PET during anticipation and receipt of monetary reward and functional magnetic resonance images collected during performance of the same task.[134]

Another approach to evaluating the possibility that increases in BOLD responses reflect changes in dopaminergic neurotransmission is to compare the response to a rewarding stimulus to that seen following injection of a drug that is known to augment dopamine neurotransmission. Observation that the same regions are activated by a rewarding stimulus and by a dopaminergic drug would support the hypothesis that BOLD responses to rewarding stimuli reflect changes in dopamine neurotransmission and this is what was found. Cocaine, a drug that increases dopamine neurotransmission by blocking the dopamine transporter, leading to prolonged action of dopamine in synapses, produced BOLD changes in the ventral tegmental area, origin of dopamine cells, and their projection areas, including the nucleus accumbens, dorsal striatum, and prefrontal cortex.[135] In work carried out in the laboratory of Bruce Jenkins at the Massachusetts General Hospital and Harvard Medical School in Charlestown, fMRI was used in *rats* to identify BOLD changes associated with amphetamine, another drug that augments dopamine neurotransmission by reversing the transporter, leading to enhanced and prolonged action of dopamine in synapses. As with humans, BOLD changes were found in the striatum and cortex. Unilateral destruction of dopaminergic cells using a specific neurotoxin led to a loss of the amphetamine-produced response in both the striatum and cortex on the lesion side but not on the intact side.[136] These findings replicated the observation with cocaine that drugs known to activate dopaminergic neurotransmission produce BOLD changes in dopamine terminal areas and confirmed that the changes depended on dopamine. The observation that drugs that are known to produce changes in dopaminergic neurotransmission lead to changes in blood oxygenation level in the same brain regions, for example striatum, where BOLD changes are produced by natural rewards and monetary rewards, as reviewed above, supports the hypothesis that natural and monetary rewards activate brain dopaminergic neurotransmission. These observations are consistent with the results of [^{11}C] raclopride displacement studies that implicate dopamine in the action of rewarding stimuli.[137]

Summary

Approaches to the experimental study of the role of dopamine in reward-related learning can be classified as those that observe the effects of stimulating the system, inactivating the system or record the activity of the system while rewarding stimuli are being presented. This chapter has focused on recording studies using postmortem biochemistry, intracerebral microdialysis, electrophysiological recording, in vivo electrochemistry, or neuroimaging, including PET and fMRI. Results from these various recording methodologies using dopamine as the dependent variable (except fMRI) converge in providing compelling evidence that dopaminergic neurons are activated by primary rewarding stimuli including food and water and by numerous conditioned incentive stimuli, including money.

Electrophysiological and in vivo neurochemical recording studies reveal that early in training, primary rewarding stimuli such as food activate dopaminergic neurons. When a cue is reliably paired with a primary rewarding stimulus it acquires an increased ability to elicit approach and other responses; over an extended series of trials, the dopamine response begins to be seen upon presentation of the cue and eventually is not seen upon presentation of the primary rewarding stimulus when it follows the cue. As a result, the cue itself acquires the ability to act as a rewarding stimulus, increasing the incentive value of stimuli that precede it. Although conditioned incentive stimuli activate dopaminergic neurons and primary incentive stimuli that follow them do not do so in well-trained animals, conditioned incentive stimuli continue to rely on the primary incentive stimulus for their ability to control responding. If conditioned incentive stimuli are repeatedly presented in the absence of primary incentive stimuli, they gradually lose their ability to elicit approach and other responses and to act as rewarding stimuli by producing incentive learning in their own right.

Chapter 6

Dopamine and inverse incentive learning

Inverse incentive learning is the loss by stimuli of their ability to elicit approach and other responses. "Other responses" could include pushing, pulling, digging, biting, and so on, depending on the situation and the natural abilities of the animal. Previous chapters have discussed how increases in dopaminergic neurotransmission are associated with incentive learning. In this chapter I will argue that the converse also appears to be the case; decreases in dopaminergic neurotransmission are associated with inverse incentive learning.

There is some unfinished business related to the material in Chapter 5 that needs to be transacted before entering into a discussion of the role of dopamine in inverse incentive learning. The large body of work on dopamine as the dependent variable incudes many studies that show changes, often increases, in measures of dopamine and/or its metabolites in association with novel, intense, or aversive stimuli. These findings have received much attention in the recent literature as they potentially pose considerable difficulty for a unitary theory of the role of dopamine in reward-related learning. Simply put, if novel, intense, or aversive stimuli produce increased activity in dopamine neurons and if increased activity in dopamine neurons leads to incentive learning, then do animals learn to approach and make other responses to novel, intense, or aversive stimuli? Unconditioned aversive stimuli by definition are those that produce pain or tissue damage and stimuli that reliably predict them become conditioned aversive stimuli. Animals naturally escape unconditioned aversive stimuli and quickly learn to avoid them by escaping from conditioned aversive stimuli. The framework of dopamine and incentive learning that was developed in Chapters 2 and 3, and the supporting evidence presented in Chapter 5 portrays dopamine as the neurotransmitter activated by rewarding stimuli and producing reward-related learning. Such a framework may seem incompatible with the activation of dopaminergic neurons by novel, intense, or aversive stimuli.

In the following, I will deal with dopamine and novel, intense, and aversive stimuli in turn, in each case reviewing some of the relevant findings and then how they can be understood within the framework of dopamine and reward-related incentive learning. At the time that I am writing this, June 2014, the effect of novel, intense, and aversive stimuli on dopamine neurons remains controversial and is not fully resolved, as I discuss. However, it is possible to understand most of the findings by attributing to dopamine a general transient orienting function to surprising or otherwise important stimuli, as well as a more enduring learning function, that of incentive learning as argued in this book. The effect of aversive stimuli on dopamine neuron firing is particularly confusing because aversive stimuli are naturally rewarding stimuli on the occasion of their offset (see Chapter 2); this aspect of aversive stimuli has made their effects on dopamine neuron firing particularly confusing and difficult to decipher.

Novel stimuli and dopamine

Beginning with novel stimuli, a number of studies, by recording from dopaminergic cell bodies in the ventral midbrain, have shown that novel stimuli lead to activation of these neurons. In 1980, Louis Chiodo and colleagues, working at the University of Pittsburgh, showed that in anesthetized rats mild tail pressure, a light flash, air puff, or the scent of ammonium hydroxide activated some (about 50%) putative dopamine neurons in the substantia nigra, the origin of dopamine cells that project to the dorsal striatum (see Chapter 11); others were inhibited.[1] In a study from Schultz's lab, by Ljungberg et al., discussed in Chapter 5, it was noted that when awake monkeys were presented with a novel stimulus, the opening of a small guillotine-type door on a panel in front of the monkey, dopamine neurons of the substantia nigra and ventral tegmental area, the origin of dopamine cells that project to the nucleus accumbens and frontal cortex, responded with a short burst of activity on the first couple of presentations; the response then faded away and with continued repeated presentations of the door-opening stimulus, no change in the firing of dopaminergic neurons was seen.[2] This showed that dopamine neurons can be activated by novel stimuli, but as the stimulus becomes more familiar and is not associated with any rewarding outcomes, the stimulus rapidly loses its ability to activate dopamine neurons.

In vivo voltammetry experiments carried out by neuroscientist George Rebec and colleagues at Indiana University in Bloomington showed that novel stimuli lead to increases in dopamine release. They habituated rats to one compartment of a box that consisted of two distinct compartments for four 30-minute periods and then removed the partition between them. They observed increases in dopamine release in the nucleus accumbens shell region when the rats entered the novel chamber. The response to novelty was brief and, like the response of dopamine neurons to a novel stimulus in the brains of the monkeys tested by Ljungberg et al., was transient, only being seen upon the first entry into the novel chamber.[3]

In microdialysis experiments, Mark Legault, working in the laboratory of Roy Wise, at the time at Concordia University in Montreal, showed that exposure to a novel environment led to increased levels of dopamine in dialysate taken from the nucleus accumbens; control animals exposed to a similar environment to which they had previously been exposed (habituated) showed no change in nucleus accumbens dialysate dopamine.[4] In a functional magnetic resonance imaging (fMRI) study, researchers at University College in London, UK, and Otto von Guericke University in Magdeburg, Germany, examined changes in blood oxygenation level-dependent responses from the dopamine cell body regions, *viz.*, substantia nigra and ventral tegmental area, of the ventral midbrain. They observed a response to novel stimuli presented in an oddball task and the magnitude of the response decreased with each subsequent exposure. They suggested the interesting idea that novelty-induced dopamine activity produces an exploration bonus, increasing the chances that the individual will find a rewarding stimulus in a novel environment.[5] If no rewarding stimulus is found, the dopamine response to novel stimuli subsides with familiarity; if a rewarding stimulus is found, the additional firing of dopamine neurons will produce incentive learning to the novel stimuli so that they will retain their ability to elicit approach and other responses even when they become familiar.

Some electrophysiological results from cats have revealed that the activation of dopamine neurons by novel stimuli is followed by a period of hyperpolarization during which it is more difficult to activate those dopamine neurons.[6] This led Jon Horvitz and colleagues from Boston College, Chestnut Hill, Massachusetts, and Columbia University, New York, to suggest that novel stimuli may produce a rapid initial excitation in dopamine neurons that takes place before the reward or non-reward status of the event can be processed and that the post-excitation inhibition serves to counteract the initial burst in cases where a rewarding outcome fails to occur.[7] In this way, novel stimuli produce a brief activation response, but if a rewarding stimulus fails to materialize, incentive learning does not occur.

These electrophysiological, in vivo voltammetry, and intracerebral microdialysis studies in rats, cats, and monkeys, and fMRI studies in humans provide convergent evidence that novel stimuli activate dopaminergic neurons and that once these stimuli become familiar, the dopamine response is no longer seen.

Intense stimuli and dopamine

Another class of stimuli that appear to activate dopamine neurons is intense stimuli. Over 30 years ago, Barry Jacobs and colleagues at Princeton University, New Jersey, recorded from putative dopamine cells in the substantia nigra of awake, freely moving cats. They observed cells that were activated by a bright flashing light or by repeated loud clicks. This response did not habituate even after 2000 trials. Like the responses recorded by Horvitz and colleagues to novel stimuli, the short-latency burst of activity was followed by a period of hyperpolarization during which the firing of dopamine cells was suppressed.[8] Christopher Fiorillo and colleagues from the Korean Advanced Institute of Science and Technology in Daejeon, South Korea, and from Stanford University in California similarly showed in monkeys that intense stimuli led to short-latency activation of substantia nigra and ventral tegmental area dopamine neurons. These activations were less than half the frequency of firing seen in dopamine neurons when a rewarding juice stimulus was presented and, unlike the response to a rewarding stimulus, were followed by hyperpolarization that suppressed responding.[9] Like novel stimuli, intense stimuli elicit an initial excitation that may alert the animal to the stimulus, but the subsequent hyperpolarization negates the effects of the initial burst of activity and, as a result, incentive learning may fail to occur to intense stimuli.

Aversive stimuli and dopamine

The effects of aversive stimuli on measures of dopamine neuron activity have been studied extensively and the large set of published papers is a challenge to summarize. There is convergent evidence from postmortem biochemical, intracerebral microdialysis, electrophysiological, and in vivo electrochemical studies that suggests that aversive stimuli lead to increases in dopamine neuron activity. On the face of it, these observations are fatal for the role of dopamine in incentive learning because they suggest that stimuli that signal dangerous or harmful events gain an increased ability to elicit approach and other responses. It would not be adaptive to be drawn to aversive stimuli! However, recall from Chapter 2 that aversive stimuli are rewarding by their offset. Thus, the offset of an aversive event activates dopamine neurons, leading to incentive learning so that the stimuli that signal *safety* have an increased ability to elicit approach and other responses in the future. Studies that evaluate evidence of dopamine neuron activity over a relatively long time scale, that is, seconds or minutes, and that observe increases, will be unable to decipher the temporal coupling between the onset or offset of aversive stimuli and changes in dopamine. The millisecond precision of electrophysiological studies provides a level of temporal resolution that allows this coupling; as you will see in the following, results from these studies are controversial. The emerging picture is that aversive stimuli, when they do activate dopaminergic neurons, do so in a manner similar to novel or intense stimuli, producing a short-latency burst of activity that is smaller than that produced by a rewarding stimulus and that, unlike the pattern of activity produced by rewarding stimuli, is followed by a period of decreased firing that may serve to cancel possible incentive learning effects of the initial burst. In the following, I review studies of the effects of aversive stimuli on dopamine as the dependent variable as measured, in turn, by postmortem biochemical, intracerebral microdialysis, in vivo voltammetry, and electrophysiological techniques.

Postmortem studies of changes in dopamine and/or its metabolites in dopaminoceptive brain areas reported that electrical shock or prolonged restraint led to increases in the nucleus accumbens or prefrontal cortex of rats and mice.[10] From among these studies, the study by Simona Cabib and Stefano Puglisi-Allegra from the National Research Council and the University of Rome in Italy is particularly informative for the present considerations. These authors exposed mice to mild electric foot shock in a shuttle box. For the experimental group, the shock lasted for four seconds and then a door opened allowing escape to the safe side of the box. They included a yoked control procedure whereby a second mouse, run in parallel to the first, received shock at the same time as the first mouse but had no control over the shock; for the yoked mouse, the shock simply started and stopped according to the experience of the experimental mouse. The animals were killed immediately after this testing and dopamine and its metabolites were measured in the nucleus accumbens. One of the metabolites, 3-methoxytyramine, was observed to increase in the experimental mice but to decrease in the yoked mice. On the basis of this and related observations, the authors concluded that exposure to controllable shock induces an increase in dopamine release and that exposure to uncontrollable shock induces a decrease. These results suggest that it is not aversive stimuli per se that lead to increases in dopamine release; instead, they suggest that it may be the reward provided by escape from controllable shock that leads to increases in dopamine release.

Many studies using intracerebral microdialysis have shown that levels of dopamine and/or its metabolites rise in a number of brain regions in animals exposed to aversive stimuli.[11] For some of the studies, aversive stimuli are confounded with novelty. Some of the studies provide little description of the behavior of the animals, making it difficult to assess possible reward resulting from escape. Others, however, provide valuable insights into the possible relationship between increases in extracellular dopamine and the behavior of the animals. For example, Assunta Imperato, Paola Casolini, and Luciano Angelucci from Sapienza University, along with Stefano Puglisi-Allegra from the National Research Council in Rome, restrained rats in a small plastic box for a two-hour test while sampling dopamine every ten minutes from the nucleus accumbens and prefrontal cortex. This novel aversive experience led to an increase in dopamine and its metabolites 3,4-dihydroxyphenylacetic acid and homovanillic acid, which peaked in about the first 30 minutes and then declined. Generally, dopamine and metabolite levels returned to baseline in the second hour of restraint. Particularly noteworthy is their observation of a second significant increase of almost the same magnitude as the first increase in dopamine and its metabolites during the 60-minute period following release from restraint. The authors suggested that "the end of restraint may be considered as a rewarding experience" (p. 115).[12] Others have reported similar findings.[13]

The observations of Imperato et al. might suggest that at the beginning of restraint, when the situation is novel and the animal is struggling to find an escape, dopamine neurons may be activated by movements that provide some relief. The tactile, visual, and proprioceptive stimuli associated with those movements may become incentive stimuli so that the next time the animal finds itself in the presence of those stimuli, it will perform similar movements to minimize the aversive input. However, as all escape attempts fail, dopamine activity subsides. Then, when the experimenter releases the animal, the end of restraint, as suggested by the authors, is a rewarding event; associated increases in dopamine release may produce incentive learning about the stimuli associated with escape from restraint. In a related study, Puglisi-Allegra and colleagues extended the period of restraint from two to four hours.[14] They observed that nucleus accumbens dopamine and metabolite levels continued to decrease to levels significantly *below* baseline for the second two hours of restraint. As before, once the rats were released, dopamine and its metabolites rose to levels significantly above baseline. The authors suggested that the period of sub-baseline dopamine activity was associated with behavioral depression and reminiscent of learned helplessness—more on this later in this chapter.

The Italian researchers went on to do another related study that is particularly elegant and informative. They restrained rats in the small plastic box for one hour each day for six consecutive days. As before, on the first day levels of dopamine and metabolites rose to a peak within the first 30 minutes and then returned to baseline by 60 minutes; when the animals were released, dopamine and metabolite levels again rose, replicating the previous findings. Over the next five days, the dopamine and metabolite signal during the first 30 minutes of restraint was less each day than the day before until by day four it was no longer significant. However, on each of these five days, the dopamine and metabolite increase following release remained intact, showing no signs of dim-inution.[15] These results are consistent with the interpretation discussed above, suggesting that the rise in dopamine and metabolites during the initial period of restraint is associated with the novelty of the situation and with futile efforts at escape. As novelty and those efforts diminish from day to day, the signal is lost. However, escape from the aversive restraint situation remains rewarding from day to day.

John Salamone, a behavioral neuroscientist at the University of Connecticut at Storrs has spent his career studying the role of dopamine in the control of behavior and he has made an important contribution to understanding the role of dopamine in incentive learning. Some of his work is cited in Chapters 2 and 5. Salamone and co-workers carried out a lever-press shock avoidance–escape experiment with rats while dialyzing their nucleus accumbens. Like Cabib and Puglisi-Allegra,[10] discussed above, who employed a yoked control procedure, Salamone and colleagues included a group that received periodic unavoidable shocks. The experimental group could press a lever to avoid imminent shock and if they failed to do so, they could press the lever to escape the shock once it had come on. The researchers found a significant increase in dopamine and its metabolites in the experimental group but no significant change in the shocked control group. Since both groups received shocks during the test session, increases in dopamine cannot be attributed to shock. Instead, it was the rewarding avoidance of shock that best predicted the increases in nucleus accumbens extracellular dopamine. In fact, they found a significant correlation between number of avoidance responses and increases in dopamine but not between number or duration of shocks and increases in dopamine.[16]

Together, the results of these intracerebral microdialysis studies make a strong case for dopamine neuron activation by the onset of aversive stimuli when they are novel; this activation declines with repeated exposure to aversive stimulus onset. Dopamine neurons are also activated by the offset of aversive stimuli and this activation endures with repeated exposures to aversive-stimulus offset; this activation may lead to incentive learning, increasing the ability of safety-related stimuli to elicit approach and other responses in the future.

In vivo voltammetry studies have likewise shown increases in extracellular dopamine following exposure to aversive stimuli. In one of the first in vivo voltammetry studies to look at possible dopamine changes associated with be-havior, Keller and colleagues reported increased dorsal striatal dopamine re-lease following exposure to novel aversive ice water or electric shock stimuli that was associated with strong behavioral activation and attempts to escape.[17] Others reported increases in nucleus accumbens and prefrontal cortical levels of dopamine or the dopamine metabolite 3,4-dihydroxyphenylacetic acid

following tail pinch or restraint in the hands of the experimenter.[18] These results are consistent with those from postmortem biochemical and intracerebral
microdialysis studies reviewed above.

A recent study from the laboratory of Joseph Cheer at the University of
Maryland in Baltimore used fast-scan cyclic voltammetry to assess changes in
nucleus accumbens core dopamine while well-trained rats were performing
a lever-press avoidance task. The rats were presented with a two-second light
stimulus and a lever extended into the chamber when the stimulus came on.
A lever press during the first two seconds was an avoidance response; it dimmed
the light, retracted the lever, and turned on a tone stimulus that signaled 20 seconds of safety. If no lever press occurred in the first two seconds, intermittent
shock came on and the next lever press was an escape response; it turned off the
shock, dimmed the light, retracted the lever, and turned on the tone signaling
20 seconds of safety. The researchers observed a decrease in dopamine when an
avoidance response failed to occur. An increase in dopamine was seen when an
avoidance or an escape response occurred; in each case, the response was rewarded by presentation of the safety-related stimuli. It was not the number of
shocks that was associated with the increase in dopamine, but rather the onset
of the safety-related stimuli.[19]

There have been many electrophysiological studies of the activity of putative dopaminergic neurons during the presentation of aversive stimuli. If the
aversive stimuli were novel or intense, brief bursts of activity in some dopamine neurons like those discussed earlier might be expected and that is what
has been reported.[20,21] In some cases, the authors stated that increases in the
activity of some dopamine neurons to aversive stimuli such as tail pressure occurred when the animal was trying to escape or was otherwise able to respond
to the aversive stimulus,[22,23] mirroring the observations from postmortem and
intracerebral microdialysis studies discussed earlier, and suggesting that it
may be the rewarding aspects of aversive stimulus offset that lead to dopamine
neurons firing.[7] In support of this idea, researchers in London, UK, reported
that dopamine neurons were excited during the half second following termination of foot shocks.[24]

In recent years the timing and intensity of bursts of action potentials in some
dopamine neurons and the suppression of tonic activity in those neurons produced by aversive stimuli have been scrutinized closely. Wolfram Schultz and
his co-worker Jacques Mirenowicz reported that about *up to 30 percent* of
dopamine neurons are activated by aversive stimuli.[25] This was the smallest
percentage compared with up to 80 percent of dopamine neurons being activated by rewarding stimuli and a high percentage by novel and intense stimuli.[26]
Fiorillo and co-workers and Joshua et al. showed that the dopamine neuron

activations produced by aversive stimuli were like those produced by novel and intense stimuli and different in several ways from those produced by rewarding stimuli.[9,23] Thus, aversive stimuli produced increases in frequency of dopamine neuronal firing that were less than half those produced by rewarding stimuli. The peak of these bursts was rapid (< 150 ms) and was followed by a period of decreased dopamine neuronal firing; the more intense bursts of firing produced by rewarding stimuli had a later peak and were not followed by a period of decreased firing. This led Fiorillo and colleagues to suggest that "The activation occurring before ~150 ms is primarily dependent on the sensory intensity of the stimulus" (2013, *Journal of Neuroscience* 33, p. 4698).[9] They suggested further that "reward value is best discriminated between ~150 and 250 ms" (p. 4698); this is the period when the peak activation by rewarding stimuli occurs and when the decrease in dopamine neuronal firing is seen following novel, intense, or aversive stimuli.

What emerges from studies of the effects of aversive stimuli on dopamine neuron firing is that aversive stimuli activate a subset of dopamine neurons, perhaps about one-third. In these neurons, aversive stimuli produce a small increase in the frequency of action potentials that peaks with a short latency (< 150 ms), the peak is less than half that produced by rewarding stimuli, and this increase is followed by a period of decreased frequency of action potentials, an effect that is not seen following rewarding stimuli. This pattern is also seen following novel and intense stimuli. This has led a number of authors to suggest that dopamine neurons serve two distinct functions. The rapid response seen to novel or intense stimuli, including aversive stimuli, serves to alert the animal and produce orientation responses; the subsequent response produces incentive learning if it involves a large increase in dopamine neuronal firing and is not followed by a suppression of firing below normal tonic baseline levels.[27]

Although up to 30 percent of dopamine neurons are activated by aversive stimuli, as just discussed, the majority is either depressed by aversive stimuli or shows no response.[26]. Mark Ungless, working with Peter Magill in the laboratory of Paul Bolam at Oxford University in the UK, observed that dopamine neurons in rats were inhibited by an aversive foot pinch,[28] and Masayuki Matsumoto and Okihide Hikosaka from the National Institutes of Health in Bethesda, Maryland, similarly observed inhibition of dopamine neurons by an air puff to the face in monkeys.[29] In a number of studies, the response of dopamine neurons to a conditioned stimulus associated with an aversive stimulus was observed to be a decrease in firing rate.[25] What might be the consequence of a decrease in dopamine neuron firing rate following an aversive stimulus? Increases in dopamine neuron firing rate (that are not immediately followed by decreases in rate) lead to incentive learning, increasing the ability of recently encountered stimuli to elicit approach and other responses in the future. I now argue that decreases in dopaminergic neurotransmission lead to inverse incentive learning, decreasing the ability of recently encountered stimuli to elicit approach and other responses.

The bar test

The discussion of inverse inventive learning will rely, in part, on studies of sensitization and conditioning in the bar test. The bar test is typically used to test catalepsy, a condition of remaining relatively motionless and detached from the environment. In the early days of drug development for the treatment of schizophrenia, discussed at more length in Chapter 7, catalepsy tests were used to identify drugs with potential antipsychotic effectiveness; drugs that produced catalepsy were good candidates.[30] In experiments with animals, catalepsy is operationalized by the amount of time an animal remains in a fixed posture. Typically, a small horizontal bar suspended between two supports is used. Some time after injection with the drug of interest, the animal is gently placed with its forepaws on the bar so that it is standing on its hind paws in an approximately vertical posture or leaning slightly forward. This is an unnatural posture for a rat and a non-drugged rat will quickly get down or, perhaps, climb onto the bar. A drug that produces catalepsy is one that causes the rat to remain in the standing posture with its paws leaning on the bar for some seconds after being placed there. The amount of catalepsy can be quantified by the duration of time the rat remains on the bar; often a maximum time, for example, three minutes, is used and if a rat remains on the bar for the full three minutes it is gently removed and returned to its home cage.[31]

Sensitization of descent latency in the bar test

Many drugs that block dopamine receptors are cataleptogenic. For example, the antipsychotic medication haloperidol blocks dopamine receptors and produces catalepsy in a dose-dependent manner.[30] It appears that there are learning components to this behavior. In groundbreaking studies carried out in the laboratory of Werner Schmidt (1950–2007) in Tubingen, Germany, rats tested in a distinct environment once a day with a *non-cataleptogenic* dose of haloperidol gradually developed increased descent latencies if they were injected and re-tested from day to day in the distinct environment. This phenomenon has been termed "catalepsy sensitization." In a sensitized animal, the sensitized response was not seen if the animal was tested in a different environment.[32] In related studies, Schmidt and colleagues showed that rats treated with a low dose of the dopamine neurotoxin 6-hydroxydopamine that failed to show catalepsy when first tested similarly developed increased descent latencies with repeated testing.[33] Researchers working in other laboratories, including mine, and sometimes using variations of the catalepsy testing procedure, have also observed sensitization to the response-reducing effects of haloperidol.[34] Jeffery Rocca, Joshua Lister (1989–2015), and I observed sensitization of descent latency in studies carried out in my lab using other dopamine receptor antagonists, including spiroperidol.[35] It is worth noting an irony in the definition of catalepsy: a condition of remaining relatively motionless and detached from the environment. Although catalepsy is defined as the period of relative motionlessness—remaining on the bar—it does not really involve detachment from the environment insofar as the phenomenon depends on the testing environment. It appears that the particular stimuli associated with the drug lose some of their ability to elicit responses from the animal.

The behavior that we typically observe in the bar test with repeated low doses of haloperidol is only superficially like catalepsy produced by high doses of haloperidol and related drugs. With high doses, the cataleptic animal is quite amenable to being placed into unusual postures and often will retain those postures for some time. With low doses, even though an animal begins to show increases in descent latency over trials, it appears quite alert, often moving its head as if looking around, but stays on the bar for increasing numbers of seconds from test to test, normally with one test a day. If this animal is handled gently and placed into an unusual posture, it will not stay there. It can also be easily distracted by extraneous noises, for example. Thus, the phenomenon that Schmidt and colleagues, and we in our first two papers on this topic, referred to as "catalepsy sensitization" does not completely correspond with what typically has been observed with high doses of dopamine receptor antagonists and termed "catalepsy." For this reason, in the following, I will refer to "increases in descent latency" and avoid the use of the term "catalepsy."

The typical experiment uses three groups of rats. Each group is tested for descent latency once a day at the same time each day in a distinct environment using the bar test described earlier. The paired group is injected with a low dose of haloperidol prior to each bar test; the unpaired group is injected with the haloperidol *vehicle* prior to each bar test. Some time after the test, for example one hour, the members of the paired group are removed from their home cage, injected with the vehicle and returned to their home cage; similarly, the members of the unpaired group are removed from their home cage but injected with haloperidol at the same dose that was used for the paired group and then returned to their home cage. The third group is a control group that is tested each day but does not receive haloperidol in the home or test environment. By using this experimental design, both drug groups have similar experience with the bar test and with haloperidol, but for the paired group, bar testing takes place while they are in the drug state; for the unpaired group, bar testing takes place while they are in an un-drugged state.

As already mentioned, researchers discovered that the paired group gradually develops increased descent latency over days.[33]. In a study done in my laboratory by Lexy Schimmel and others, on the first test day, the paired group, in spite of having been injected with haloperidol, descended or otherwise moved almost immediately upon being placed on the bar and was indistinguishable from the unpaired and control groups. However, gradually over days, the groups began to separate, with the paired group, on average, spending longer and longer periods of immobility, the rats remaining with their forepaws on the bar and not stepping down after being placed there by the experimenter. Even on days two or three a small difference is often observed between the paired and the other two groups, and by day four of testing the paired group is clearly different (Figure 6.1).[36] One explanation for the observation of sensitization of descent latency might be that the drug is building up in the system of the rat with repeated daily dosing; if the drug is not entirely secreted from one injection to the next, it is possible that each injection results in a slightly higher circulating level of the drug so that the dose experienced by the rat is gradually increasing and the descent latency sensitization reflects this putatively elevating dose. The fact that the unpaired group had the same number of injections of haloperidol but never developed increased descent latency and did not differ from the control group mitigates this concern but does not eliminate it because the unpaired group was never tested following an injection of haloperidol. However, additional experiments ruled out the escalating-dose explanation. I discuss those studies in the following three paragraphs, then studies showing that increases in descent latency can be conditioned to environmental stimuli associated with decreased dopamine neurotransmission. This leads to a conceptualization of increases in descent latency as a gradual loss of responding to a set of stimuli analogous to what is seen in habituation. Before developing this conceptual framework, it is important to fully examine the phenomenon of sensitization of descent latencies in the bar test.

In some studies, descent latency sensitization was demonstrated as described earlier. On the next day, rats in both the paired and unpaired groups were injected with haloperidol and then tested. Results revealed the expected sensitized descent latency response in the paired group. The unpaired group showed no increase in descent latency, moving from the leaning posture on the bar almost immediately after being placed there (Figure 6.2).[36]. This observation eliminates the argument that the sensitized response might result from a build-up of the drug with repeated daily injections. If the sensitized response in the

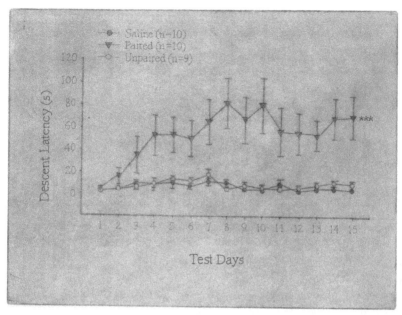

Figure 6.1 *Increased mean (± standard error of the mean) descent latencies (seconds) in the bar test with haloperidol:* Rats in the paired group received haloperidol (0.25 mg/kg) 60 minutes prior to each of 15 test sessions, one per day; they received saline in the home cage an hour after testing. Rats in the unpaired group were tested one hour after an injection of saline and received haloperidol (0.25 mg/kg) in the home cage 60 minutes later. Rats in the saline group received saline one hour before and after testing. ***Analysis of variance revealed significant main effects of group and group × day interaction. Post-hoc comparisons showed the descent latencies of the paired group to be significantly longer than those of the unpaired and saline groups.

Adapted from *Behavioural Brain Research*, 293 (1), Lexy N. Pezarro Schimmel, Tomek J. Banasikowski, Emily R. Hawken, Eric C. Dumont, and Richard J. Beninger, Brain regions associated with inverse incentive learning: c-Fos immunohistochemistry after haloperidol sensitization on the bar test in rats, pp. 81–8, doi.org/10.1016/j.bbr.2015.06.041, Copyright 2015, with permission from Elsevier.

paired group resulted from a drug build-up, then the unpaired group, when tested with haloperidol, might be expected to show an elevated descent latency to the low dose of haloperidol because it, too, had received daily injections of haloperidol for the same number of preceding days. The observation that the unpaired group did not show increased descent latency when tested with haloperidol confirms that the descent latency sensitization response in the paired group is not simply the result of repeated drug injections.

The failure to observe increased descent latency in the unpaired group when tested with haloperidol cannot be the result of it being the first bar test because this group was tested for descent latency each day following a saline injection

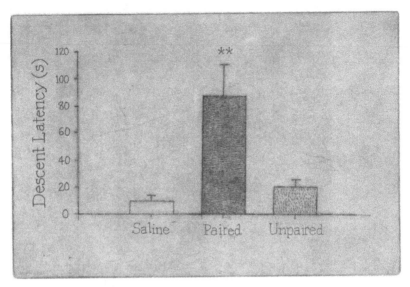

Figure 6.2 *Increased mean (± standard error of the mean) descent latencies (seconds) only in the paired group when all groups are tested with haloperidol (0.25 mg/ kg):* Both the paired and unpaired groups had received an injection of haloperidol (0.25 mg/kg) on each of the preceding 15 days (see Figure 6.1). The paired group received the injection prior to bar testing and the unpaired group received the injection in their home cage one hour after being tested in the bar test following an injection of saline; the saline group had never received haloperidol previous to this test. **Significantly different from saline and unpaired in pairwise comparisons following a significant group effect in analysis of variance.

Adapted from *Behavioural Brain Research*, 293 (1), Lexy N. Pezarro Schimmel, Tomek J. Banasikowski, Emily R. Hawken, Eric C. Dumont, and Richard J. Beninger, Brain regions associated with inverse incentive learning: c-Fos immunohistochemistry after haloperidol sensitization on the bar test in rats, pp. 81–8, doi.org/10.1016/j.bbr.2015.06.041, Copyright 2015, with permission from Elsevier.

in parallel with the paired group that was tested each day following an injection of a low dose of haloperidol. How can the observation of no increase in descent latency in the unpaired group tested with haloperidol be understood? It might be argued that the first treatment with haloperidol in the test situation was relatively novel and, as a result of this putative novelty, increased descent latency was not seen. The results of a further experiment conducted in my laboratory make this explanation unlikely.[37] This experiment used four groups and two distinct testing environments: two paired groups received haloperidol each day before bar testing and then saline later in the home cage, and two unpaired groups received saline each day before bar testing and then haloperidol later in the home cage. One of the testing environments was painted white, the horizontal bar was held by black Plexiglas supports, and the surface of the horizontal bar upon which the rats' forepaws were placed was smooth; the other testing environment was painted black, the horizontal bar was held by clear Plexiglas supports, and the surface of the horizontal bar was rough (with spiraling ridges; it was, in fact, a bolt). Half of the rats in each of the four groups were tested in the white box and half in the black box. As expected, the two paired groups showed sensitization of descent latency and the two unpaired groups did not over ten days of testing. The environment in which the rats were tested made no difference to the results; what mattered was whether the haloperidol was paired or unpaired with the test environment.

On the following day, all animals were tested with haloperidol. One paired group was tested in the environment in which it had always been tested (the white box for half of this group and the black box for the other half). The other paired group was tested in the environment it which it had never been tested. Rats from the two unpaired groups were similarly assigned, one group being tested in the familiar environment and the other in the unfamiliar environment. If we begin by focusing on the paired and unpaired groups that were tested in the same environment that was used during training trials results reveal that the paired group showed increased descent latency to haloperidol and the unpaired group did not, even though both groups had previously received the same number of haloperidol injections; this replicates the effect already described and shown in Figure 6.2. Neither the paired nor the unpaired groups that were tested in the different environment from the one used for training showed increased descent latency. This result eliminated the argument that the failure to observe increased descent latency in the unpaired group in the experiment described resulted from the putative novelty of haloperidol while actually being tested for descent latency. The paired group that was tested with haloperidol in the new environment had a history of bar testing while under the influence of haloperidol yet failed to show increased descent latency when injected with haloperidol and tested in a new environment. What's more, this group had shown descent latency sensitization in the original environment. Clearly, descent latency sensitization is not simply a result of repeated injections of haloperidol and bar testing. Environmental stimuli play a critical role in the control of this behavior.

Conditioned increases in descent latency

A phenomenon related to sensitization of descent latency is conditioned increases in descent latency; it has been reported by a number of researchers.[32,37]. In this paradigm, a paired and an unpaired group, like those already described, undergo repeated bar testing over ten days, for example, and then both groups are tested following a *saline* injection. Greater descent latency is observed in the paired group that previously had haloperidol paired with testing in the bar test environment than in the unpaired group that previously had saline before being placed on the bar in the test environment and haloperidol later in their home cage. It is worth noting again that the drug history of both groups is similar; both the paired and the unpaired group had received ten injections of haloperidol prior to the saline test day. In spite of this, the groups differed significantly in the amount of time they remained motionless with their paws resting on the bar; the paired group showed increased descent latency, whereas the unpaired group did not. The observed increase in descent latency is not simply a result of repeated injections of haloperidol.

A further demonstration of the importance of the testing environment for a conditioned increase in descent latency was seen in animals from the two-environment version of the experiment discussed earlier.[37] As already described in the sensitization of descent latency section, this experiment originally employed four groups of rats. I will focus on two groups here; they are the paired and the unpaired groups originally tested in the same environment where they had received sensitization sessions. Both groups had been tested for descent latency each day for ten days. Half of each group was tested in the white environment and half in the black. The paired group had received haloperidol before testing each day and saline later in the home cage and vice versa for the unpaired group. On each of two test days, all animals were tested for descent latency following an injection of saline. On the first day, half of each group was tested following saline in the environment originally used for bar testing and the other half was tested in the other environment; on the next day, all the animals were tested again but in the environment not used on the first day. The results combined over the two test days show conditioned increases in descent latency only in the paired group that was tested in the same environment that had been used during descent latency sensitization sessions. This shows that conditioned increases in descent latency do not occur once sensitization has taken place unless the test for conditioned effects is conducted in the presence of the same environmental stimuli that were present when sensitization was established. This result further emphasizes the critical role played by environmental stimuli in the conditioned-increase-in-descent-latency effect.

We conducted one additional experiment to evaluate the nature of the conditioned descent latency effect. The paired and unpaired groups from the previous experiment continued to be tested for conditioned increases in descent latency in the chamber originally used for sensitization sessions. We observed extinction of the conditioned response in the paired group tested in the original chamber. The observation of extinction, a gradual decline in the strength of the conditioned response with repeated exposure to the conditioned stimulus (the test environment) in the absence of the original unconditioned stimulus (halo-peridol), confirms that the observation of increased descent latency following saline injections and placement in the chamber originally used for sensitization sessions is a learning phenomenon.

Habituation

Descent latency sensitization can be defined as the gradual loss of responding to a set of stimuli and resembles the phenomenon of habituation. Habituation is often described as a form of non-associative learning.[38] Habituation is termed "non-associative" because it does not involve the learning of an association between two or more stimuli. Rather, habituation refers to the gradual diminution of responding to a stimulus or stimuli that do not signal anything of importance to the animal. Habituation can be observed experimentally by introducing a novel object into an animal's environment and measuring the amount of time the animal spends exploring the object, for example by counting number of contacts or amount of time spent oriented to the object. Initially, the animal, for example a rat, will investigate the object by sniffing it, touching it, and, if the object is small enough, manipulating it. If it is a large object, a rat may climb onto it. If the object is placed into the animal's environment each day, say for 15 minutes each time, and these measures are taken, a learning curve will be seen. The animal will engage in less and less exploration of the object from day to day as defined by the responses used to quantify exploration. This learning curve defines habituation.

The learning curve for descent latency sensitization shows increased latency from day to day, whereas the learning curve for habituation shows decreased responding from day to day. Increased descent latency, however, is a sort of non-response that can be contrasted with the rat's normal response towards the bar and associated stimuli. One way to think about increased descent latency is that it is time spent not exploring the environmental stimuli. In the experiments described above, bar testing sessions had a maximum duration of three minutes or 180 seconds. Descent latency scores could be plotted as the difference between 180 seconds and the amount of time spent immobile on the bar (Figure 6.3) to better reflect the inactive nature of the increased descent latency response. When plotted this way, it is clear that the overall activity level of the paired animal in the bar test situation is decreasing from test to test.

When descent latency scores are plotted as mobility time, shown in Figure 6.3, they resemble habituation. This led us to ask the question, "Will descent latency sensitization progress even faster if the animals are first

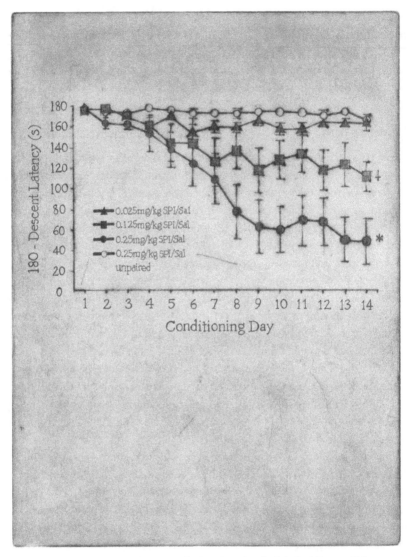

Figure 6.3 *Inverse incentive learning, the loss by stimuli of their ability to elicit approach and other responses*: Mean descent latencies subtracted from 180 (seconds) for rats tested in the bar test one hour after injection of the dopamine receptor blocking drug spiroperidol (SPI; 0.025, 0.125, 0.25 mg/kg, filled symbols) or following an injection of the drug vehicle (open symbols); the unpaired group received SPI (0.25 mg/kg) and the paired groups received drug vehicle in the home cage one hour following testing. Mean data are shown for a single test performed each day for 14 days. "Sal" refers to saline injections that were given prior to the bar test on day 15 (data not shown). *Significantly different from the other three groups and ✛ significantly different from the 0.25 mg/kg SPI/SAL unpaired group in Tukey testes

habituated to the bar testing apparatus and its associated environmental cues?" The answer turned out to be "Yes." In this study, conducted by Kathleen Xu in my laboratory, we had three groups: a paired group like that already described and two additional groups, one paired and one unpaired, but both groups received one exposure each day for six days to the bar and bar-test environment, five minutes each time. The usual paired group also was handled and exposed to a novel environment like the bar test environment but with the bar oriented differently, the walls a different color and a different floor texture each day for six days to control for the handling and related experiences of the habituated groups. When bar testing with a low dose of haloperidol began, increased descent latency developed in the paired groups but not in the unpaired group, as seen before. However, the paired group that had been habituated to the bar test environment prior to the beginning of testing developed increased descent latency at a significantly faster rate (Figure 6.4).[39] It appears that the effects of habituation added to those of haloperidol; in agreement with this finding, a previous researcher reported more rapid habituation to a tone in cats treated with the dopamine receptor blocker chlorpromazine.[40] Results might suggest that the phenomena of descent latency sensitization in haloperidol-treated rats and habituation in drug-free rats are related.

Understanding sensitization and conditioning of descent latency

The phenomena of descent latency sensitization and conditioned increases in descent latency induced by a low dose of the dopamine receptor-blocker haloperidol are a form of learning not to respond. Each day, exposure to a set of environmental stimuli in association with haloperidol apparently lessened the ability of those stimuli to engage the animal. From this point of view, the bar, its supports, and the other environmental stimuli lose their ability to activate responding or, perhaps, to interest the rat. The increased descent latency response per se is not so much a conditioned response to the haloperidol-paired stimuli

performed following a significant group effect in simple effects analysis of variance of groups on day 14 following a significant interaction of group × day in analysis of variance.

Modified with permission from Jeffery Rocca, Joshua Lister, and Richard Beninger, Spiroperidol, but not eticlopride or aripiprazole, produces gradual increases in descent latencies in the bar test in rats, *Behavioural Pharmacology*, 28 (1), p. 30–36, Figure 1a, doi: 10.1097/FBP.0000000000000264, Copyright © 2017, Wolters Kluwer Health, Inc.

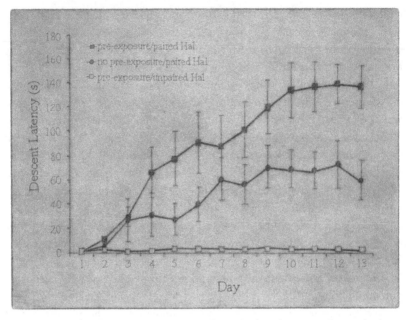

Figure 6.4 *Effects of habituation on inverse incentive learning*: Mean (± standard error of the mean) descent latencies (seconds) of three groups (ns = 10) of rats in the bar test over 13 days of testing. The no pre-exposure/paired haloperidol (Hal) group was not pre-exposed to the test environment (they were pre-exposed to a different environment five minutes per day for six days as a control) and received Hal (0.25 mg/kg) one hour prior to each test session. The remaining two groups were pre-exposed to the test environment for five minutes per day for six days prior to the onset of sensitization testing. The pre-exposed/paired Hal group received haloperidol (0.25 mg/kg) one hour prior to each test and saline one hour later in their home cage; the pre-exposed/unpaired Hal group was tested one hour following an injection of saline and received haloperidol one hour later in their home cage. Pre-exposure/paired Hal is significantly different from the other two groups on days 10–13 and no pre-exposure/paired Hal is significantly different from the pre-exposure/unpaired Hal group on days 9–13 in pairwise comparisons following simple effects analyses of variance of groups on each day following observation of a significant group × day effect in analysis of variance.
Data from studies completed by Kathleen Xu in my laboratory.

as it is a manifestation of the loss of the ability of those stimuli to engage the animal. In Chapter 3 I spoke about how activation of dopaminergic neurotransmission by rewarding stimuli led to incentive learning, increasing the ability of previously neutral stimuli to elicit approach and other responses. In the case of descent latency sensitization and conditioned increases in descent latency, it appears that the opposite is happening. *Stimuli associated with decreased dopaminergic neurotransmission lose their ability to elicit approach and other responses.*

For many years I had thought that dopamine plays two roles in the control of behavior.[41] One was a consequence of tonic dopamine activity that was related to the general level of activation or responsiveness. On the low end of this putative continuum of tonic dopamine activity was relative lethargy and disinterest, but within a functional range, not yet Parkinsonism, and on the high end was hypomania characterized by strong interest and high energy. The other role for dopamine was a consequence of transient increases in synaptic concentrations that took place when rewarding stimuli were encountered, and resulted in incentive learning. I envisioned tonic dopamine activity as a sort of clutch, engaging the interface between sensory–perceptual systems and motor systems. In this sense, the putative tonic function of dopamine was somewhat mechanical; as long as there were sufficient levels of tonic dopamine activity, motor responding to stimuli was possible. When tonic levels of dopamine dropped below a critical threshold, responding to environmental stimuli was no longer possible and the symptoms of Parkinson's disease ensued (see Chapters 7 and 9). The observations of descent latency sensitization and conditioned increases in descent latency suggest an elaboration of this conceptual framework.

Descent latency sensitization and conditioned increases in descent latency associated with repeated pairings of particular environmental stimuli with reduced levels of dopaminergic neurotransmission suggest that the ability of environmental stimuli to produce responding depends in part on dopamine-mediated synaptic plasticity. As long as tonic levels of dopamine are above a critical threshold, the ability of environmental stimuli to engage the organism and elicit responding remains intact. If an animal repeatedly encounters particular stimuli when tonic dopamine levels are reduced, those stimuli gradually lose their ability to elicit responding. Thus, the role of tonic dopamine in the control of general activity and engagement with environmental stimuli, like the role of dopamine in incentive learning, involves dopamine-mediated plastic changes in the brain. Dopamine may not serve simply a clutch-like function operating between sensory-perceptual systems and motor systems; low dopamine may actively modify the ability of stimuli to engage behavior. Not only do increases in dopaminergic neurotransmission lead to incentive learning, increasing the ability of neutral stimuli to elicit approach and other responses in the future, but, conversely, decreases in dopaminergic neurotransmission produce an opposite effect, decreasing the ability of stimuli to elicit approach and other responses in the future. It is difficult to know what to call this anti-incentive learning effect. One possibility is to follow from the use of the term "inverse agonist" in pharmacology: a drug that activates a receptor but produces postsynaptic consequences opposite in direction to the agonist, not simply blocking the agonist effect like a receptor antagonist.[42] By analogy, the descent latency sensitization and conditioned increases in descent latency effects of decreased dopaminergic neurotransmission might be termed "inverse incentive learning." Inverse incentive learning refers to the loss of the ability of neutral stimuli to elicit approach and other responses.

With the discovery of inverse incentive learning, it appears that dopamine does not simply act as a clutch so that when dopamine is present at sufficient concentrations stimuli can elicit approach and other responses and when its concentration is too low, stimuli cannot elicit approach and other responses. Just as incentive learning is acquired gradually through repeated pairings of environmental stimuli with rewarding stimuli, so it appears that inverse incentive learning is acquired gradually with repeated pairing of stimuli with non-reward. In the case of incentive learning, the effects of rewarding stimuli are to increase activity in dopaminergic neurons; in the case of inverse incentive learning the effects of non-reward are to decrease activity in dopaminergic neurons. The inescapable conclusion from the observation of descent latency sensitization and conditioned increases in descent latency is that dopamine is not only involved in incentive learning, but also in inverse incentive learning.

New insights into how to think about stimuli are provided by the discovery that dopamine plays an important role in both incentive learning and inverse incentive learning. For any given individual rat or human, all stimuli are novel when they are encountered for the first time. Novel stimuli activate dopaminergic neurons, as discussed earlier in this chapter, and tend to elicit exploratory responses consisting of approach and inspection. If the novel stimuli are intense, they may initially elicit immobility or even flight. Some stimuli have an innate ability to elicit immobility or flight, for example a looming stimulus for some avian species,[43] but many stimuli are simply objects in the environment producing no strong innate response other than exploration. Exploration will lead to at least two separable consequences in terms of memory systems (see Chapter 3). Declarative memory will record the sensory/perceptual features of the object so that in the future it will be recognized, and it will record relationships of the object with other objects and events in the environment as the animal builds its cognitive map of its environment. As we saw in Chapter 3, this type of learning appears to take place independently of dopamine. The animal will also discover whether or not the stimulus signals a biologically important outcome. If the animal is an urban raccoon and the stimulus is a garbage can, it may discover by its approach and inspection of the garbage can that it contains tasty food scraps. Eating the food will activate dopamine neurons and produce incentive learning, increasing the ability of the garbage can and related stimuli to elicit approach and other responses in the future. If the same raccoon encounters and investigates a clay flowerpot, it will not find anything of biological import (assuming there is no food or water stored in the flowerpot). We know from observation and behavioral research that the raccoon will respond less and less to the flowerpot if it is repeatedly introduced into the raccoon's environment. This contrasts with the garbage can that can repeatedly elicit approach and other responses. Novel stimuli initially produce a burst of activity in dopaminergic neurons that is followed by a brief period of suppression of firing if no rewarding stimuli are encountered. With repeated exposures, those previously novel stimuli lose their novelty and they lose their ability to activate dopamine neurons.

There clearly is a continuum of stimuli with respect to incentive value. Novel stimuli are inherently incentive stimuli insofar as they have an innate ability to elicit approach and other responses. Familiar stimuli can be conditioned incentive stimuli if they signal biologically important outcomes or they can be habituated stimuli if they are associated with no biologically important outcomes. The role of dopamine in incentive learning is now well established, as discussed in this book. The role of dopamine in habituation learning is not well established, but the observations of descent latency sensitization, conditioned increases in descent latency, and additive effects of habituation to descent latency sensitization suggest that dopamine is also involved in this type of learning. Once stimuli have been encountered by an animal and are no longer novel, they either become conditioned incentive stimuli through dopamine-mediated incentive learning or they become habituated stimuli putatively through dopamine-mediated inverse incentive learning. Perhaps habituated stimuli should be termed "conditioned inverse incentive stimuli," to reflect the apparently active mechanism that is involved in their establishment.

Inverse incentive learning may be involved in the phenomenon of latent inhibition.[44] Latent inhibition is demonstrated by the reduced ability of a previously experienced stimulus to control responding. For example, if an animal is exposed to a tone stimulus 30 times and then that stimulus is used to signal a biologically significant stimulus such as food, the tone will acquire incentive value more slowly than in a non-pre-exposed group. Repeated presentation of the tone alone would be like pre-exposure to the bar-testing environment insofar as both procedures would putatively lead to inverse incentive learning. In the case of descent latency, the pre-exposure leads to augmented descent latency sensitization perhaps as a result of inverse incentive learning; in the case of tone–food pairings, the pre-exposure may also lead to inverse incentive learning, retarding subsequent incentive learning.

The effects of manipulations of dopaminergic neurotransmission on latent inhibition have been investigated. The latent inhibition procedure normally involves a pre-exposure, conditioning, and test phase. During pre-exposure animals are exposed to the to-be-conditioned stimulus a number of times; subsequently, that stimulus is paired with a biologically important stimulus such as mild electric foot shock or sickness. In the test, the strength of conditioning is indicated by the strength of responding to the conditioned stimulus. Pre-exposure lessens the strength of responding to the conditioned stimulus, revealing the latent inhibition effect. Treatment with haloperidol during the pre-exposure phase increased the strength of conditioning showing the additive effects of stimulus pre-exposure and dopamine receptor blockade. Treatment with the dopamine-enhancing drug amphetamine during pre-exposure had the opposite effect, mitigating latent inhibition.[45] These results implicate dopamine-mediated inverse incentive learning in latent inhibition.

I remember having a conversation with Roy Wise when I was a graduate student at McGill University back in the 1970s and Roy was a young professor at Concordia University in Montreal. He suggested that dopamine may not only mediate reward-related learning, but that it may mediate learning about all stimuli that affect an animal. By then it was already well known that animals depleted of dopamine showed very low responsiveness to environmental stimuli, so the suggestion made sense. At the time I was studying with my PhD supervisor Peter Milner and through my discussions with him was beginning to have some idea of a possible dopaminergic mechanism for reward-related learning, but there was no suggestion at the time that dopamine may also play a role in habituation learning. It therefore seemed more parsimonious to conceptualize dopamine as having two functions, one the clutch-like role in behaviorally engaging with the environment already mentioned above, and the other the now well-known incentive learning role. With the emergence of these new data implicating dopamine in inverse incentive learning, it appears that Roy may have been right after all. I return to a discussion of the role of dopamine in learning versus the general control of motor activity in Chapter 7.

In electrophysiological studies, Schultz and his co-workers observed that the withholding of an expected rewarding stimulus led to a brief depression in the firing of dopaminergic neurons. They termed this observation "negative prediction error."[46] If decreases in dopamine produce inverse incentive learning as just discussed, it follows that negative prediction errors that result in decreases in dopamine neuron firing may produce inverse incentive learning. Conditioned stimuli that reliably predict a rewarding stimulus become conditioned incentive stimuli with an enhanced ability to elicit approach and other responses. If those stimuli are encountered but are not followed by the expected rewarding stimulus, a negative prediction error occurs leading to a decrease in dopaminergic neuron firing and a transient drop in dopamine concentrations in dopamine terminal areas.[47] This drop in concentration of dopamine may produce inverse incentive learning about the stimuli preceding the drop, reducing the incentive value of the reward-predicting stimulus. In this way, inverse incentive learning may work to reduce responsiveness to stimuli that previously predicted a rewarding stimulus but no longer do so.

Studies of the effects of aversive stimuli on dopamine concentrations and neuron firing, like those discussed earlier in this chapter, provide some observations that may be understood from the point of view of inverse incentive learning. For example, Italian researchers working at the Universities of Siena and Sassari exposed rats to restraint and inescapable tail shock for 30 minutes a day over several days. Subsequent microdialysis of dopamine in the nucleus accumbens showed a significant decrease.[48] These findings are in agreement with those of Puglisi-Allegra and colleagues discussed earlier. Recall that when Puglisi-Allegra and colleagues extended a period of restraint from two to four hours, they observed that nucleus accumbens dopamine and metabolite levels decreased to levels significantly *below* baseline for the second two hours of restraint.[14]. The stimuli associated with decreased dopamine might be expected to become conditioned inverse incentive stimuli with a reduced ability to serve as incentive stimuli in a conditioning procedure. This is what the researchers from the Universities of Siena and Sassari found; animals preexposed to restraint and inescapable shocks were impaired in their ability to learn to avoid shocks when given the opportunity. This finding was similar to the phenomenon of learned helplessness that originally grew out of the work of psychologist Richard Solomon (1918–1995) at the University of Pennsylvania in Philadelphia and was further developed by his students, Martin Seligman and Bruce Overmier.[49] Results might suggest that animals' failure to learn to avoid may result from inverse incentive learning about the shock-associated stimuli resulting from exposure to those stimuli while dopaminergic neurotransmission is depressed.

Electrophysiological studies of the effects of aversive stimuli on the firing of dopamine neurons sometimes found evidence suggestive of excitation, as discussed earlier. However, as already discussed, these studies frequently revealed that dopamine neurons were inhibited by aversive stimuli.[26, 28,29] If this inhibition by the *onset* of aversive stimuli produces inverse incentive learning, environmental stimuli associated with aversive stimuli should have a weakened ability to elicit approach and other responses. This would be an adaptive response—do not go near that place because danger may be lurking there. At the same time, the *offset* of aversion may lead to increases in the firing of dopamine neurons and incentive learning about stimuli that signal safety. In this way, dopaminergic neurotransmission may work constantly to mold the incentive features of the environment into those that are neutral, those that are attractive and those that are not attractive.

Summary

I remember Roy Wise once saying that the term "neutral stimulus" is an oxymoron. If something is a stimulus, how can it be neutral? From within the incentive learning/inverse incentive learning framework outlined in this chapter, a neutral stimulus can be understood as one that has neither an enhanced ability to elicit approach and other responses nor a decreased ability to elicit approach and other responses. The framework suggests that dopamine determines a continuum of incentive value and that stimuli can lie somewhere on that continuum. Novel and intense stimuli are innately able to activate dopamine neurons but the activation is rapid and followed by decreased dopamine neuron firing. As a result, novel or intense stimuli produce little incentive learning if they do not signal biologically important outcomes. In the case of novel stimuli, their repeated presentation leads to a loss of their ability to produce both the rapid activation and the subsequent decrease of dopamine neuron firing. Biologically important appetitive stimuli (e.g., food, water, social partners, safety, etc.) activate dopamine neurons and produce incentive learning, leading to conditioned incentive stimuli with increased ability to elicit approach and other responses in the future. Aversive stimuli, biologically important by definition, often deactivate dopamine neurons and may produce inverse incentive learning, leading to conditioned inverse incentive stimuli with decreased ability to elicit approach and other responses in the future. The offset of aversion may lead to increases in the firing of dopamine neurons and incentive learning about stimuli that signal safety. The observation that habituation to stimuli enhances the ability of those stimuli to produce inverse incentive learning suggests that some level of inverse incentive learning may take place during the habituation process, as a stimulus moves from being novel to neutral to becoming a conditioned inverse incentive stimulus. In the end, there may be no "neutral" stimuli, just stimuli that lie on a continuum of incentive value from strong conditioned positive incentive stimuli to strong conditioned inverse incentive stimuli with most of the things we encounter in our day-to-day lives falling somewhere in between.

Chapter 7

Dopamine receptor subtypes and incentive learning

When neurotransmitters are released from neurons, they influence the electrical and chemical activity of other neurons by occupying receptors on those neurons.[1] The receptors for dopamine were gradually identified through the research efforts of many scientists around the world and it is challenging to try to construct the story of their discovery. At least two lines of work converged in the 1970s to support the existence of two subtypes of dopamine receptors, now referred to as D1-like and D2-like, but further advances in molecular biological techniques in the 1980s led to the identification of five major dopamine receptor subtypes but still within the two families that were identified earlier. Thus, the D1-like receptor family includes the D1 and D5 receptor and the D2-like receptor family includes the D2, D3, and D4 receptors.

This chapter reviews work leading up to identification of the two dopamine receptor families and then the subsequent work identifying family members. Interwoven in this story is the discovery of the site of action of antipsychotic medications. The chapter reviews behavioral studies of the role of D1- and D2-like receptors in the control of locomotor activity and incentive learning. Some differences between the behavioral effects of dopamine receptor subtype-specific agents in intact and chronically dopamine-depleted animals are discussed. I review behavioral studies of genetically modified animals with one of five dopamine receptor subtypes knocked out. Psychopharmacological studies, particularly those with agents relatively specific for D3 receptors, are covered followed, finally, by a brief consideration of receptor heteromers that contain a dopamine receptor.

Discovery of D1 and D2 receptors

D1-like receptors are characterized by their ability to activate the enzyme adenylyl cyclase leading to the formation of cyclic adenosine monophosphate (cAMP), an important enzyme for intracellular chemical signaling. This line of research can be traced to discoveries made by Earl Sutherland (1915–1974) while working at Western Reserve University (now Case Western Reserve

University) in Cleveland, Ohio, and later at Vanderbilt University in Nashville, Tennessee. Sutherland and his colleague, Ted Rall, discovered that hormones such as glucagon and epinephrine activated liver enzymes by first activating cAMP, and they showed further that cAMP was synthesized when a hormone activated adenylyl cyclase.[2] It appeared that different hormones had unique receptors but that each was coupled with adenylyl cyclase. cAMP became known as a second messenger, intervening between the hormone receptor and downstream enzymes known to be affected by the hormone. Sutherland's discovery was recognized with the 1971 Nobel Prize in Physiology or Medicine. Some years later Edwin Krebs (1918–2009) and co-workers at the University of Washington in Seattle discovered a protein kinase that was one of the downstream targets of cAMP; this cAMP-dependent protein kinase became known as protein kinase A (PKA)[3]. Subsequently, Paul Greengard and co-workers at Yale University in New Haven, Connecticut, showed that PKA was prominent in the brain.[4]

In 1971, John Kebabian, Paul Greengard, and co-workers at Yale discovered that dopamine, like the hormones studied by Sutherland and Rall, activated adenylyl cyclase and increased levels of cAMP in neural tissue.[5] Paul Greengard went on to identify further signaling molecules downstream of cAMP; this work led to the Nobel Prize in Physiology or Medicine in 2000. The importance of Greengard's work for understanding the molecular mechanisms of incentive learning is discussed in Chapter 12. In a short article published in 2011, Solomon Snyder of Johns Hopkins University in Baltimore, Maryland, explains how Kebabian, Greengard, and their co-workers made the leap from the discoveries of Sutherland and Rall to investigate dopamine's effects on the adenylyl cyclase–cAMP second messenger system in neural tissue.[6] Kebabian, Greengard, and co-workers were influenced by the discovery in 1958 of Arvid Carlsson and colleagues at the University of Lund in Sweden that the caudate nucleus of the brain contained very high levels of dopamine—higher levels than would have been expected if dopamine was present simply as the metabolic precursor of another neurotransmitter.[7] This observation suggested a possible role for dopamine as a neurotransmitter in the brain. During the same period, neurologists Herbert Ehringer and Oleh Hornykiewicz, working at the University of Vienna, Austria, in 1960, discovered dopamine depletion in the caudate nucleus of postmortem brain tissue from patients with Parkinson's disease (see Chapter 9),[8] further implicating dopamine as a neurotransmitter.

Kebabian, Greengard, and co-workers carried out their pioneering work on the mammalian sympathetic ganglion. Histochemical studies had reveled that the sympathetic ganglion contained interneurons with dopamine in them.[9] This finding, coupled with the reports of Carlsson, and Ehringer and

Hornykiewicz, suggested that dopamine may function as a neurotransmitter in the sympathetic ganglion. In March of 1971, Greengard and co-workers reported that electrical stimulation of the preganglionic nerve fibers of the sympathetic ganglion led to an increase in the content of cAMP, showing for the first time that synaptic activity can change the content of cAMP in nervous tissue.[10] Then, in December of the same year, Kebabian and Greengard reported that dopamine stimulated adenylyl cyclase in the mammalian superior cervical ganglion and suggested that the existence of the enzyme may be responsible for the observed increases in cAMP produced by stimulation of preganglionic fibers.[5] The authors suggested that the physiological effects of dopamine in the nervous system may be mediated through the adenylyl cyclase–cAMP second messenger pathway. Their subsequent observation that dopamine similarly activated adenylyl cyclase in brain tissue from the caudate nucleus led them to suggest that dopamine-sensitive adenylyl cyclase "may be the *receptor* for dopamine in mammalian brain" (Kebabian et al. 1972, p. 2145, my italics).[5]

In their 1972 paper, Kebabian et al. made another important observation. They showed that two antipsychotic drugs, haloperidol and chlorpromazine, were able to dose-dependently block the ability of dopamine to stimulate cAMP formation in brain tissue from the caudate nucleus.[5] Around about the same time, researchers were finding that these same antipsychotic agents blocked the behavioral effects of pharmacological compounds that increase dopaminergic neurotransmission,[11] and earlier studies had shown that brain levels of dopamine were altered by antipsychotic drugs.[12] Since antipsychotic drugs are used to treat schizophrenia and they appear to block the effects of dopamine in the brain, it was suggested by Jacques van Rossum at the Catholic University of Nijmegen (now Radboud University of Nijmegen) in the Netherlands that schizophrenia results from overactive dopamine in the brain;[13] this dopamine hypothesis of schizophrenia has been very influential and enduring, as discussed further in Chapter 9.

The finding of Kebabian et al. that antipsychotic drugs blocked the ability of dopamine to stimulate cAMP formation led to the hypothesis that the therapeutic effect of antipsychotic drugs is correlated with their ability to inhibit cAMP formation. Kebabian, Greengard, and co-workers found that a number of antipsychotic drugs, especially those in the phenothiazine class, for example chlorpromazine, inhibited cAMP formation; however, other non-phenothiazine antipsychotic drugs, for example haloperidol and pimozide, although effective as antipsychotics at *lower* doses than phenothiazines, required *higher* concentrations to block cAMP formation.[14] Furthermore, the concentrations of antipsychotic drugs, even phenothiazines, that were needed to inhibit cAMP formation in vitro were orders of magnitude higher than the concentrations that would be achieved in vivo when the drugs were administered at their usual clinical doses.[15] These findings presented a disconnect for the hypothesis that the therapeutic effect of antipsychotic drugs is mediated by their ability to inhibit cAMP formation.

Resolution of this dilemma came within the next few years with the development of radio-receptor binding techniques for dopamine receptors. These techniques can be traced directly to the discovery of artificial radioactivity by the Joliot-Curies in the 1930s, discussed in Chapter 5. As a result, more and more radioactive compounds were being synthesized for use in medical diagnostics and research. For example, in a 1965 study, William Paton (1917–1993) and Humphrey Rang of Oxford University used tritium-labeled atropine ([3H]-atropine), a drug known to block muscarinic cholinergic neurotransmission, to identify the site of action of atropine, providing the first evidence of the muscarinic cholinergic receptor.[16] Following from this observation and further refinement of receptor-binding technology,[17] in 1973 Candace Pert and Solomon Snyder at Johns Hopkins University identified the binding site for tritiated naloxone in the brain and thereby discovered the brain's opioid receptors.[18] These discoveries heralded what Humphrey Rang, now at University College London, termed the great "'grind and bind' era of the 1970s and 1980s" (p. S13).[1]

Philip Seeman and colleagues working at the University of Toronto in Canada first identified the receptor for dopamine using receptor-binding techniques in 1975.[19] Seeman and his co-workers were able to obtain a radioactive version of the antipsychotic drug haloperidol, that is, [3H]haloperidol, with sufficient specific activity to be detectable in tissue samples. They also used [3H] dopamine and showed that the stereoselective component of [3H]haloperidol and [3H]dopamine binding was inhibited by various antipsychotic drugs. The clinical potency of antipsychotic drugs correlated with their ability to inhibit this binding. This groundbreaking work led the way to a characterization of dopamine receptors and provided compelling evidence that the locus of action of antipsychotic medications was dopamine receptors, further supporting the dopamine hypothesis of schizophrenia proposed by van Rossum a decade earlier.

Bertha Madras of the Harvard Medical School in Southborough, Massachusetts, has compiled the history of the discovery of the antipsychotic dopamine receptor.[20] In her excellent paper she describes the exciting findings that led up to the discovery by Seeman and his colleagues. She describes how, in the lobby of a convention hotel in Paris in July 1975, Phil Seeman informed Solomon Snyder that he had been able to obtain custom-made [3H]haloperidol with appropriate specific activity. That year and the next, Snyder and his colleagues published results that confirmed those of Seeman et al.[21]

In the following years, extensive receptor binding and neurochemical studies of dopamine receptors presented a dilemma that was eventually resolved by the insight that "dopamine receptors are two different populations of which only one is directly coupled to the activation of adenylate cyclase" (p. 163).[22] Pier Franco Spano, Stefano Govoni, and Michele Trabucci, working at the time (1978) at the Universities of Cagliari and Milan in Italy wrote this in the concluding remarks of their paper. They showed: (i) stereoselective binding of [³H]haloperidol and [³H]dopamine in the pituitary gland but undetectable dopamine-stimulated adenylyl cyclase activity; (ii) a number of ergot derivatives (e.g., bromocriptine) well known to affect dopamine-mediated behaviors had no significant effect on striatal or pituitary adenylyl cyclase activity; (iii) sulpiride, a drug with antipsychotic activity, had no effect on adenylyl cyclase in striatal homogenates; and (iv) sulpiride displaced stereospecific binding of [³H]haloperidol in rat striatal tissue. Results presented a strong case for the conclusion that there were at least two subtypes of dopamine receptors, one that stimulated adenylyl cyclase and another that did not stimulate the enzyme.

In 1979, John Kebabian and Donald Calne at the National Institutes of Health in Bethesda, Maryland, published their now-classic paper suggesting the nomenclature for dopamine receptors: D1 receptors stimulate adenylyl cyclase, D2 receptors do not.[23] (It was subsequently found that D2 receptors actually inhibit adenylyl cyclase.[24]) Another distinction between D1 and D2 receptors was the difference in the potency of dopamine; at D1 receptors dopamine is effective in *micro*molar concentrations, whereas at D2 receptors dopamine is effective in *nano*molar concentrations. This differentiation may contribute importantly to the differential role of dopamine receptor subtypes in incentive learning and is discussed further in Chapter 12. Kebabian and Calne showed great insight in their 1979 paper when they stated that "This is only the first level of division in the classification of dopamine receptors; it is likely that with further examination… subcategories of each type of receptor will be discerned" (pp. 95–96).[23]. They anticipated that the new classifications might come from pharmacological evidence. It turned out that a number of developments in molecular neuroscience revealed the five subtypes of dopamine receptors.

Discovery of D1- and D2-like receptor families

In the same years that Seeman and his co-workers were using [³H]haloperidol to identify dopamine receptors in brain homogenates, Robert Lefkowitz and co-workers, working at Duke University in Durham, North Carolina, were using tritiated compounds to identify α- and β-adrenergic receptors, receptors for the neurotransmitter noradrenaline or norepinephrine.[25] Lefkowitz and his co-workers went on to develop chromatography techniques that allowed them to isolate the adrenergic receptor molecules. They showed that these isolated glycoproteins could be inserted into cells that would then respond to β-adrenergic drugs by producing cAMP, proving that the isolated proteins were β-receptors. The link between the receptor molecule and the enzyme for producing cAMP, adelylyl cyclase, was made with a small protein known as a guanine nucleotide regulatory protein or G protein.[26] Thus, β-receptors were referred to as G protein-coupled receptors (GPCRs). Their next step was to work backward from the isolated receptor protein to design oligonucleo- tide probes that allowed them to clone the β_2-adrenergic receptor, something they achieved in 1986.[27] Lefkowitz and his co-workers immediately noticed something curious about the β-receptor. The long molecule snaked across the cell membrane, first inward, then outward until it had made seven trans- membrane crossings, analogous to another molecule, rhodopsin, that had recently been sequenced. Remarkably, the β-receptor also showed sequence homology with rhodopsin, that is, it shared some of the same amino-acid sequences. As additional adrenergic receptors and a serotonin receptor were cloned, they were all found to conserve the seven transmembrane-spanning domains organization and they were all GPCRs.[28] Lefkowitz and co-workers began to think that all GPCRs were members of a superfamily of seven trans- membrane receptors; this turned out to be the case. For the discovery of this receptor superfamily and some of their mechanisms of cell signaling, Robert Lefkowitz, along with his colleague, Brian Kobilka, received the Nobel Prize in Chemistry in 2012.

Additional GPCRs were quickly found. This research was greatly aided by the invention of polymerase chain reaction technology.[29] Among those that were cloned during this time were the five dopamine receptors. Robert Civelli and co-workers at the Oregon Health and Science University and Veterans Administration Medical Center in Portland, Oregon, first cloned the dopa- mine D2 receptor in 1988 and from the amino-acid sequence, identified it as a member of the GPCR superfamily.[30] Using similar techniques in 1990, Civelli's group, simultaneous with a group at Duke University in Durham, North Carolina, a multicenter group and a group at the National Institutes of Health in Bethesda, Maryland, cloned the D1 receptor,[31] and similarly found it to be a GPCR. In the same year, Pierre Sokoloff and colleagues at the Centre Paul Broca and University René Descartes in Paris cloned the D3 receptor.[32] In the following year, the remaining two members of the dopamine receptor family were cloned: Civelli's group cloned the D4 receptor,[33] and researchers at the University of Toronto, Canada, cloned the D5 receptor.[34] The dopamine receptor families were now complete: D1-like receptors included D1 and D5; D2-like receptors included D2, D3, and D4.

Differential locomotor function of D1- and D2-like receptors

After the delineation of D1 and D2 receptors by Kebabian and Calne in 1979, there was extensive interest by behavioral neuroscientists in the possible differential function of the two dopamine receptor subtypes. Pharmacological tools became available that made it possible to compare D1-like versus D2-like receptor agonist and antagonist effects in standard behavioral tests of incentive learning. I was intensely engaged in this line of research at the time and wrote a number of reviews of the emerging picture of differential roles for the two major dopamine receptor subtypes.[35] In the following I will summarize some of the findings and focus on results that were particularly instructive for identifying different roles for D1-like and D2-like receptors in incentive learning.

Learning, especially of the non-declarative type, such as incentive learning, is, by definition, gradual (see Chapter 4). Some manipulations of dopaminergic neurotransmission, such as high doses of the stimulant amphetamine, or treatments with doses of dopamine neurotoxins, such as 6-hydroxydopamine that produce severe (greater than 85%) depletions of dopamine,[36] have large and immediate effects on behavior that appear to be unconditioned. For this reason, in my early reviews of dopamine and behavior, I divided experimental results into two categories: the role of dopamine in locomotor activity and the role of dopamine in learning.[37] As discussed in Chapter 6, it appears that environmental stimuli repeatedly associated with relatively minor decreases in dopaminergic neurotransmission *gradually* lose their ability to elicit approach and other responses leading to inverse incentive learning, and, as outlined in Chapter 3 and elsewhere in this book, stimuli associated with a rewarding stimulus that increases dopaminergic neurotransmission *gradually* acquire an increased ability to elicit approach and other responses leading to incentive learning. Insofar as manipulations of dopaminergic neurotransmission have *immediate* effects, these effects cannot be attributed to learning, although they may lead to learning, increased descent latencies to the effects of dopamine receptor antagonists, for example (discussed in Chapters 6 and 9). These considerations suggest that dopamine plays a role in unconditioned behavior, as well as in the learning that underlies conditioning.

In looking at the role of D1- and D2-like receptors in the control of locomotor activity, it appears that both families are involved. In otherwise-normal rats, increases in locomotor activity are produced by injections of D1-like agonists, such as SKF 38393 (the prototypical D1-like receptor agonist, although it is only a partial agonist[38]).[39] Some authors found that these compounds also increase the frequency of other behaviors, such as grooming.[40] Treatments with the prototypical D2-like receptor agonist quinpirole (originally known as LY 171555),[41] or other D2-like receptor agonists, including bromocriptine, also increase locomotor activity.[42] With high doses of D2-like receptor agonists, stereotyped behavior is seen, with the animal remaining in one location for extended periods of time and making repetitive movements such as head bobbing or licking; stereotypy, although it does not involve extensive whole-body movements, is seen as the upper end of the locomotor activity continuum.[43] D1- and D2-like agonists have synergistic effects when co-administered; sub-threshold doses of a D1- and a D2-like receptor agonist lead to locomotor stimulation, even though neither dose on its own has an effect.[44] Generally, the locomotor effects of D2-like receptor agonists are larger than those of D1-like receptor agonists, but both families of receptors appear to be involved and to work cooperatively in the control of locomotion.

The locomotor effects of D1- and D2-like receptor antagonists support the conclusion that both families of receptors are involved. The prototypical D1-like receptor antagonist SCH 23390,[45] and other D1-like receptor antagonists, for example R-SKF 83566,[46] and D2-like receptor-preferring antagonists such as haloperidol decrease locomotor activity, and both D1- and D2-like receptor antagonists produce unconditioned catalepsy at high doses.[47] Just as stereotypy can be seen as the upper extreme of the continuum of locomotor activity, catalepsy can be seen as the lower extreme of the continuum. The apparent contribution of both receptor families to the control of locomotor activity is further supported by the observation that either D1- or D2-like receptor antagonists block the stimulant effects of either D1- or D2-like receptor agonists.[48]

The results just discussed are for intact animals. In chronically dopamine-depleted animals a different picture emerges. Dopamine depletions can be made with neurotoxins such as 6-hydroxydopamine, already mentioned earlier, or 1-methyl-4-phenyl-1,2,3,6-tetrahydropyridine, also known as MPTP; the dopamine neurotoxicity of this compound was discovered tragically when recreational drug users who thought they were injecting pure desmethylprodine, an opioid compound, were actually injecting desmethylprodine contaminated with MPTP as a result of botched synthesis.[49] The young drug users came down with the symptoms of Parkinson's disease, a disease normally found in the elderly and a rarity in young people. Parkinson's disease is caused by a loss of dopamine cells in the midbrain and postmortem examination of one of the young men who had used MPTP, developed Parkinson's symptoms, and died some months later as a result of a drug overdose, showed a major loss of dopamine cells. The effects of D1- and D2-like agonists were subsequently studied in animals that had undergone 6-hydroxydopamine- or MPTP-induced dopamine depletions.

In chronically dopamine-depleted rats, D1- *or* D2-like receptor agonists produce locomotor stimulation, at least partially reversing the locomotor loss resulting from the dopamine depletion. Unlike what is seen in intact rats, the effects of dopamine receptor subtype-specific antagonists are specific to the type of agonist used. Thus, in chronically dopamine-depleted rats, the locomotor stimulant effects of D1-like receptor agonists are blocked by D1-like receptor antagonists but not by D2-like receptor antagonists, and the locomotor stimulant effects of D2-like receptor agonists are blocked by D2-like receptor antagonists but not be D1-like receptor antagonists.[50] In chronically dopamine-depleted primates, the story is different again. The resultant Parkinson's-like symptoms in marmosets or *Macaca fascicularis* monkeys were reversed by D2-like receptor agonists but not by D1-like receptor agonists.[51] Similar results have been reported in humans with Parkinson's disease.[52] When dopamine is chronically depleted, changes in the number, location, and molecular organization of dopamine receptors take place. These include a proliferation of postsynaptic D2 receptors and possible changes in dopamine receptor hetero-oligomerization.[53] However, the exact mechanisms underlying changes in dopamine receptor function in dopamine denervation conditions such as Parkinson's disease are largely unknown.

Taken together, results from studies of the effects of D1- and D2-like receptor agonists and antagonists in normosensitive and dopamine-depleted animals suggest the following picture. In normosensitive animals, D1- and D2-like receptors work cooperatively in the control of locomotor activity; stimulation of either receptor family alone can increase locomotion and sub-threshold doses of agonists for each receptor family produce synergistic effects. Receptor antagonists for either receptor family can reverse the locomotor stimulant effects of receptor agonists for either receptor family. In chronically dopamine-depleted animals, this interdependency of D1- and D2-like receptors seems to be lost. Agonists at either receptor family can increase locomotion in rats and only family-specific receptor antagonists block the effects of receptor agonists. In primates, including humans, D2- but not D1-like receptor agonists appear to be effective in treating Parkinsonian symptoms. The apparent cooperation between D1- and D2-like receptors seen in normosensetive animals is lost in chronically dopamine-depleted animals.

Differential incentive learning function of D1- and D2-like receptors

I will begin with the effects of receptor antagonists. In my 1993 review,[35] based on results from studies of incentive learning in animals lever pressing for food, brain stimulation reward or drugs of abuse, or conditioned place preference based on stimulant drugs that activate dopaminergic neurotransmission, I concluded that both D1- and D2-like receptor antagonists block the usual effects of rewarding stimuli on behavior. In two subsequent reviews we focused on studies that made direct comparisons between D1- and D2-like receptor antagonists in a number of incentive learning paradigms and concluded from those studies that D1-like receptors played a more important role in the mechanisms of incentive leaning. These review papers were published in 1996 with graduate student Patricia Nakonechny and in 1998 with my colleague and collaborator Robert Miller, working at the time at the University of Otago in Dunedin, New Zealand (I return to Robert's pioneering work on dopamine and schizophrenia and the mechanisms of dopamine-related learning in Chapters 9 and 12, respectively).[35] I will discuss one study from those reviews that strongly differentiated the role of D1- and D2-like receptors in incentive learning and then review some more recent studies on the same theme.

Stephen Fowler, at the time working at the University of Mississippi in Oxford, Mississippi, and his co-worker, Jiing-Ren Liou, observed the effects of the dopamine D1-like receptor antagonist SCH 23390 and D2-like receptor antagonists, including raclopride, on the lever-press responding of trained rats. Antagonists at both receptor families produced a dose-dependent decrease in responding. The authors also measured the duration of lever-press responses and the duration of nose entries into the water-reward alcove and they found that doses of D2-like receptor antagonists had a greater tendency than doses of SCH 23390 to increase the duration of both of these measures. Although both types of antagonists dose-dependently decreased lever pressing for water, Fowler and Liou concluded from the duration data that D2-like receptor antagonists were having a greater impact on motor responses and that SCH 23390 was having a greater impact on the effects of the rewarding stimulus.[54] These data supported a greater role for D1- than D2-like receptors in reward-related incentive learning.

John Horvitz, at the time from City College of the City University of New York, is a leading behavioral neuroscientist whose studies have contributed importantly to understanding the role of dopamine in reward-related learning.[55] Working with colleagues at Columbia University in New York and Boston College, Chestnut Hill, Massachusetts, Horvitz carried out a study similar to that of Fowler and Liou. Rats were trained to make a cued approach response or a cued lever press for food and then the effects of a range of doses of SCH 23390 and racolpride were tested. Like Fowler and Liou, they found that both compounds decreased responding but only raclopride increased the duration of head entries into the food compartment. By using a discrete-trial procedure, they were able to show further that SCH 23390 but not raclopride decreased the proportion of trials during which an approach and operant lever-press response was seen. Thus, results revealed a double dissociation: SCH 23390 but not raclopride decreased the proportion of responses to the conditioned cue; raclopride but not SCH 23390 increased the duration of responses.[56] Results suggest that treatment with SCH 23390 led to a decrease in the ability of the cue-light stimulus to elicit approach and other responses and support a greater role for D1- than D2-like receptors in reward-related incentive learning.

Another pair of City University of New York researchers, Anthony Sclafani at Brooklyn College and Richard Bodnar at Queen's College, has shown the relative importance of D1-like receptors in incentive learning. Their research has focused on the control of feeding behavior and one theme has been the contribution of conditioning factors. Rats and mice, like people, prefer high-fat and high-sugar foods. Sclafani, Bodnar, and their co-workers have shown a conditioned flavor preference in rats for flavors that have been paired with these foods. From an incentive learning point of view, the flavor paired with the preferred food will acquire an increased ability to elicit approach and other responses; incentive learning will be manifested by increased choice of the bottle containing the paired flavor in two-bottle tests. They found that treatment with the D1-like receptor antagonist SCH 23390 but not the D2-like receptor antagonist raclopride during pairing trials (acquisition) blocked the learning of a preference for the flavor paired with the preferred food. They showed further that neither SCH 23390 nor raclopride blocked the expression of a preference in rats conditioned without drug treatments.[57] These, and related,[58] results show that D1-like receptors play a greater role than D2-like receptors in the acquisition of incentive learning and that once incentive learning has taken place it is, at least transiently, resistant to the effects of D1- or D2-like receptor blockade (see Chapter 3). Further studies by Sclafani, Bodnar, and colleagues, and others, have reported similar findings and localized the role of D1-like receptors in this flavor-preference phenomenon to the amydgala.[59]

The effects of D1- and D2-like receptor-specific agonists on the acquisition of incentive learning also reveal a more important role for D1-like receptors. In the late 1980s there were a number of puzzling findings from studies using dopamine receptor family-specific agonists that made it difficult to discern the contribution of D1- and D2-like receptors to incentive learning. I had findings from my own laboratory during that time that puzzled me for a couple of years and then, finally, I realized their meaning. I will begin by describing those results and then discuss why it was puzzling and how it finally made sense.

We were studying the effects of D1- and D2-like receptor-specific agents on responding for conditioned reward. The basic procedure is fairly simple and is quite similar to the procedure used for testing conditioned place preference described in Chapter 3. Rats receive five 40-minute pre-exposures to a test box outfitted with two levers; one produces a three-second tone and the other a three-second lights-off period when pressed. We record the number of presses on each lever. Then the levers are removed from the chamber and over the next four days the lights-off stimulus is presented 80 times at random intervals averaging 45 seconds, followed intermittently by a food pellet delivered into a food magazine located on one of the walls of the test chamber.[60] For the two-session test phase, the levers are replaced in the chamber and again the number of presses on each is recorded during 40-minute sessions. The lights-off stimulus is considered to have become a conditioned rewarding stimulus if the animal now presses the lever that produces that stimulus more than it did in the pre-exposure phase and if this ratio if significantly higher than the corresponding ratio for the tone lever.[61]

From an incentive learning point of view, what is happening in the conditioned reward procedure is as follows. During the pre-exposure phase the animal will learn the layout of the test chamber, the location of the levers and the relationship between the levers and the tone and lights-off stimuli; this learning appears to be relatively independent of dopamine systems, as discussed in Chapter 4. During the conditioning phase, the rats will learn the association of the lights-off stimulus with food and incentive learning will lead to the lights-off stimulus acquiring the ability to elicit approach and other responses. From Chapter 5 we know that the lights-off stimulus itself will acquire the ability to produce dopamine release; we know further that if the conditioned lights-off stimulus is presented repeatedly without being followed by food, it will initially produce dopamine release but will gradually lose this ability. During the test phase (when no food is presented), delivery of the lights-off stimulus following lever presses on the lights-off lever will initially produce dopamine release leading to incentive learning, the acquisition by the lever and lever-related stimuli of an increased ability to elicit approach and other responses. This learning will lead to increased presses on the lights-off lever. My former mentor, Anthony Phillips, at the University of British Columbia, and I showed previously that blocking dopaminergic neurotransmission during the pairing phase blocked the conditioned reward effect,[62] and several researchers have shown that blocking dopaminergic neurotransmission during the test phase also blocked the conditioned reward effect,[63] demonstrating the important role for dopamine in incentive learning in this paradigm.

The studies that produced puzzling results used D1- and D2-like receptor agonist in the test phase of the conditioned reward procedure. We found that the D1-like receptor agonist SKF 38393 given during the test phase dose-dependently *blocked* the conditioned reward effect; by contrast, the D2-like receptor agonists quinpirole or bromocriptine at moderate doses *enhanced* the effect.[64] On the face of it, these results seemed to suggest that D2-like receptors were more important for conditioned reward and that enhanced stimulation of D1-like receptors impaired reward-related learning. It was difficult to make sense of these findings and they remained unpublished for some time.

To unravel the meaning of the results with dopamine receptor subtype-specific agonists on responding for conditioned reward, the effects of non-specific agonists with different mechanisms of action are instructive. Apomorphine is a direct-acting dopamine receptor agonist that mimics the effects of dopamine at the receptor.[65] Amphetamine and related drugs, however, are indirect-acting; amphetamine reverses the dopamine transporter so that when an action potential arrives at the neurotransmitter-releasing terminal of a dopamine neuron, more dopamine is released and that dopamine remains in the extracellular space longer.[66] In conditioned reward studies, Trevor Robbins from Cambridge University, UK, a prolific and influential neuroscientist and a pioneer of the study of the role of dopamine in learning, and colleagues showed that apomorphine and amphetamine-like drugs produced different effects on responding for conditioned reward. Both apomorphine and amphetamine produced increases in responding, but, whereas the effect of apomorphine was not specific to the conditioned reward lever, in fact obscuring the conditioned reward effect, the effect of amphetamine was specific to the conditioned reward lever and as a result enhanced the conditioned reward effect.[67]

To understand the results with apomorphine and amphetamine it is important to remember from Chapter 5 that dopamine neurons show brief, phasic activation when a rewarding stimulus is presented. The transient increase in synaptic concentrations of dopamine produced by the phasic burst will increase the incentive properties of the most recently encountered stimuli. In the case of responding for conditioned reward, the presentation of the conditioned stimulus immediately following depression of the relevant lever will lead to that lever and lever-related stimuli (e.g., that location in the chamber) acquiring an increased ability to attract the animal in the future. The close temporal contiguity between the lever-press response and the lever-related stimuli assures that it is the lever and lever-related stimuli and not other stimuli in the test chamber that become strong incentive stimuli.

Now consider the effects of apomorphine. Apomorphine will occupy dopamine receptors mimicking the action of dopamine. This effect of apomorphine will be temporally indiscriminate with respect to presses on the lever that produce conditioned reward. Since increases in dopamine produce incentive learning, in the presence of apomorphine incentive learning will occur not only to the conditioned reward lever and lever-related stimuli, but also to other stimuli in the chamber. As a result, the conditioned reward will no longer control responding. Apormorphine essentially *masks* or *occludes* the reward signal.

With amphetamine the situation will be different because of its mechanism of action. Thus, amphetamine will not indiscriminately enhance synaptic concentrations of dopamine but rather will do so when a reward signal is generated, thereby augmenting the reward signal. When a rat is acquiring responding for conditioned reward while under the influence of amphetamine, the *signal* generated by dopamine neurons will remain intact and be enhanced because amphetamine will increase the amount of dopamine released and that dopamine will remain longer in the extracellular space.

One final thing: the dose–response curve for the effects of amphetamine on responding for conditioned reward is an inverted U-shaped function. At low doses (e.g., 0.01 mg/kg) there is no effect, at moderate doses (e.g., 0.1–1.0 mg/kg) enhanced responding for conditioned reward is seen, and at high doses (e.g., 2.0 mg/kg) the enhancement is no longer seen and the conditioned reward effect itself is eventually lost with increasing dose. This can be understood if the high doses of amphetamine lead to sufficiently elevated extracellular concentrations of dopamine that the reward-related signal is masked or occluded much as it is by apomorphine. In this way the failure of high doses of amphetamine to enhance the rewarding effect of conditioned rewarding stimuli can be understood.

How can the results with apomprphine and amphetamine help to explain the results with D1- and D2-like receptor-specific agonists? Recall that a D1-like receptor agonist impaired responding for a conditioned rewarding stimulus and a D2-like receptor agonist enhanced responding for conditioned reward. Both types of agonists are apomorphine-like insofar as they are direct-acting; they mimic the effects of dopamine at the receptor, but SKF 38393 acts specifically at D1-like receptors, and qunipirole and bromocriptine act specifically at D2-like receptors. The fact that SKF 38393, like apomorphine, blocks the conditioned reward effect, whereas quinpirole and bromocriptine enhance it strongly, implies that the conditioned reward-blocking effects of apomorphine reside in its action at D1-like receptors. This suggests further that the critical site of action of dopamine for producing reward-related learning is D1-like receptors.

When quinpirole or bromocriptine are used, their action at D2-like receptors stimulates motor activity as discussed earlier, but the control of behavior by the conditioned rewarding stimulus is intact because the dopamine signal at D1-like receptors remains temporally linked to pressing the conditioned reward lever. As a result the conditioned reward effect remains intact and is enhanced. Like amphetamine, quinpirole and bromocriptine have inverted U-shaped dose–response curves. When the doses get into the high range, above about 1.0 mg/kg for quinpirole and above 10 mg/kg for bromocriptine, perhaps the intensity of locomotor stimulation is so high that the control of behavior by incentive learning is overwhelmed and responding on the two levers becomes indiscriminate.

Studies of the role of D1- and D2-like receptors in locomotor activity showed that both were involved, but generally the effects of D1-like receptor agonists were smaller (see earlier). The same was seen in responding for a conditioned rewarding stimulus where D2- but not D1-like agonists elevated overall responding. Thus, the conditioned reward results and the locomotor activity results agree. The observation that SKF 38393 and a number of other D1-like receptor agonists blocked the conditioned reward effect,[68] whereas D2-like receptor agonists at moderate doses did not further show a critical role for D1-like receptors in reward-related incentive learning.

D1- and D2-like receptor agonists produce a conditioned place preference.[69] Why would they produce differential effects on responding for conditioned rewarding stimuli but similar effects in conditioned place preference? This is an important question. The answer has to do with the stimuli that become conditioned incentive stimuli and control responding. In the case of lever-press responding, the lever and lever-related stimuli are a *subset* of the stimuli within the test environment. If an animal is exposed to those stimuli while D1-like receptors are being tonically stimulated, the dopamine signal associated with reward for lever pressing is putatively masked and the rewarding stimulus does not lead to incentive learning that is specific to the lever and related stimuli, as just discussed. However, in place conditioning, the animal is confined to one side of a chamber consisting of two distinct sides connected by a tunnel. With D1-like receptor stimulation during confinement, the stimuli from that environment will become incentive stimuli. There is no need for a particular subset of stimuli within that environment to come to control responding; the putative masking effect of an agonist on a particular subset of stimuli, as observed in the lever-pressing situation, is not an issue here. The other side is paired with saline. Then, when the preference test is carried out, more time is spent on the drug-paired side because the stimuli there have become incentive stimuli. In this case, the incentive learning produced by a D1-like agonist is complementary to the test procedure and a conditioned place preference is seen. My colleague in psychology at Queen's University, Mary Olmstead, and I have discussed these apparently paradoxical effects of D1-like receptor agonists in a chapter that we co-authored in the book *Brain Dynamics and the Striatal Complex.*[70]

Dopamine receptor-knockout mice and incentive learning

The studies reviewed so far used pharmacological tools to evaluate the possible differential role in incentive learning of D1- and D2-like receptors. Advances in molecular genetics in the last two decades of the twentieth century led to the development of mice that lacked one of the specific dopamine receptor sub-types. Thus, it became possible to target and knock out a particular gene in a mouse. Working independently, Mario Capecchi and colleagues, at the time at the University of Wisconsin in Madison, and Oliver Smithies and colleagues at the University of North Carolina in Chapel Hill discovered how to insert foreign DNA into a specific place in a chromosome of a mammalian cell using a tech-nique that took advantage of a natural process called homologous recombin-ation.[71] Around the same time, Martin Evans and colleagues at the University of Cambridge, UK, learned to grow embryonic stem cells from mouse embryos.[72] They found that they could insert these cultured embryonic stem cells into a mouse embryo and the result was a chimera, that is, an animal with some tis-sues derived from the original embryo and some from the injected stem cells. By mating offspring that had sperm or ova derived from the injected embryonic stem cells, Evans and his co-workers could derive a line of mice that carried the stem cell genes in all of their tissues.[73] Capecchi and Smithies were able to take advantage of this system to create mouse lines with specific genes knocked out. Capecchi, Smithies, and Evans received the 2007 Nobel Prize in Physiology or Medicine for this groundbreaking work.[74]

There quickly followed multiple different lines of mice with various individual genes knocked out that needed to be tested to identify their behavioral pheno-type. Among these were D1-, D2-, D3-, D4-, and D5-knockout mice. They would appear to be a perfect tool for isolating the role of individual dopamine receptors in the acquisition and expression of incentive learning. However, there is a catch. To appreciate this catch, it is helpful to consider the results of studies of dopamine-depleted rats.

As mentioned earlier in this chapter, 6-hydroxydopamine is a neurotoxin that, when injected into the brain kills monoaminergic cells, including those that use dopamine or norepinephrine as their neurotransmitter.[75] By injecting 6-hydroxydopamine into the brains of rats that have been pretreated with a norepinephrine uptake-blocking drug, it is possible to selectively destroy dopaminergic cells.[76] This approach was used extensively in research carried out in the last decades of the twentieth century and the behavioral consequences of dopamine depletion in *adult* rats were well characterized. These treatments produced effects that were often described as Parkinson-like. Rats depleted of dopamine in adulthood neglected sensory stimuli in their environment and were severely hypokinetic, showing almost no movement. They were unable to feed themselves, did not drink, and would have died if they were not fed by the experimenters.[77] Function gradually recovered in some of the lesion rats if the lesion spared at least ten percent of the striatal dopamine content,[78] and the recovery depended on compensatory changes in the dopamine system.[79] However, similar 6-hydroxydopamine treatments in *neonates* had far less severe effects. Treated pups still nursed and they ate solid food after they were weaned.[80] In adulthood, rats treated with 6-hydorxdopamine as neonates did not show the severe sensorimotor deficits observed in adult-lesion rats; they were able to feed themselves, to move about, and, in fact, showed more signs of hyperactivity than non-lesion control rats (more on this in Chapter 9).[81] Perhaps not surprisingly, neonatal-lesion rats showed deficits in incentive learning when tested as adults.[82] Unlike adult-lesion rats, behavioral abilities in neonatal-lesion rats tested as adults were less dependent on compensatory changes in the dopamine system.[83] Both adult-lesion and neonatal-lesion rats were found to have similar and large losses of dopamine neurons. What could account for the difference?

The apparently milder effects of neonatal versus adult 6-hydroxydopamine lesions suggest that behavior in adulthood of rats that received lesions as neonates is relatively less dependent on dopamine and that compensatory processes that take place in neonatal-lesion rats involve systems other than the dopamine system. Jeffrey Joyce of the University of Pennsylvania in Philadelphia and co-workers provide a thorough review of the differential effects of neonatal versus adult 6-hydroxydopaine lesions on behavior and brain chemistry. They argue that dopamine plays a role in development of the striatum and that development of the striatum is altered in neonatal-lesion rats. The differential severity of neonatal versus adult lesions of dopamine neurons reflects these developmental alterations in neonatal-lesion rats.[84] Generally, the long-term outcomes of various forms of damage to the nervous system in humans are more severe in adulthood than in childhood, with childhood damage often followed by substantial recovery of function; the mechanisms of this recovery continue to be the topic of extensive research.[85] For the purposes of the present discussion, these findings with 6-hydroxydopamine lesions in neonates versus adults sound a cautionary note. They warn that developmental compensatory processes that are different in young animals versus adult animals might mitigate the effects of neonatal treatments such as genetic alterations.

D1 receptor-knockout mice show deficits in incentive learning. They are slower to learn a lever-pressing task for food or sucrose reward,[86,87] and rate-frequency functions show that the rewarding effects of brain stimulation are reduced in D1 receptor-knockout mice.[88] They were reported to show no deficit in incentive learning based on cocaine in conditioned place preference experiments,[89] but, compared with wild-type control mice, failed to learn a place preference based on brain stimulation.[88] D1 receptor-knockout mice failed to learn to self-administer cocaine,[90] and showed evidence that incentive learning based on ethanol was reduced.[91] Learning to traverse a maze for food involves incentive learning (see Chapter 5); this type of learning was impaired in D1 receptor-knockout mice.[92] As discussed in Chapters 2 and 3, learning to escape and avoid aversive stimuli involves incentive learning, safety-related stimuli acquiring an increased ability to elicit approach and other responses. D1 receptor-knockout mice are deficient in learning a water maze,[93] or an analogous dry-land task involving escaping from an open field by entering a small dark chamber recessed below the surface.[94] As might be expected, D1 receptor-knockout mice are deficient in conditioned avoidance learning.[94]. Using sophisticated molecular genetics approaches, Bryan Gore and Larry Zweifel of the University of Washington in Seattle showed that reconstruction of D1 receptor signaling in the nucleus accumbens of D1 receptor-knockout mice could rescue deficits in incentive learning observed in approach and instrumental response tests.[86] Taken together, results from genetic knockout of dopamine D1 receptors make a strong case for a role for D1 receptors in incentive learning.

D2 receptor-knockout mice took longer to learn to lever press for food or water,[95,96] and showed changes in rate-frequency functions for brain stimulation indicative of reduced reward-related learning.[97] They failed to show a conditioned place preference for morphine,[96,98] and were slower to learn to go to a place where they received rewarding brain stimulation.[99] Intravenous cocaine was a less rewarding stimulus in D2 receptor-knockout mice and they failed to self-administer the D2 receptor-specific agonist quinelorane.[95]. They also showed lower rates of acquisition of a rewarded alternation.[99]. These findings complement those from psychopharmacological experiments reviewed earlier, implicating D2 receptors in reward-related incentive learning.

Fewer studies have investigated the possible effects on incentive learning of knockout of D3, D4, or D5 receptors. D3 receptor-knockout mice showed normal or *enhanced* cocaine or morphine reward in conditioned place preference tests.[100,101,102] However, when they were trained using the conditioned place preference procedure based on cocaine, then tested for preference repeatedly over several days, D3 receptor-knockout mice showed a more rapid reduction of the conditioned place preference effect than wild-type control mice;[100] the implications of these findings for a role for D3 receptors in the expression of incentive learning are discussed in the next section. D4 receptor-knockout mice showed reduced exploration of a novel stimulus but increased rates of lever pressing for food.[103,104] They showed no significant change in their ability to learn food-rewarded lever-press tasks,[104,105] and little change in incentive learning in a conditioned place preference task based on the dopamine indirect agonists methylphenidate, amphetamine, or cocaine.[106] They did not differ significantly from wild-type mice in their ability to learn to self-administer cocaine.[107] The dopamine D4 receptor has been implicated in novelty seeking and in several neuropsychiatric disorders, including attention deficit hyperactivity disorder;[108,109] this aspect of dopamine function is discussed further in Chapter 9. Dopamine D5 receptor knockout appeared to have little effect on conditioned place preference based on cocaine.[110] Further studies are needed to fully characterize the effects of D3, D4, and D5 receptor knockout on reward-related learning. In summary, results from studies with D1 and D2 receptor-knockout mice are in fairly good agreement with results from psychopharmacological studies implicating both receptors subtypes in incentive learning.

Psychopharmacology of D3 and D4 receptors

In recent years, new pharmacological agents that are relatively specific for dopamine D3 or D4 receptors have started to become available. At present, D5 receptor-preferring pharmacological agents are not available. The D3 and D4 receptor-preferring agents make it possible to conduct psychopharmacological experiments to assess the possible role of D3 and D4 receptors in incentive learning. In the following, I will review these studies, beginning with those that used D3 receptor-preferring agents.

In 2008, along with one of my doctoral students I reviewed the studies that had evaluated the effects of D3 receptor-preferring agents, all receptor antagonists at the time, in incentive learning paradigms.[111] We drew a number of conclusions that I summarize here and in each case I review the related studies that have been published since the time of our review. The results reported in almost all of the more recent papers support the conclusions from our earlier review.

One focus of our review was the effects of D3 receptor antagonists on drug self-administration. We concluded that when the maintenance of self-administration depended heavily on conditioned incentive cues, D3 receptor-preferring antagonists generally decreased responding. When responding was relatively less dependent on conditioned incentive cues, because the density of primary reward was high, D3 receptor-preferring antagonists usually had little effect. Self-administration on fixed-ratio-one or fixed-ratio-two schedules, where each response or every other response produces an intravenous drug infusion, respectively, are examples of high-density primary reward schedules. The studies we reviewed showed that D3 receptor-preferring antagonists or partial agonists, that would also serve as partial antagonists, had little effect on responding for cocaine or nicotine, but the one study available reported that responding for ethanol was decreased.[111]. In agreement with this general picture, more recent studies have reported that D3 receptor-preferring antagonists fail to affect self-administration responding on a fixed-ratio-two schedule for methamphetamine.[112] One paper reported that the D3 receptor-preferring antagonist S33138 decreased the rewarding effects of cocaine on a fixed-ratio-two schedule, but the authors suggested that this effect was seen at doses that likely also affected D2 receptors (as reviewed earlier, it is well known that D2 receptor antagonists or D2 receptor knockout decreases incentive learning produced by primary rewards).[113] Most of the studies examining the effects of D3 receptor-preferring antagonists on self-administration on high-density reward schedules have used a relatively high single dose of the reward substance. When a dose–response curve was generated, rats and mice were found to take fewer infusions of cocaine at lower doses following treatment with D3 receptor-preferring antagonists, but the antagonists had no significant effect at higher doses.[114] The findings with higher doses are consistent with those from previous studies that used a single dose. The decrease in responding for lower doses of cocaine reward seen following D3 receptor-preferring antagonists might reflect the relatively greater reliance of low-dose responding on incentive cues rather than the primary rewarding effects of the drug; from this point of view, the results are consistent with a more prominent role of D3 receptors in the control of responding by conditioned incentive cues.

Self-administration protocols that depend heavily on conditioned incentive cues for the maintenance of behavior include second-order schedules and progressive ratio schedules. Second-order schedules are best conceptualized as having a simple schedule of reward as the unit response. For example, in a study by Patricia Di Ciano, a former undergraduate student from my laboratory, working at the time as a postdoctoral researcher at the University of Cambridge in the UK, instead of the unit response being a single lever press, the unit response was a fixed-ratio-ten. At the end of each fixed-ratio-ten, the animal received a brief presentation of a conditioned incentive stimulus previously associated with cocaine reward. In one version of the second-order schedule, the requirement was a fixed-ratio-ten of the unit response to receive the primary reward of an intravenous cocaine infusion. Thus, the second-order schedule was a fixed-ratio-ten (fixed-ratio-ten: conditioned incentive stimulus), indicating in parentheses the unit response of a fixed-ratio-ten rewarded with a conditioned incentive stimulus and, outside parentheses, the requirement that ten unit responses be completed for primary cocaine reward; primary reward is signaled by the conditioned incentive stimulus. Di Ciano also employed a fixed-interval-15 minutes (fixed-ratio-ten: conditioned incentive stimulus) second-order schedule. According to this schedule, the first unit response completed after the passage of 15 minutes resulted in the presentation of primary drug reward signaled by the incentive stimulus.[115] Prior to the first drug reward, responding is maintained by conditioned incentive stimuli. The study by Di Ciano and a number of related studies reviewed in our 2008 paper show that treatment with D3 receptor-preferring antagonists or partial agonists decreased responding in the first component of a second-order schedule of cocaine reward.[111]. One recent paper reported no effect of a D3 receptor-preferring antagonists on responding of monkeys on a second-order schedule of cocaine reward, but they did not analyze the first component separately.[116]

Another self-administration protocol that depends heavily on conditioned incentive stimuli for the maintenance of behavior is the progressive ratio schedule. These are ratio schedules requiring a specified number of responses for each rewarding stimulus but have the added twist that the ratio requirement increases after each reward. In our previous review we observed that D3 receptor antagonists decreased progressive ratio responding for cocaine or nicotine.[111]. Additional papers that have appeared since our review report corroborative findings from progressive ratio studies of responding for cocaine, nicotine, and methamphetamine.[112,114,117] As progressive ratio values increase, responding relies more and more on conditioned incentive stimuli for its maintenance. The observation that D3 receptor antagonists decrease progressive ratio responding is consistent with a role for D3 receptors in the control of responding by conditioned incentive stimuli.

Some additional observations from studies using multiple schedules that included drug reward and food reward components generally support the findings from studies using second-order and progressive-ratio schedules. Multiple schedules have two or more components, each signaled by a unique stimulus. Within each component, responding is controlled by a particular simple schedule. For example, the component schedule could be a variable interval of 60 seconds, providing a rewarding stimulus for the first response that takes place after a variable interval has elapsed with the average of the intervals being 60 seconds. Researchers in the laboratory of Janet Neisewander at Arizona State University in Tempe, Arizona, trained rats on a multiple variable interval 60-second variable interval 60-second schedule, with cocaine available for self-administration in one component and sucrose in the other, components alternating and being in effect for 15 minutes. They observed that D3 receptor partial agonists decreased responding in both components,[117,118] consistent with a role for D3 receptors in the control of responding by conditioned incentive stimuli. They also observed that a D3 receptor agonist, WC44, decreased responding on the multiple schedule. This latter result might reflect a masking effect of the D3 agonist like that seen with the non-specific dopamine receptor agonist apomorphine in conditioned reward experiments discussed earlier in this chapter.

With respect to the reinstatement of responding for self-administered drugs that is produced by exposure to conditioned incentive stimuli previously associated with the drug, we concluded that D3 receptor "antagonists or partial agonists generally reduced the response-reinstating effects of cues associated with self-administered cocaine or ethanol" (p. 62).[111] With the exception of one study using monkeys,[116] more recent studies have similarly shown that D3 receptor antagonists block the response-reinstating effects of conditioned incentive cues for methamphetamine,[119] cocaine,[120] and nicotine.[121]

In our review of the role of D3 receptors in the control of responding by conditioned incentive stimuli, we also covered studies that used natural rewards. We concluded that D3 receptor antagonists affect responding maintained by conditioned incentive stimuli based on food or sucrose but that non-significant effects have also been reported.[111] Studies that have appeared since our review was published reported no effect of D3 receptor antagonists on fixed-ratio-two responding for sucrose,[114,119] a finding consistent with the general lack of effects of these agents on responding on high-density drug-reward schedules, reviewed earlier. One study reported that the D3 receptor antagonist S33138 decreased fixed-ratio-two responding for sucrose; this was the same study that reported that S33138 decreased fixed-ratio-two responding for cocaine but attributed the effect to a blockade of D2 receptors at the observed dose.[113] The same study that reported no effect of a D3 receptor antagonist on responding on a second-order schedule for cocaine in monkeys found no effect of the D3 receptor antagonist on responding on a second-order schedule for sucrose pellets but, as mentioned above, this study did not isolate the first component as had been done in previous studies.[116] Two recent studies reported decreased progressive ratio responding for sucrose following treatment with a D3 receptor antagonist.[117,119]

The effects of D3 receptor antagonists have also been tested on brain stimulation reward presented according to a fixed-ratio-one schedule. No significant effect was reported.[120,122] This finding is consistent with the general finding of no effect of D3 receptor antagonists on responding for high-density drug or food reward.

A recent study reported that some monkeys well trained to self-administer cocaine continued to self-administer the D3 receptor-preferring agonists quinpirole, ropinirole, and pramipexole when these compounds were substituted for cocaine in the infusion syringe. The authors made the following comment: "It is therefore possible that quinpirole, ropinirole, and pramipexole were not serving as primary reinforcers in any monkeys in the current study, but rather were serving to enhance the motivational effects of the stimulus conditions that were associated with the administration of cocaine" (p. 336).[123] This conclusion is in good agreement with our conclusion about the effects of D3 receptor antagonists on the ability of conditioned incentive stimuli to control responding. Thus, D3 receptor antagonists decrease the ability of conditioned incentive stimuli to control responding and D3 receptor-preferring agonists may increase the ability of conditioned incentive stimuli to control responding. From the studies discussed so far, it would appear that this is the case whether the primary incentive stimulus is a drug or a natural reward.

After reviewing conditioned place preference studies in our 2008 paper, we concluded that D3 receptor antagonists and partial agonists consistently block *expression* of conditioned place preference based on cocaine, nicotine, d-amphetamine, morphine, and heroin but not food. In these studies, the D3 receptor agents were given during the testing phase after pairing sessions without treatment with D3 receptor agents. When the D3 receptor-blocking agents were given during *acquisition*, results were mixed: cocaine-conditioned place preference was either blocked or there was no effect of D3 receptor agents; there was no effect of D3 receptor agents given during acquisition on amphetamine-conditioned place preference; one study showed a block and another no effect on conditioned place preference based on opioid drugs; a D3 receptor partial agonist had no effect on acquisition of a conditioned place preference based on food.[111] Since we published this review, one additional paper has reported that a D3 receptor antagonist blocked the expression of morphine-conditioned place preference when given on the test day but had no significant effect when given during pairing (acquisition) sessions.[124]

Earlier in this chapter when discussing results from studies with dopamine receptor-knockout mice, I referred to a study with D3 receptor-knockout mice that were trained using the conditioned place preference procedure based on cocaine. Recall that they were tested repeatedly over several days and that the D3 receptor-knockout mice initially did not differ from their wild-type controls, but they showed more rapid loss of the conditioned place preference effect over days. In the same study, the effects of a D3 receptor antagonist were tested in a similar protocol using wild-type mice. The authors observed a dose-dependent increase in the loss of the conditioned pace preference effect in the drug-treated group.[100] These results implicate D3 receptors in the expression of incentive learning and, along with other studies of the effects of D3 receptor antagonists or partial agonists on acquisition and expression of incentive learning, generally support a more prominent role for D3 receptors in expression.

Conditioned activity in an environment previously paired with a rewarding stimulus such as cocaine or food can be understood as a manifestation of conditioned incentive learning. In our review, we concluded that results from the few available studies suggest that D3 receptors may not be necessary for the establishment but are implicated in the expression of conditioned activity based on rewarding drugs.[111]. Along with colleagues from AbbVie (formerly Abbott Laboratories) in Ludwigshafen, Germany, and Abbott Park Illinois, we published a more recent paper examining the effects of the D3 receptor antagonist AB-127 on conditioned activity. We found that AB-127 blocked expression of conditioned activity based on cocaine at doses that did not block acquisition. We also showed a double dissociation with the effects of the D2 receptor-preferring antagonist haloperidol that blocked acquisition at doses that did not block expression.[125] The locomotor response to a number of drugs increases from day to day when the drug is repeatedly given in the same environment, a phenomenon termed sensitization. Insofar as sensitization is specific to the drug-paired environment, it is a conditioned response and can be understood as resulting from the additive (or possibly multiplicative) effects of the unconditioned stimulant properties of the drug and the conditioned incentive properties of the environmental cues.[126] Researchers from China and the USA showed that a D3 receptor antagonist injected into the dopamine terminal region, the nucleus accumbens, significantly reduced the conditioned sensitization of locomotor activity produced by morphine.[127] This finding and those from conditioned activity studies support a greater role for D3 receptors in expression than acquisition of incentive learning.

We have recently found that D3 receptors also seem to play a greater role in the expression than in the acquisition of inverse incentive learning. The D3 receptor antagonists nafadotride and NGB 2904 failed to significantly affect the development of increased descent latencies in the bar test when they were given prior to haloperidol on conditioning days. When the same doses were given prior to a saline test day following conditioning with haloperidol alone, the normally observed conditioned increase in descent latencies was attenuated.[128] Although this is the only study that has investigated the possible role of D3 receptors in inverse inventive learning, the results are consistent with those from studies of incentive learning in more strongly implicating D3 receptors in expression than in acquisition. Researchers at Cambridge in the UK and at GlaxoSmithKline in Verona, Italy, have recently reported that humans treated with a D3 receptor antagonists showed reduced approach bias to incentive cues based on food, tested using a computer-based task.[129] These findings complement those reviewed here from studies with non-human animals and suggest that the stronger role for D3 receptors in the expression of conditioned incentive motivation than in the establishment of incentive conditioning extends across a number of mammalian species.

In 2002, Bernard Le Foll, working at the time at the Centre Paul Broca, and colleagues in Paris trained mice using a conditioned activity protocol based on cocaine. On the drug-free test day, they observed conditioned activity in the paired group as expected. They killed the mice after testing and assessed their brains for D1, D2, and D3 receptor messenger RNA (mRNA) and D3 receptors; they found significantly elevated levels of D3 but not D1 or D2 receptor mRNA and increased levels of D3 receptors in the nucleus accumbens of the paired but not the unpaired mice. They found this difference even though both groups had had a similar history of cocaine injections, but injections had been paired with the test environment for the paired group but not for the unpaired group.[130] This showed that it was exposure to the cocaine-paired cues that affected the expression of D3 receptors, not simply having had a number of injections of cocaine. The conditioned-sensitization-to-morphine study mentioned included assessment of mRNA for D1, D2, and D3 receptors and found, like Le Foll et al., an increase in D3 but not D1 or D2 receptors in the nucleus accumbens only in the group that had had morphine paired with the test environment.[127] These studies show that exposure to conditioned incentive stimuli leads to an upregulation of D3 receptors and are consistent with a role for D3 receptors in the expression of incentive learning. The underlying mechanism for this putative role of D3 receptors is unknown but is considered further in Chapter 12.

There are few psychopharmacological studies of the possible role of D4 receptors in incentive learning. Perhaps not surprisingly, because it would also act as a partial antagonist, the D4 receptor partial agonist ABT-724 was not self-administered by monkeys.[123] Nicotine or cocaine self-administration on a high-density schedule of reward was not significantly affected by the D4 receptor blocker L-745,870,[95,131] results in agreement with the finding, discussed earlier in this chapter, that D4 receptor-knockout mice showed no significant difference from wild-type mice in cocaine self-administration.[107] The D4 receptor agonist A-412997 failed to show a conditioned place preference in rats.[132] There is one report that D4 receptor blockade decreased the response-reinstating effectiveness of nicotine-associated conditioned incentive stimuli but did not affect the response-reinstating effects of food-associated conditioned incentive stimuli.[131] This finding might suggest a role for D4 receptors in the control of responding by conditioned incentive stimuli, but further studies are needed.

As discussed further in Chapter 9, in humans the D4 receptor gene is highly polymorphic and allelic variation has been associated with drug dependence, novelty seeking, and impulsivity.[133] Psychopharmacological studies with rats have used models of risk-based decision-making or impulsivity to evaluate the possible contribution of D4 receptors. Working at the University of British Columbia in Vancouver, Jennifer St Onge and Stan Floresco found no significant effect of the D4 receptor agonist PD168,077 or antagonist L745,870 on risk-based decision-making.[134] Others found that the D4 receptor partial agonist ABT-724 decreased the choice of a large delayed rewarding stimulus versus a small immediate one, possibly implicating D4 receptors in the control of impulsivity.[135] The effects of receptor partial agonists often are similar to the effects of receptor antagonists; the finding with ABT-724 might suggest that D4 receptors play a role in the ability of stimuli to control responding over a delay period. From this point of view, diminished D4 receptor function might lead to a loss of the ability to withhold responding during a delay period, a behavioral index of impulsivity (see Chapter 9).

At the time of this writing (December 2014), I know of no pharmacological agents that prefer or are selective for D5 receptors. A psychopharmacological characterization of D5 receptor function will have to await the development of relevant compounds.

Receptor heteromers that include dopamine receptors

"A receptor is a signal transducing unit, a cellular macromolecule or an assembly of macromolecules that is concerned directly and specifically with chemical signaling between and within cells" (p. 131).[136] Beginning with a report in 1999,[137] it has been found that some neurotransmitter receptors, including dopamine receptors, can form receptor heteromers. These are receptor complexes consisting of two or more receptor subtypes. The subtypes can be members of the same receptor class, for example dopamine receptors, or they can be receptors for different neurotransmitters. Although not without controversy, a fascinating feature of receptor heteromers is that their signaling properties can be different from those of the two or more receptor subtypes that have combined into the heteromer.[136]

Although this book is about dopamine, clearly dopamine does not act alone in its effects on behavior and learning. How dopamine functions within brain circuits consisting of multiple neuronal pathways that use different neurotransmitters is discussed in Chapters 11 and 12. This already-complex circuitry is further complicated by the existence of receptor heteromers.

Receptor heteromers can be made up of two receptors for the same neurotransmitter. For example, a D1–D2 receptor heteromer has been identified. As discussed near the beginning of this chapter and also in Chapter 12, D1 and D2 receptors affect the signaling molecules adenylyl cyclase and cAMP and their downstream targets. A fascinating feature of D1–D2 receptor heteromers is that they influence calcium signaling through the phospholipase C pathway.[138] This is a novel cellular function for dopamine receptors and demonstrates the importance of receptor heteromerization. An obvious question that arises from the discovery of D1–D2 receptor heteromers concerns their possible contribution to incentive learning. Almost no work has been done to explore this question, but some results are beginning to appear. Recent findings suggest that blockade of D1–D2 receptor heteromers in rats with an antagonist specific to the heteromer produced a conditioned place preference; stimulation of the heteromer with an agonist, however, produced a conditioned place aversion and blocked the conditioned place preference produced by cocaine.[139] These findings suggest that although stimulation of D1 and D2 receptors is important for the establishment of incentive learning, as discussed above, stimulation of their heteromers produces the opposite effect with *antagonism* of the heteromer apparently leading to incentive learning. Further work is needed to eventually integrate these observations into a cohesive understanding of the role of dopamine in incentive learning.

Many other heteromers have now been identified,[140] and they are too numerous to list them all here. D1–D3 receptor heteromers have been found where stimulation of the two receptors produces a synergistic effect; D1 receptor stimulation of cAMP formation is augmented by stimulation of D3 receptors within the heteromer.[141] D1 receptors have been found to heteromerize with glutamatergic *N*-methyl-D-aspartate (NMDA) receptors and the stimulation of cAMP by D1 receptors within the D1–NMDA receptor heteromer is enhanced when glutamate stimulates NMDA receptors.[142] D1 and D2 receptors form heterodimers with adenosine A2A receptors; within the A2A–D2 receptor heteromer, adenosine stimulation of the A2A receptor decreased the affinity of the D2 receptor for dopamine.[143] Mice lacking A2A receptors showed diminished conditioned place preference based on cocaine, revealing a possible contribution of adenosine to incentive learning mediated by dopamine (see Chapter 12).[144] Recently, D2 receptor heteromers with the ghrelin receptor GHSR1a have been identified in mice; the authors found that the anorexic effects of D2 receptor agonists were blocked by a GHSR1a receptor antagonist or in mice with the GHSR1a receptor gene knocked out.[145] Both ghrelin and dopamine have been found to play an important role in the control of appetite and the D2–GHSR1a receptor heteromer reveals one site of their interaction.

From these examples, it is clear that the influence of receptor heteromers will have to be factored into considerations of the role of various neurotransmitters in the control of behavior.

Summary

Dopamine receptors are GPCRs and form two families: the D1-like receptors, including D1 and D5, stimulate adenylyl cyclase, cAMP formation, and PKA; the D2-like receptors, including D2, D3, and D4, inhibit cAMP formation. Antipsychotic medications used to treat patients with schizophrenia are dopamine receptor antagonists and their clinical potency is strongly correlated with their ability to block D2 receptors; this observation suggested the hypothesis that psychosis in schizophrenia is associated with overactivity of dopamine at D2 receptors. Both D1- and D2-like receptors appear to be involved in the control of unconditioned locomotor activity with increased stimulation of dopamine receptors leading to increased locomotion and decreased stimulation of dopamine receptors leading to decreases in locomotion. Studies with pharmacological compounds relatively specific for D1- or D2-like receptors implicate both receptor families in incentive learning: antagonists at either receptor family produce a gradual decrease in operant responding for food and agonists at either receptor family produce a conditioned place preference. Careful studies with receptor antagonists implicate D1-like receptors more strongly in incentive learning and D2-like receptors more strongly in the control of locomotor responses. Studies investigating the acquisition of responding for conditioned reward in rats treated with agonists relatively specific for D1- or D2-like receptors similarly implicate D1-like receptors more strongly in incentive learning. Genetically modified mice with D1 or D2 receptors knocked out show decreases in incentive learning. D3 receptors may play a relatively greater role in the expression of incentive learning than its acquisition. The discovery that dopamine receptor subtypes form heteromers with each other and with the receptors of other neurotransmitters (e.g., NMDA, A2A, GHSR1a) and that the signaling properties of these heteromers can differ from those of either receptor in isolation has opened up a new area of investigation. A complete understanding of the role of dopamine receptor subtypes in the control of locomotor activity and learning will require the integration of new findings from studies of dopamine receptor subtype-containing heteromers.

Chapter 8

Dopamine and social cooperation

We interact extensively with other people. Sometimes the interaction is co-operative in nature and sometimes it is not. It is possible to imagine a range of cooperative social interactions with highly cooperative interactions involving formation of a strong bond between two individuals and highly beneficial outcomes for both individuals on one end, and minimal interactions where the two people barely notice each other on the other. There are also social interactions that result in outcomes (e.g., loss of resources, injury) that are costly for one individual; in this case, the interaction is not cooperative and the victim's best recourse may be to avoid the dominant interlocutor. This chapter focuses not only on cooperative social interactions, but also touches on agonistic interactions. Research suggests that cooperative social interactions may activate dopamine and lead to incentive learning.

Dopamine and social cooperation in humans

Suggestive observations come from functional magnetic resonance imaging (fMRI) studies. A participant's brain is scanned while he or she is performing a task that involves a social interaction and the areas of the brain that are using the most oxygen during the task can be identified. In a study done at Princeton University in New Jersey, in the laboratory of cognitive neuroscientist Jonathan Cohen, postdoctoral fellow James Rilling and colleagues had the participants play a social game called the prisoner's dilemma. The game is played by two people. The first person decides whether she will cooperate with, or not cooperate with, that is, defect from the second person. The second person then chooses to cooperate or defect. If both people cooperate, each wins a fixed amount, for example $5. If the first person opts to cooperate and the second defects, the second person, the defector gets $6 and the first person, the cooperator, gets nothing. In the opposite scenario, that is, defect–cooperate, the payoff would be $6 to the first person and nothing to the second. If both players defect, each will be paid $1. As you can see, a strategy of cooperation is most beneficial for both players combined, but if you look at the profits of each individual, one who defects regularly when playing with a cooperator can gain more.

The game was set up so that the participant who was being scanned thought she was playing the game with another person in another room whom she had met before being placed into the scanner and whose picture she could see on a computer screen; in reality, she was playing with the computer. The participant was shown a picture of the person she thought she was playing and then decided to cooperate or defect. There was a brief delay and then the other player chose to cooperate or defect. Then the result of the game was shown on the computer screen. The comparison of interest for the researchers was cooperate–cooperate versus cooperate–defect. During the scanning session, the participant played the game one time with each of a series of other individuals, each depicted on her computer screen (although none was actually in the other room). The researchers were able to average the blood oxygenation level-dependent (BOLD) response for each trial of the same type.

Rilling and his associates found that comparison of the BOLD responses associated with cooperate–cooperate with those for cooperate–defect revealed that the nucleus accumbens was more strongly activated by cooperate–cooperate. This brain area receives a strong input from the dopamine neurons of the ventral midbrain, as discussed in Chapter 11. Importantly, Rilling et al. included trials where the participant was told that she was playing the game with a computer rather than with another person; when the cooperate–cooperate versus cooperate–defect contrast was derived for those trials, no difference was found. This control procedure confirmed that the two scenarios only produce a contrast in the nucleus accumbens when the game is being played with another person. The results imply that dopamine neurons may have been more active in the social cooperate–cooperate situation than in the cooperate–defect situation.[1] In a similar, earlier study Rilling and co-workers observed that the cooperate–cooperate outcome led to activation in "the caudate nucleus and nucleus accumbens ... , both of which receive midbrain dopamine projections known to be involved with processing reward" (p. 397).[2] These studies do not provide knockdown evidence that dopamine is involved in cooperative social interactions because fMRI studies do not measure dopamine activity, they measure BOLD responses. However, as discussed in Chapter 5, if a person is given cocaine, a drug that increases dopaminergic neurotransmission, while his brain is being scanned in a fMRI machine, a BOLD response is seen in the nucleus accumbens.[3] This shows that enhancement of dopaminergic neurotransmission can produce a BOLD response in the nucleus accumbens and provides some support for the suggestion that the response seen during the cooperate–cooperate scenario does represent a dopamine response.

A further observation of interest from the Rilling et al. studies is that the dopamine terminal areas that were activated by a cooperate–cooperate outcome were deactivated by a cooperate–defect outcome. As discussed below, a cooperate–cooperate outcome may lead to incentive learning about the cooperator and related environmental stimuli, making that person and related stimuli more likely to elicit approach and other responses in the future. A cooperate–defect outcome may lead to inverse incentive learning, decreasing the ability of the defector and related stimuli to elicit approach and other responses in the future.

In studies done elsewhere, increased BOLD responses were seen in the caudate nucleus during cooperative social interactions in a fMRI study involving two people playing a game that required social exchange. The two people played a multi-round trust game; one person was identified as the investor and the other as the trustee. The game began with the investor receiving a stake ($20) that he could use to invest and he decided how much of the stake he wanted to invest. According to the rules that had been communicated to both players, the trustee automatically received three times the invested amount (e.g., if the investor decided to invest $9 from the stake, the trustee received $27). The round was completed when the trustee decided how much of the money to return to the investor. Multiple rounds were played allowing the investor and the trustee to form expectations about each other's social cooperation. This made it possible to identify trials where the investment was better than expected by the trustee (benevolent reciprocity) and trials where the investment was worse than expected by the trustee (malevolent reciprocity). Using images from the trustee's brain, the authors evaluated the contrast between these two types of trials and found that on benevolent-reciprocity trials versus malevolent-reciprocity trials there was a greater BOLD response in the caudate nucleus.[4] This result showed that a brain area that receives a strong dopamine input was activated when a cooperative social interaction took place and agreed with the findings from Rilling and associates discussed earlier.

Possible activation of dopamine neurons has been found to be associated with intense romantic love. Reciprocated romantic love would certainly qualify as an example of social cooperation. In a fMRI study, one of the main investigators was Rutgers University anthropologist Helen Fisher, who has written extensively on the biology of romantic love. She worked with colleagues, including psychologist Arthur Aron from the State University of New York in Stony Brook and neuroscientist Lucy Brown from Albert Einstein College of Medicine in the Bronx, NY. The brains of participants who were in the early stages (first six months) of intense romantic love were scanned while they were viewing a picture of their beloved and thinking about a pleasant, non-sexual experience that the two of them had shared. Scans were also made when the participant was viewing a picture of someone they knew well who was the same age and sex as their beloved. The researchers were then able to subtract the results of one scan from the other to identify areas of the brain that were uniquely activated when the participants viewed the picture of their beloved. Results revealed a stronger BOLD response in the caudate nucleus and in the ventral midbrain region, where dopaminergic cell bodies are located.[5] Results suggest that dopamine neurons may be activated when a person who is in love is viewing and thinking about their beloved.

The same authors carried out a more recent study where they investigated BOLD changes in the brains of men and women who had been in love on average for more than 20 years. They contrasted the signal from when the participants viewed a picture of their beloved to that produced when they viewed a picture of a highly familiar acquaintance or a close long-term friend. Consistent with the results from their study with people in the early stages of romantic love, they found increased BOLD responses in the dopamine terminal area, the caudate nucleus, and in the location of dopamine cell bodies in the ventral midbrain. Moreover, the intensity of romantic love correlated positively with BOLD responses in the caudate and ventral midbrain.[6] These results may implicate dopamine in the maintenance of long-term pair bonds.

Maternal love also involves activation of brain areas that receive a strong dopamine input. Researchers at University College in London collected functional magnetic resonance images from mothers when they viewed photographs of their own child and when they viewed photographs of another child of the same age and sex with whom they were acquainted. Results of contrasts between the BOLD responses to the two types of stimuli revealed activations in a number of brain areas when the mothers were viewing photographs of their own child. These areas included the dopamine-rich caudate nucleus, putamen, and substantia nigra;[7] the last structure is the origin of the dopamine cell bodies that project to the first two structures (see Chapter 11). With the necessary caveats from fMRI studies involving BOLD responses rather than direct measurement of dopamine neuron activity, these results suggest that dopaminergic system activation may be a component of the brain activations produced by social cooperation involved in a mother–child interaction. A mother's interactions with her newborn child influence brain levels of the hormone oxytocin, which, in turn, may modulate the activity of dopamine systems or circuits that involve dopamine and thereby influence dopamine-mediated incentive learning; oxytocin is discussed in more detail later in this chapter.

Activation of the caudate nucleus was found to be associated with being persuaded by an expert. This may represent another form of social cooperation. A group of Dutch researchers used fMRI to scan the brains of participants while they were viewing pictures of everyday items, each paired with a particular celebrity. Sometimes the pairings were congruent (e.g., a well-known tennis player with a tennis racquet) and sometimes not (e.g., a well-known hockey player with a soccer ball). In a later part of the experiment, carried out after the brain scanning part of the study was finished, the participants were asked to rate the products they had seen during the scanning session for purchase incidence, that is, the likelihood that someone would purchase that item. As expected, participants showed what is known in social psychology as the "expert persuasion effect." The products that were paired congruently with a celebrity were given higher purchase-incidence scores by the participants than the products that were paired incongruently. Of course, the participant had to recognize the celebrity and his or her specialty for the effect to take place. Note that it was not simply the particular celebrity who produced the effect because products paired with a known celebrity that were incongruent with that celebrity's specialty were not scored as high for purchase incidence.

Armed with the knowledge about purchase incidence, the authors went to their fMRI data and organized the scans into two sets. One set was those scans associated with viewing a congruent celebrity–product pair that included a product that was subsequently given a high purchase-incidence score and the other set of scans was associated with viewing an incongruent celebrity–product pair that included a product that was not subsequently given a high purchase-incidence score. The scans were subtracted from each other. Results allowed identification of areas of the brain that were uniquely activated by persuasion by an expert; this analysis identified the dopamine-rich caudate nucleus.[8]

What might dopamine be doing in the brain in these situations? Activation of dopamine neurons produces incentive learning, leading to an increase in the ability of previously neutral stimuli to elicit approach and other responses. The stimuli that become conditioned incentive stimuli are those that are encountered just before the dopamine neurons are activated. When social cooperation takes place, one of the stimuli most recently encountered in the context of increased firing of dopamine neurons is the social cooperator, the other person. The activation of dopamine neurons may lead to that other person having an increased ability to elicit approach and other responses in the future. When I say "that other person" what I really mean is the pattern of neuronal activity that is produced in the brain of the participant by that person (see Chapter 11). It is that pattern of neuronal activity that becomes the conditioned incentive stimulus. From the point of view of the person undergoing the incentive conditioning, the other person will appear to be more attractive—not "attractive" in the Hollywood sense but "attractive" in the sense of being more able to attract attention or draw the person towards her in the future. When playing the prisoner's dilemma or multi-round trust game, partners who cooperate may become more attractive because the cooperative social interaction with them led to putative increases in dopaminergic neuron activity and incentive learning.

The same sort of thing might be part of what is taking place in intense romantic love. When the person being scanned is viewing a picture of her beloved and thinking about a pleasant experience that they shared, dopamine neurons appear to be activated in her brain. The most recently encountered stimulus was the picture of the beloved so the neuronal pattern of activation produced by the image of the beloved will acquire an increased ability to elicit approach and other responses. Thus, the person in love is strongly attracted to her beloved.

In the expert persuasion experiment, it is important to remember that the caudate signal was detected by subtracting the scan for celebrity-plus-congruent-object from the scan for celebrity-plus-incongruent-object. Celebrities are often people who embody characteristics that we admire or aspire to. Given their obvious ability to attract people, celebrities would appear to already be conditioned incentive stimuli to many people. The comparison of the two scans does not provide an answer to the question of how much evidence there is that a celebrity leads to dopamine activation; there is a celebrity in the picture that was viewed prior to each scan. The comparison provides evidence of additional brain areas that are uniquely activated by pairing the celebrity with a congruent versus incongruent object. Results showed that celebrity-plus-congruent-object was associated with indirect evidence of increased dopamine activity in the caudate. This suggests that the pattern of neuronal activation produced by the congruent object acquired incentive value, making the object more likely to elicit approach and other responses in the future. This incentive value of the congruent object was reflected in its higher purchase-incidence rating.

These examples suggest that activation of dopamine neurons that project to the nucleus accumbens or caudate nucleus in conjunction with social stimuli may change the incentive value of those social stimuli (and other stimuli associated with them). Some people become more (or less) attractive depending on the nature of the interaction we have with them. Dopamine appears to sculpt the incentive contours of the social landscape (see Figure 8.1).

Human genetic studies have found that dopamine-relevant genes are associated with level of social cooperation. Catechol-O-methyltransferase is a dopamine-degrading enzyme that influences dopamine function predominantly in the frontal cortex and is encoded by the gene *COMT*. The level of activity of catechol-O-methyltransferase varies depending on the amino acid, valine or methionine, at codon 158 of *COMT*. The met/met allele leads to about 30–40% less catechol-O-methyltransferase activity (and therefore higher levels of dopamine) than the val/val allele with the heterozygotes in between. Further variation in dopamine function is associated with polymorphisms of the gene

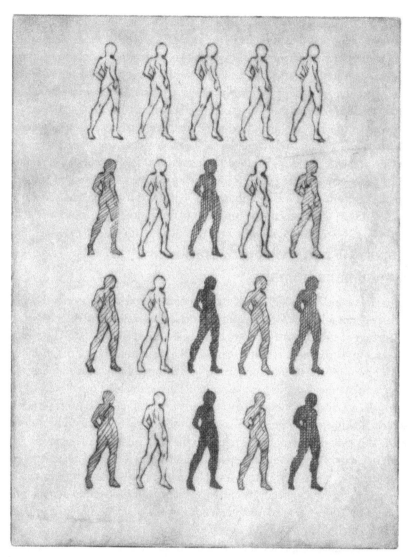

Figure 8.1 *Incentive learning underlying social cooperation*: Social cooperators gradually (top to bottom in each column) acquire incentive value—an increased ability to elicit approach and other responses; the gradual darkening of the figure is a heuristic devise used to show how incentive learning strengthens with repeated social cooperation. The different levels of shading in the columns suggest different levels of social cooperation: the individual indicated in column three is a strong social cooperator, no social cooperation has occurred with the individual depicted in column two, and the incentive value of the remaining individuals is intermediate between the two.

DRD2, which codes for the dopamine D2 receptor. Researchers in Bonn, Germany, reported that variants of the *COMT* and *DRD2* genes were associated with increased performance in a teamwork situation.[9] These were among the first data from genetic studies of an association between dopamine-related genotypes and social cooperation. Results are consistent with other studies suggesting a role for dopamine in social cooperation.

Recall from Chapter 4 that dopamine-mediated learning is non-declarative and that non-declarative memories are not conscious. This suggests the following: (i) as we go through our social environment, the extent of cooperation we encounter with other people is influencing our dopamine systems and producing incentive learning, modifying the ability of those people to "attract" us in the future; (ii) we may not be conscious of this process taking place.

Dopamine and social cooperation in non-humans animals

In the following I discuss findings from studies of a variety of species that provide evidence for a role for dopamine in social cooperation and the subsequent formation of stronger attraction to conspecifics. Researchers at the University of Texas at Austin have recently reviewed the neuroanatomy of the social behavior network and its interconnection with the mesolimbic dopamine reward system in mammals, birds, reptiles, amphibians, and teleost fish. They provide compelling evidence for homology of these systems and related function across vertebrate lineages, supporting a comparative approach to the study of dopamine and social cooperation.[10] I return to the neuroanatomy of dopamine systems in Chapter 11. Some of the species that have been studied include the rat, vole, hamster, songbirds, lizards, amphibians, and fish. In every case, as with the human examples already discussed, evidence links activation of dopamine systems by cooperative social interactions to the formation of strengthened social bonds.

In a wide range of species, the hormones oxytocin and vasopressin have also been implicated in sociality. I begin the discussion with a brief introduction to studies of the role of oxytocin and vasopressin in complex social behavior and social cognition and the possible role of dopamine. I then discuss the role of dopamine in social cooperation in the various species mentioned above.

Oxytocin and vasopressin are nonapeptides that differ by only two amino-acid positions; they are found in most mammals. Similar peptides that vary by a single amino acid are found in non-mammalian vertebrates and arthropods. In mammals, oxytocin- and vasopressin-synthesizing and oxytocin- and vasopressin-releasing neurons are located in hypothalamic brain regions.

They project to the posterior pituitary where their peptides are released into the bloodstream; peripheral oxytocin is involved in uterine contractions at childbirth and milk ejection during lactation, and peripheral vasopressin influences fluid retention by the kidney. Oxytocin neurons also project to several dopaminoceptive brain regions including the nucleus accumbens and to the origin of dopamine neurons in the ventral tegmental area. Besides those in the hypothalamus that release vasopressin into the bloodstream via the pituitary, vasopressin neurons that release vasopressin centrally are found in limbic structures.[11] These peptides play a key role in facilitation of species-typical social and reproductive behaviors. In vertebrates, oxytocin generally influences female sociosexual behavior and vasopressin influences corresponding male behaviors.[12]

Oxytocin release during parturition induces maternal behavior in female rats. For example, experiments showed that central infusion of oxytocin into virgin females stimulates maternal behavior towards pups that they normally would ignore or even attack.[13] In humans, oxytocin released during childbirth is similarly thought to induce mother–infant attachment.[14] Oxytocin is implicated in pair bonding in the small percentage of mammals (3–5%) that show selective preference for a particular mate. In prairie voles (*Microtus ochrogaster*), for example, central administration of oxytocin to a female while she is exposed to a male induces a partner preference that normally would not come about unless the pair copulated (see later).[15] Some authors have suggested that the oxytocin system was originally specialized for maternal behavior and mother–infant attachment but was co-opted to modulate mate preference in monogamous species.[16] Oxytocin can stimulate dopamine release,[17] and, as I discuss later, oxytocin is thought to influence mother–infant attachment and pair bonding through a mechanism involving modulation of dopamine-mediated incentive learning. Variations in the gene that encodes oxytocin have been reported and, as you might have guessed, these variations lead, in turn, to alterations in dopamine function that may affect incentive learning related to social stimuli.[18]

Vasopressin administered centrally to sexually naïve male prairie voles leads to monogamy-associated behaviors, including mate preference and mate guarding, manifested as aggression towards conspecific males.[19] If the expression of vasopressin receptors in dopamine-innervated brain areas of another vole species that is normally polygamous, the meadow vole (*Microtus pennsylvanicus*) is increased using a viral vector to enhance gene expression in those areas, monogamy-associated behaviors are observed, including mate preference.[20] This observation suggests that the effects of vasopressin on the incentive value of social stimuli might also depend on dopamine.

A number of authors, noting the strong evidence for a role for oxytocin, vasopressin and dopamine in social cooperation, have suggested that oxytocin and vasopressin modulate incentive learning processes that build social relationships including mating pair bonds, parent–child bonds, and interactions that require trust.[21] Prairie voles are monogamous, but montane voles (*Microtus montanus*) and, as mentioned earlier, meadow voles are not. If dopamine is activated by copulation in any of these three species, why does it lead to monogamy in the case of prairie voles but not the other two species? Helen Fisher and colleagues suggest that in monogamous species, oxytocin release in the nucleus accumbens and vasopressin release in the ventral pallidum (another dopamine terminal area) triggered during copulation increase dopamine release and incentive learning, leading to attachment and pair bonding. They suggest that incentive learning also occurs in promiscuous species but that the conditioned incentive stimuli are those from a mating partner in general, not those from a *specific* mating partner. Thus, courtship attraction (attraction between a male and female) and partner attachment (strong attraction between a specific male and specific female) can occur independently in non-monogamous species. Fisher et al. suggest that such a mechanism would enable "individuals to prefer specific mating partners yet avoid long-term attachments" (p. 2179).[22] It appears that oxytocin and vasopressin modulation of dopamine-mediated incentive learning contributes to the differences between monogamous and promiscuous species; however, in both cases, dopamine may mediate incentive learning.

Dopamine and social cooperation in monkeys

There are relatively few studies of dopamine and social cooperation in monkeys because most approaches to measuring dopamine are highly invasive. One group of researchers carried out positron emission tomographic imaging of cynomolgus monkeys (*Macaca fascicularis*) who were members of small female groups that formed social hierarchies. They found increased dopamine D2 receptors in the dominant female versus a subordinate female.[23] As discussed below, similar findings have been made in a variety of species (e.g., hamsters) and suggest that the rewarding consequences of winning a dyadic social interaction may include increased dopaminergic neurotransmission and incentive learning about the responses that are instrumental in dominating the conspecific.

Dopamine and social cooperation in rats

Recall from the beginning of Chapter 5 that the methods of behavioral neuroscience can be seen as fitting into three broad categories: stimulation, lesion, and record. There is a convergence of evidence from these different approaches, supporting a role for dopamine in cooperative social interactions in rats (*Rattus norvegicus*). In females, maternal behavior is not normally seen in the absence of high levels of the hormones estrogen and progesterone. However, maternal behavior can be activated when these hormone levels are low by injection of a dopamine D1 receptor agonist into the nucleus accumbens and exposure to pups.[24] Neuroscientist Michael Meaney from McGill University in Montreal, Quebec, has studied maternal behavior extensively and has identified molecular genetic mechanisms mediating the intensity of maternal care; Meany and co-workers reported that injection of a dopamine uptake-blocking drug that elevated levels of dopamine in the nucleus accumbens led to high levels of licking and grooming behavior in mothers that normally showed low levels of licking and grooming,[25] supporting the previous finding that stimulation of dopamine receptors in the nucleus accumbens can activate maternal behavior. Maternal behavior was significantly disrupted by injections of the dopamine neurotoxin 6-hydroxydopamine into the nucleus accumbens or the ventral tegmental area, the origin of dopamine inputs to the nucleus accumbens.[26] Similarly, injection of dopamine receptor antagonists into the nucleus accumbens decreased maternal behavior.[27] In vivo voltammetry and microdialysis[28] studies showed elevated levels of dopamine in the nucleus accumbens of lactating female rats upon presentation of pups and when they licked and groomed their pups.[25,28] Thus, there is convergent evidence from studies using different methods, suggesting that maternal behaviors depend, at least in part, on dopaminergic neurotransmission in the nucleus accumbens and other striatal regions.

Alison Fleming from the University of Toronto campus at Mississauga, Ontario, has extensively studied the brain mechanisms of maternal behavior. With her co-workers, she found that mother rats performed an operant response to receive their pups, clearly demonstrating that the pups act as rewarding stimuli, increasing the ability of pup-related stimuli to elicit approach and other responses.[29] The work of Janet Neisewander and colleagues from Arizona State University in Tempe revealed that juvenile male rats showed a conditioned place preference based on social interaction with another male. The experimental rats were housed singly. Using the place-conditioning paradigm described in Chapter 3, the researchers placed rats in one side where they could interact socially with another male rat alternating with placements in the other side without a conspecific. They noted that the interactions between rats during conditioning sessions were playful in nature and did not include aggression. On the test day, experimental rats showed a preference for the place associated with social interaction.[30] This simple, but elegant, procedure clearly shows that social interaction acts as a rewarding stimulus; results are consistent with a number of earlier studies using different procedures cited in the paper from Neisewander's lab.

In a technological *tour de force*, researchers at Stanford University in California used fiber photometry to examine the activity of identified dopaminergic neurons during social interaction in mice. Fiber photometry is an optical tool that allows real-time recording of the activity of genetically identified neurons using calcium indicators. Gunaydin et al. observed increased activity in ventral midbrain dopaminergic neurons during social interaction.[31] Increased dopamine concentrations produce incentive learning; in the case of cooperative social interactions, the increase in dopamine may increase the ability of the cooperative interlocutor and other associated environmental stimuli to elicit approach and other responses in the future.

In a provocative recent paper from the University of Chicago, researchers claimed to observe empathy and prosocial behavior in rats. They placed a free rat in a test arena along with a cage-mate rat that was trapped in a restrainer, a small plastic box that restricted movement. Over several trials, the free rat learned to open the restrainer door, freeing its cage mate. Free rats did not learn to open empty restrainers or restrainers that contained inanimate objects. Unfortunately, the researchers did not use an unfamiliar rat in the restrainer to see if there was a difference in the willingness of the free rat to work to release an unfamiliar versus familiar (cage mate) conspecific.[32] The finding that the free rat learned to open the restrainer door when the restrainer held a cage mate might reveal the rewarding qualities of social cooperation. Previous cooperative social interactions between the free and restrained rat in their home cage might have led to the restrained rat becoming a conditioned incentive stimulus for the free rat. Conditioned incentive stimuli can induce dopamine release that can produce incentive leaning about other stimuli (see Chapter 5), in this case the door apparatus that could be manipulated to open the restrainer. These results might suggest that seeing a restrained familiar conspecific provided the motivation to try to find a way to free the conspecific and that succeeding produced reward-related learning; reward-related learning involves activation of dopamine neurons and the acquisition by recently encountered stimuli of the ability to elicit approach and other responses.

The University of Chicago researchers noted that the restrained rats emitted ultrasonic vocalizations of approximately 23 kHz. The human hearing range is 20–20,000 Hz (i.e., 0.02–20 kHz) so these rat vocalizations are termed "ultrasonic" because they are of a higher frequency than those heard by humans. Neuroscientist Stefan Brudzynski from Brock University in St. Catharines, Ontario, has extensively studied rat ultrasonic vocalizations. These vocalizations include calls in the 22 kHz and 50 kHz range that communicate the animal's "emotional state" to conspecifics. The 22-kHz calls are indicative of a negative or aversive state and the 50-kHz calls indicate a positive or appetitive state.[33] When I discussed the University of Chicago experiment with my colleague at Queen's University, Vernon Quinsey, he wondered if the operant door-opening responses of the free rats were being maintained by negative reinforcement provided by offset of the 22-kHz vocalizations of the restrained rats. Previous studies have shown that 22-kHz vocalizations are avoided by rats; researchers including Stefan Brudzynski from Brock University and Jaak Panksepp (1943–2017), a prolific researcher from Washington State University in Pullman who studied animal communication for decades, observed that rats nose-poked to produce playback of 50-kHz vocalizations but avoided making nose-pokes when they produced playback of 22-kHz vocalizations.[34] These results suggest that 22-kHz vocalizations may be aversive and raise the possibility that the door-opening responses of the free rats were being maintained by the offset of aversive 22-kHz vocalizations of the restrained rats. You may recall from the discussion of avoidance learning in Chapter 3 that avoidance responses are maintained by the offset of aversive stimuli; this suggests that the offset of 22-kHz vocalizations might be a rewarding stimulus to rats and might provide a dopamine signal that mediates incentive learning about stimuli that signal their offset. More studies are needed to fully evaluate the controlling stimuli in the University of Chicago study.

Klaus Miczek from Tufts University in Boston is an influential and productive neuroscientist who has served as a principal editor of the journal *Psychopharmacology* for many years. He is a leading researcher of agonistic social interactions in rats. One procedure involves introducing an intruder rat into the home territory of a resident rat. What ensues is a fairly stereotyped social interaction involving the resident rat threatening and attacking the intruder rat. The intruder rat signals social defeat by lying on his or her back. Miczek and co-workers recorded the electrical activity of mesencephalic dopamine neurons and dopamine concentrations in the nucleus accumbens of intruder rats during social defeat. They observed a significant increase.[35] This might seem contradictory to a role for dopamine in reward-related incentive learning. However, recall the discussion in the first part of Chapter 6 about dopamine and novel, intense, and aversive stimuli. Among other things, results showed that although aversive stimuli strongly activated dopamine neurons upon their first presentation, their ability to do so lessened with repeated exposure to the aversive stimuli if no escape was possible. In a number of studies, Miczek and colleagues have evaluated the effects of repeated exposures to the resident-intruder test on measures of dopamine in the intruder rat. Results revealed a diminishing dopamine signal with repeated testing.[36] These results are consistent with other findings of an initial dopamine response to an aversive stimulus followed, on repeated testing, with a diminished and finally no dopamine response. As suggested in Chapter 6, perhaps the initial elevation of dopamine neuron firing alerts and activates the animal in a dangerous situation. If an effective escape response is made, the stimuli associated with safety may become conditioned incentive stimuli; if no escape is possible, the dopamine response subsides.

Dopamine and social cooperation in voles

I mentioned prairie voles in the earlier brief discussion of oxytocin and vasopressin. These are small rodents found in the grasslands of the central USA and Canada. As I mentioned earlier, they are among the small percentage of mammals that are monogamous. After copulation, a male–female pair forms a pair bond, a stable relationship that involves sharing a territory and parental duties. They aggressively repel unrelated intruders. If one member of the pair disappears, the other will not accept a new mate.[37]

Numerous studies implicate dopamine in pair bonding. Many excellent studies in this area have come from the laboratories of Thomas Insel who was at Emory University in Atlanta, Georgia, and Zuoxin Wang from Florida State University in Tallahassee. In the laboratory, if a male–female pair of prairie voles is allowed to cohabitate for one day and copulation takes place during that time, a pair bond is formed. This is quantified using a choice test where a male can choose to spend time in side-by-side contact with either the female he previously cohabitated with or with a novel female. The male choses his partner almost every time after one day of cohabitation with copulation, but if he has spent only six hours with a female without copulation, no preference is seen for that female. If a low dose of the dopamine receptor agonist apomorphine is infused into the nucleus accumbens, a dopamine terminal area, during the six-hour cohabitation session, the male subsequently shows a preference for that female in the choice test.[37] If the dopamine receptor antagonist haloperidol is infused into the nucleus accumbens of the male during the day-long cohabitation period, no partner preference is observed in the choice test; similarly, if haloperidol is infused into the nucleus accumbens of the female during the cohabitation period, no partner preference is observed in the choice test.[38] When dopamine levels were recorded using intracerebral microdialysis of the nucleus accumbens, increased levels were seen during mating in female prairie voles.[39] These findings converge to support a critical role for dopamine in the formation of pair bonds. Dopamine released during cohabitation and copulation may produce incentive learning, increasing the incentive value of the mate. Subsequently, the mate may be a strong conditioned incentive stimulus with an increased ability to elicit approach and other responses.

Dopamine and social cooperation in hamsters

Studies of male Syrian hamsters (*Mesocricetus auratus*) implicate dopamine in social reward. Adult male hamsters show a conditioned preference for a place previously associated with the scent of female hamster vaginal secretions. Juvenile males and gonadectomized adult males fail to show a conditioned place preference but can be induced to do so by injecting testosterone before pairing sessions, showing the dependence of sexual responses on this steroid hormone. Low doses of the dopamine receptor-blocking drug haloperidol given during pairing sessions blocked the development of a place preference to the female scent.[40] Postmortem studies show increased dopamine metabolites in the medial preoptic area of adult but not juvenile male Syrian hamsters exposed to the scent of female vaginal sectetions.[41] Female Syrian hamsters show a preference for a place previously associated with sexual behavior with a male, and dopamine receptor antagonist attenuates this learning.[42] These findings are consistent with many previous studies showing that incentive learning in place conditioning depends on dopamine and extend the role of dopamine to incentive learning based on sociosexual cues. They also show a strong convergence of findings from humans, rats, voles, and hamsters implicating dopamine in social cooperation.

In the discussion of dopamine and social defeat in rats, the resident–intruder test was used and the focus was on the intruder rat (see earlier). What, if anything, happens to dopamine in the resident animal when he or she defeats an intruder? A recent study looked at this in the Syrian hamster. The authors noted that "animals with a history of winning aggressive interactions are more likely to succeed in future agonistic encounters" (p. 290),[43] a phenomenon termed the "winner effect." The authors found increased optical density of markers for the dopamine-synthesizing enzyme tyrosine hydroxylase in the nucleus accumbens shell of the male hamsters that had a history of winning aggressive interactions. Aggressive behavior is rewarding in many species; individual mice will learn to make an operant response for the introduction of an intruder conspecific that they can fight,[44] the rewarding effect of aggression in mice is reduced by dopamine receptor antagonists injected into the nucleus accumbens,[45] and aggressive behavior increases nucleus accumbens and prefrontal cortical dopamine measured by intracerebral microdialysis in rats.[46] These observations from mice and rats converge with the findings from hamsters to suggest that the winner effect may be associated with increased dopamine and incentive learning.

What is learned in the winner effect? The authors suggested that the winning hamsters "learned through training to display a behavioral repertoire that favored the likelihood of winning a dominant status" (p. 297).[43] This introduces an aspect of incentive learning that I have not yet discussed but cover more extensively in Chapter 11. Up until now, incentive learning has been defined as an increased ability of stimuli to elicit approach and other responses. The above quote focuses on the "other responses" part of incentive learning. Responses can be seen as having an efference copy in the brain;[47] at the same time that output signals are sent to the muscles to effect a response, a copy of those signals is sent to cortical sensory–motor areas. In those areas, this copy of responses is associated with the sensory, afferent inputs from environmental stimuli that are encountered when those responses are made. Incentive learning may act not only on environmental stimuli to increase their ability to elicit responses, but also on the efference copy of various associated responses to increase their likelihood of occurring in conjunction with the conditioned incentive stimuli in the environment. In this way, repeated aggressive encounters and winning might activate dopamine and increase the ability of stimuli from a subordinate conspecific to elicit specific responses from the dominant animal that are instrumental in favor of the likelihood of winning.

Recall from Miczek's work discussed in the section on dopamine and social cooperation in rats that defeated animals show elevated dopamine too. However, recall further from the same section that in defeated animals the dopamine signal decreases with repeated encounters with a dominant conspecific and social defeat (also see Chapter 6). As already discussed, the initial dopamine signal in defeated animals may be a response to novel or intense stimuli associated with being placed into another animal's territory. If social defeat occurs, the dopamine signal diminishes on subsequent encounters. The dominant animal that wins the encounter, however, may continue to have elevated dopamine associated with social encounters that it wins, leading to incentive learning about subordinate conspecifics and the responses that defeat them. This learning can maintain not only the incentive value of subordinate conspecific stimuli and effective fighting responses, but also operant responding for exposure to subordinate conspecifics and the opportunity to defeat them.

Dopamine and social cooperation in avians

Male, but not female, songbirds sing socially *directed* songs; these songs are produced in response to another individual or serve to influence the behavior of another individual, normally to attract females or to repel male competitors. Directed song may be rewarded by the successful attraction of a mate or by threat reduction resulting from successfully repelling an intruder. Male songbirds also sing *undirected* song that may have a social function, but it remains poorly understood.[48] Some authors refer to the situations that result in directed versus undirected song as "social context." I will focus on directed song.

Lauren Riters at the University of Wisconsin in Madison has studied male European starlings (*Sturnus vulgaris*). In the medial preoptic area, a dopamine terminal region, the optical density of tyrosine hydroxylase, a marker for dopamine, was found to be correlated with the proportion of time spent in female-directed song but not undirected song. Song took place during a 45-minute test period and the birds were sacrificed immediately afterward.[49] In a related study in zebra finches (*Taeniopygia guttata*), Riters and her colleagues found increased optical density of tyrosine hydroxylase in the nucleus accumbens of birds paired with an opposite-sex partner versus those paired with a same-sex partner. Tyrosine hydroxylase optical density in the ventral tegmental area, location of dopamine cell bodies, was positively correlated with number of directed songs and the quantity of courtship behaviors received from the partner during the observation periods before sacrifice.[50] These finding reveal the influence of social context on birdsong and implicate dopamine specifically in directed song.

Researchers at Duke University in Durham, North Carolina, used intracerebral microdialysis of a region of the striatum in zebra finches; they found that singing directed song increased dopamine levels more than undirected song,[51] further implicating dopamine in directed song. Electrophysiological studies at the RIKEN Brain Science Institute in Wako City, Saitama Prefecture, Japan, revealed evidence of increased activity in dopamine neurons located in the ventral tegmental area of male zebra finches that had seen a female or had seen and sung to a female (directed song) in the previous hour. Finches that had engaged in undirected song did not show this effect.[52] Although none of these studies provides high temporal resolution that would allow activity in dopamine neurons to be linked to a specific event, they provide evidence for a link between activity in dopaminergic neurons and directed song.

Midbrain dopamine neurons were found to reflect different affiliation phenotypes in five species of estrildid finches. Two of the species were territorial, two were highly gregarious, and one was moderately gregarious. Birds were individually exposed to a same-sex conspecific for 90 minutes and then sacrificed for immunohistochemical studies. Results revealed a larger number of dopamine cells in the caudal region of the ventral tegmental area of the three gregarious species that form relatively large groups versus the two territorial species that form smaller groups.[52] These findings reveal a link between dopamine and sociality with more social species having more dopamine cells. The authors of this paper also observed that individual male birds that were identified as "courters" (displaying high levels of directed singing to females) in observational studies had more dopamine cells in this brain region than "noncourters." Referring to the link between dopamine neurons and reward-related learning, they suggested that "divergent social phenotypes may arise due to the differential assignment of 'incentive value' to conspecific stimuli" (p. 8737).[53]

It follows from these observations of dopamine as the dependent variable that interfering with dopaminergic neurotransmission will affect directed song and that is what has been found. In one study, a dopamine receptor antagonist was infused during song learning, that is, the sensitive period for song memorization, in juvenile male zebra finches. As adults, these males showed less courtship and copulatory behavior, implicating dopamine during the development of song in the subsequent effectiveness of directed song.[54] Male adult zebra finches treated with a dopamine receptor antagonist sang less directed song and showed fewer courtship displays.[55] Further work from Lauren Riter's lab showed that female European starlings were less responsive to male directed song when the females had been injected with a dopamine receptor agonist.[56] Recall from the discussion in Chapter 7 that dopamine receptor agonists can occlude the normal dopamine signal produced by rewarding stimuli, thereby interfering with incentive learning about specific reward-related stimuli. In fact, Riters and her colleague reported that the impairment they observed in their female starlings treated with a dopamine receptor agonist resulted from increased responses to purple martin songs, song stimuli that usually have low incentive value and elicit little approach. It has been found that the variability of birdsong is lower when a female is present. Arthur Leblois from the University of Paris Descartes showed that a dopamine receptor blocker infused into Area X, an avian brain region that receives dopamine inputs and is homologous with the dopaminoceptive striatum in mammals, increased the variability of directed song in zebra finches, making it more like undirected song.[57] The important role of dopamine in controlling the variability of directed song was recently confirmed in studies using distorted feedback; recordings from ventral tegmental area dopaminergic neurons projecting to Area X showed that they fired when an expected distortion failed to occur.[58] These results further show the importance of dopamine for context-dependent, directed song.

Perhaps the way to think about birdsong is to begin with a male bird's natural motivation to find a mate. Song can be instrumental in attaining an unconditioned stimulus (a female) that mitigates that motivation, in an analogous manner to how operant responses like manipulating environmental stimuli can be instrumental in attaining food stimuli by hungry rats. Directed song is normally elicited by the presence of a female and sometimes results in mate attraction and copulation. As discussed in Chapter 5, copulation may lead to increased dopamine neuron firing and incentive learning about the sexual and related stimuli that preceded copulation. Those stimuli would be the specific female encountered and the efference copy of the song that was successful in attracting her. This might have the effect of decreasing the variability of directed song compared to undirected song, as has been observed. Also, as discussed in Chapter 5, conditioned incentive stimuli acquire the ability themselves to activate dopamine neurons. Subsequent sightings of the particular female might be expected therefore to activate dopamine and the motor responses that produce directed singing that is instrumental in attracting the female. Supporting this suggestion, the results from the RIKEN Brain Science Institute study discussed earlier showed that just the sight of a female was sufficient to activate dopamine neurons. Another alternative is that the sight of a female for a male songbird, like the taste of food for a rat, has the unconditioned ability to activate dopamine neurons.[59] Incentive learning produced by increased dopamine would increase the ability of stimuli associated with that specific female to elicit approach and other responses (directed singing) in the future. This system may contribute to the formation of monogamous pair bonds in songbirds like those seen in prairie voles.

On a broader group level, members of species that form larger flocks have more dopamine cells than members of species that form smaller flocks. The gregarious species that form larger flocks may release more dopamine when exposed to a conspecific male or female, making conspecific stimuli incentive stimuli, increasing the ability of conspecifics to elicit approach responses and facilitating large aggregations of individuals. As discussed later, a similar mechanism may underlie shoaling in fish.

Simonyan et al., a group of American researchers, review the role of dopamine in birdsong and human speech. They provide an excellent overview of the comparative anatomy of vocal control systems in songbirds and humans; both have a strong dopamine neuron component. They review some of the evidence from songbirds already discussed here implicating dopamine in social context-dependent (directed) song that depends on the presence of a female. They review the limited evidence implicating dopamine in human speech. Evidence comes mostly from neurological and psychiatric patients. For example, patients with Parkinson's disease, suffering from a loss of dopamine neurons (Chapter 9), show profound changes in voice quality, including limited pitch range, decreased amplitude, and reduced accuracy of articulation. As the disease progresses, many patients develop further speech-related problems, including difficulties with phonological processing, complex syntax, and language comprehension. The authors make no mention of dopamine and incentive learning.[60] In this chapter, I have discussed evidence from a range of species that implicates dopamine in social rewards produced by social cooperation. The studies with songbirds are particularly interesting because they provide evidence that social rewards, that activate dopamine neurons and produce incentive learning, contribute to the acquisition of birdsong by juveniles, and alter the structure of birdsong in adults, for example by decreasing its spectral variability. If there is strong homology between song control systems in songbirds and language control systems in humans, as argued by Simonyan et al., it follows that in humans dopamine-mediated incentive learning may also contribute to the acquisition and maintenance of language. In 1957, BF Skinner published his book, *Verbal Behavior*.[61] In it, he provides a reinforcement-learning account of language acquisition. In 1959, linguist Noam Chomsky from the Massachusetts Institute of Technology famously criticized Skinner's work, arguing that Skinner's framework could not account for the novel utterances observed in language, suggesting instead that language is controlled by innate organizational structures. Chomsky discusses many examples of learning in the absence of explicit rewarding stimuli, for example latent learning, as further evidence against a role for reinforcement in language learning;[62] at the time the concept of multiple memory systems discussed in Chapter 4 was in its infancy. If dopamine-mediated incentive learning, produced by rewarding stimuli including those provided by social cooperation, eventually is found to contribute to language acquisition and maintenance, Skinner may yet be vindicated.

Dopamine has been implicated in social cooperation in non-passerine avian species too. In male galliform Japanese quail (*Coturnix japonica*), exposure to a receptive female led to increases in extracellular dopamine in the medial preoptic area, a dopamine terminal region. Increases were seen only in males that subsequently copulated with the female.[63] In this case the female served as an incentive stimulus in sexually motivated males. Injection of dopamine receptor antagonists into the medial preoptic area decreased measures of sexual interest and behavior in Japanese quail.[64] Results implicating dopamine in sexual reward are consistent with the findings from many studies with mammals some of which are reviewed in Chapter 5. Increased dopamine activity during exposure to a female and during sexual activity may increase the incentive value of female-related stimuli and associated environmental stimuli, enhancing their ability to elicit approach and other responses in the future.

Dopamine and social cooperation in reptiles

Reptiles engage in cooperative sexual interactions and dopamine has been implicated. In two species of whiptail lizards, desert grassland (*Cnemidophorus uniparens*) and little striped (*C. inornatus*), treatment with a dopamine receptor agonist increased the proportion of individuals mounting and decreased the latency to mount.[65] Tyrosine hydroxylase is a dopamine-synthesizing enzyme; greater levels of tyrosine hydroxylase were found in the dopamine cell-body regions of little striped whiptail lizards that were more sexually vigorous.[66] In leopard geckos, a dopamine receptor antagonist decreased the display of court-ship behavior in males.[66] Although these studies did not evaluate incentive learning, results are consistent with those from mammals and birds and, as the authors suggest, the "similar distributions of dopaminergic cells between mam-mals, birds, and reptiles may have similar functions across taxa" (p. 487).[65]

Reptiles form dominance relationships and dopamine has been implicated in the underlying brain mechanisms. Researchers at Stanford University in California and at the University of South Dakota in Vermillion evaluated dom-inance relationships in Carolina anoles (*Anolis carolinensis*). In a natural agon-istic interaction between two males, activity in the sympathetic nervous system darkens the postorbital skin (eyespot) and the darkness of the eyespot serves as a signal that inhibits opponent aggression. By artificially coloring the eyespot black in one member in a dyadic interaction and green in the other member, it was observed that in every case, the anole with the black-colored eyespot won the interaction and became the dominant male. Postmortem evaluation of dopamine and its metabolite 3,4-dihydroxyphenylacetic acid (DOPAC) re-vealed elevated levels in a number of regions, including the striatum and nu-cleus accumbens, dopamine terminal areas, and in the substantia nigra and ventral tegmental area, location of dopaminergic cell bodies with afferents to the striatum and nucleus accumbens, in the dominant anoles. Submissive anoles showed increased dopamine and metabolite in the medial and lateral amygdala.[67] Elevated dopamine in the amygdala in defeated animals may reflect a first-encounter effect that would gradually diminish with repeated encounters as observed in rats, discussed earlier, and as discussed in Chapter 6. Evidence of increased dopamine in the striatum and nucleus accumbens in dominant anoles is consistent with findings in dominant rats and may reflect incentive learning about stimuli from and associated with the submissive male. The authors stated that dopamine may "be associated with maintenance of an increased readiness to perform contextually appropriate stereotypical movements associated with dominant status" (p. 98).[67] Although they did not mention it by name, incentive learning is the acquisition by stimuli (context) of an increased ability to elicit approach and other responses (stereotypical movements associated with dom-inant status). Perhaps dopamine produces incentive learning in reptiles.

There are some further data suggesting a relationship between dopamine and incentive learning in reptiles. Jon Sakata and David Crews from the University of Austin at Texas exposed male leopard geckos (*Eublepharis macularius*) in their home cage to sexually receptive females each day for ten days. Each day the test period began by removing materials from the geckos' home cage (e.g., water dish, brick, shelter) and observing their behavior for five minutes before introducing the female. The female remained for five minutes unless the male initiated sexual activity in which case the session was extended to allow for copulation. Control males had the materials from their home cages removed, were observed for five minutes, and were then observed for another five minutes but they were never exposed to a female. The researchers observed increases in scent marking during the pre-female introduction period in the experimental group compared to the controls,[68] revealing clear evidence of conditioning. In a subsequent paper, Crews and collaborators showed that leopard geckos with a similar incubation temperature to those that showed conditioned responding to cues signaling a sexually receptive female have higher levels of dopamine in the nucleus accumbens.[69] Although these data are correlational, they are consistent with a role for dopamine in incentive learning in reptiles.

Dopamine and social cooperation in amphibians

Few studies of dopamine and social cooperation in amphibians have appeared. In a field study, male green tree frogs (*Hyla cinerea*) were captured, injected with a dopamine D2 receptor agonist and released. Decreased advertisement calling, used to attract females, was observed in these frogs compared with control frogs that were captured, injected with saline, and released.[70] This finding implicates dopamine in song production in male frogs. Neurotoxic lesions of dopamine cells in female gray treefrogs (*H. versicolor*) decreased approach to a loudspeaker playback of a standard mating call;[71] as dopamine depletions are known to decrease motor behavior even in frogs,[72] this result does not allow an unequivocal conclusion about dopamine and incentive learning, but results are consistent with a decreased incentive motivational effect of the male call in treated females. Juvenile Mexican spadefoot toads (*Spea multiplicata*) of both sexes normally approach male mating calls. They were exposed to male mating calls and then their brains were assayed for dopamine and other monoamines. Significant increases of dopamine were observed in the tegmentum, a brain region that contains dopamine cell bodies, of toads that were exposed to male mating song prior to sacrifice compared with similarly handled control toads that did not hear calls. Increases in the neurotransmitters norepinephrine and epinephrine and the serotonin metabolite 5-hydroxyindoleacetic acid were also observed.[73] Results are consistent with a role for dopamine and incentive learning in social communication, but further studies are needed.

Dopamine and social cooperation in fish

Fish shoal and school for protection from predation,[74] suggesting that conspecific proximity may serve as a rewarding stimulus by providing relative safety from an external threat. In zebrafish (*Danio rerio*), recent hatchlings do not shoal, but shoaling behavior develops gradually during the first several weeks post-fertilization. The average nearest-neighbor distance in groups of ten fish is used to quantify shoaling. Christine Buske and Robert Gerlai at the Mississauga Campus of the University of Toronto observed that average nearest-neighbor distance decreased over the first ten weeks after fertilization. During the same period, whole-brain levels of dopamine, its metabolite DOPAC, and serotonin and its metabolite, 5-hydroxyindoleacetic acid, increased.[75] Although these results are only correlational and both dopamine and serotonin changed over the same period, the correlation between dopamine and shoaling is consistent with a role for dopamine in social behavior. As discussed earlier for flocking in various estrildid finch species, perhaps dopamine released by proximity to a conspecific zebrafish produces incentive learning about conspecific stimuli that promotes shoaling. In a related study, researchers observed that zebrafish showed a preference for conspecifics of the same color variant as those they were exposed to during development,[76] suggesting that incentive learning may have been occurring during the development of shoaling behavior. Incentive learning has been observed in zebrafish. Lina Al-Imari and Robert Gerlai presented a colored cue card paired with a small group of conspecifics to individual zebrafish and then observed that the individual zebrafish had a preference for the colored cue card in a maze task.[77]

A dopamine receptor antagonist disrupts social preference in zebrafish. Gerlai and his collaborators exposed individual zebrafish to a choice between two computer screens at opposite ends of a rectangular aquarium. One screen showed a small shoal of conspecifics and the other was dark. Untreated fish moved closer to the synthetic shoal and approached it more than fish treated with a dopamine receptor antagonist that showed a dose-dependent decrease in these measures.[78] Results implicate dopamine in the maintenance of incentive learning about conspecific fish. In a related study, Gerlai and his associates made postmortem measures of dopamine and DOPAC in several brain areas following exposure to animated images of other zebrafish. They observed an increase and the magnitude was greater with longer exposure time (15 vs. 5 minutes). They also measured serotonin and one of its metabolites and found no significant changes.[79] Their results suggest that exposure to a conspecific leads to enhanced dopaminergic neurotransmission in the brain of the zebrafish.

Dopamine has been implicated in agonistic behavior in fish. Juvenile Arctic char (*Salvelinus alpinus*) form social hierarchies. Researchers at Uppsala University in Sweden studied pairs of char placed together in a tank. Prior to placement in the tank, one individual was injected with 3,4-dihydroxyphenylalanine (L-DOPA), a precursor of dopamine that is made into dopamine in the brain.

In a significant proportion of tests, the L-DOPA-injected fish won the aggressive interaction, becoming the dominant fish.[80] This result was found with a low dose of L-DOPA but not with higher doses, suggesting that a small increase in dopaminergic neurotransmission may provide an advantage in social interactions but not a large increase. This relates to the possible occlusion of dopamine signals by high levels of dopamine receptor activation as discussed in Chapter 7 and this idea is developed further in Chapter 9, where I discuss the implications of elevated levels of dopaminergic neurotransmission in humans for effective social functioning. One of the authors of the Arctic char paper co-authored a more recent paper with three researchers from Portugal evaluating the effects of winning or losing a dyadic social encounter on telencephalic monoaminergic neuronal activity in zebrafish. Winners showed elevated serotonin and dopamine activity. The authors suggested that dopamine activity in the telencephalon "may be representative of social reward" (p. 17 in Teles et al.).[81] As discussed earlier for hamsters, mice, rats, and voles, winning an agonistic social interaction may produce reward-related learning, increasing the incentive value of stimuli from, and associated with, the defeated conspecific.

Dopamine and social cooperation in insects

Insects show reward-related learning and dopamine has been implicated.[82] Furthermore, dopamine appears to be involved in social cooperation in insects. Insects are invertebrates and are part of the phylum Arthropoda, which also includes arachnids (e.g., spiders), myriapods (e.g., centipedes), and crustaceans (e.g., lobsters). As I discuss in Chapter 11, dopamine systems are found in arthropods. Nicholas Strausfeld from the University of Arizona in Tucson and Frank Hirsh from the Institute of Psychiatry at Kings College London in the UK have provided an in-depth review of the arthropod central complex, showing its strong homology with the basal ganglia of vertebrates, including a strong dopaminergic innervation. They conclude that the arthropod central complex, like the vertebrate basal ganglia, underlies "the selection and maintenance of behavioral actions" (p. 157).[83] A number of studies have implicated dopamine in the social behavior of arthropods.

Neurogenetic methods were used to manipulate dopamine in the fruit fly (*Drosophila melanogaster*). Acute disruption of dopamine was found to almost eliminate social interactions in tests using pairs of dopamine-altered flies; this was observed in male–male pairs that normally engage in aggressive interactions and develop a dominance relationship and in male–female pairs where males normally engage in courtship behaviors.[84] Results might suggest that dopamine normally contributes to the establishment of social relationships through incentive learning and that disruption of dopaminergic neurotransmission interferes with this process. In the solitary large carpenter bee (*Xylocopa appendiculata*), dopamine was implicated in the territorial flight behavior of males, an important element of mating.[85] In recent studies by researchers at the Chinese Academy of Sciences in Beijing, dopamine was implicated in behavioral aggregation in migratory locusts (*Locusta migratoria*). Locusts switch between gregarious and solitary phases depending on environmental and genetic factors. The Chinese researchers identified some of the molecular genetic mechanisms underlying the phenotypic switch and showed that decreases in dopamine were associated with the transition from the gregarious to the solitary phase and, conversely, increases in dopamine were associated with the transition from solitary to gregarious.[86] As discussed in this chapter, dopamine was implicated in the flocking behavior of estrildid finches and the shoaling behavior of zebrafish, and it was suggested that dopamine may mediate incentive learning about conspecific stimuli that increases their ability to elicit approach and other responses that lead to aggregation. Perhaps a similar mechanism operates in migratory locusts to produce swarms.

Summary

In humans, brain areas that receive strong dopaminergic inputs, for example nucleus accumbens, dorsal striatum, and brain areas where dopaminergic cell bodies are located, for example ventral midbrain, are activated during cooperative social interactions, when viewing a picture of the person who is a romantic love partner or in a mother when she views a picture of her child. These findings suggest that these social stimuli are primary incentive stimuli with the ability to activate dopaminergic neurons and produce incentive learning. In non-human animals, nucleus accumbens dopamine is released during maternal behavior and dopamine neuron-specific lesions of this structure or the ventral tegmental area, the origin of dopaminergic projections to the nucleus accumbens, decrease maternal behavior. Lactating female rats will lever press for access to their pups and this access leads to increased dopamine release in the nucleus accumbens. These results suggest that pups may be primary incentive stimuli to their mothers and that dopamine-mediated incentive learning may contribute to maternal care; dopamine appears to interact with the neurohormones oxytocin and vasopressin in producing these effects. Animals will learn a conditioned preference for a place where they have previously engaged in social interaction with a conspecific. Adult male Syrian hamsters will learn a preference for a place associated with the scent of female vaginal secretions; microdialysis studies show that the scent increases dopamine release in the nucleus accumbens of males and a dopamine receptor antagonist given during pairing blocks the learning. These results implicate dopamine in incentive learning in sexually mature males to cues associated with a female. In songbirds dopamine release in striatal regions appears to be associated with directed song that is used, in part, to attract a mate; dopamine may influence the incentive value of the mate, increasing his or her ability to elicit approach and other responses in the future. Dopamine neuron number is higher in social species that form large groups compared with similar species that form small groups. Various observations link dopamine to social behavior in reptiles, amphibians, fish, and insects. Taken together, there is mounting evidence that dopamine-mediated incentive learning contributes to the organization of socially cooperative behavior in a wide range of species.

Chapter 9

Schizophrenia, Parkinson's disease, and attention deficit hyperactivity disorder

Schizophrenia and Parkinson's disease are both diseases of the dopamine system, and attention deficit hyperactivity disorder (ADHD) has a strong link to dopamine. In the case of schizophrenia, evidence suggests hyperfunction of dopamine, sometimes termed "hyperdopaminergia." In Parkinson's disease, dopamine neurons gradually die off, leaving the patient with too little dopamine, termed dopamine *hypo*function. Dopamine hypofunction may also be a feature of ADHD. A consideration of the symptomatology of these disorders should provide some insight into the normal function of dopamine in humans. They provide natural experiments in the effects of increased dopamine and decreased dopamine, respectively. By recognizing the role of dopamine in incentive learning and inverse incentive learning, we can begin to understand how extremes in these forms of learning may account for some of the symptoms of schizophrenia, Parkinson's disease, and ADHD

Schizophrenia is a psychiatric illness described in the early twentieth century by German psychiatrist Emil Kraepelin (1856–1926), who named the illness "dementia praecox" in his famous textbook on psychiatry.[1] Swiss psychiatrist Eugen Bleuler (1857–1939) subsequently coined the term "schizophrenia" and described the characteristics of the syndrome in young adults.[2] Schizophrenia is characterized by a number of symptoms that are often grouped into three categories, termed positive, negative, and cognitive. Positive symptoms include delusions and hallucinations and are perhaps the best-known features of schizophrenia. Negative symptoms include a loss of emotional expression and motivation, neglect of personal hygiene, and social withdrawal. Cognitive symptoms include impairments of verbal and visuospatial (declarative) memory, attention, executive function, and processing speed. Cognitive symptoms were not included in the *Diagnostics and Statistical Manual (DSM) IV-TR* of the American Psychiatric Association,[3] which for years was the gold standard in North America for psychiatric diagnoses. However, cognitive symptoms are now broadly seen as a central feature of schizophrenia, they are included as associated features of schizophrenia in the *DSM V*,[4] and research and therapeutic efforts are being directed towards the amelioration of these symptoms.[5]

Parkinson's disease is a progressive neurological illness first identified by James Parkinson's in 1817.[6] It is characterized by motor and mental slowing, sometimes termed "bradykinesia" and "bradyphrenia," respectively. Motor symptoms often begin in patients on one side of the body, that is, unilaterally, as a relative weakness in an arm or leg. Symptoms progress over months and years to both sides of the body, leaving the patient with Parkinson's disease with difficulty initiating movements. Muscles show rigidity when moved passively. The rate and auditory volume of speech is lessened and writing becomes smaller and smaller, eventually micrographic. Often there is tremor of the hands, showing the classic pill-rolling movements. Sometimes a patient with Parkinson's disease who is trying to begin to walk will find himself stuck, unable to move. Sensory input, such as a parallel series of lines painted on the floor, have been found to facilitate walking in such patients. Patients with Parkinson's disease show mental slowing, too, but remain aware of their environment.

ADHD is characterized by inattention and/or hyperactivity and impulsivity.[4] It was originally described in children but in the latter half of the twentieth century began to be recognized as a disorder that persists into adulthood.[7] Many authors credit Scottish physician Sir Alexander Crichton (1773–1856) with the first description of the disorder in his 1798 publication on the "*nature and origins of mental derangement* ... "[8] In the 1930s it was serendipitously discovered by US physician Charles Bradley (1902–1979) that children with learning and behavioral problems, possibly some with ADHD, when treated with Benzedrine, showed marked improvement in school performance and were better able to focus on a task.[9] Benzedrine is racemic amphetamine, a psychomotor stimulant drug, known now to augment monoaminergic (including noradrenergic and dopaminergic) neurotransmission. This was a puzzling finding because a well-known stimulant drug had an apparently calming effect. After dopaminergic neurons were discovered in the brain (see Chapter 11) and it was recognized that amphetamine augmented dopaminergic neurotransmission, Bradley's finding provided one of the first possible links between ADHD and dopamine.

In this chapter, I discuss schizophrenia and Parkinson's disease with regard to the role of dopamine in incentive learning. You will see that this perspective provides unique insights into these dopamine diseases and their response to medication. I also discuss ADHD, its dopamine and incentive learning links, and its possible relationship to Parkinson's disease.

Schizophrenia and dopamine

If schizophrenia results from hyperdopaminergia, do sufferers of this debilitating condition have excessive incentive learning? The evidence suggests that they do. Recall that incentive learning is the acquisition by neutral stimuli of an increased ability to elicit approach and other responses; "other responses" could include pushing, pulling, digging, biting, and so on, or even particular vocalizations, depending on the situation and the natural abilities of the animal (Chapters 2–4 and 8). If people with schizophrenia have excessive incentive learning, too many stimuli will become incentive stimuli, appearing attractive to the individual. Recall also that there are multiple memory systems (Chapter 4) and that although dopamine is important for incentive learning, it is not necessary for declarative memory formation. Declarative memory includes memory for facts and events and how they are associated with one another. Considering this information, it is possible to begin to understand the underlying brain processes that lead to schizophrenia.

First, I will review the evidence for dopamine hyperfunction in schizophrenia.[10] The dopamine hypothesis of schizophrenia is built on three pillars (Figure 9.1).[11] They are: (i) there is a strong positive relationship between the average daily dose of antipsychotic drugs used to treat schizophrenia and their ability to block dopamine D2 receptors; (ii) drugs that enhance dopaminergic neurotransmission are psychotogenic, that is, they produce psychotic symptoms indistinguishable from those seen in patients with schizophrenia; and (iii) postmortem neurochemical studies and imaging studies suggest elevated dopaminergic neurotransmission in schizophrenia.

The first pillar of the dopamine hypothesis comes from the now-classic finding of Phil Seeman and others, discussed in Chapter 7, that there is a strong positive relationship between the average daily dose of antipsychotic drugs used to treat schizophrenia and their ability to block dopamine D2 receptors in the dopamine projection brain region known as the striatum. In fact, the first modern antipsychotic medication to be widely used, chlorpromazine, was introduced into psychiatry in the 1950s,[12] but its ability to block dopamine receptors was not discovered until some years later (see Chapter 7). Since the discovery of this relationship, many newer antipsychotic medications have been developed and brought into use; all of them continue to share the common quality of blocking dopamine D2 receptors.[13]

The second pillar of the dopamine hypothesis is that drugs that enhance dopaminergic neurotransmission are psychotogenic.[14] Psychotogenic drugs include amphetamine and cocaine, both of which enhance dopaminergic neurotransmission by augmenting the amount of dopamine in synapses. Psychiatrists

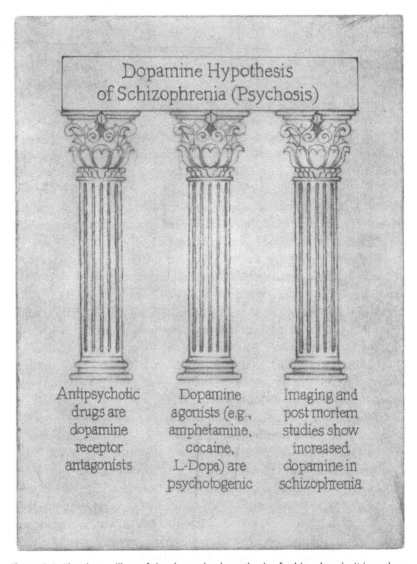

Figure 9.1 *The three pillars of the dopamine hypothesis of schizophrenia*: It is perhaps more accurate to refer to this as the "dopamine hypothesis of psychosis", the positive symptoms of schizophrenia, as negative and cognitive symptoms are generally refractory to the effects of dopamine receptor antagonist antipsychotic medications.

who work in emergency medicine sometimes treat patients who are in an acute psychotic state that is indistinguishable from that seen in schizophrenia. The treatment is often to prescribe antipsychotic medications that, as just described for the first pillar, are dopamine receptor blockers. Most psychotic patients respond to these medications. It is sometimes only after the patient is stabilized and a history can be taken that it is learned that the patient had been abusing a psychomotor stimulant and that the psychosis was related to that drug abuse. A related phenomenon is seen in patients with Parkinson's disease who are treated with drugs such as L-3,4-dihydroxyphenylalanine that enhance dopaminergic neurotransmission. Some patients develop hallucinations and delusions when taking these medications.[15] In this case, as in the case of psychomotor stimulant abuse, it appears that enhanced dopaminergic neurotransmission leads to symptoms like those seen in schizophrenia, supporting the second pillar of the dopamine hypothesis.

The third pillar is evidence from postmortem neurochemical studies and imaging studies suggesting elevated dopaminergic neurotransmission in schizophrenia. In postmortem studies, when brain tissue from dopamine terminal regions, including the striatum (caudate and putamen), was assayed to evaluate the density of dopamine D2-like receptors it was found that the density was higher in the brains of patients with schizophrenia compared with age- and sex-matched controls who did not have a diagnosis of schizophrenia.[16] This was an exciting finding but it came into question because of the possible influence of antipsychotic medications on dopamine receptor density. It had been found from animal studies that a period of daily treatment with an antipsychotic drug, a known dopamine receptor blocker, led to an apparently compensatory elevation in the level of dopamine D2-like receptors.[17] If patients with schizophrenia had been treated with antipsychotic medications, and most of them had, perhaps the elevated density of dopamine receptors was a consequence of treatment and did not reflect a state that existed prior to treatment. One solution to this complication is to try to do the same study using postmortem brain tissue from people who had a diagnosis of schizophrenia or probable schizophrenia in their lifetime but who had not taken medication for a substantial period of time, for example one year, before their death. If these people still showed elevated dopamine-receptor density, the concern about treatment effects would be assuaged. Such studies were carried out by psychiatrist Tim Crow and co-workers at the Medical Research Council Clinical Research Centre located at Northwick Park Hospital in North London, UK, and they found a significantly elevated density of dopamine receptors in the striatum and substantia nigra, the origin of dopamine cells, compared with age- and sex-matched controls.[18] These were promising results for the dopamine hypothesis, but the nagging possibility that the effect was still linked to medication history remained. One solution is to find brains from those rare people who had a diagnosis of schizophrenia or possible schizophrenia but who had not received medication up to the time of their death (often at a young age and frequently by suicide). In a review paper, Phil

Seeman reports that Tim Crow and his colleagues presented dopamine receptor binding data from individuals with schizophrenia or probable schizophrenia who had never received antipsychotic medication at a professional meeting in 1981. Again they found elevated dopamine-receptor densities in the striatum.[19] The reliability of the findings from this study may be limited by questions about the possible influence of death by suicide on brain neurochemistry. Although findings generally appeared to support the dopamine hypothesis, doubts about their interpretation remained.

A far more direct approach to evaluating the status of dopamine receptors in the brains of people with schizophrenia is to look at those receptors in the brains of living participants, especially in individuals who have never before received antipsychotic medication. The advent of neuroimaging techniques, including positron emission tomography (PET), in the 1970s afforded this possibility (see Chapter 5). In one study, Anissa Abi-Dargham and her co-workers from Columbia University in New York used a variation of PET known as single-photon computerized emission tomography that made it possible to evaluate the occupancy of dopamine D2-like receptors by dopamine in the brain. They recruited patients with schizophrenia symptoms but who had never received antipsychotic medication and imaged them twice. The first imaging session provided a measure of binding of a dopamine D2 receptor ligand in the striatum, a dopamine terminal region. Prior to a second imaging session, they treated the patients with a drug that depletes endogenous brain dopamine. This treatment leads to an increase in binding of the D2 receptor ligand because the ligand can now bind to D2 receptors that were previously occupied by endogenous dopamine. The researchers found that the increase for the schizophrenia group was significantly greater than the increase for the control group.[20] This showed that in the normal, non-depleted state, more D2 receptors are occupied by dopamine in people with schizophrenia than in matched controls. This excellent work, and a number of related studies that have now been done,[21] provide strong evidence for the third pillar of the dopamine hypothesis stating that the brains of people with schizophrenia will have significantly higher levels of dopaminergic neurotransmission.

In the early part of the twenty-first century I had added a fourth pillar to the evidence for the dopamine hypothesis based on findings from genetics studies using linkage analyses and candidate gene association approaches. Some findings appeared to identify an association between genes (e.g., *DRD1*, *DRD2*) coding for molecules that are involved in dopamine signaling and schizophrenia.[22] However, in recent years these findings have been repudiated.[23] One of the problems that dogged genetics research for many years was a general failure to replicate. It is now clear that candidate gene studies suffered from limited power because of small sample sizes and low density of genetic markers, contributing to this failure. A further difficulty relates to clinical heterogeneity and the need for endophenotyping;[24] a number of authors commented that Bleuler's notion of the disease as the "Group of Schizophrenias" may better reflect the reality of the situation.[25] Modern genetic approaches involve genome-wide association studies that have begun to produce replicable findings. These studies can analyze up to five million genetic markers that tag a high proportion of single-nucleotide polymorphisms (SNPs) in the human genome. They can also identify copy number variants, that is, chromosomal deletions and duplications. This approach has led to the discovery of a number of SNPs that are reliably associated with schizophrenia.[26] For example, the gene *MIR137* is associated with schizophrenia as are four other loci that contain predicted *MIR137* target sites. *MIR137* codes for a microRNA that regulates neuronal maturation and adult neurogenesis; this may reveal developmental mechanisms contributing to the etiology of schizophrenia.[27] How the genetic evidence eventually links to the hyperdopaminergia observed in schizophrenia awaits further study. At present, it is premature to include a genetics pillar in the evidence for the dopamine hypothesis, although it may eventually be possible to do so.

In Chapter 3, I discuss incentive learning in rats; learning was based on food presentations in an operant chamber, dopamine-enhancing drug presentations in conditioned place preference and conditioned activity procedures, and shock avoidance. In each case it is possible to see that through the action of dopamine a particular subset of environmental stimuli acquired an enhanced ability to elicit approach and other responses. In Chapter 8 I discuss the role of dopamine in social cooperation and there, too, it is possible to see that through the action of dopamine, a particular subset of social stimuli, that is, stimuli from conspecifics, acquires an increased ability to attract. How can this information help us to understand schizophrenia?

For many years I have lectured at my home university and at other universities and conferences about dopamine, incentive learning, and schizophrenia. In the early years before imaging studies had linked dopamine projection brain areas to social cooperation and romantic love, and perhaps because my own thinking about these topics was not as clear as it is now, I struggled with the jump from the findings of animal studies to the understanding of schizophrenia. I would go over the results of animal studies showing that dopamine receptor antagonist drugs blocked the acquisition of incentive leaning and that these drugs produced a gradual loss of incentive learning in pre-trained animals. I would discuss conditioning produced by dopamine enhancers such as amphetamine or cocaine. Then I would review the evidence for hyperactive dopamine in schizophrenia. This would lead to making the critical link between incentive learning and schizophrenia, as I suggested in some publications in the 1980s.[28]

I often felt that the leap from incentive learning to schizophrenia was the weakest part of my presentation, and in the next paragraph I will explain why. However, before doing that, it is noteworthy that there is now accumulating evidence from imaging studies of altered blood oxygenation level-dependent (BOLD) changes in dopamine-innervated brain areas associated with incentive learning in schizophrenia. Earlier evidence had come from studies that used medicated patients with schizophrenia; since it has been found that antipsychotic medications themselves affect reward signaling in imaging studies, those studies did not provide unequivocal evidence.[29] Some studies using unmedicated patients avoided this problem. German researchers from universities in Berlin and Bochum trained people with schizophrenia to perform a reaction-time task with visual cues signaling target stimuli that could be responded to for monetary gain or loss avoidance. The researchers observed that patients—compared with controls—showed reduced activation in the ventral striatum, including the nucleus accumbens, during reward-indicating cues. They suggested that elevated dopamine in patients with schizophrenia led to a partial occlusion of the reward signal (see Chapter 7), leading to the observed reduction in BOLD changes associated with monetary reward.[30] These results are consistent with elevated dopamine in schizophrenia and a resultant impairment of incentive learning.[31]

There are at least two reasons why I had not found the linking of incentive learning and schizophrenia completely satisfactory or felt that it was not as convincing as it could be in the earlier years of studying this fascinating topic. One reason is that most of the examples of incentive learning that I used came from animal studies.[32] Although the commonalities among species are well recognized and similar functions of homologous brain systems from species to species have been identified and integrated into evolutionary explanations, it still remained difficult to see immediately how a rat pressing a lever for food could have anything to do with understanding schizophrenia. The other reason is that memories created by incentive learning are non-declarative. I used to try to think of incentive learning in people. It seemed clear that people went to the kitchen for food when they were hungry, but it was difficult to imagine incentive learning in that situation, perhaps because it all seems to involve learning that relies on declarative memory. I have thought that the wide availability of food items in our rich, Western, urban world makes it very difficult to identify specific food-related stimuli that have an increased ability to attract. It is easier to think of incentive learning taking place in an ancestral environment where food sources were less numerous and food, in general, was less plentiful, especially during some times of the year. There it might be easier to identify particular environmental stimuli that have acquired an increased ability to attract.

What did seem to resonate better with my audiences was the idea that incentive learning is also involved in our attraction to certain people. As I discuss in Chapter 8, dopamine neurons appear to be activated by cooperative social interactions and, as a result, certain other individuals and the stimuli associated with them attain incentive value, having an increased ability to elicit approach and other responses. Remember that this form of learning relies on non-declarative memory, meaning that it takes place outside of conscious awareness. In this manner, dopamine insidiously molds our social landscape, creating peaks and valleys of social attractiveness of other people, as well as producing incentive learning about non-social-reward-related stimuli.

What would happen if the dopamine system were overactive in a social situation? When dopamine functions normally, it is activated by cooperative social interactions and the cooperators putatively acquire incentive value. Perhaps dopamine neuron firing is inhibited by non-cooperative social interactions producing inverse incentive learning and decreasing the ability of some people to attract. If dopamine is overactive, it is possible that excessive incentive learning takes place, resulting in other individuals, as well as non-social stimuli (i.e., objects in the environment), inappropriately acquiring increased incentive value. What would this be like for the affected individual? Recall that incentive learning is non-conscious—the affected individual might feel drawn or attracted to people in a social situation, as well as to other stimuli and not know why. They may not even know the people to whom they are attracted. Diagnosticians might identify this phenomenon as "overinclusive thinking" or "imagination out of control."[33]

It is here that recalling multiple memory systems (Chapter 4) helps to understand what might be taking place in the brain of the affected individual. The individual is finding himself in a social situation where he is attracted to other individuals (i.e., those individuals have become incentive stimuli); he may not even know some of them. As Kraepelin put it, "The patient notices that he is looked at in a peculiar way ... " (p. 27); a patient said, "I feel myself referred to here" (p. 31).[1] This is putatively occurring because of faulty dopamine function. The individual's declarative memory capacities, however, may be relatively intact. Thus, he may formulate an interpretation of the world as it is appearing to him. For example, "These other individuals must think I am an extraordinary person," or "These other individuals are all out to get me." You may recognize these as the bare bones of respective delusions of grandeur or persecution. In either case, the affected individual is attributing importance to stimuli, in this case social stimuli from other people, who ought to be ignored. I do not mean to imply that anyone "ought" to be ignored. Everyone has inherent dignity and equal and inalienable rights. But each of us benefits from our individual social incentive learning, making some individuals more attractive than others, in the incentive-learning sense, because those individuals cooperate with us and are important for our survival. If the system that mediates that social incentive learning is overactive, too many individuals may become attractive. Other non-social stimuli also may inappropriately acquire incentive value. The "delusions" that follow can be reasonable interpretations of the world as the affected individual experiences it.

Yesterday morning I went by the beer store to pick up a case of beer (at the time of this writing there is a near monopoly in Ontario so that beer is only available at specified outlets). I parked my car, collected my empties from the trunk, and walked up to the door only to realize that the store did not open until 10:00 a.m.; it used to open at 9:30 a.m. As it was 9:50 a.m., I decided to wait. A few other people gathered in the ensuing minutes. One of them looked at another and quite demonstratively exclaimed how good his old friend looked and that his friend was Jesus. They hugged and high-fived. Then the first one began to proclaim quite loudly that he was the Father and Jesus was his son. "I am the Father of all of you," he loudly proclaimed. I was pleased that his delusion was grandiose rather than persecutory. I could not help but notice how he was apparently attributing excessive importance to stimuli that normally would be deemed unremarkable, in this case his friend and the other people, myself included, waiting for the store to open. His delusion may have provided a way to make sense of that putatively ill-attributed importance. He was sorting his empties from bags into cases in a coordinated manner and did not seem to be drunk. I do not know if the person I witnessed yesterday morning had schizophrenia, but his behavior suggested to me that he might have that disorder.

Researchers have studied the content of delusions in patients with schizophrenia from different cultures and found that the content differs. For example, a group from Hanyang University of Medicine in Seoul, South Korea, Taiwan National University School of Medicine in Taipei, and Shanghai Medical Health Center in China compared the content of delusions in patients with schizophrenia from Seoul, Taipei, and Shanghai. They found similar frequencies of persecutory delusions or delusions of being controlled among the different patient groups. However, the themes of the delusions differed. Religious and supernatural themes were significantly more frequent in patients from Seoul and Taipei than those from Shanghai, perhaps reflecting the different frequency of religious beliefs in South Korea and Taiwan compared with mainland China. Patients from Shanghai were significantly more likely to have ideas of being poisoned or being pricked by poisonous needles than those from Seoul or Taipei, perhaps reflecting the widespread use of acupuncture in China.[34]

A related study from researchers at Government College Lahore in Pakistan and University of Birmingham in the UK compared three groups of patients with schizophrenia: British whites, British Pakistanis who had lived in Britain for an average of 17 years, and Pakistanis living in Lahore. They found similar frequencies of delusions of control and delusions of reference among the three groups, but they also found some differences. For example, the Lahore sample had a significantly higher frequency of delusions of persecution. The authors suggested that paranoid beliefs develop in a climate of suspicion where victimization is common and protection by government institutions is relatively poor; in such a climate it is common to be mistrustful towards others.[35] If excessive incentive learning takes place in such a social environment, delusions of persecution may be the most reasonable explanatory framework to formulate. This may account for the greater frequency of persecutory delusions in Lahore where the level of political, economic, and social turmoil was higher than in the UK at the time this study was done. By contrast, the British Whites and British Pakistanis had significantly higher frequencies of delusional explanations based on physical sources or machines than the Pakistanis from Lahore. The British individuals were surrounded by television, radio, electricity, computers, radar, and related technologies; many people have limited understanding of how these technologies work and of their limitations. Devices like televisions, radios, and mobile phones pick up messages from thin air. From these observations the authors comment that "perhaps [it is] not difficult to understand why this technology has found its way into delusions" (p. 135 in Suhail and Cochrane).[35] At the time that this work was published, that is, 2002, these electronic technologies were more present in the UK than in Lahore. Results suggest that stimuli in the immediate environment contribute most strongly to the content of psychotic delusions.

Researchers from the University Psychiatric Hospital at the University of Ljubljana, Slovenia, carried out a retrospective study of the content of delusions of patients with schizophrenia (or patients with a similar disorder under a different name before "schizophrenia" came into use) using case notes during the period 1881– 2000. They randomly sampled ten records, of five males and five females, from each decade for a total of 120 records. They found significant changes in the frequencies of delusions involving persecution, self-reference, and religion/magic over time. For example, they found an increase in outside influence and control delusions following the spread of radio in the 1920s and again following the spread of television in the 1950s. Delusions with religious or magical content decreased from 1881 until 1980, perhaps reflecting a general decrease in religiosity over that period, as also seen in other parts of Europe and North America. Delusions with religious or magical content increased again after 1980, perhaps reflecting the waning influence of communism and a resurgence of religious openness.[36] Although retrospective studies of this sort are fraught with challenges, for example changing diagnostic categories, and the sample size was small, these results are consistent with the suggestion that the content of psychotic delusions reflects the content of declarative memory producing a credible framework to explain the apparent importance of environmental stimuli that normally should be ignored.

Many cultural norms are represented as semantic knowledge in declarative memory. Observations of culturally specific themes in the delusions of patients with schizophrenia are consistent with the suggestion that delusions are generated by information from declarative memory to formulate reasonable interpretations of a world distorted by excessive incentive learning.

Hallucinations are another feature of psychosis in schizophrenia. They can occur in all sensory modalities but are frequently auditory. Kraepelin describes the hearing of voices as a characteristic symptom of schizophrenia but says hallucinations of voices are usually preceded in the disease process by hearing simpler noises such as "rustlings, buzzing, ringing in the ears, tolling of bells ... " (p. 7).[1] These simpler hallucinations may be linked to excessive incentive learning. Stimulus events such as sounds in the environment may begin to take on apparent importance, making them appear to be louder or otherwise more salient than they really are. As suggested by Robert Miller, an ex-patriot Briton, who is a prolific and insightful theoretical neuroscientist living in New Zealand, perhaps excessive incentive learning similarly enhances the thoughts of a person with schizophrenia and this leads to their being heard as voices.[37] The linking of hallucinations to incentive learning mediated by dopamine finds support in the common observation that in many cases hallucinations quickly subside with the commencement of treatment with dopamine receptor-blocking antipsychotic medications.[38]

Like delusions, the nature of hallucinations in schizophrenia is influenced by the cultural context of the sufferers. The collaborative study from Lahore and Birmingham, UK, mentioned earlier showed a similar frequency of verbal hallucinations in the three patient groups but a significantly greater frequency of visual hallucinations in the Pakistani group from Lahore compared with the Pakistani and white groups from Birmingham. Visual hallucinations contained significantly more images of people and spirits or ghosts. The authors state that their findings corroborated those of others reporting a greater frequency of visual hallucinations in non-Western cultures. They suggest that one possibility is "that a greater acceptance of 'seeing spirits' in traditional Pakistani culture may lead either to a lower threshold for the experience of visual hallucinations, or to an increased willingness to report them" (p. 137).[39] In a related study from Turkey, researchers found a greater frequency of visual hallucinations involving goblins and religious figures, including God, the Prophet, saints, and the devil, in a group from the middle region compared with a group from the western region of Turkey; the group from the western region was urban and less traditional, from Istanbul and surrounding regions, and the group from the middle region was from the environs of two smaller cities, Ankara and Afyon Province—more traditional regions.[40] Results show that the nature and content of hallucinations in schizophrenia is influenced by cultural background.

Putative hyperdopaminergia underlying excessive incentive learning in schizophrenia may contribute to an enhanced salience of thoughts, leading to hallucinations as suggested by Robert Miller.[37] Results from cross-cultural studies suggest that cultural factors may influence the nature of hallucinations in patients from different regions. Like in the case of delusions, results suggest the combined influence of non-declarative incentive learning and declarative memory systems on the content of hallucinations.

The underlying abnormality in schizophrenia appears to be hyperactive dopaminergic neurotransmission leading to excessive incentive learning. Observations implicating cultural and local stimulus factors in the content of delusions and hallucinations provide a means for understanding some of the variability in the symptoms. Another factor that may influence the nature of symptoms in schizophrenia is the age of onset. Excessive incentive learning may lead to different manifestations in young people with schizophrenia who do not yet have well-integrated declarative knowledge about the world compared with older sufferers who have a more integrated foundation of declarative knowledge to construct a reasonable interpretation of a world where excessive stimuli are acquiring incentive value. This consideration may provide a better understanding of some schizophrenia subtypes.

In the fourth version of the *Diagnostic and Statistical Manual of Mental Disorders* (DSM-IV) of the American Psychiatric Association there is a schizophrenia diagnosis that was often applied to people in their late teens and early 20s;[3] this diagnosis is classified as "disorganized" and refers to the previous classification, "hebephrenia."[41] The first part of the word derives from the Greek goddess of youth, "Hebe," and has its origin in Greek for "young adult" or "reaching puberty." Disorganized schizophrenia is characterized by disorganized behavior and speech. Although fragmentary delusions may be present, more elaborate delusional frameworks like those seen in patients with later onset usually do not occur. Kraepelin, for example, stated that "their delusions ... appear mostly as sudden thoughts, which are not further worked up or retained" (p. 96).[1] Sometimes the patient may laugh inappropriately, or emotion may be generally absent, described as flat affect. The characteristic symptoms of disorganized schizophrenia may reflect the stage of learning of the afflicted individual. Like in an older patient, hyperdopaminergia in a young individual putatively leads to excessive incentive learning about environmental stimuli that normally should be ignored. Whereas the older patient can use her more elaborated and integrated framework for understanding the world to interpret the apparent importance of environmental stimuli, including other people, by formulating a complex delusion, the afflicted individual who has not yet developed an integrated framework for understanding the world may fail to formulate an integrated and elaborate delusion. Instead, the patient seems disorganized, responding inappropriately to many stimuli and generally being ineffective in the usual activities of daily living. In the pre-phenothiazine era of Kraepelin, the prognosis for these patients was the worst, perhaps because they were deprived of the opportunity to formulate an integrated understanding of the world before the onset of their illness. Although responding less well than other forms of the disease, disorganized schizophrenia is remediated somewhat by antipsychotic drugs, implicating enhanced dopaminergic neurotransmission in the disorder.

The observations from animal studies of disrupted acquisition of learning while under the influence of a dopamine-enhancing drug (Chapter 7) and disrupted behavioral functioning in people with disorganized schizophrenia suggest that dopamine-mediated (non-declarative) incentive learning and declarative learning are not entirely independent. Although declarative and non-declarative memory have been shown to depend on different neurotransmitter networks and brain regions (Chapter 4), dopamine-mediated incentive learning influences the content of declarative memories. We see this clearly in the case of schizophrenia developing in older individuals (adults) who begin to formulate elaborate interpretative frameworks of the world as it appears to them; to the rest of us it is seen as a delusion. In younger individuals (teens, early adulthood), overactive dopamine and excessive incentive learning before they have an integrated framework for understanding the world may deprive them of the ability to formulate such a framework. Instead, their thoughts become a mishmash of poorly organized and poorly integrated individual ideas. Kraepelin described Hecker's hebephrenia under the classification "silly dementia" (p. 94).[1] It is perhaps not surprising, therefore, to learn that the poorest prognosis for patients with schizophrenia is for those with the disorganized type. Even after treatment with antipsychotic medications and the suppression of inappropriate incentive learning, these individuals may have a relatively poorly organized framework for viewing the world upon which to try to build an effective and fulfilling life.

Before turning to Parkinson's disease, it is important to acknowledge that no neurotransmitter works alone. It is very unlikely that dopamine alone is the culprit in schizophrenia. A number of other neurotransmitters have been implicated, including glutamate and γ-aminobutyric acid. Neuropathological studies of postmortem brains from people with schizophrenia have identified abnormalities in a subtype (parvalbumin-positive) of γ-aminobutyric acid neurons found in the hippocampus and frontal cortex.[42] Other researchers found evidence suggesting enhanced glutamatergic neurotransmission in schizophrenia.[43] An influential and convincing synthesis has been formulated by Anthony Grace, a prominent neuroscientist from the University of Pittsburgh, Pennsylvania. Using animal models and a variety of techniques, including electrophysiology, Grace and his co-workers have shown that a loss of parvalbumin-positive neurons in the ventral hippocampus leads to increased activity in glutamatergic neurons projecting to the ventral tegmental area, a midbrain region containing many dopaminergic cells. Glutamate is an excitatory neurotransmitter and increased activity of glutamatergic inputs to the dopamine cell region results in increased activity of dopamine neurons.[44] Grace's formulation provides a means of reconciling the changes in several neurotransmitter systems with the apparent hyperdopaminergia of schizophrenia. The neuroanatomy of dopamine and the situation of dopamine neurons within brain circuits involving a number of neurotransmitters is discussed in Chapter 11.

There is a "revised dopamine hypothesis" of schizophrenia positing hyperactive dopaminergic neurotransmission in brain structures, including the caudate, putamen, and nucleus accumbens, and *hypo*active dopaminergic neurotransmission in the prefrontal cortex.[45] As discussed in Chapter 11, dopamine neurons project to a number of brain regions, including the prefrontal cortex. I have not focused on this projection because, as the revised hypothesis suggests, dopamine does not appear to be hyperactive in the prefrontal cortex in schizophrenia. The original dopamine hypothesis presented here focuses on subcortical regions. The frontal cortex has been more strongly implicated in working memory than in incentive learning and there is good evidence that dopamine in the prefrontal cortex plays a critical role in working memory.[46] There is also good evidence of impaired working memory in schizophrenia,[47] and possible remedial effects on working memory of enhancing prefrontal dopaminergic neurotransmission.[48] Many years ago, researchers showed that manipulations that decreased prefrontal cortical dopamine function produced an increase in subcortical dopamine function in rats, suggesting a possible reciprocal interaction between prefrontocorticopetal and striatopetal dopamine neurons.[49] The integration of these findings into a full understanding of the neurocircuitry abnormalities underlying schizophrenia awaits further study. Many prominent schizophrenia researchers continue to pursue that understanding and their efforts continue to contribute to that end.

Parkinson's disease and dopamine

I will turn now to Parkinson's disease. Parkinson's disease is a progressive neurological disorder. The central symptoms are often described as the Parkinson's triad: bradykinesia, rigidity, and tremor. "Brady" comes from the Greek word for "slow" and "kinesis" from the Greek for "movement" or "activity." Instead of "bradykinesia" sometimes the word "hypokinesia," "hypo" from the Greek for "beneath" ("less than normal"), is used. In other words, people with Parkinson's disease are slow moving. They show rigidity of the limbs. One of the diagnostic tests used by neurologists to detect rigidity is to have the patient hold her arm out with the elbow flexed at 90 degrees and the forearm extending upward. The neurologist then places one hand under the elbow and with the other pulls on the wrist of the vertically extended forearm, attempting to move it passively. If this is done to a normal person who is relaxed, the arm moves smoothly and without resistance. In a patient with Parkinson's disease, the movement is resisted, even when the patient is asked to relax and let the doctor move the limb. The resistance builds up but then suddenly dissipates and the limb moves a short distance. Then the limb resists again and again suddenly gives way, and so on. As a result the limb moves in a jerky, stepwise manner termed "cogwheel rigidity." Tremor in Parkinson's disease usually starts in the periphery, for example, the hand, and early in the disease can be unilateral. It is present at rest. The tremor in the hand is sometimes called "pill-rolling tremor" because the fingers and thumb move in opposing directions as if the patient is rolling a small pill between her fingers and thumb. Tremor of larger muscle groups such as those of the arms or legs may be seen as the disease progresses, hence James Parkinson's description of the disease as the "shaking palsy (*paralysis agitans*)."[6]

Unmedicated patients with Parkinson's disease eventually have great difficulty initiating movements and, prior to the development of effective dopaminergic medications, were doomed to unproductive lives in the back wards of hospitals where they needed extensive care. One of the unusual features of Parkinson's disease is that even though patients have great difficulty or are apparently unable to initiate movements on their own volition, they are observed to move under some circumstances, a phenomenon termed "*kinesia paradoxa*." A commonly used example is that of patients with chronic Parkinson's disease running out of a burning building only to resume their akinetic state upon reaching safety out of doors. Another example is that of a grandfather with

Parkinson's disease sitting in a beach chair watching his grandson swimming when the boy begins to have difficulty. The patient leapt from his chair, ran to the water, swam to his grandson, brought him to safety, and then quickly returned to his bradykinetic state.[50] I knew a patient with Parkinson's disease who could help himself begin to walk by chanting to himself. For example, he would begin a football cheer such as "One, two, three, four, who are we for ... ," and as he got the beat he would begin to step. Beyond these anecdotes, *kinesia paradoxa* was systematically studied beginning in the late twentieth century. Patients with Parkinson's disease who had great difficulty initiating walking were observed to walk if parallel lines or wooden slats were placed on the ground in front of them that they could step over.[51] These observations tell us that Parkinson's disease does not exclusively involve a dysfunction of the muscles or of the capacity to actually move. Instead, it may better be seen as a disorder that includes a diminished ability of environmental stimuli to elicit approach and other responses.

The faces of people with Parkinson's disease often show little expression, a symptom that is referred to as "masked *facies*." A related phenomenon to the impaired ability of patients with Parkinson's disease to initiate whole-body movement is an impaired ability to volitionally smile or make other facial expressions when asked to do so.[52] Just as patients with Parkinson's disease are impaired in their ability to initiate walking, they are impaired in their ability to use their facial musculature. This means that patients with Parkinson's disease cannot easily smile socially, that is, will a smile in a social situation. I have occasionally given talks to groups of patients with Parkinson's disease and found it more challenging than usual to look into a sea of faces when many of them appear detached and uninterested. I have also found that it is very gratifying to see these faces smile. And they do smile if the patients are genuinely amused by something they hear. Here may be another example of the paradoxical ability to use muscles under some circumstances. The driving force for the facial movement may be stronger when it comes from outside of the individual with Parkinson's disease just as it did for walking and related movements as described earlier.

In his excellent 1967 book on the role of the basal ganglia in posture, Ireland-born physician James Martin (1893–1984), working at the National Hospital for Nervous Disease, Queen Square, London, describes how patients with Parkinson's disease can apparently overcome their "motor" deficits under certain conditions, for example the placing of lines on the floor, as already mentioned earlier. From these observations, Martin comments that "the executive mechanism for these reactions [i.e., walking] ... is sufficiently intact" (p. 35) and goes on to say that the neuronal circuits controlling walking must have been interrupted at the "afferent" end.[53] The "afferent" end is the input end. Martin's conclusions about Parkinson's disease are that it is a disease characterized by apparent motor dysfunctions but not by a loss of motor capacity per se; what appears to be impaired is the effect of stimuli (inputs) on motor circuits.

There is strong evidence implicating a loss of dopaminergic neurons in Parkinson's disease. Arvid Carlsson and colleagues, working at the University of Lund in Sweden in 1957, reported observations from mice and rabbits treated with the monoamine-depleting drug reserpine; they found that the Parkinsonism-like tranquilizing effect of reserpine was rapidly reversed by injection of the dopamine precursor L-3,4-dihydroxyphenylalanine (L-DOPA).[54] In the following year Carlsson and colleagues reported the presence of dopamine in the brains of rabbits at a concentration high enough to suggest that it existed as a neurotransmitter in its own right rather than as a precursor for another neurotransmitter.[55] Two years later, Herbert Ehringer and Oleh Hornykiewicz, working at the University of Vienna in Austria, reported dopamine depletion in the caudate nucleus of postmortem brain tissue from patients with Parkinson's disease.[56] This set the stage for the first test of L-DOPA in patients with Parkinson's disease carried out in Vienna by Walther Birkmayer and Oleh Hornykiewicz. The remarkable effect was seen within minutes of intravenous injection—previously akinetic patients were able to get up and walk around.[57] Arvid Carlsson was a co-recipient of the Nobel Prize in Physiology or Medicine in 2000 along with Paul Greengard and Eric Kandel. Carlsson received the Prize for his pioneering work on dopamine and Parkinson's disease.[58]

Earlier, we considered the possibility that people with schizophrenia that appears to arise from hyperdopaminergia may suffer from excessive incentive learning. In the case of Parkinson's disease, the corresponding question is: As Parkinson's disease results from *hypo*dopaminergia, do patients suffer from deficient incentive learning? If Parkinson's patients suffer from deficient incentive learning, exposure to conditioned incentive stimuli will result in the gradual loss of their ability to elicit approach and other responses. By conceptualizing Parkinson's disease within this framework, it is possible to understand that patients do not lose their ability to act on their environment but rather that environmental stimuli have a diminished ability to control responding, as discussed in Chapter 6. An explanation based on (1) reduced ability to respond to environmental stimuli or (ii) reduced ability of stimuli to elicit responding would equally account for the loss of responsiveness to environmental stimuli seen in Parkinson's disease. However, the first explanation does not explain *kinesia paradoxa*. If the patient's ability to respond is reduced, why is he sometimes observed to make responses? The second explanation provides for the possibility that some stimuli appear to retain the ability to elicit responses. Thus, the view that patients with Parkinson's disease suffer from diminished incentive learning provides a more complete understanding of the illness than the view that the patient's ability to respond is greatly reduced or lost.

In Chapter 2, I discussed some results from experiments with animals that showed that the decrease in responding for a rewarding stimulus, produced by dopamine receptor-blocking drugs, could not be attributed simply to a loss of motor ability. Recall the study by Franklin and McCoy from McGill University.[59] They trained rats to respond for brain stimulation reward that was presented in alternating six-minute components, each signaled by a different stimulus. Trained rats were treated with the dopamine receptor-blocking drug pimozide and placed back into the test chamber where they could lever press for brain stimulation reward in the presence of the first of the two cues that signaled the components. In this test, the duration of the first component was extended to the point where no responding was observed for two minutes. As expected, pimozide-treated rats showed a gradual decline in responding for brain stimulation reward presumably because the reward-related learning effects of the stimulation depended on dopaminergic neurotransmission that was blocked by the drug. After responding ceased, the researchers turned on the second cue that signaled the alternative component where brain stimulation previously had been available. They observed that the rats resumed responding.[59] This result showed that the cessation of responding in pimozide-treated rats did not reflect simply a motor incapacitation. The rats clearly were able to respond as demonstrated when the second cue was presented. It is too simplistic to suggest that dopamine receptor blockade decreases motor ability. The behavioral observations can be understood better from the incentive learning point of view. A conditioned incentive stimulus loses its ability to control responding when it is encountered in the absence of primary reward (either because the reward has been withheld or because dopaminergic neurotransmission has been reduced), but a second conditioned incentive stimulus that has not been encountered in the absence of primary reward retains its ability to control responding. If the second conditioned incentive stimulus is encountered in the absence of primary reward, it will initially control responding, but its ability to do so will be lost gradually. The point here is that the observation of diminished responding for a rewarding stimulus seen in animals treated with a dopamine receptor-blocking drug is not simply a motor impairment.

Jon Horvitz, working at Boston College, and co-workers were interested in the observation of *kinesia paradoxa* in Parkinson's disease. In animal studies, they showed that increased training led to increased resistance to the response-reducing effects of a dopamine receptor-blocking drug. They simply fed rats periodically each day in a testing cubicle outfitted with a feeder cup and recorded when the rat's nose was in the feeder cup. Each intermittent pellet delivery was signaled by the click of the feeder apparatus. They found that dopamine receptor blockade produced a greater decrease in feeder cup responses following the click after three days of training than after 17 days of training. They concluded that acquisition of incentive learning was dependent on dopamine neurons but that once strong learning had taken place, the incentive learning was manifested even under conditions of reduced dopaminergic neurotransmission.[60] The authors relate these findings to *kinesia paradoxa* observed in Parkinson's disease.

How can the characterization of Parkinson's disease as resulting from deficient incentive learning account for the ability of lines on the floor to facilitate walking as described by James Martin (above)? I can only speculate here. If *kinesia paradoxa* results from previous incentive learning as I have just suggested, the lines on the floor must be conditioned incentive stimuli. Perhaps during early childhood when walking is learned, incentive learning plays a role. If walking is attempted for the purposes of attaining a goal, obstacles that impede the walking, causing falling, for example, will frustrate the goal attainment. The successful avoidance of obstacles (e.g., by stepping over them) may be rewarding, leading to increased dopamine release and incentive learning related to obstacles (i.e., the obstacles acquire an increased ability to elicit stepping-over responses). In the future, stimuli associated with avoidance of obstacles will have an increased ability to elicit response adjustments that are successful in avoiding the obstacle. Lines on the floor that resemble obstacles may have enough conditioned incentive value to activate walking (stepping-over) responses in patients with Parkinson's disease. It is well known that these so-called "tricks," such as lines on the floor or generating a rhythm using a chant, work only for a time in patients with Parkinson's disease; the patients eventually become refractory to their response-energizing effects.[61] This latter observation would be consistent with the point of view that the response-energizing effects of these stimuli were conditioned. *Conditioned incentive stimuli gradually lose their ability to elicit responses with repeated exposure to those stimuli in the absence of primary reward.* Thus, the (transient) ability of lines on the floor to facilitate walking may result from the activating effects of conditioned incentive stimuli.

Parkinson's disease is associated with a loss of over 80 percent of the dopaminergic innervation of some striatal terminal regions.[62] As shown in psychopharmacological, optogenetic, and lesion studies in animals, decreases in dopamine are associated with a loss of incentive learning; new incentive learning does not take place or is significantly slowed and previous incentive learning is lost *upon repeated exposure to conditioned incentive stimuli.* This suggests the hypothesis that patients with advanced Parkinson's disease who are generally nonresponsive to familiar stimuli will respond to conditioned incentive stimuli that have not been encountered since before the onset of the illness. To my knowledge, this hypothesis has not been tested. A friend once told me about her mother with Parkinson's disease who was in the advanced stages of the illness, no longer responsive to anti-Parkinson's medication, and confined to bed. She and her siblings were visiting their mother and the siblings were having a conversation among themselves about old times. The memory of a family event came up and the siblings were trying to recall the name of an old friend who was part of the memory. The mother, who had not spoken for weeks, spontaneously and clearly said the name and then lapsed again into her mute state. This is another example of *kinesia paradoxa* that can be understood from within the incentive-learning framework. This friend from long ago may not have come up in conversations for many years and perhaps was still a conditioned incentive stimulus in the brain of the mother. The mother could understand the conversation she was hearing (having relatively intact declarative memory; see later) and was able to contribute when a particular memory activated the neurons representing the old friend's name, neurons that still had an increased ability to elicit responses. I discuss the possible mechanism for this learning in Chapter 12. I once discussed with a graduate student the idea of trying to show patients with advanced Parkinson's disease old family photographs that they had not looked at for years to see if some of the photos could elicit responses as a way to test the above hypothesis. To my knowledge, this hypothesis has never been systematically tested.

As dopamine levels drop in Parkinson's disease, they eventually reach a level below the threshold for incentive learning. At that point, new incentive learning will no longer take place and previous incentive learning will be weakened with exposure to conditioned incentive stimuli in the absence of a sufficient dopamine signal. The patient will become less and less responsive to her environment with repeated exposure to the stimuli there. When conditioned incentive stimuli, that have not yet been encountered since reaching the dopamine level that is below the threshold for incentive learning, are subsequently encountered, apparently paradoxical responses may occur as already described. As dopamine levels continue to fall, they may reach the threshold for inverse incentive learning. Recall from Chapter 6 that inverse incentive learning is the loss by stimuli of the ability to elicit responses and is associated with reduced levels of dopamine. At this point, the nervous system may actually be engaged in actively down-regulating the ability of environmental stimuli to elicit responses. This might suggest that in advanced Parkinson's disease, not only is new incentive learning deficient and the ability of previous incentive stimuli to control responding being lost with exposure to those stimuli, but also that the ability of environmental stimuli, in general, to control responding gradually may be lost through excessive inverse incentive learning.

The findings from a study published by neuroscientist Michael Frank and colleagues, working at the time at the University of Colorado in Boulder and the Colorado Neurological Institute Movement Disorder Center in Englewood, may provide some insight into inverse incentive learning in patients with Parkinson's disease. They trained medicated patients with Parkinson's disease on a probabilistic selection task. Each trial involved choosing between two stimuli and there were three pairs of them. For each pair, one of the stimuli more often was correct than the other and the probabilities of the stimuli being correct varied across pairs: 80 percent and 20 percent, 70 percent and 30 percent, and 60 percent and 40 percent, respectively. After training, patients with Parkinson's disease were tested with novel pairs, that is, the 80 percent stimulus along with one of the stimuli from the other two pairs or the 20 percent stimulus along with one of the stimuli from the other two pairs. During these novel-pair tests, no feedback was given. Patients were tested twice, once when on medication and once when off medication. When the patients were tested on medication, they were more likely than age-matched controls to choose the 80 percent stimulus; when they were tested off medication, they were more likely than controls to *avoid* the 20 percent stimulus.[63] On-medication results suggest that enhanced dopamine seen soon after taking dopaminergic medication led to increased incentive learning about the 80 percent stimulus and more choices of that stimulus when it was presented in the novel pairs. Off-medication results suggest that reduced dopamine, seen several hours after the last dose of medication, increased avoidance of the 20 percent stimulus when it was presented in novel pairs. The off-medication results may reflect inverse incentive learning. Stimuli associated with decreased dopamine lose their ability to elicit responses; in the off-medication condition, the 20% stimulus may be even less likely than usual to be selected. Frank and co-workers referred to the negative prediction error results of Schultz (see Chapter 5) in hypothesizing that patients off medication would choose the 20 percent stimulus less often. These results support the suggestion in the previous paragraph that the loss of dopamine associated with Parkinson's disease may lead to excessive inverse incentive learning.

As I discuss in Chapter 4, my former doctoral student Danielle Charbonneau, who is now at the Royal Military College in Kingston, Ontario, studied learning and memory in patients with Parkinson's disease for her PhD thesis research. Recall that she evaluated acquisition of a non-declarative memory-dependent point-loss avoidance task in patients and controls and found that patients with Parkinson's disease learned significantly more slowly. In the same experiment, she included a declarative memory task involving learning associations between pairs of words and found no significant difference in the learning rate of patients and controls.[64] These results showed a clear dissociation between memory that depends on non-declarative incentive learning and declarative memory, the former more than the latter being compromised in Parkinson's disease. Also, as I discuss in Chapter 4, in the same year that Danielle published her study, the eminent memory researcher Larry Squire from the University of California in San Diego and colleagues reported impaired learning of a non-declarative probabilistic classification task in patients with Parkinson's disease who showed no deficit compared with controls on a declarative memory questionnaire. In that study, amnesic patients who did poorly on the declarative memory questionnaire learned the probabilistic classification task as well as controls.[65] It is still amazing to me that patients with Parkinson's disease who can clearly learn associations and remember details of the probabilistic classification task cannot learn it and that amnesic patients, who, in spite of being unable to remember elements or details of the probabilistic classification task, nevertheless learn it! These findings remind us that there are multiple memory systems and that the loss of dopamine in Parkinson's disease is associated with a relatively greater impairment of memory that relies on non-declarative incentive learning than of declarative memory for facts and events. They also remind us that patients with Parkinson's disease who are generally unresponsive to the stimuli around them nevertheless understand and remember declarative aspects of what is going on.

Incentive learning and inverse incentive learning in patients with Parkinson's disease will be influenced by a number of variables. Parkinson's disease is progressive, so the stage of the illness is an important consideration. The impact of decreased dopamine on incentive learning may be expected to increase as the disease progresses. Putative excessive inverse incentive learning may also be more pronounced later in the course of the disease. The possible activating effects of conditioned incentive stimuli depend on whether or not those stimuli have been encountered by the patient while in a dopamine-depleted state. Recent findings have shown seasonal variations in striatal dopamine synthesis capacity in Parkinson's disease,[66] identifying season as another variable that needs to be considered in studies of patients with Parkinson's disease. The medication state of the patient influences her responses to environmental stimuli as shown, for example, in the work of Frank and colleagues discussed earlier. In the following, I expand on possible behavioral effects associated with medications used to treat schizophrenia and Parkinson's disease.

Dopamine receptor antagonist medications

I begin with schizophrenia; as I discuss in Chapter 7, the first evidence that some of the symptoms were linked to dopamine was the finding that the effective antipsychotics were dopamine receptor blockers. The therapeutic effectiveness of the prototypical antipsychotic medication, chlorpromazine, was discovered in 1952 at Sainte-Anne's Hospital in Paris by French psychiatrists Pierre Deniker (1917–1998) and Jean Delay (1907–1987);[12,67] many related phenothiazine compounds, including trifluoperazine, thioridazine, and fluphenazine, were discovered subsequently and came into use in the treatment of schizophrenia. Paul Janssen (1926–2003) at Janssen Pharmaceutica in Beerse, Belgium, developed the butyrophenone antipsychotic haloperidol in 1958.[68] Additional classes of antipsychotics soon appeared. The strong correlation between the average daily dose of individual antipsychotic medications taken by patients and their ability to block dopamine D2-like receptors (see Chapter 7) supported the dopamine hypothesis of schizophrenia that first appeared in 1966.[69]

The response to antipsychotic medications was remarkable. More than 60 years after their introduction, it is difficult to appreciate the impact these medications had on the care of the mentally ill. Prior to chlorpromazine, patients with schizophrenia were generally kept in insane asylums. Today we refer to buildings housing the mentally ill as psychiatric hospitals or mental health services, and many patients are no longer institutionalized. Asylums were noisy places, where the moans, laments, yelling, and screams of patients were frequently heard. These were often patients with schizophrenia responding to their hallucinations and delusions. Frequently, there was little that could be done for these poor souls who, like unafflicted individuals, were sometimes dangerous to themselves and others. Restraint was often necessary and sometimes provided the only means of preventing human injury. All this changed with the advent of chlorpromazine. The superficially most apparent effect of chlorpromazine on the asylums was that they fell silent.[70]

At first chlorpromazine was seen to be a tranquilizer, a classification that stuck as chlorpromazine and related compounds are still sometimes referred to as major tranquilizers. These compounds had a calming effect. But Deniker and Delay also noticed that features of schizophrenia such as delusions began to resolve over days. For example, they described a patient who had been engaging in behaviors such as giving improvised political speeches on the street and getting into fights with strangers who was able to maintain a normal conversation after a nine-day course of treatment with chlorpromazine and who was discharged from the hospital after three weeks of treatment. They also reported that chlorpromazine was ineffective in the treatment of depression and that it did not relieve many of the negative symptoms of schizophrenia.[71] Chlorpromazine launched the effective use of pharmacological compounds to treat psychiatric illnesses and heralded the rise of biological psychiatry.

An important caveat is that people today who have experience with anti-psychotics might not agree for several reasons that these medications are as remarkable as I have suggested. Antipsychotic medications are effective in re-ducing the positive symptoms of schizophrenia, that is, delusions and hallu-cinations. They are, however, less effective at treating the negative symptoms, including the loss of emotional expression and motivation, neglect of personal hygiene, and social withdrawal. Schizophrenia has also been associated with cognitive impairments, including impaired working memory.[47] Patients who are treated with antipsychotics may be less affected by their hallucinations and delusions and, as a result, may be easier to manage in a hospital or community setting, but they often do not regain the quality of life that many of us experi-ence. This is one of the reasons people today may not see antipsychotics as a panacea for the treatment of schizophrenia. There is another.

A further problem with the early antipsychotics was their side effects. Drugs that were effective in treating schizophrenia also produced side effects known as "extrapyramidal side effects" or "EPS." Sometimes these side effects were re-ferred to as "Parkinsonian" because they included rigidity, bradykinesia, and tremor. Here we begin to see the continuum of dopaminergic activity. For ef-fective functioning, dopamine levels need to be in a window somewhere in the range of levels that can be too high or too low. If dopaminergic neurotransmis-sion is too high, symptoms of schizophrenia begin to emerge, and if it is too low, symptoms of Parkinson's disease begin to emerge. If people with schizo-phrenia are treated with drugs that excessively block dopamine receptors, they experience side effects with symptoms resembling those of Parkinson's disease. The trade name for chlorpromazine when it first became available in the USA was "Thorazine." Patients with schizophrenia treated with this drug would sometimes develop the stooped posture and shuffling gait character-istic of Parkinson's disease, a condition that became known as the "Thorazine shuffle." When psychiatrists first began subscribing chlorpromazine to patients, they would titrate the dose to try to find the dose that was just on the threshold of producing EPS.[72] It was believed that this was the optimal dose for treating the positive symptoms while producing minimal side effects. Thus, chlorpro-mazine was a boon to psychiatry in its efforts to reduce the suffering of patients with schizophrenia and to try to provide them with a more fulfilling life while at the same time it brought with it iatrogenic side effects that to some patients presented a whole new set of problems.

Chlorpromazine and related phenothiazines, haloperidol, and several additional drugs that are used to treat schizophrenia and that have a relatively high liability for producing EPS are known as "first-generation antipsychotics" or "typical antipsychotics." Second- and third-generation antipsychotics are referred to as "atypical." The prototypical second-generation compound is clozapine,[73] and other second-generation compounds include olanzapine, risperidone, quetiapine, ziprasidone, and lurasidone;[74] additional second-generation antipsychotics are being developed and marketed. The prototypical third-generation compound is aripiprazole.[75] What distinguishes the atypical from the typical antipsychotics is their liability for producing EPS. The atypicals, by definition, have low EPS liability. EPS are produced by atypical antipsychotics but often at higher doses than those that are typically used therapeutically. Thus, the therapeutic window is wider for atypicals and for this reason they are deemed safer than typicals with respect to EPS liability.

Atypical antipsychotics are not without side-effect risk. Although they have come into wide use, they have brought with this use their own suite of side effects that make them less than perfect medications. The prototypical atypical, clozapine, first came into use in some European countries in 1972, surprisingly early in antipsychotic history, but was soon removed because of the risk of the blood disorder agranulocytosis. This condition involves the loss of white blood cells and proved to be fatal in a number of patients. Years later clozapine was reintroduced for use as an antipsychotic (clozapine was introduced in the USA in 1990), but treated patients undergo regular blood monitoring for the detection of possible agranulocytosis. As a result, clozapine is more complicated to use than other antipsychotic medications. Clozapine is now used for the treatment of patients who are refractory to other antipsychotic medications. Clozapine is an effective antipsychotic medication with low EPS risk.[76]

Weight gain is a major side effect of several atypical antipsychotics. One recent study reported that 64% of people treated with antipsychotic medications showed increased waist circumference and 44% showed metabolic syndrome; this is a condition defined by elevated waist circumference, fasting blood glucose, triglycerides, and blood pressure, and reduced low-density lipoprotein. Clozapine and olanzapine produce the largest effects and ziprasidone and aripiprazole the smallest. Compared with the general population, people with mental illness have an increased risk for cardiovascular disease, and weight gain related to the use of antipsychotic medications contributes to this risk. Weight gain is associated with type 2 diabetes. First-generation antipsychotics, for example haloperidol, are associated with weight gain but to a lesser extent than second-generation drugs such as clozapine.[77] Although atypical antipsychotics reduce the risk of EPS, they increase the risk of cardiovascular disease. Ameliorating the side effects of antipsychotic medications continues to be a challenge to scientists and clinicians.

When clozapine use with blood monitoring began and other atypical anti-psychotics began to emerge in the 1990s, many studies compared the anti-psychotic efficacy of the typicals and atypicals. Some studies concluded that the atypicals were superior to the typicals because they reduced not only positive symptoms, but also negative symptoms. There were claims, for example, that patients, who had been treated with typical medications such as haloperidol, when switched to clozapine, began to show emotional responses when their mood previously had been flat. However, more extensive and better-controlled studies failed to corroborate these claims. It was suggested that some of the negative symptoms of schizophrenia observed in medicated patients were themselves iatrogenic.[77] Recall that patients with Parkinson's disease, suffering form a loss of dopamine, showed masked *facies*. Some patients treated with high doses of antipsychotic medications that block dopamine receptors simi-larly show a loss of facial expression. This medication side effect may contribute to the negative symptom score of patients with schizophrenia. There is no good evidence that atypical antipsychotics are more effective than typicals at treating negative symptoms.

Returning to the therapeutic effects of antipsychotic medications, both the typicals and atypicals proved to be effective at reducing the positive symptoms of schizophrenia. However, one aspect of their action is perplexing and con-tinues to be poorly understood: antipsychotic medications have a gradual onset of action, often requiring several weeks of treatment before their full therapeutic effect is seen.[78] Their tranquilizing effects are seen within minutes and hours of treatment, but the reduction of hallucinations, and especially delusions, does not respond as quickly but rather gradually takes place over days and weeks. There have been a number of biological hypotheses as to why antipsychotics have a delayed onset of action, including a gradual depolarization-induced inactivation of dopaminergic neurons,[79] and long-term changes in recep-tors and other proteins.[80] As argued masterfully by theoretical neuroscientist Robert Miller, working at the time at the University of Otago Medical School in Dunedin, New Zealand, the inactivation hypothesis predicts that high doses of antipsychotics that block postsynaptic dopamine receptors should have a rapid therapeutic effect in the treatment of schizophrenia; available data, how-ever, do not support this prediction.[81] The idea suggested by Michael Kuhar and Andrew Joyce from Emory University in Atlanta, Georgia, that the slow onset of therapeutic action of antipsychotics may be related to gradual changes in effector or signaling proteins downstream from dopamine receptors is not incompatible with the incentive learning framework developed in this book and used to understand the symptoms and responses to medication of schizophrenia patients,[80] as I show in Chapter 12.

Recall the proposed sequence of events in developing psychosis. I suggested that it begins with hyperdopaminergia producing excessive incentive learning. Thus, too many stimuli acquire an increased ability to elicit approach and other responses. The declarative memory system formulates an interpretation of the world that is consistent with the apparent importance of people and things that normally would not appear important. To others this appears to be a delusion. Elaborate delusions are not formed overnight; especially in people who already have a well-formed worldview, it takes some time to formulate a logical re-interpretation of the world that incorporates the apparent importance of many stimuli. Now suppose that this deluded individual begins treatment with an antipsychotic medication. These agents are dopamine receptor blockers and will reverse the underlying hyperdopaminergic condition. However, the learning underlying the delusion did not take place overnight and it does not go away overnight. Once antipsychotic treatment is begun, it takes some time for previous incentive stimuli to lose their ability to elicit approach and other responses, gradually extinguishing as incentive stimuli *with repeated exposure to those stimuli in the absence of elevated dopaminergic neurotransmission*. As excessive incentive learning is gradually lost, it will take more time for the patient to again adjust his worldview to incorporate the loss of importance of stimuli that previously seemed important. As my former student Brenda Hahn and I suggested in our 1983 paper in *Science*,[82] this provides a basis for understanding the delayed onset of action of antipsychotic medications.

This perspective on the development of positive symptoms of schizophrenia and their gradual remission after the beginning of treatment with antipsycotic medications provides a basis for understanding additional phenomena seen in patients with schizophrenia. It is important to remember that conditioned incentive stimuli retain their ability to attract until they are experienced repeatedly in the absence of elevated dopaminergic neurotransmission. Recall again the experiment of Franklin and McCoy.[59] Rats were trained to respond in the presence of two different stimuli. They were then injected with a dopamine receptor-blocking drug and exposed to the first stimulus. Responding to that stimulus gradually declined to a low level. Then the second stimulus was presented and responding resumed. I discuss the same phenomenon in Chapter 10 on drug addiction: a previously addicted individual who undergoes rehabilitation and has not taken drugs for weeks or months is seen to relapse when exposed to conditioned incentive stimuli previously associated with drug taking. All of this suggests that patients with schizophrenia who have undergone treatment and whose positive symptoms have begun to remit may still be susceptible to the incentive properties of stimuli that have not been experienced while under treatment with an antipsychotic medication. For example, if a patient is treated in a hospital—a rather austere environment lacking many of the stimuli encountered on a daily basis in a busy urban and home environment—and then released into the environment where she previously developed positive symptoms, symptoms may transiently worsen until those stimuli can lose their conditioned incentive value. It might follow that substantially improved patients relapse when they are sent home, even if they are continuing with their medication. The high relapse rate of apparently remitted and drug-compliant patients with schizophrenia upon release is well documented.[83] This suggests that the best therapeutic results will be achieved with antipsychotics when they are used in the presence of the stimuli that were encountered when the psychotic symptoms emerged.

Much has been written about relapse in schizophrenia. As might be expected, the strongest predictor of relapse is withdrawal of medication. In the late twentieth century, an additional factor that was studied was termed "expressed emotion." This refers to the content of the verbal communications of family and friends in the home environment of the patient with schizophrenia. High expressed-emotion families make more negative and critical comments, show more hostility, and are emotionally overinvolved in the patient's life than low expressed-emotion families. Some results showed that apparently remitted and drug-compliant patients who were returned to home environments with high expressed emotion were more likely to relapse than those returning to homes with low expressed emotion. These findings spawned new practices, termed "family psychoeducation" or "family therapy," aimed at working with the family of patients with schizophrenia with the goal of reducing expressed emotion and thereby reducing relapse.[84] These therapeutic practices, although varying considerably in form and content across different sites, proved to be effective at reducing relapse rates and family interventions continue to be a component of many schizophrenia treatment programs.[85] In spite of theses findings, some research results have questioned whether expressed emotion is predictive of relapse.[86] The incentive learning perspective may shed some light on these findings.

I have argued that hyperdopaminergia in schizophrenia leads to excessive incentive learning and emphasized that the conditioned incentive value of stimuli is not lost even after the commencement of antipsychotic medication until those stimuli have been repeatedly encountered. If schizophrenia developed in the home environment and medication was begun in a treatment facility, the conditioned incentive stimuli from the home environment will retain their ability to elicit approach and other responses (and the delusions that make sense of them) until those stimuli are encountered while the patient is medicated. Exposing the apparently remitted and drug-compliant individual to those stimuli might lead to relapse. The initiation of family therapy, involving bringing together the family members from the home environment and the patient, sometimes in the home environment, may institute precisely those conditions that are conducive to remission. By encountering family members while under medication, putatively excessive incentive value associated with those individuals (see Chapter 8) may be gradually lessened. It is possible that expressed emotion in families contributes to the development of schizophrenia symptoms and that therapeutics aimed at reducing expressed emotion effectively mitigate its effect; it is also possible that efforts to address expressed emotion have the unintended consequence of reducing the impact on patients of aberrant incentive learning associated with family members. After a patient has been treated with medication and experiences family therapy involving exposure to individuals from the home environment, returning to the home environment may be less likely to lead to relapse because the putative excessive incentive value of stimuli (e.g., people) from that environment will have had a chance to weaken.

I return briefly to subtypes of antipsychotic medications. Typical and atypical antipsychotic medications have been found to affect different parts of the brain that are major dopamine terminal areas. Evidence from several different research approaches suggests that typicals and atypicals alike affect the dopamine-terminal area, the nucleus accumbens, but, whereas typicals generally also affect the striatum, another dopamine terminal area, the atypicals affect the medial prefrontal cortex, also a dopamine terminal area.[87] This distinction led some of my students to investigate the performance of patients with schizophrenia on two tasks that had been shown previously to depend differentially on the striatum or the medial prefrontal cortex. As I discuss in Chapter 4, the probabilistic classification task involves predicting the weather based on a set of visual stimuli that, unbeknownst to the participant, are probabilistically associated with each outcome. Learning of the probabilistic classification task appears to depend on intact striatal functioning.[88] The Iowa gambling task involves choosing from a set of four decks that have payoffs and penalties associated with them with the aim of maximizing payoffs. Two decks produce a positive overall payoff and are the advantageous or good decks and the other two produce an overall loss and are the disadvantageous or bad decks. Neurological patients with damage to the medial prefrontal cortex are impaired on the Iowa gambling task.[89]

Working in a team of students and colleagues, we recruited patients with schizophrenia who were treated with typical or atypical antipsychotics and tested them on these two tasks. We found a double dissociation. The group treated with typicals was impaired on the probabilistic classification task but not the gambling task; the group treated with atypicals was impaired on the gambling task but not the probabilistic classification task. Recalling that the typicals generally affect the striatum but not the medial prefrontal cortex and that the atypicals generally affect the medial prefrontal cortex but not the striatum, these results corroborate previous findings implicating the striatum in learning of the probabilistic classification task and the medial prefrontal cortex in learning the Iowa gambling task. These results further suggest that some of the cognitive (non-declarative memory) impairments seen in patients with schizophrenia treated with antipsychotic medications may be iatrogenic.[90] The nature of the cognitive impairment may be related to the type of medication being used: drugs that more strongly affect striatal function may impair incentive learning needed to learn the probabilistic classification task; drugs that more strongly affect the medial prefrontal cortex may impair decision-making and planning needed to learn the gambling task. These results reveal a complex relationship between the therapeutic and undesirable side effects of antipsychotic medications.

To further complicate matters, not all atypical antipsychotic medications have the same effects on the brain. In particular, the so-called atypical risperidone has been shown to have a different profile of effects on the brain than other medications classified as atypical. Risperidone is classified as an atypical because it has lower EPS liability than most of the typical antipsychotics, but in some tests of its effects on the brain and behavior, it appears to affect the striatum rather than the prefrontal cortex.[91] In an extension of the work described in the previous paragraph, several of my students, my colleague, psychiatrist Nicholas Delva, and I recruited a group of patients with schizophrenia treated with risperidone and compared them with patients treated with the prototypical atypical antipsychotic clozapine, the atypical olanzapine, or typical antipsychotics. Similar to the previous study, we found evidence that the effects of the atypicals clozapine and olanzapine were doubly dissociable from those of the typicals, patients treated with the former performing less well on the Iowa gambling task and patients treated with the latter performing less well on the probabilistic classification task. Patients treated with risperidone performed like those treated with typicals, showing significant learning of the Iowa gambling task but not the probabilistic classification task.[92] This work shows that antipsychotic medications that have good effects at reducing the positive symptoms of schizophrenia bring with them a suite of motor and cognitive side effects that vary depending on the class of antipsychotic and, to some extent, on the individual member of the class.

The discovery of chlorpromazine marked the birth of modern psychiatry, sometimes called biological psychiatry. Prior to the introduction of chlorpromazine, much of psychiatry had been dominated by the psychodynamic theories of Sigmund Freud (1856–1939). Often little could be done for patients with schizophrenia and many were tormented by their delusions and hallucinations with little respite.[70] All that changed with chlorpromazine. When it was subsequently discovered that chlorpromazine and other antipsychotic medications that followed were dopamine D2 receptor blockers, the dopamine hypothesis of schizophrenia was born. It has proven to be the most enduring and influential hypothesis in the history of psychiatry. The antipsychotic medications freed patients from a non-functional life filled with suffering. For many patients, they brought the ability to have a fruitful and fulfilling life. They brought with them their own suite of side effects that for some patients replaced one set of problems with another. Compared with the prospects of patients before chlorpromazine to their prospects after, chlorpromazine can justifiably be called a miracle drug.

Dopamine agonist medications

The treatment of Parkinson's disease involves the discovery of another miracle drug. As mentioned earlier in this chapter, in 1957 future Nobel laureate Arvid Carlsson injected mice and rabbits that had been made cataleptic by treatment with the dopamine-depleting drug reserpine with the dopamine precursor L-DOPA and they regained their ability to move,[54] ushering in the era of treatment of Parkinson's disease with L-DOPA.[57] Prior to Carlsson's discovery, patients with Parkinson's disease were doomed to a lifetime of dependency and often were kept in the back wards of hospitals, sometimes for decades. Just like the dopamine-depleted mice and rabbits that Carlsson injected, these patients woke up when injected with L-DOPA. People who had hardly moved and not conversed sometimes for years regained their old personalities and began to move and speak. For friends and family, and indeed for the patients themselves, L-DOPA was certainly a miracle drug. The stories of some of these patients and their transitions back to a more active life after years of suffering from untreated Parkinson's symptoms are told in a captivating and sensitive manner by neurologist Oliver Sacks in his extraordinary book, *Awakenings*.[93]

Like antipsychotic medications, L-DOPA appears to have an immediate action and a further action that is delayed by days or weeks. These actions have been termed respectively the "short-" and "long-duration response to L-DOPA." Thus, upon initiation of L-DOPA therapy, there is an activating response within minutes of taking the drug. Over subsequent days there is further improvement.

If the patient takes a drug holiday, there is an immediately observable effect, sometimes termed the "off" state, followed over days with further deterioration of motor function. Several possible mechanisms of the long-duration response to L-DOPA have been proposed; a number of pharmacokinetic hypotheses were found to be untenable.[94] An alternative mechanism involves motor learning. If inverse incentive learning takes place during a period when dopamine levels are reduced, as discussed in Chapter 6 and earlier in this chapter, it follows that treatment with L-DOPA will lead to a gradual reversal of this learning, accounting for the long-duration response. It also follows that skills training while off medication could exacerbate rather than ameliorate motor deficits in Parkinson's disease. Although they did not call it inverse incentive learning, this consideration led neurobiologist Jeff Beeler and associates, working at the time at University of Chicago, to make the intriguing suggestion that skill practice during low medication periods "might degrade rather than improve motor skills" (p. 1759 in Beeler et al.).[63]

Patients with Parkinson's disease are often treated with medications that directly stimulate dopamine receptors (e.g., pramipexole, ropinirole). A small percentage of these patients (up to, perhaps, 7%) develop pathological gambling; pathological gambling is observed in up to about two percent of the general population.[95] The greater frequency of pathological gambling in patients with Parkinson's disease treated with dopamine receptor agonsits may reflect enhanced reward-related learning and/or impaired inverse incentive learning in affected individuals.[96] There appears to be greater loss of dopaminergic innervation of the dorsal striatum than the ventral striatum in Parkinson's disease;[97] treatment with dopamine receptor agonists may improve dorsal striatal function while leading to hyperfunction of ventral striatal dopamine,[98] possibly contributing to enhanced incentive learning that might contribute to the enhanced ability of gambling-related stimuli to control behavior. Disorders such as binge eating, hypersexuality, and compulsive shopping also have been observed in a small subset of patients with Parkinson's disease treated with dopamine receptor agonists; these and pathological gambling are sometimes classified as "impulse control disorders," characterized by a failure to resist an impulse, drive, or temptation to perform an act that may be harmful to the self or others.[99] Excessive incentive learning may also contribute to these related impulse control disorders. Cortical–basal ganglia–thalamic–cortical circuit abnormalities have been implicated in pathological gambling in patients with Parkinson's disease (also see references and discussion in Santangelo et al.),[95,96] but the possible role of dopamine-mediated incentive learning in the functioning of these circuits has yet to be specified. The possible role of dopamine in altering frontal cortical synaptic plasticity is mentioned near the end of Chapter 12, but how frontal cortical dopamine might contribute to incentive learning is not yet clear.

Just like patients with schizophrenia who take too high a dose of an antipsychotic and develop extrapyramidal symptoms that resemble those of Parkinson's disease, so it is with patients suffering from Parkinson's disease who take too high a dose of L-DOPA or other pro-dopamine anti-Parkinson's medications and develop symptoms that resemble those of schizophrenia. Schizophrenia-like symptoms, including hallucinations and delusions, have been observed in up to 40 percent of patients with Parkinson's disease.[100] The hallucinations in patients with Parkinson's disease are more often visual in contrast to the more frequently reported auditory hallucinations in schizophrenia. I have occasionally spoken to Parkinson's disease groups and had patients speak to me about fantastic things they have seen while taking L-DOPA that sounded like hallucinations, and I have heard patients with Parkinson's disease describe suspicions about being followed or otherwise persecuted that resemble paranoid delusions. A group of researchers from the University of Athens in Greece describe delusions in several medicated patients with Parkinson's disease. One patient developed persecutory paranoid delusions, believing he was under constant surveillance. "He would identify members of the public as his persecutors" (p. 550).[101] Another claimed that "the other patients in her room had cameras in their fingers and were recording her" (p. 551).[101] These delusions can be understood as reasonable explanations of stimuli that have acquired inappropriate or excessive incentive value. Apparently, effective dopaminergic neurotransmission requires tuning to a level within a window of activity that is high enough to avoid Parkinson's-like symptoms and low enough to avoid the positive symptoms associated with schizophrenia.

Attention deficit hyperactivity disorder and dopamine

I turn now to another neuropsychiatric disorder that may have links to dopamine. ADHD is characterized by inattention and/or hyperactivity and impulsivity; ADHD includes behaviors such as failing to pay close attention to details, difficulty organizing tasks and activities, excessive talking, fidgeting, or difficulty remaining seated in situations that require sitting quietly. About five percent of children and 2.5 percent of adults suffer from ADHD. It is effectively treated with the drugs methylphenidate or d-amphetamine, both pro-dopaminergic compounds (although they also affect noradrenergic neurotransmission).[102] As already mentioned, the therapeutic effectiveness of amphetamine was discovered by American physician Charles Bradley (1902–1979), working at what is now eponymously named "Bradley Hospital" in East Providence, Rhode Island, in 1937, when he observed the paradoxical calming effect of this psycho-motor stimulant drug on children with learning and behavioral problems that fit many of today's criteria for a diagnosis of ADHD.[103] Although two to three decades passed before Bradley's treatment came into wide use, the intervening years did not mitigate the dilemma of how drugs that are known to be psycho-motor stimulants can have a calming effect.

The first step to resolving this dilemma is to recall the differential behavioral effects of dopamine depletions in young versus adult animals. As mentioned in Chapter 7, while dopamine depletions in adult rats (age six months (about 180 days) or older) produce Parkinson's-like symptoms, including decreased re-sponsiveness to the environment and hypokinesia, similar treatments in young animals do not produce hypokinesia. Research by the influential University of Chicago neuroscientist Lewis Seiden (1934–2007) and colleagues shows that dopamine cell-destroying 6-hydroxydopamine lesions lead to *hyper*kinesia in young rats. They showed that treatments given to rats at several ages up to about 23 days (corresponding to the period of human childhood) led to hyper-activity that persisted into early adulthood (they measured up to 60 days of age), whereas similar 6-hydroxydopamine treatments given around the age of 47 days, approximate sexual maturity in rats, did not significantly alter the level of motor activity; as already mentioned, 6-hydroxydopamine lesions in adults lead to decreased levels of activity. Seiden and colleagues additionally observed that injections of *d*-amphetamine significantly *reduced* locomotor hyperactivity in young lesion rats while having the usual stimulant effect on locomotor ac-tivity of age-matched, non-lesion, control rats.[104]

The observation by Seiden and colleagues that amphetamine reversed hyper-activity in young rats is in good agreement with the original observation of Bradley that amphetamine reversed the hyperactivity of children. It appears that the amphetamine-induced augmentation of dopaminergic neurotransmission ameliorated the hyperactive behavior.[102] This suggests further that hyperactive children may be suffering from underactive dopaminergic neurotransmission. Is there any additional evidence?

Some observations from the epidemic of encephalitis lethargica that lasted roughly from 1917 to 1925 hint at a link between low dopaminergic neuro-transmission and ADHD. (As an aside, note that the encephalitis epidemic overlapped with the 1917 flu epidemic and there continues to be much interest in a possible link between them. Recently researchers have used modern tech-niques of molecular biology to examine preserved brain tissue from patients known to have suffered from encephalitis lethargica and found no evidence of the flu virus (H1N1 influenza A). However, limitations of those experiments have been identified and the cause of encephalitis lethargica remains un-known[105].) Encephalitis lethargica may have killed half a million people world-wide, up to 40 percent of those infected. Although it affected people of all ages, the highest incidence was in people in the age range of 10–29 years. Perhaps half of those who survived went on to develop post-encephalitic Parkinson's disease. Of the children who survived, an estimated one-third exhibited behavioral disorders.[106] Austrian neurologist and psychiatrist Constantin von Economo (1876–1931) described many of the symptoms of children who survived en-cephalitis lethargica. These included a range of behaviors, for example annoying strangers, making faces, writing on walls, misconduct at school, impulsiveness, and so on, that today contribute to the diagnosis of ADHD.[107] Encephalitis leth-argica is often referred to as von Economo disease, reflecting his original char-acterization of the illness. The coincidence of ADHD-like symptoms in many children survivors and of Parkinson's-like symptoms in many adult survivors of encephalitis lethargica may reveal a common insult to the brain's dopamine systems in affected individuals.

The brain pathology associated with encephalitis lethargica is consistent with damage to dopaminergic neurons. von Economo concluded that a major region of damage in victims was the midbrain;[107] this is the region where many dopa-minergic cell bodies are located, although at the time the dopamine systems were unknown. In their 1926 review of post-encephalitic behavior disorders in boys, psychiatrist Earl Bond (1879–1968) and psychologist George Partridge (1870–1953), working at the Pennsylvania Hospital in Philadelphia, concluded that the changes observed were most probably due to damage to the basal ganglia;[108] these are major projection areas of the brainstem dopaminergic neurons. These observations suggest that hyperactivity in post-encephalitic children may have arisen as a result of damage to dopaminergic neurons early in life analogous to the hyperactivity effects observed in neonatal 6-hydroxydopamine-treated rats by Seiden and colleagues (see earlier).

Results from neuroimaging studies hint at a possible link between decreased dopaminergic neurotransmission and hyperactivity in children. In a magnetic resonance imaging (MRI) study of post-stroke children who became hyper-active, the size of the lesion in the ventral putamen, a ventral striatal region and part of the dopaminergically innervated basal ganglia, correlated significantly with the risk for ADHD traits.[109] A functional MRI study of ADHD adoles-cents showed that when unmedicated, they had reduced activation in left ven-tral basal ganglia regions during performance of a divided attention task; when the same adolescents were given the same task after receiving a dose of the pro-dopaminergic medication methylphenidate, the level of basal ganglia activa-tion no longer differed from that of control adolescents.[110] Other neuroimaging studies have reported reduced activation of areas of the basal ganglia that receive dopaminergic input in participants with ADHD tested at rest or while performing tasks that require attention and that methylphenidate regularizes striatal BOLD responses in participants with ADHD.[111] These findings imply that reduced basal ganglia activation observed in unmedicated participants with ADHD may be related to low dopaminergic neurotransmission that is remediated by pro-dopaminergic medication.

A 2009 study by psychiatrist Nora Volkow, current director of the National Institute of Drug Abuse in Bethesda, Maryland, and colleagues evaluated, using PET, dopamine synaptic markers in unmedicated adults with ADHD. They observed significantly lower binding of [^{11}C]cocaine, a marker for the dopamine transporter and [^{11}C]raclopride, a marker for D2/D3 receptors, in dopamine-innervated brain regions. Brain regions included the left nucleus accumbens, ventral midbrain, caudate, and hypothalamus. Ratings of attention correlated with the measure of [^{11}C]raclopride binding in these areas.[112] These results implicated low dopaminergic neurotransmission in these brain regions in people with ADHD.

Are people with ADHD more likely to develop Parkinson's disease? It appears that low dopamine in children leads to ADHD symptoms and that low dopamine in adults leads to Parkinson's symptoms. It follows that as children who suffer from low dopamine grow older they may reach the threshold for Parkinson's disease at an earlier age than unaffected children. This inference is based on the well-known age-related decrease in dopamine levels in the brain;[113] as people age they often begin to show Parkinson's-like symptoms and the incidence of Parkinson's disease increases with age.[114] It is important to note, however, that the regional pattern of dopamine loss in aging is somewhat different from that seen in Parkinson's disease.[113,114]

Neuroscientist Manfred Gerlach from the University of Würzburg in Germany and colleagues investigated a possible link between ADHD in childhood and Parkinson's disease in adulthood. They administered questionnaires to patients with Parkinson's disease and age- and sex-matched controls, retrospectively evaluating ADHD-like symptoms in childhood. Results revealed that the patients with Parkinson's disease scored significantly higher on the questionnaires, suggesting greater ADHD-like symptoms.[115] Although the patients with Parkinson's disease scored below the ADHD range on the questionnaires, obviating the conclusion that they suffered from ADHD in childhood, the finding that they scored higher than controls on items assessing attention deficit and hyperactivity in childhood is consistent with a possible relationship between childhood ADHD-like characteristics and the development of Parkinson's disease later in life. This paper also mentions the interesting anecdote that in his autobiography, the well-known actor Michael J. Fox, who developed Parkinson's disease at an early age, reported ADHD-like symptoms in childhood.

I have thought that there must be epidemiological studies looking at the history of ADHD in patients with Parkinson's disease to see if there is a possible link but have been unable to find any. One problem is that the diagnosis of ADHD has not been around that long so that such studies may have to rely on retrospective diagnosis like those inferred in the study from Gerlach and associates referred to earlier. Such studies are eagerly awaited.

If the attention deficits of ADHD are related to decreased dopamine function, it might be expected that patients with Parkinson's disease, who suffer from a decrease in dopaminergic neurotransmission, will suffer from attention deficits. Some findings support this idea. For example, researchers from the University of Otago in Dunedin, New Zealand, reported that patients with Parkinson's disease, versus age-matched controls, showed increased distractibility in a task that required focused attention.[116] This and related findings support a relationship between decreased dopamine and attention deficit.

There have been many studies aimed at identifying possible genes associated with ADHD. One of the most consistent findings has been a possible association between ADHD and a variant of the gene *DRD4*, which codes for the dopamine D4 receptor. In exon three of *DRD4* a 48-base pair variable-number tandem repeat has been found with the number of repeats ranging from two to 11.[117] The seven-repeat variant, sometimes referred to as coding for the D4.7 receptor, has been associated with ADHD in a large number of studies,[118] but genome-wide association studies have failed to identify a role for this gene.[119] The D4.7 receptor is less sensitive to dopamine than the D4.4 or D4.2 receptor,[120] raising the possibility that part of the mechanism underlying a putative below-normal level of dopamine function in ADHD relates to the D4.7 receptor morph.

Genetic studies have found another association with the seven-repeat allele of *DRD4*. In 1996, Israeli researchers reported that the gene that codes for the D4.7 receptor variant is associated with the human personality trait of novelty seeking.[121] In spite of reports of failures to replicate this finding,[122] including a meta-analysis co-authored by the senior author of the original paper,[123] published papers continue to suggest an association between D4.7 and novelty seeking or a related trait. For example, frequency of the D4.7 allele increased with distance travelled out of Africa following the migrations of our species, thought to have begun at least 50,000 years ago; successful migration may have been facilitated by a phenotype with relatively low reactivity to novelty and increased exploration and risk taking.[124] US researchers suggested that natural selection operated on the gene encoding the D4 receptor and that there was selection for all of the alleles but in different environments. In resource-depleted, time-critical, or rapidly changing environments selection might have favored the D4.7 allele because it provided a more "response-ready" adaptation. Resource-rich, time-optimal, or little-changing environments might have selected against the gene encoding D4.7 in favor of one of the other alleles. The authors suggested that the presence of the D4.7 allele in a classroom setting may reflect an environmental mismatch; children with the response-ready adaptation are not well suited to a classroom setting and are diagnosed as having ADHD.[125]

From these various considerations, it appears that in ADHD and Parkinson's disease there is low dopaminergic neurotransmission. How can the symptoms be so different? Incentive learning may provide the answer. Early in life, many stimuli are novel. Recall from Chapter 5 that novel stimuli are activating and they produce a dopamine signal. Recall further that repeated exposures to a novel environmental stimulus that does not signal a biologically important outcome results in the loss by that stimulus of its ability to activate dopamine neurons; it becomes habituated perhaps through a process that involves inverse incentive learning, as discussed in Chapter 6. Some environmental stimuli do signal biologically important outcomes that produce a dopamine signal and those stimuli become conditioned incentive stimuli with an increased ability to elicit approach and other responses in the future. Recall from Chapter 8 that biologically important stimuli can be social stimuli, such as cooperation by a conspecific. This paints a picture of a young individual navigating her environment and gradually learning that responding to some stimuli leads to rewarding outcomes and responding to others does not. Now consider another individual who has low dopaminergic neurotransmission perhaps subsequent to a childhood disease. For her, novel stimuli may be as activating as they are for any young individual but those that are followed by a biologically important outcome may fail to become conditioned incentive stimuli. According to this scenario, the low-dopamine individual will fail to stay on a task. Perhaps relatively fewer stimuli acquire the ability to elicit approach and other responses. The result may be above-normal locomotor activity, constantly moving from stimulus to stimulus perhaps because few stimuli have the ability to control responding.

Conditioned incentive stimuli, with their ability to elicit approach and other responses, could be said to control attention. A number of authors have written about the role of dopamine in attention,[126] and experimental results have shown apparent impaired attention in animals with reduced dopamine function. However, others have shown that dopamine depletions do not lead to a loss of attention. In an ingenious study carried out in the Cambridge laboratory of one of the UK's leading behavioral neuroscientists, Trevor Robbins, it was found that rats with unilateral depletions of striatal dopamine detected equally well brief stimuli presented to either hemisphere. The rats were impaired in responding to the side contralateral to the lesion. These results show that dopamine depletions do not result in sensory inattention but rather in impairment in ability to use sensory information to guide motor responses.[127] This reflects dopamine's incentive learning function.

In the operant conditioning laboratory, researchers speak of rewarding stimuli *shaping* responding. As a child grows up, its behavior is constantly shaped by the outcomes associated with its action towards various stimuli in its environment. If dopamine is low, outcomes may have less of an impact on the behavior of the child. The discipline problems often reported in children with ADHD can be understood as resulting from a failure of environmental stimuli (including social stimuli) to shape their behavior. Treatment with prodopaminergic drugs such as *d*-amphetamine or methylphenidate may increase the ability of positive outcomes to produce incentive learning. As a result, the medicated child may stay on task longer, be more responsive to social rewards, and experience fewer behavioral problems.

In later years, an unmedicated adolescent with low dopamine may be less hyperactive because fewer stimuli are novel, but he may continue to have difficulty staying on task or planning, he may appear impulsive—showing the defining symptoms of ADHD. In adulthood, hyperactivity may be absent but attention deficits may persist. Pro-dopaminergic medications are expected to provide some therapeutic benefit in these individuals, as has been reported.

This framework provides a means of understanding the paradoxical effects of stimulant drugs that enhance dopaminergic (and other monoaminergic) neurotransmission on children with ADHD,[128] and normal children or adults. In ADHD children, possibly with low dopamine, psychomotor stimulant drugs may increase the dopamine signal, increasing incentive learning and leading to environmental stimuli that can control behavior; as a result, hyperactivity gives way to more normal levels of activity. In normal children and in adults, the same drugs may lead to too many stimuli acquiring the ability to attract and hyperactivity may ensue.

Summary

Converging evidence from several lines of investigation suggests that hyperactivity of dopaminergic neurotransmission underlies the positive symptoms of schizophrenia. Further evidence shows that an extensive loss of dopaminergic neurons in adulthood leads to Parkinson's disease and suggests that dopaminergic hypofunction may underlie the symptoms of ADHD in children. Enhanced dopaminergic neurotransmission leads to incentive learning, suggesting that the positive symptoms of schizophrenia, which are particularly responsive to dopamine D2 receptor-blocking drugs, may arise from excessive incentive learning. The gradual remission of positive symptoms over days observed in people with schizophrenia after the commencement of antipsychotic drug therapy may result from the gradual loss of incentive value of stimuli that inappropriately acquired incentive value while the patient was in an unmedicated hyperdopaminergic state. The neurocircuitry underlying declarative learning and memory may be relatively intact in adults with schizophrenia and may contribute to the formulation of delusions based on the excessive attribution of incentive value to stimuli that normally would be ignored. In adolescent or young adult individuals who experience excessive incentive learning, less developed and less integrated declarative learning and memory neurocircuitry may produce disorganized symptoms rather than well-formulated delusions.

The loss of dopaminergic neurotransmission in Parkinson's disease is associated with a general loss of responsiveness to environmental stimuli that may result from a decrease of conditioned incentive value of environmental stimuli encountered while in a state of decreased dopaminergic neurotransmission or even inverse incentive learning about those stimuli. Previously learned conditioned incentive stimuli not encountered while in a state of decreased dopaminergic neurotransmission may retain their ability to elicit approach and other responses; those stimuli may produce *kinesia paradoxa* in otherwise bradykenetic of akinetic patients with Parkinson's disease. Treatment of patients with Parkinson's disease with L-DOPA remediates to some extent the loss of dopamine associated with the loss of dopaminergic neurons and may prevent or at least mitigate for a time the loss of conditioned incentive value by environmental stimuli and the associated decrease in ability to respond to those stimuli. Excessive dosing with L-DOPA may excessively elevate levels of dopaminergic neurotransmission leading to inappropriate incentive learning and the formulation of delusions based on that learning.

The loss of dopaminergic neurons in juvenile animals does not lead to hypokinesia as seen in adults, but, instead, and perhaps paradoxically, can lead to hyperkinesia. Novel stimuli have an unconditioned ability to elicit approach and other responses, and the relatively high level of novelty in the environments of young animals may contribute to their maintenance of normal activity levels even in the face of diminished dopaminergic neurotransmission. Enhanced dopamine neuron activity produced by rewarding stimuli and leading to an increased ability of associated stimuli to elicit approach and other responses may serve to focus an animal on particular aspects of its environment. Low dopamine may result in a diminution or loss of this function. As a result, an affected animal may constantly move from stimulus to stimulus, resulting in hyperactivity. This may provide a basis for understanding the behavior of young humans with ADHD. The remarkable finding that psychomotor stimulant drugs that get their name from their ability to energize animals actually have a calming effect on sufferers of ADHD supports this suggestion. This presumably occurs because psychomotor stimulants enhance synaptic concentrations of dopamine to a level that permits normal incentive learning. In early adulthood, as the psychomotor drive provided by novelty in the environment declines, it might be expected that people with ADHD become less hyperactive, ADD without the H. However, the putative impairment of incentive learning associated with low dopamine will remain and with it the difficulty in focusing on particular stimuli in the environment; in these people, psychomotor stimulants continue to have a therapeutic effect, presumably through increasing incentive learning.

Chapter 10

Drug abuse and incentive learning

People abuse many drugs. In most cases these drugs produce dopamine-mediated reward-related learning.[1] Dopamine receptor antagonist agents or other techniques that decrease dopaminergic neurotransmission block the reward-related learning effects of nicotine, ethanol, marijuana, amphetamine, cocaine, morphine, heroin, and numerous related drugs.[2] If drugs of abuse activate dopaminergic neurotransmission they should produce incentive learning resulting in an increased ability of drug-related stimuli to elicit approach and other responses. This may help in understanding the development of drug craving and addiction. There is one thing in particular that sets drug rewards aside from natural rewards such as food or water and perhaps social stimuli. As discussed in Chapter 5, a stimulus, for example a tone, that reliably predicts reward, for example food, itself gradually develops the ability to activate dopaminergic neurons. Once this happens, the conditioned tone stimulus activates dopaminergic neurons and the predicted unconditioned food stimulus no longer does so. This can be contrasted with what happens when stimuli come to signal drugs of abuse. Like stimuli that signal food, stimuli that signal a drug of abuse gradually begin themselves to activate dopamine neurons.[3] However, in the case of drugs of abuse, the unconditioned drug stimulus retains its ability to enhance dopaminergic neurotransmission. As a result, *repeated drug users experience two activations of dopaminergic neurotransmission, one upon exposure to the conditioned stimuli signaling the drug and another upon actually taking the drug.* This unnatural and excessive activation of dopaminergic neurotransmission associated with drug abuse may lead to long-term compensatory changes in the neurochemical mechanisms that underlie dopamine-mediated learning that may contribute to the development of withdrawal symptoms and addiction.

The ability of drugs to produce reward-related learning can be evaluated in a number of ways. Two of the most common are intravenous self-administration and conditioned place preference. I describe these methodologies in Chapter 3 and only briefly describe them here. For the former, animals are outfitted with a chronically indwelling intravenous catheter that can be connected to tubing coming from a syringe mounted in an infusion pump. Animals are tested in a chamber outfitted with a lever that they can press to operate the infusion pump producing a small infusion of solution containing the drug. For place conditioning, a test apparatus consisting of two distinct chambers connected by a tunnel is typically used. With access to the tunnel blocked, one chamber is paired with the drug over several days by injecting the animal with the drug and confining it there. On alternate days the animal is injected with the drug vehicle and confined to the other chamber. The animal is then tested while drug-free with the tunnel open. If it spends more time in the chamber previously paired with the drug, a conditioned place preference is observed, demonstrating the rewarding properties of the drug.

Using these techniques, it has been discovered, perhaps not surprisingly, that the drugs that humans abuse also produce reward-related learning in animals. Self-administration and conditioned place preference have been observed for nicotine,[4] ethanol,[5] Δ^9-tetrahydrocannabinol (THC; the active ingredient of marijuana),[6] amphetamine,[7] cocaine,[8] morphine,[9] heroin,[10] and numerous related drugs.[11]

Drugs of abuse activate dopaminergic neurotransmission

The primary action of amphetamine and cocaine is to increase synaptic concentrations of dopamine. This has been shown in a number of ways, including postmortem in vitro biochemistry,[12] intracerebral microdialysis,[13] in vivo voltammetry,[14] and, in humans or non-human primates, using positron emission tomography (PET).[15] The other drugs of abuse that I have listed are not considered dopaminergic drugs. Their actions are on other neurotransmitter systems; however, they appear to produce reward-related learning by affecting dopamine.

Nicotine is one of the active ingredients of tobacco. It is a receptor agonist that affects neurotransmission by acetylcholine, an important neurotransmitter in the brain. Nicotine acts at a subtype of cholinergic receptors, the nicotinic receptor, which got its name from the ability of nicotine to effect a subset of physiological responses known now to be mediated by acetylcholine.[16] In studies using intracerebral microdialysis in rats, nicotine was shown to increase concentrations of dopamine in brain areas that receive an input from dopaminergic neurons.[17] In vivo voltammetry studies in rats showed that nicotine increased the level of dopamine metabolites in dopamine terminal areas.[18] PET studies with monkeys revealed that nicotine modulated dopamine synthesis.[19] In humans, PET studies showed that nicotine led to displacement of

[11C]raclopride binding in dopamine terminal areas.[20] Raclopride binds to dopamine D2 and D3 receptors; a decrease in binding is taken as evidence that levels of endogenous dopamine have risen and the dopamine is competing with [11C]raclopride for binding to dopamine receptors (see Chapter 5). Although nicotine's primary site of action is at cholinergic nicotinic receptors, it indirectly influences dopaminergic neurotransmission.

Ethanol, like nicotine, may not directly affect dopaminergic neurotransmission. One of its actions is to decrease neurotransmission mediated by the inhibitory neurotransmitter γ-aminobutyric acid (GABA) in the ventral midbrain, the origin of dopaminergic cells projecting to the forebrain.[21] Through this action, ethanol may disinhibit dopaminergic neurons; this suggestion is supported by the observation that, like nicotine, ethanol increases dopamine concentrations in its terminal areas in the brain,[22] and increases the firing rate of dopamine neurons.[23] In PET studies in humans, ethanol reduced [11C]raclopride binding, providing further evidence that ethanol leads to activation of dopaminergic neurons.[24] Dopaminergic neurons are under inhibitory control by γ-aminobutyric-acid; when ethanol reduces the strength of γ-amino-butyric-acidergic inhibition, dopamine neurons fire and dopamine levels increase in terminal areas. In this way, ethanol can activate dopamine neurons.

The active ingredient of marijuana, THC, discovered in 1964 by Y. Gaoni and Raphael Mechoulam at the Weizmann Institute in Rehovoth Israel,[25] acts on cannabinoid receptors in the brain. People have been smoking marijuana for centuries, but it was only in the last decades of the twentieth century that the site of action of its active ingredient was discovered. In 1988, American researchers at St. Louis University Medical School, Missouri, and Pfizer Central Research in Groton, Connecticut, discovered the endogenous cannabinoid receptor,[26] now termed the CB1 receptor; THC acts at this receptor. In 1992 Raphael Mechoulam and colleagues discovered that the brain has its own endogenous cannabinoid, anandamide,[27] and in 1995 they found a second endogenous cannabinoid, 2-arachidonoyl glycerol.[28] The name "anandamide" was derived from the Sanskrit word *ananda*, meaning "bliss." The discovery of an endogenous cannabinoid system in the brain is a good example of the progress of brain science in the past decades and represents an important advance in understanding the underlying mechanisms mediating the effects of marijuana abuse.

In vitro studies,[29] intracerebral microdialysis, and in vivo voltammetry studies[30] show that THC, like nicotine and ethanol, increases dopamine concentrations in dopamine terminal areas of the brain. I remember meeting a researcher, Lakshmi Voruganti, at a conference many years ago, who told me a story about an imaging study he was doing. He and his colleagues were imaging an antipsychotic medication-free patient with schizophrenia using single-photon emission computerized tomography with a dopamine D2 receptor ligand, iodobenzamide. After acquiring several scans, the patient complained of anxiety and asked for a break. He used the washroom and returned in 15 minutes. They repositioned him in the scanner and acquired several additional scans. When analyzing the results, the researchers found that there was about a 20 percent decrease in ligand binding in dopamine terminal areas after the break versus before. Upon questioning the participant, they learned that he had smoked a joint (marijuana cigarette) during his bathroom break. This single-case observation suggested that THC may have increased dopamine release in the brain; this dopamine would then have competed with the radioactive ligand for dopamine receptors, leading to the observed decrease in binding. Voruganti and colleagues from the University of Toronto and Western University in London, Ontario, published this interesting case study in 2001.[31] Since then, PET studies have corroborated this finding in groups of participants.[32] Although none of nicotine, ethanol, and THC is classified as a dopamine agonist, these compounds increase dopamine release in the brain.

The 1980s and 1990s were the decades of the discovery of the endogenous cannabinoid system, whereas the 1970s was the decade of the discovery of the endogenous opioid system. Like marijuana, humans have abused opiates for centuries, but little was known about how they affected brain function. In 1973, Candace Pert and Solomon Snyder, working at John's Hopkins University in Baltimore, Maryland, discovered the binding site of the opiate receptor antagonist naloxone in the brain, revealing that there are stereospecific opiate binding sites in the central nervous system.[33] Subsequently, researchers working at several sites in the UK in 1975 and 1976 identified the endogenous ligands for opioid receptors, the enkephalins and β-endorphine.[34,35] Like the cannabinoid discoveries that followed in the next decades, the discovery of the endogenous opioid systems was an amazing breakthrough that ushered in a new level of understanding of the neural mechanisms underlying the action of opioids in the brain. Opiates, including morphine and heroin, act on opioid receptors in the brain to produce their psychoactive effects. However, in vivo microdialysis studies show that they increase dopamine concentrations in dopamine terminal areas,[36] opening the door to the possibility that the ability of opiates to produce reward-related learning is mediated by dopamine.

Drugs of abuse produce incentive learning

Dopamine receptor antagonist drugs, many of the same drugs that are used to treat psychosis in patients with schizophrenia discussed in Chapters 7 and 9, block reward-related learning produced by drugs of abuse. We have already seen that drugs of abuse, although acting on diverse systems in the brain, share the ability to increase the concentration of dopamine in its terminal areas. If blocking dopaminergic neurotransmission blocks the rewarding effects of nicotine, ethanol, marijuana (or its active ingredient), amphetamine, cocaine, and opiates, results would suggest that activation of dopaminergic neurotransmission may be a common mechanism for reward-related learning produced by all of these compounds. Data suggest that it is.

Studies carried out in the laboratory of neuroscientist Gaetano Di Chiara at the University of Cagliari in Sardinia, Italy, were the first to show that a dopamine receptor antagonist blocked the ability of nicotine to produce reward-related learning in the conditioned place-preference paradigm.[37] Subsequent studies corroborated this finding and implicated dopamine in the shell region of the nucleus accumbens, a dopamine terminal area, in nicotine-induced place preference.[38] In studies of intravenous self-administration of nicotine, neurotoxic destruction of dopaminergic neurons in the nucleus accumbens decreased responding.[39] Related studies in rats and mice showed that nicotine acts on specific subtypes of nicotinic receptors located on dopaminergic cell bodies in the ventral tegmental area to stimulate dopamine release in the nucleus accumbens and to produce reward-related learning maintained by intravenous or intracranial self-administration of nicotine.[40] Recent studies reveal some of the complex neurotransmitter interactions involved in the rewarding effects of nicotine in conditioned place preference. Thus, mice with glutamatergic N-methyl-D-aspartate receptors knocked out specifically on dopamine neurons in the ventral tegmental area,[41] and mice with the δ subtype of opioid receptors knocked out,[42] failed to show a conditioned place preference to nicotine. These results suggest that the effect of nicotine on dopaminergic neurotransmission is modulated by glutamatergic and opioidergic influences. At the same time, nicotine appears to rely on dopamine for its ability to produce reward-related learning.

Dopamine D1-like or D2-like receptor antagonists significantly attenuated conditioned place preference produced by ethanol.[43] A later study in mice reported that a D1-like receptor antagonist or the use of small interfering RNA to knock down D1 receptor function in the nucleus accumbens blocked the acquisition of a conditioned place preference based on ethanol.[44] Home-cage ethanol drinking by rats was decreased by the dopamine receptor antagonist pimozide,[45] and operant responding maintained by oral ethanol was decreased by the dopamine receptor antagonist haloperidol; the pattern of the decrease in operant responding resembled that observed when ethanol was no longer available,[46] suggesting that treatment with haloperidol produced effects like those resulting from removal of the rewarding stimulus. Results implicate dopamine in reward-related learning produced by ethanol. As was the case with nicotine, the ability of ethanol to produce reward-related learning, although dependent on dopaminergic neurotransmission, probably also involves other neurotransmitters, including opioids and GABA. (The eminent neuroscientist George Koob, current director of the National Institute of Alcohol Abuse and Alcoholism in the USA, and his many students and colleagues, have carried out much of the critical research examining the mechanisms of ethanol use and abuse and written extensively about the neurotransmitter systems involved in ethanol addiction.[47] I return to these mechanisms later in this chapter.)

A group of Italian researchers reported that a synthetic cannabinoid receptor agonist—WIN 55,212-2—was self-administered by rats; they used intracerebral microdialysis of the nucleus accumbens and showed that dopamine levels rose during self-administration sessions, suggesting that the maintenance of responding for intravenous injections of a cannabinoid receptor agonist may involve activation of dopaminergic neurotransmission.[48] I was unable to find any published reports of the effects of direct manipulations of dopaminergic neurotransmission on cannabinoid-induced conditioned place preference. However, one group of researchers reported that the conditioned place preference produced by THC was blocked by SL327, a specific inhibitor of mitogen-activated protein kinase/extracellular signal-regulated kinase.[49] This kinase is activated by D1-like dopamine receptors. Its activation is inhibited by dopamine receptor antagoinsts,[49] and, as I discuss in Chapter 12, my former doctoral student, Todor Gerdjikov, colleague Gregory Ross, and I found that its inhibition blocks conditioned place preference produced by intra-nucleus accumbens microinjections of the dopamine-activating drug amphetamine.[50] These results indirectly link conditioned place preference produced by THC to dopamine by showing that inhibition of an intracellular signaling molecule influenced by dopamine (see Chapter 12) blocks reward-related learning produced by THC. A recent paper reported that a drug thought to block endocannabinoid release reduced reward-related learning produced by nicotine in conditioned place preference and nicotine-induced dopamine elevations in the nucleus accumbens shell in rats.[51] These findings implicate endocannabinoids in reward-related learning produced by nicotine, which has been shown to depend on dopamine. Overall, results show that the reward-related learning effects of endocannabinoids depend on dopaminergic neurotransmission.

Amphetamine and cocaine are self-administered by animals.[52] A particularly attractive feature of the self-administration paradigm is that manipulations that produce decreases in the magnitude of drug reward lead to *increases* in responding. For example, if the concentration of the self-administered drug is halved, animals will self-administer more injections of the drug by pressing the lever more often to achieve the same level of dopamine receptor activation.[53] This is attractive from an experimental point of view because it pits two possible interpretations of the effects of dopamine receptor antagonists against one another. Within an appropriate dose range, if a receptor antagonist is having an effect on motor capacity, it will produce a decrease in responding, whereas if it is affecting reward-related learning, it will produce an *increase*. In 1975, Robert Yokel and Roy Wise, working at the time at Sir George Williams (now Concordia) University in Montreal found that the dopamine receptor antagonist pimozide produced a dose-dependent increase in responding for amphetamine,[54] and two years later Harriet De Wit and Roy Wise found that pimozide similarly produced an increase in self-administration rates of cocaine in rats.[55] These results show that decreasing dopamine receptor stimulation leads to increased intake of amphetamine and cocaine, and suggest that reward-related learning produced by these psychomotor stimulants is dependent on dopamine.

Roy Wise, along with his student at the time, Michael Bozarth, at Concordia University in Montreal found that a conditioned place preference based on the opiate drug heroin was blocked by the dopamine receptor antagonist pimozide.[56] This finding was consistent with earlier reports that the dopamine receptor antagonist haloperidol decreased opiate self-administration,[57] but, as pointed out by Bozarth and Wise, those results were not unequivocal because the decrease could be attributed to a sedation effect of the dopamine receptor antagonists leading to the reduction in responding. The observation that pimozide blocked conditioned place preference based on heroin provided strong evidence for a role for dopamine in reward-related learning produced by opiate drugs.[58]

Role of conditioned incentive stimuli in drug abuse

The results reviewed in the previous section reveal that drugs of abuse activate the dopamine system and produce incentive learning, the acquisition by neutral stimuli of an increased ability to elicit approach and other responses. The stimuli that become incentive stimuli are those that were encountered immediately prior to the activation of the dopamine system. Nicotine, the psychomotor stimulants amphetamine and cocaine, and the synthetic opiate heroin (diacetylmorphine) are fast acting, whereas the onset of action of ethanol, marijuana, and morphine is more gradual (although still within minutes of intake). For the fast-acting drugs of abuse, the increase in synaptic concentrations of dopamine will occur in close temporal proximity to the stimuli associated with taking the drug and those are the stimuli that are most likely to become the strongest incentive stimuli. Perhaps for the slightly slower-acting drugs, other drug-state-related cues, for example friends with whom the drug is taken, may initially become strong incentive stimuli, but with repeated use, stimuli that are antecedent to those will also gradually acquire incentive value so that eventually stimuli associated with taking the drug will also become strong incentive cues.[59]

In the case of nicotine, most commonly taken by inhaling the smoke of cured tobacco leaves, the stimuli most proximal to intake of the drug will frequently be those produced by drug delivery. Those stimuli will most commonly be cigarettes and their packages, but could also be other delivery systems, such as pipes. During the period of nicotine intake, the delivery system cues are present. Nicotine rapidly activates the dopamine system; as a result, the delivery system cues would be expected to become strong conditioned incentive stimuli, attaining an increased ability to elicit approach and other responses in the future. Nicotine is often taken in multiple environments ranging from the home, car, and workplace to recreational locations, including, for example, sport-fishing boats and athletic fields. As a result, for an individual who regularly consumes nicotine, many additional stimuli would be expected to become conditioned incentive stimuli. These additional conditioned incentive stimuli will also have strong associative links to the cues of the delivery system. Thus, nicotine users will find themselves drawn to many stimuli and those stimuli will have a strong association with taking the drug.

Incentive learning produced by drugs of abuse such as nicotine may work the same as that produced by food-related stimuli. Food activates dopaminergic neurotransmission (see Chapter 5) and environmental stimuli associated with finding food become conditioned incentive stimuli. There is an aspect of incentive conditioning based on food that may be particularly relevant to understanding drug abuse. Studies have shown that even in the absence of a strong biological need for food, food-related conditioned incentive stimuli can still control responding, a phenomenon termed "resistance to satiation."[60] Thus, animals trained to lever-press for food while food-restricted, when tested following a period of access to free food, initially press the lever a number of times, but responding gradually lessens as the animals receive food pellets, many of which they do not consume.[61] If testing of previously trained animals following access to free food is repeated over several days, responding is seen each day, but it decreases from day to day. The within- and across-day pattern resembles the extinction of responding seen in food-restricted animals tested during sessions when food pellets are no longer presented.[62] These results show that *even in the absence of a primary biological need, conditioned incentive stimuli can control responding*. In the case of reward-related learning produced by drugs such as nicotine, this suggests that conditioned incentive stimuli based on nicotine will have the ability to elicit approach and other responses, even in the absence of any biological need for nicotine.

There are a couple of aspects of these conditioning paradigms to consider briefly before going on. One is that if conditioned incentive stimuli based on nicotine are repeatedly encountered in the absence of nicotine, those stimuli should gradually lose their incentive properties just as conditioned incentive stimuli based on food lose their incentive properties when they are repeatedly encountered in the absence of food. As discussed in Chapter 9 with respect to treating excessive incentive learning in people with schizophrenia, this has clear implications for the treatment of people with drug addictions; specifically, it suggests that the best therapeutic effects will result from repeated exposure to the conditioned incentive stimuli in the absence of the primary incentive stimulus, in this case nicotine (see below). Another aspect of these conditioning paradigms is to consider how it might feel to encounter conditioned incentive stimuli. Conditioned incentive stimuli come about by their association with rewarding stimuli such as food or drugs. Encountering conditioned incentive stimuli based on nicotine might be expected to activate memories of nicotine, including, for example, its smell, taste, and other sensory/perceptual effects. Perhaps the activation of these memories in conjunction with the increased approach and other responses elicited by conditioned incentive cues based on nicotine is the condition we describe as "craving." The possible relationship between activation of various brain regions and circuits, on the one hand, and mental experiences, on the other, is discussed in Chapter 13.

From the above, it is possible to see how incentive conditioning can lead to approach and consumption of drugs such as nicotine, even in the absence of a primary biological need for the drug. However, recall the italicized sentence in the opening paragraph of this chapter: *repeated drug users experience two activations of dopaminergic neurotransmission, one upon exposure to the conditioned stimuli signaling the drug and another upon actually taking the drug.* In the case of incentive conditioning based on food, the food stimulus itself gradually loses its ability to activate dopaminergic neurons when it is reliably predicted by a conditioned stimulus; in tandem with this change, the conditioned stimulus gradually acquires the ability to activate dopaminergic neurons (see Chapter 5). In the case of incentive learning based on drugs such as nicotine, however, conditioned stimuli that reliably predict the drug acquire the ability to activate dopaminergic neurons, but nicotine itself retains the ability to activate dopaminergic neurons.[63] The double activation of dopaminergic neurons may lead to compensatory changes in the brain that form part of the substrate of a biological need state for the drug. Nicotine withdrawal leads to symptoms, including, but not limited to, depressed mood, anxiety, and distractibility. Drugs may then be consumed to slake the appetite created by this need. Drugs of abuse activate dopaminergic neurons and ameliorate the need state; they also produce incentive learning, perpetuating the incentive value of drug-related cues. Upon withdrawal, drugs of abuse perpetuate the very need state they are taken to ameliorate. The development of a need state for the drug may considerably complicate the biological underpinnings of drug addiction (see Chapter 12).

These considerations of incentive learning based on nicotine abuse suggest that one way to reduce nicotine use might be to reduce the number of conditioned incentive stimuli associated with nicotine. Recent social policies that restrict the smoking of tobacco products to specified areas may actually help nicotine users to reduce their drug use. Smoking is no longer permitted on many passenger airplanes. Many company and public buildings in many parts of the world are now designated as no-smoking areas and those who wish to smoke must use specific rooms set aside for smoking or go outdoors. For tobacco smokers, these policies will limit the number of environmental stimuli that are conditioned incentive stimuli associated with nicotine intake. The nicotine need state will still develop gradually as blood levels of nicotine drop and associated physiological responses will continue to take place, but this need state will not be augmented by exposure to conditioned incentive stimuli associated with nicotine if the individual is in a work or public environment that is not associated with nicotine use.[64] This may be analogous to hunger in the absence of food-related cues. An individual may be in a need state for food, but that state may not be strongly influencing behavior until she smells the aroma of food cooking or sees food-related messages; the combination of the need state and these conditioned incentive stimuli for food may elicit approach and other responses to the food-related cues. Similarly with nicotine, the need state may influence behavior, particularly in the presence of conditioned incentive stimuli based on nicotine.

As reviewed above, ethanol produces reward-related learning in conditioned place preference, increases dopaminergic neurotransmission, and dopamine receptor antagonists block its reward-related learning effects, strongly implicating dopamine in learning produced by ethanol reward. If the increase in dopamine produced by ethanol leads to incentive learning, ethanol-associated stimuli will acquire an increased ability to elicit approach and other responses. Similar to the situation with nicotine discussed earlier, the range of stimuli that may come to be incentive stimuli and to be associated with ethanol will be as broad as the range of stimuli that is encountered while taking ethanol. The delivery system cues, for example bottle, brand name on the label, the scent of the alcohol, and so on, would be expected to become conditioned incentive stimuli. If ethanol is regularly taken in a particular place, that place may acquire conditioned incentive value. In the future, these conditioned incentive stimuli will elicit approach and other responses and associated memories of alcohol and related cues. As discussed earlier, incentive conditioning itself, even in the absence of a need state, can control behavior. However, as was the case with nicotine, chronic use of alcohol leads to physiological changes that can serve as the need state for more alcohol.[47] The combination of the need state and incentive cues associated with alcohol provides those cues with a strong ability to elicit approach and other behaviors, including consummatory responses.

Some drugs have a much stronger effect on dopamine release than others; for example, amphetamine and cocaine increase dopamine levels to a greater extent than alcohol and alcohol increases dopamine release to a greater extent than THC.[65] Chronic use of some drugs produces a more intense need state than others; for example, alcohol withdrawal is more severe than marijuana withdrawal.[66] In the case of alcohol, in addition to incentive conditioning, the need state produced by withdrawal from chronic alcohol use may be strong, providing a strong motivation to seek and take alcohol. Thus, incentive conditioning will not be the only variable contributing to drug abuse and addiction. The need state created by withdrawal from chronic drug use will interact with incentive conditioning to determine the strength of drug seeking and taking.

Of the drugs being discussed here, marijuana may be the least difficult to stop taking. This may be because marijuana creates the least uncomfortable need state. Although the active ingredient of marijuana, THC, increases dopaminergic neurotransmission and produces incentive learning, the incentive stimuli associated with marijuana may not have a strong accompanying need state produced by withdrawal from the drug like that seen in chronic nicotine and alcohol use; however, newer forms of marijuana are more potent and may produce more prominent withdrawal effects.[67] Whatever the strength of the need state, there is good evidence that conditioned incentive stimuli, in the absence of a need state, can control behavior (see earlier), suggesting that marijuana users will be attracted to cues associated with marijuana-taking. Additionally, those cues will have associations with memories of the stimulus properties and effects of the drug. This learning may contribute to further drug use.

Amphetamine and cocaine both strongly activate dopaminergic neurotransmission and produce strong incentive learning. Stimuli associated with amphetamine- or cocaine-taking will become conditioned incentive stimuli. If cocaine is taken by snorting lines of the powdered drug from a mirror through a rolled up bank note or a straw, those stimuli may become conditioned incentive stimuli with an increased ability to attract in the future. Similar learning may take place to the people associated with drug taking and the place where it is taken. Withdrawal from chronic use of amphetamine or cocaine leads to symptoms characterized by loss of energy, depressed mood, and sleep disturbance,[66] creating the need state for the drug that may enhance the incentive motivational effects of conditioned incentive stimuli when they are encountered. The more people, places, and things associated with taking amphetamine or cocaine, the more conditioned incentive stimuli the individual will encounter. Some of these stimuli may be temporally removed from actually taking the drug, especially in the case of amphetamine because of its relatively long half-life.[68] These stimuli will be attractive but may not necessarily have strong associations with drug taking. In this situation the apparent importance of stimuli, for example other people, encountered while under the influence of amphetamine or cocaine may lead to the development of persecutory or grandiose cognitive interpretations of what is being experienced. To others these will appear to be delusions (see Chapter 9). This paints the picture of the amphetamine or cocaine addict as someone who is in a need state induced, at least in part, by the double activation of dopaminergic neurotransmission by conditioned incentive stimuli and the drug itself,[69] who is attracted by many conditioned incentive stimuli induced by enhanced dopaminergic neurotransmission produced by the drug, and who may have developed delusional beliefs based on excessive incentive learning.

Morphine and heroin enhance dopaminergic neurotransmission that would be expected to produce incentive learning, stimuli associated with drug taking coming to control behavior. Conditioned incentive stimuli based on heroin will also activate dopaminergic neurotransmission.[70] With chronic use, opiates produce well-known withdrawal effects characterized by, but not limited to, anxiety, fatigue, nausea, muscle pain, and cramping,[66] which will provide the need state for continued drug seeking and taking, and will augment the behavioral impact of conditioned incentive stimuli associated with drug taking. The relative severity of opiate withdrawal symptoms created by chronic use may contribute to the maintenance of opiate abuse but the influence of this need state may itself be modulated by conditioning factors as discussed in the next section.

Mechanisms of the need state

One of the consequences of chronic use of drugs of abuse is a down-regulation of dopaminergic neurotransmission. This has been shown in a number of ways. For example, researchers evaluated learning produced by brain stimulation reward in rats that had previously experienced a period of daily administration of cocaine or amphetamine; they found that brain stimulation reward thresholds were elevated even a week later (elevated thresholds indicate reduced sensitivity to the rewarding brain stimulation).[71] Neuroscientists Athena Markou (1961–2016), George Koob, and their collaborators and students at the Scripps Research Institute in La Jolla, California, extended these findings to additional drugs; they found elevations in brain stimulation reward thresholds in rats after chronic treatment with nicotine,[72] ethanol,[73] and morphine.[74] In related studies, extracellular dopamine concentrations measured with microdialysis of the nucleus accumbens in rats following chronic cocaine were observed to decrease.[75] Researchers at the University of Cagliari in Italy showed similar depressions of extracellular dopamine in the nucleus accumbens of rats following chronic amphetamine, ethanol, or morphine.[76] In general agreement with these findings, Francis White (1952–2006) and coworkers, at the time at Wayne State University in Detroit, Michigan, reported results from electrophysiological studies showing decreased activity in dopaminergic neurons located in the ventral tegmental area, the origin of dopaminergic projections to the nucleus accumbens (see Chapter 11), in rats following chronic cocaine administration.[77] Similar decreases in dopaminergic neuronal activity have been reported for up to 14 days following chronic nicotine,[78] ethanol,[79], THC,[80] and morphine.[81] Mexican-American psychiatrist Nora Volkow, current director of the National Institute of Drug Abuse in Bethesda, Maryland, and collaborators review human imaging studies of drug-addicted individuals during a period of withdrawal; they report a decrease in dopamine D2 receptors and a blunted response to a dopaminergic challenge, evidence of reduced dopamine functioning.[82] All of these findings implicate decreased dopaminergic neurotransmission in the need state that develops following chronic use of drugs of abuse; this decrease is manifested as withdrawal during a period of abstinence from the drug.

George Koob and a leading French neuroscientist, Michel Le Moal, from the Université Victor Ségalen Bordeaux 2 in Bordeaux, in their 2006 textbook on the *Neurobiology of Addiction*, comment that "Decreases in reward neurotransmitter function have been hypothesized to contribute significantly to the negative motivational state associated with acute drug abstinence ... " (p. 430).[83] As you have seen in the results reviewed earlier, there is extensive evidence supporting this hypothesis. Koob and Le Moal review additional evidence showing that other brain systems are also involved in the need state associated with withdrawal from drugs of abuse. They refer to these as stress systems that include the brain's corticotrophin-releasing factor system and dynorphin-κ opioid system, located in forebrain regions, including the nucleus accumbens.[84] The engagement of these systems contributes to symptoms such as anxiety and fatigue that occur in withdrawal from drugs of abuse. Koob describes how extended access to drugs of abuse, including nicotine, methamphetamine, cocaine, and heroin, leads to an escalation of intake. One of the functions of the dynorphin-κ opioid system may be to negatively regulate the dopamine system;[85] thus, escalations of activation of dopaminergic neurotransmission are accompanied by escalations of activation of an opponent system that suppresses the activity of dopamine possibly contributing to the dopamine hypofunction associated with withdrawal.

By taking the drug when withdrawal symptoms are present, the user elevates dopaminergic neurotransmission and reduces the symptoms of withdrawal. Recall from Chapter 2 that some stimuli produce reward-related learning by their offset and that such stimuli were said to produce negative reinforcement. Chapters 3 and 6 include a discussion of learning conditioned avoidance responses and outline how the offset of aversive stimuli putatively activates dopaminergic neurotransmission producing incentive learning to the stimuli that signal safety. From these considerations, it is possible to see that taking an abused drug while in the withdrawal state should produce reward-related learning for two reasons: (i) it reduces the aversive symptoms (e.g., anxiety, fatigue, depression) that form part of the withdrawal state; and (ii) it augments dopaminergic neurotransmission. The reward signal would be expected to maintain incentive learning about the drug-associated cues. It will also lead to the double activation of dopaminergic neurons, by conditioned incentive cues and by the drug itself, putatively perpetuating compensatory changes in dopaminergic and related systems that lead to subnormal levels of dopamine neuron activity and the need state for continued drug taking.

Treating drug abuse

Consideration of drug abuse within the framework of incentive learning provides insights into important aspects of rehabilitation of drug abusers. Drug abuse rehabilitation programs often involve a combination of drug abstinence and education about lifestyle changes and the hazards of drug taking. From the above discussion it is clear that there are at least two important elements in drug abuse: conditioned incentive stimuli and the need state created by physiological adjustments to the drug. A drug rehabilitation program that combines abstinence and education will do a good job in reducing the need state by allowing the body to detoxify, re-adjusting its physiology to a more natural state in the absence of the drug of abuse. However, all those conditioned incentive stimuli retain their ability to elicit approach and other responses until they are encountered repeatedly in the absence of the drug. I return to rehabilitation programs later.

A relevant anecdote may be useful here. The fictional book *Trainspotting* (1993), by Irvine Welsh,[86] follows the lives of a number of heroin addicts in

Edinburgh, UK. One character, Mark Renton, went through a drug intervention program and was detoxified. He then moved to London where he continued to abstain from heroin use, managed to build up a successful career, and he also developed a relationship with a woman he knew in Edinburgh. While in London, Renton at one point found himself at a party with a number of Londoners who were smoking marijuana that also had some opium mixed in with it. He commented (in his phonetically transcribed Edinburgh Scots dialect) on how out of place he felt at the get together, "Now ah'm oot ay place here, still in ma suit n tie, sitting in this comfortable flat . . . " (p. 299).[86] He was handed the joint and urged by his new friends to try it. He held it, sniffed it but then handed it back. He mused,

> Ah look again at the joint burning away in her hand. Ah try tae feel something. Anything. What ah'm really looking for is the demon, the bad bastard, the radge inside ay me who shuts down ma brain, who propels hand to joint and joint to lips and sucks and sucks like a vacuum cleaner. He's not coming oot tae play. Maybe he doesnae live here any mair. All that's left is the nine-to-five arsehole (p. 300).[86]

These comments suggest that, for Renton, the usual incentive stimuli for drug taking were not present. The stimuli in this relatively novel, non-drug-taking-associated environment, including the non-drug-taking-associated people, were not strong conditioned incentive stimuli for drug taking and he abstained. Later in the narrative, Renton gave up his job in London, returned to Edinburgh, and began again to associate with his former friends with whom he had injected heroin in the past. Renton relapsed. The narrator made the following comment:

> Renton, who has now been clean for ages, since long before he packed in his London job and came back up (to Edinburgh), could not resist the uncut Columbian brown Seeker had supplied them with. It was the real thing, he had argued, a once-in-a-lifetime hit for an Edinburgh junky used to cheap Pakistani heroin (p. 328).[86]

Here, many of the usual incentive cues for drug taking were present. Renton was with his old drug-taking friends, he was in a situation where the drug was being delivered, and it was reputedly high-quality heroin. The ability of the cues to elicit approach and other responses was strong and Renton, even though it meant throwing away the months of success he had experienced since going through rehabilitation and even though he was not in a state of withdrawal, resumed drug taking. Not long after this scene in the book, Renton was on a bus and began to experience mild withdrawal from the heroin he had taken. He went into the toilet on the bus and injected himself with another hit. He was once again a junkie.

I realize this book is fiction but assume that Welsh's characters are based on people he knew in the council houses of Edinburgh, where he grew up.

I remember being astounded at how immediately and apparently thoughtlessly Renton was willing to throw away the promising life he had built up for himself. From the point of view of conditioned incentive stimuli, it is easier to understand. Renton's former drug-taking mates and all the associated conditioned incentive stimuli in Edinburgh would still have a strong ability to control his behavior. It is only after elimination of the need state through detoxification *and* mitigation of the incentive value of conditioned incentive stimuli that he will be relatively free from the behavioral control exerted by the drug and associated stimuli.[87] In support of this view, a recent study by a group of European researchers used affective-state modulation to show that heroin-related cues retained their incentive value in former users who had been abstinent for over a year.[88]

The putative role of conditioned incentive stimuli in the control of drug-seeking and drug-taking behavior may also be elucidated by another example, this one from real life. It concerns US veterans from the war in Vietnam (1955–1975). There was something of a stir in US medical circles when it began to be apparent that a high percentage, perhaps as high as 95 percent, of US veterans returning from Vietnam who had been heroin users in Vietnam stopped taking heroin when they returned home to the USA.[89] In 1971, Barry Rosenbaum, a doctor at the United States Air Force Hospital at Tachikawa, Japan, a way station on the trip home, reported in a letter to the editor of the *New England Journal of Medicine* that heroin users from among US servicemen returning from Vietnam were experiencing extremely mild withdrawal symptoms compared with the usual suite of symptoms observed in withdrawal from heroin use.[90] This was a surprising finding that led Dr. Rosenbaum to speculate in his letter that the severity of withdrawal might be related to the method of use: heroin was usually sniffed or smoked in Vietnam rather than injected, as was more common in the USA. An alternative hypothesis, not suggested at the time, is that the severity of withdrawal symptoms and the ability to abstain from further drug use are related to exposure to conditioned incentive stimuli associated with drug taking.

The study of drug use in returning Vietnam veterans was taken up by psychiatric epidemiologist, Lee N. Robins (1922–2009), at Washington University in St. Louis, Missouri, in the early 1970s. She was invited to undertake her study by Jerome Jaffe, who had been appointed by President Richard Nixon (1913–1994) as the chief of the Special Action Office for Drug Abuse Prevention, set up after two congressmen who travelled to Vietnam announced that many servicemen were addicted. It was Robins who found that a very high percentage of returning Vietnam veterans who had been dependent on heroin in Vietnam stopped using heroin on a daily basis when they returned to the USA.[89] In follow-up studies she found further that half of the men who had been dependent on heroin in

Vietnam occasionally used heroin again in the USA, but only half of them became addicted again. This contradicted the common belief that to recover from heroin addiction the user must avoid any further contact with heroin. Robins' findings can be understood from an incentive learning point of view, as I discuss in the following.

Before considering the role of incentive learning in the transition of addicted US Vietnam veterans back to the USA it will be useful to review a related finding about the role of conditioning in withdrawal from heroin use. In a now classic study carried out by Shepard Siegel and colleagues from McMaster University in Hamilton, Ontario, and Western University in London, Ontario, it was found that heroin overdose death in rats was related to environmental cues associated with drug injections. Rats received heroin injections every other day for 15 days and doses escalated over days. The rats received a vehicle injection on the alternate days. Heroin injections and vehicle injections were given in different and distinct environments using a counterbalanced design. On the test day, both groups were injected with a high dose of heroin, but one group received the heroin in the usual environment and the other in the alternate environment not previously associated with heroin. Remarkably, even though both groups had identical drug histories, there was significantly higher mortality in the group injected with heroin in the environment not previously associated with heroin compared to the group injected with heroin in the environment previously associated with heroin.[91] These results show that conditioned stimuli associated with heroin contribute to heroin tolerance.

The following picture emerges from the results of Siegel et al., the finding that dopaminergic neurotransmission is decreased during withdrawal from opiates, and the role of dopamine in incentive learning produced by opiates. Once heroin taking begins, the activation of dopaminergic neurotransmission by heroin leads to incentive learning, heroin-related cues acquiring an increased ability to elicit approach and other responses. Simultaneously, heroin-related cues develop the ability to activate compensatory physiological responses (e.g., down-regulation of cellular signaling) that lead to tolerance to the drug's effects. As long as heroin is taken in the presence of conditioned cues and the compensatory physiological responses occur, higher doses will be tolerated. If the same, higher doses are taken without the usual cues present and compensatory responses fail to occur, the higher doses may lead to overdose symptoms (e.g., respiratory depression) and death as shown by Siegel et al. Even in the absence of drug-associated cues, withdrawal symptoms may begin to appear within as little as six hours after last taking heroin. These withdrawal symptoms (e.g., anxiety, fatigue, agitation, somatic symptoms) may be associated with similar physiological changes to those produced by exposure to drug-associated cues that contribute to tolerance. This implies that withdrawal will be more severe in the presence of drug-associated cues or, conversely, less severe in the absence of those cues.

From this picture, some of the observations regarding returning Vietnam veterans who had been addicted to heroin in Vietnam can be understood. Thus, the mild withdrawal symptoms observed by Rosenbaum in veterans coming through Tachikawa on their way home might be partly attributed to the absence of drug-associated cues. The absence of those cues in the USA might have contributed importantly to the unusually high rate of quitting heroin abuse observed by Robins. Robins also found that half of the smaller number of previously addicted Vietnam veterans who used heroin when they returned to the USA did not become dependent. This contrasted with the general observation of very high relapse rates in domestic heroin users who had become abstinent but then tried heroin again after some time;[92] perhaps the absence of the original conditioned incentive cues associated with heroin taking in Vietnam contributed to the relative resistance of these individuals to relapse into daily heroin use and addiction. All of this had led me to think that if previously heroin-addicted veterans returned to Vietnam, they may be susceptible to relapse because of re-exposure to conditioned incentive stimuli for heroin taking. However, many of those cues, for example, an American military compound, young comrades-in-arms, sandbags, barbed wire, bullets, weapons, perhaps various odors, may no longer be there. Perhaps the more likely scenario is that relapse might have occurred if the Vietnam veteran had returned to another military conflict zone where many stimuli like those that may have supported heroin use in Vietnam were present.

The idea that environmental cues associated with drug taking may contribute to dependence and relapse was suggested in an influential paper published by Abraham Wikler (1910–1981) of the University of Kentucky Medical Centre at Lexington in 1973.[93] In it he suggested that relapse to opiate abuse observed long after detoxification may be attributed to "whatever the neural processes may be that underlie operant conditioning of drug-seeking behavior" (p. 612).[93] We know now that those processes involve dopamine-mediated incentive learning about the cues that signal drug rewards. Wikler suggested further that drug-associated cues may trigger counteradaptations to the original effects of the drugs. Shepard Siegel's work discussed above shows the important role of environmental stimuli in controlling counteradaptations that form the basis of tolerance. In a former addict who has been drug-free for a long period of time, exposure to drug-associated cues may activate conditioned counteradaptive responses that reinstate the drug-related need state and contribute to the resumption of drug seeking and taking.

Wikler showed a deep understanding of the dynamics of drug dependence that is clearly instructive for the treatment of drug dependence. As he said,

> ... mere detoxification with or without conventional psychotherapy and prolonged retention in a drug-free environment does not result in extinction of the conditioned responses any more than satiating a rat with food (ie, reducing its hunger drive) and keeping it away from the operant cage for a period of time will cure it of the lever pressing habit acquired previously under conditions of food deprivation. Rather, what is needed (for) post-detoxification treatment are repeated elicitation of the conditioned responses by appropriate conditional stimuli and *active* extinction of them by programmed self-injection of the drug of dependence under conditions that preclude its reinforcing effects (pp. 614–615).

This approach, however, has not been used extensively in the years following Wikler's insightful article.

Just over a decade after Wikler's article, in 1985 leading American drug addiction researchers Anna Rose Childress, A. Thomas McLelland, and Charles O'Brien, working at the Veterans Affairs Hospital and University of Pennsylvania in Philadelphia, reported some of their results from the use of extinction techniques in drug addicts along the lines of those proposed by Wikler. In several studies, they established a hierarchy of drug-related stimuli for opiate users and then undertook extinction training. Exposure to drug-related stimuli without the drug produced signs of withdrawal in a number of participants as expected. They incorporated a relaxation period after these sessions to help the participants get through the uncomfortable state. For some of the participants the strength of the withdrawal response diminished over non-reward trials, providing evidence in support of the use of this approach.[94] Childress et al. concluded that the use of extinction techniques shows promise but needs to be more fully explored. Twenty-five years later, researchers at McLean Hospital and Harvard Medical School in Belmont, Massachusetts, Karyn Myers and William Carlezon Jr., in their review of the use of extinction of drug-associated cues in the treatment of addiction, commented that "this work is still in the early stages."[95] They identified additional variables that may be important in the use of these techniques. For example, extinction of conditioned responses to drug-related cues might be more effective if exposure therapy was conducted in multiple environments. They review additional variables such as knowledge of drug availability that may modulate the intensity of the need state elicited by drug cues. Terry Robinson, a prolific researcher from the University of Michigan in Ann Arbor, who has specialized in the study of reward-related learning, along with Benjamin Saunders identified individual differences in predilection to incentive learning that may be related to susceptibility to drug addiction.[96] The prominent British neuroscientist Barry Everitt from the University of Cambridge has emphasized the promise of better success in treating drug addiction by using extinction methods to reduce the impact of conditioned stimuli on drug seeking.[97] Collectively, these authors identify some of the important challenges faced by efforts to bring theoretical understanding of the learning mechanisms of drug addiction to practical use in its treatment.

Summary

Drugs of abuse, including nicotine, ethanol, marijuana, amphetamine, cocaine, morphine, heroin, and numerous related drugs, depend on dopamine for their ability to produce reward-related learning. Amphetamine and cocaine act to increase synaptic concentrations of dopamine by interfering with the process for removing dopamine from synapses. Nicotine acts through cholinergic receptors, alcohol through GABA receptors, THC (the active ingredient of marijuana) acts through endogenous cannabinoid receptors, and morphine and heroin through opioid receptors; however, in every case, by acting through a variety of mechanisms, these substances also augment dopaminergic neurotransmission. They all produce conditioned place preference and all are self-administered by animals, demonstrating their ability to produce reward-related incentive learning; dopamine receptor antagonists or other manipulations that reduce their ability to augment dopaminergic neurotransmission block the rewarding effects of drugs of abuse. When an environmental stimulus becomes a reliable predictor of a natural rewarding stimulus such as food, increased burst firing of dopaminergic neurons begins to take place when that stimulus is presented and the burst of activity normally seen in dopaminergic neurons when the predicted food stimulus is presented begins to abate. Environmental stimuli that become reliable predictors of drug reward likewise acquire the ability to produce burst firing in dopaminergic neurons, but the drug retains its ability to activate dopaminergic neurons. As a result, *repeated drug users experience two activations of dopaminergic neurotransmission, one upon exposure to the conditioned stimuli signaling the drug and another upon actually taking the drug.* This unnatural and excessive activation of dopaminergic neurotransmission associated with drug abuse may lead to long-term compensatory changes in the neurochemical mechanisms that underlie the action of abused drugs and dopamine-mediated learning; these putative changes may contribute to the development of withdrawal symptoms and addiction. Many of the neurobiological changes that contribute to withdrawal symptoms can be remediated by a period of abstinence from the addictive agent. However, diminution or elimination of withdrawal symptoms does not reduce the conditioned incentive value of cues associated with drug taking. Exposure to those cues can lead to relapse, even in a person who no longer suffers from withdrawal symptoms. These observations suggest that effective treatment for drug abuse will include detoxification *and* systematic exposure to conditioned incentive stimuli associated with drug taking in the absence of the drug itself so that those stimuli gradually lose their ability to elicit approach and other responses.

Chapter 11

Neuroanatomy and dopamine systems

Neuroanatomy is dizzyingly complex. Even after decades of brain and behavior studies, it is not uncommon to read about a brain region or circuit that is entirely new. For example, in 2009, Daniel S. Zahm at the St. Louis University School of Medicine, along with co-workers at Johns Hopkins University in Baltimore, Maryland, and Rosalind Franklin University in Chicago, Illinois, described in detail a region of the brainstem now known as the mesopontine rostromedial tegmental nucleus.[1] This nucleus seems to play a key role in regulating the activity of dopaminergic neurons and therefore is integral to incentive learning. I have studied and written about incentive learning for many years but have never referred to this nucleus in my writing until recently. If you are relatively new to neuroanatomy, it may be reassuring to know that the connections of the brain, recently referred to as the *connectome*,[2] is very much a work in progress.

Another phenomenon I have observed regarding neuroanatomy is that even apparent specialists often have lacunae in their knowledge of the brain. For example, I remember attending a meeting of the Society for Neuroscience many years ago and listening to an oral presentation by a young postdoctoral fellow from the southern USA. I was very impressed by the polish of the presentation and of the speaker's obvious detailed knowledge of the anatomy of the brain region he was discussing. This struck me as something to aspire to. Then, during the question period, someone asked him about the possible relationship of the anatomic region he was discussing to another region located slightly more caudally in the brain. In the same clear and articulate manner that he used to make his impressive presentation, he looked at the questioner and said that he did not study that region of the brain and was unaware of its connections. This left me with as an important lesson. Neuroanatomy is so complex that few individuals will have a working knowledge of all of it. With this in mind, I will chart a course through some parts of the brain with the aim of establishing a framework for beginning to understand how incentive learning leads to the increased ability of reward-related stimuli to elicit approach and other responses.

There are crucial physiological functions such as respiration that are controlled by the brain. These functions notwithstanding, one of the main functions of the nervous system is to detect stimuli in the environment and to produce, through the musculature, appropriate responses. Simple nervous systems, for example those of the nematode worm *Caenorhabditis elegans*, detect light (without eyes!), chemicals, osmotic gradients, and contact, and use this input to steer the organism away from harmful stimuli that may produce tissue damage and towards beneficial stimuli that may satisfy biological needs.[3] The highly complex mammalian brain had its humble beginnings in a nervous system like this. Millions of years of evolution have elaborated the sensory organs and especially the processing of sensory information between the input side and the output side of the nervous system. As I discuss in Chapter 13, evidence suggests that all of our experiences and everything that constitutes our conscious life resides in the connections of those billions of neurons that have evolved to elaborate sensory input in aid of better controlling the output side of the system.

Functional anatomy of vision

Studies of vision form a large part of the neuroscience enterprise, with thousands of vision scientists probing the functions of the retina, its projection pathway into the brain and the neuronal circuits that process visual information. Among the most influential studies is the now iconic work of Torston Wiesel and David Hubel (1926–2013) who worked at Harvard Medical School in Boston, Massachusetts; they received the Nobel prize in Physiology or Medicine in 1981 for their electrophysiological studies of the visual system. Hubel and Wiesel recorded from neurons in the optic nerve, the cable that carries information from the retina to the brain. For this work they used deeply anesthetized spider monkeys with their heads fixed and their eyes directed forward towards a large illuminated screen. As an electrode was lowered into the optic nerve, they took the electrical signal they were picking up and passed it through an amplifier to a speaker. With this arrangement they could listen to the electrical activity of brain cells. As the electrode was lowered into the optic nerve, the speaker produced a sound referred to as white noise, a mixture of many frequencies a bit like the sound of wind in trees in a forest or a waterfall. As they slowly lowered the electrode, it would eventually be positioned adjacent to the axon of a cell so that the signal from that cell was discernable from the background noise. They found cells that seemed to have action potentials at fairly regular intervals. At this point, they have isolated a cell.

By projecting spots of light onto the screen towards which the monkey's eyes were directed, they were able to identify a region of that screen where the projected light affected the firing rate of the isolated cell from which they were recording. Using this technique, they mapped the visual field of the cell, that is, the region on the screen where light affected the firing rate of the cell. If light fell within the visual field, the firing rate of the cell changed in predictable ways; if it fell outside of the visual field, the firing rate of the cell remained unchanged.

The visual fields of cells within the optic nerve turned out to have specific characteristics. They were circular. They consisted of two regions, an outer annulus and an inner circle. The two regions had different and opposing effects on the firing rate of the cell so that either light projected onto the annulus had an excitatory effect and light projected onto the center had an inhibitory effect or vice versa. Thus, the cells were found to have circular excitatory fields characterized by excitatory centers and inhibitory surrounds or inhibitory centers and excitatory surrounds.[4]

In subsequent studies using cats, Hubel and Wiesel placed their recording electrodes into the primary visual cortex, a region of the cerebral cortex that is one of the destinations of visual inputs to the brain. Axons comprising the optic nerve do not project directly there but make synaptic contacts with cells in the thalamus or thalamus then superior colliculus on the way. This is already an example of the complexity I referred to at the beginning of this chapter and if we were to explore this complexity we would soon find that there are additional layers of anatomical complexity that will soon envelope us so that we can no longer see the bigger picture that I am trying to draw. So let's jump from the optic nerve to the visual cortex. In the visual cortex, Hubel and Wiesel used the same set-up that they used for recording cells in the optic nerve and were able to isolate the signal from individual cells in just the same way. Once a single cell was identified, the process began again to map its field—first its boundaries and then its characteristics.

What they found was that the fields of these cells were different from those in the optic nerve. For one thing they were larger. They were roughly rectangular in shape instead of circular. The cells in the visual cortex responded with either excitation or inhibition, as did the cells in the optic nerve. It turned out that in some cells the excitatory region was a band across the field running orthogonally to one of its sides and this excitatory region was flanked on either side with an inhibitory region; Hubel and Wiesel termed the line orientation running through the center of the excitatory band as the "receptive-field axis." Alternatively, the central band was inhibitory and was flanked by two excitatory bands. Perhaps the most striking thing about the fields of these cells in the primary visual cortex was that they responded maximally to a band or line of light in a particular orientation. If the band of light was parallel to the receptive field axis, if it was the right width, and if it fell directly onto the excitatory band in the field of the cell, the cell fired maximally. If there were two bands of light appropriately oriented and of the right width that fell directly onto the inhibitory surrounds in the field of the cell, the cell was maximally inhibited. If the entire field of the cell was illuminated, the firing rate of the cell did not show much change, presumably because the influence of light falling in the excitatory region was cancelled by the influence of light falling in the inhibitory region. Unlike the cells recorded in the optic nerve that seemed to be sensitive to points of light in the visual field, cells in the primary visual cortex seemed to be sensitive to bars or lines of light in their visual field. These latter cells were named "simple cells" by Hubel and Weisel. Simple cells could detect edges and they could detect spatial frequencies. Many also had a preferred direction of movement of the stimulus through the field.[5]

The groundbreaking work of Hubel and Wiesel precipitated an avalanche of electrophysiological studies aimed at identifying the fields and characteristics of cells in many regions of the brain that receive signals originating in the eyes. More complex fields were found in regions downstream from the primary visual cortex.[6] These observations supported the concept of hierarchical processing of information within the visual system. Beginning with cells that have small visual fields and respond strongly to a light/dark edge that covers the center but not all of the surround, it is possible, through convergence of individual optic nerve axons onto single cells at the next level of the system, to build line detectors like the simple cells described above. Sets of simple cells can detect spatial frequencies. Further convergence can produce cells that detect more complex features of visual stimuli including corners or angles. Color is embedded in all of these features; cells that are differentially affected by three different types of cones in the retina, so called red, green, and blue cones, carry the information. As you know from the three types of color cartridges for color printers, three primaries are all that is needed to produce the range of colors we normally see.

Polish neurophysiologist Jerzy Konorski (1903–1973), working in Warsaw, presciently postulated the existence of what he called "gnostic neurons" in his 1967 book;[7] these cells would be at the pinnacle of information processing and would be maximally activated by complex stimuli such as faces, for example. In a region of the cortex in the temporal lobe known as the fusiform gyrus, electrophysiologist Charles Gross from Princeton University, New Jersey, and colleagues subsequently (in 1972) identified cells that seemed to respond maximally to complex stimuli such as hands or faces;[8] others have confirmed the presence of face-selective cells in this area.[9] These cells would need to receive information about the features of a face, including, for example, in the facial plane, its generally overall round or oval shape, the horizontal and relatively parallel lines that define the eyes, inter-eye distance, oblique lines that define the eyebrows, the presence and position of nose and mouth, and so on. It is possible to imagine adding additional features of contours around the eyes or mouth, or idiosyncratic features such as scars, and color, to get to the point of identifying individual faces.[10] We are all aware of this ability to identify individual faces as we do it almost every day, but some individuals lack the ability to identify individual faces. People with damage to the fusiform gyrus have prosopagnosia, a neurological deficit characterized by this inability. These individuals can see, read, and find their way through complex environments but they cannot identify people by their faces.[11] This condition provides further support to the idea of hierarchical processing of visual information towards cells that represent complex stimuli.

The hierarchical processing model led to the idea that there may be individual cells that are activated by very specific stimuli and the discovery of cells that seemed to respond specifically to faces supported this view. However, it is generally accepted now that stimuli such as individual faces are probably represented by a number of cells. Harvard neurobiologist Margaret Livingstone and colleagues concluded that "The mechanism for distinguishing between individual faces appears to rely on a division of labor among cells tuned to different subsets of facial features" (p. 1194).[10] All of these cells do not need to be located together in a particular area, although regions of the cortex seem to be specialized for certain kinds of information. This distributed-representation point of view does not abrogate the value of the hierarchical model; instead, it adds to its complexity. In the end, it may not be the activity of a single cell that represents a particular stimulus in the environment but perhaps the activity of a set of cells. These putative sets of cells are reminiscent of Donald Hebb's (1904–1985) cell assemblies,[12] and Bindra's gnostic-assemblies and pexgos.[13] Some of the features of a particular stimulus may be common to other stimuli. What makes a stimulus unique is the specific *set* of cells it activates.

Functional anatomy of audition

The hierarchical model seems to apply to other sensory systems, too, but is not as well worked out as it is for vision. One of the challenges is the difficulty in identifying features and how they combine to make the percept. In audition, for example, we hear frequencies in the range of 20–20,000 Hz and those frequencies can vary in intensity. If we record from neurons in the auditory nerve using techniques like those described above for recording from the optic nerve, we find individual units that respond to a range of frequencies but that are tuned optimally to a particular "best" frequency; at that frequency they respond to a lower intensity of sound than at other frequencies.[14] Deriving these tuning curves is not simple. Once a neuron is isolated, the experimenter will play a tone of a particular frequency to see if the neuron responds to it. Once a frequency is found to which the neuron fires, the minimum intensity of that frequency that will activate the neuron needs to be found by presenting it at a range of different intensities. Then adjacent frequencies need to be tested in a similar manner until the entire tuning curve of the neuron is found. Using this approach, researchers have found that the tuning curve plotting frequency on the horizontal axis and intensity on the vertical axis is roughly V-shaped with the best frequency being the one that activates the neuron at the lowest intensity.

Electrophysiologists have recorded from different levels of the auditory system, ascending from the first nucleus in the brainstem, the cochlear nucleus, to the next synapse, the superior olive, then the inferior colliculus, medial geniculate, and cortical regions that receive auditory input. By analogy to the visual system, it might be expected that the preferred stimulus for cells at ever-higher levels of the auditory system will get progressively more complex. A 1974 review of the frequency selectivity of single cells at various levels of the auditory system found that as one ascends the system, frequency selectivity is gradually *lost*.[15] This might be expected if the preferred stimulus for activating cells at higher levels of the system was getting progressively more complex. Perhaps at the highest levels of the system in humans, cells that represent complex speech sounds or even short sentences, for example "Run for it," might be found. Electrophysiologists cannot do these sorts of experiments in humans, but some studies in non-human primates provide data supportive of this general idea. European researchers have found "voice" cells, by analogy to face cells, in the supratemporal plane, a region of auditory cortex of the rhesus monkeys; voice cells respond more strongly to conspecific voices than to the voices of other animals or non-voice sounds. Among the voice cells were some that showed selectivity to the call type (e.g., grunt, bark, scream, coo) and some that showed selectivity to the particular individual voice.[16] The calls are often short in duration but differ in their frequency structure. If the axons from cells lower in the auditory system that respond to specific frequencies in a call converged on a cell in the auditory cortex, that cortical cell might be maximally activated by the call. It may be partially activated by other sounds that contain some of the frequencies of the call, but it will *prefer* a very specific spectrum of frequencies, making it a specific call detector.

Audition depends on a flow of information in a way that vision does not. If you are watching a movie and stop it at any particular point, a complex visual image remains. It is possible to isolate a particular element of the scene, for example a face, and to identify the features that make up the face. Then the convergence of feature detectors onto specific cells in the fusiform cortex can be seen as the underlying wiring of the nervous system that makes that perception possible. In the case of audition, if you stopped the soundtrack of the movie, assuming you could keep playing the slice of sound at the time you stopped the soundtrack, it would probably be meaningless. Suppose there was a busy urban scene playing in the movie at the moment it stopped. The slice of sound that was playing might be a mix of frequencies from cars, buses, and voices, but none might be identifiable. Audition depends a lot more than vision on sequential processing; the meaning of sounds comes from transitions of multiple frequencies over time. This has made the study of the processing of auditory information more challenging than the study of vision (although I do not mean to imply that studies of the visual system have been easy). In spite of these challenges, results are beginning to emerge showing that the complexity of stimuli to which cells in the auditory system respond increases as one ascends the system from the auditory nerve to the cortex. As was the case in the visual system, and this point bears repeating, it is probably not the case that a particular stimulus in the environment leads to the unique activation of a single cell but rather that a particular stimulus leads to the unique activation of a set of cells. Some of the features of a particular stimulus may be common to other stimuli. What makes a stimulus unique is the total set of cells it activates.

Functional anatomy of olfaction

The principle of hierarchical processing of information from sensory receptors through the various nuclei of the system to the cortex is a general one that applies to all sensory systems. I have briefly discussed the visual and auditory systems and it is possible to apply the same reasoning to olfaction, gustation, and somatosensation. The study of olfaction has proven challenging because of the difficulty in identifying the primary stimuli. In the case of vision, the frequencies of light that maximally activate each of the sensory cells, one type of rod and three types of cones in humans, are well characterized. The synaptic organization of the retina is beginning to be understood.[17] As a result, we have a pretty good idea of how visual information is parceled and sent towards the brain and, as I have discussed briefly earlier, how it is processed. The hair cells of the auditory receptor apparatus, the organ of Corti, have been extensively studied,[18] as has their synaptic organization within the organ of Corti.[19] The organization of frequency and intensity information carried by the axons of the auditory nerve is quite well characterized and, as already discussed, many studies have examined the response characteristics of cells at higher levels of the auditory system. In the case of olfaction, it now appears that there is a large number, many hundreds, of primary stimuli that are detected by different olfactory receptors. This was discovered late in the twentieth century by Richard Axel and Linda Buck at Columbia University in New York,[20] and earned them the 2004 Nobel Prize in Physiology or Medicine. Axel and co-workers showed further that the receptors for a single odorant converge onto cells in a single glomerulus of the second-order olfactory neurons in the olfactory bulb.[21] The high level of convergence may allow amplification of weak olfactory signals.[22]

Glomerular cell axons that form the lateral olfactory tract project to the olfactory cortex and to the olfactory tubercle, a striatal structure; the olfactory cortex includes the piriform cortex, anterior olfactory nucleus, and parts of the amygdala and entorhinal cortex. These areas are densely interconnected. The response characteristics of cells in the olfactory cortex have received relatively little attention compared with those in visual and auditory areas. Odor coding has been studied in the piriform cortex and it has been found that an odor stimulus elicits activity in a small fraction of the neurons recorded,[23] and that those neurons only respond to a limited number of odors.[24] Piriform cortex neurons are also strongly influenced by previous learning via additional cortical–cortical inputs from other regions of the piriform cortex and from other olfactory cortical regions.[25] The response characteristics of cells in the primary olfactory cortex are reminiscent of those seen in the visual and auditory systems and are consistent with a hierarchical model of processing that posits feature extraction.[26] Presumably, various first-order telencephalic olfactory neurons send converging projections to higher-order neurons that represent complex odors such as the scent of an edible plant, the scent of a predator or prey, or the bouquet of a fine wine. As was the case with the other sensory systems, there is probably not a single neuron that represents the aroma of, for example, a specific fruit, but rather an ensemble of neurons the activity of which collectively represents the scent of that stimulus. Furthermore, as discussed in the next section, other sensory modalities influence olfactory processing leading to neuronal activity that is best characterized as multisensory.

Functional anatomy of gustation

The perception of taste begins at taste receptors located on the tongue, palate, epiglottis, and esophagus of mammals. Five different receptor types specialized for salt, sweet, bitter, umami (a savory taste), and sour (acidic) encode taste as action potentials in gustatory neurons that travel in the seventh (facial), ninth (glossopharyngeal), and tenth (vagal) cranial nerves to the nucleus of the solitary tract in the medulla of the brainstem. From there (in some, but not all, mammals), gustatory information is relayed to the parabrachial nucleus located dorsally at the midbrain–pontine border before projecting to the ventral posterior medial nucleus of the thalamus, on to the primary gustatory cortex located in the insular region, and then to the secondary gustatory cortex, part of the orbitofrontal cortex. Additional projections from the parabrachial nucleus go to the bed nucleus of the stria terminalis and amygdala.

One of the ongoing discussions about taste perception has been whether taste is encoded by labeled lines, that is, axons carrying specific information about a particular primary, or by the integration of signals from across multiple fibers.[27] Electrophysiological recordings from individual primary taste afferents reveal that they often respond to several primary tastes, for example sweet, salt, and bitter, but when a range of concentrations is used, each fiber shows greater sensitivity to one particular taste.[28] Some fibers are fairly narrowly tuned so that they respond minimally to other than one stimulus, but other fibers are more broadly tuned. Broadly tuned fibers have been identified as, for example, "salt best" or "sucrose best." With respect to these broadly tuned fibers, if the signal from only one gustatory nerve fiber was available it would not be possible to know if the stimulus was a low concentration of the "best" stimulus for that neuron or a higher concentration of another stimulus that also affects that neuron. However, by reading the signal from multiple fibers simultaneously, it would be possible to identify the nature of the stimulus. The same would be the case for neurons in the auditory nerve that have a preferred frequency but are affected by a range of frequencies, as already discussed. Results suggest that some "lines" in the gustatory system appear to be labeled insofar as they are narrowly tuned but many individual "lines," although being, for example, "salt best" or "sucrose best," respond to several primaries. For these lines it is only by reading the signals from across fibers that the stimulus can be decoded. As is so often the case when opposing views are presented, there is good evidence for both labeled-line and across-fiber coding of tastes.[28],[29]

Neurons of the nucleus of the solitary tract that receive input from primary gustatory afferents are broadly tuned.[30] The same has been found for responses to tastes by individual neurons in the gustatory cortex.[31] In spite of this broad tuning, Takashi Yamamoto and co-workers from Osaka University in Suita, Japan, have shown that sub-regions of the parabarchial nucleus and insular cortex are specialized for specific primary tastes, showing a "chemotopy" by analogy to the tonotopic organization of auditory input.[32] Results of studies where populations of insular cortical neurons were recorded simultaneously suggest that flavor perception is best encoded by the spatial and temporal across-fiber pattern of activity.[33] As in the case of other sensory systems, results are consistent with the idea that more specific aspects of sensory input are identified at each level of processing. As mentioned in the case of olfaction, there are also influences of other sensory/perceptual information (e.g., physiological state, previous learning) that converge onto gustatory neurons even at the level of the nucleus of the solitary tract and parabrachial nucleus that further complicate neuroscientists' efforts to unlock the code for gustatory processing.[34] I consider multimodal cells after a brief discussion of the anatomical pathways mediating the sense of touch and related body sensations.

Functional anatomy of somatosensation

Somatosensation begins with stimulation of a range of different receptors found in the skin, epithelium, muscles, bones, joints, organs, vestibular system, and cardiovascular system (note that the vestibuar system can be treated as a sensory system in its own right; for present purposes I am including it as part of somatosensory systems). Many primary afferent neurons carry somatosensory information to the brain via two main pathways: the dorsal-column medial-lemniscal system and the anterolateral system. Primary afferents of the dorsal-column medial-lemniscal system synapse in the dorsal column (gracile and cuneate) nuclei and the trigeminal nucleus, from there project to the ventral posterior nucleus of the thalamus, and thalamic afferents project to the somatosensory cortex on the postcentral gyrus. Primary afferents in the anterolateral system contact dorsal horn spinal cord neurons and the axons of those neurons form the spinoreticular, spinotectal, and spinothalamic tracts, terminating, respectively, in the reticular formation of the medulla and pons, collicular region of the tectum, and thalamic nuclei, including the ventral posterior lateral nucleus. Thalamic efferents project to cortical regions, including the somatosensory cortex. Additional somatosensory information is carried via the spinocerebellar tracts to the cerebellum. Afferents of the vestibular system project via the auditory (vestibulocochlear) nerve to the vestibular nuclei; they project to the cerebellum and to the ventral lateral nucleus of the thalamus. The ventral lateral nucleus projects signals originating in the vestibular system to cortical regions, including the region of the somatosensory cortex.

Somatosensation includes mechanoreception, thermoreception, and nociception. Mechanoreception takes place when specialized receptors are mechanically deformed, leading to the generation of action potentials in primary afferents that project to the spinal cord or cranial nerve nuclei. A familiar sensation from mechanoreception is touch. Mechanoreceptors found in muscles, tendons, and joints convey information about the amount of stretch. Mechanoreceptors in the semicircular canals and vestibules of the vestibular system convey information about body position and acceleration. (The hair cells of the organ of Corti that sense auditory signals are also mechanoreceptors; audition is covered earlier in this chapter.) Thermoreception is performed by free nerve endings that respond to hot or cold temperatures. The term "nociception" was coined by Nobel laureate Charles Sherrington (1857–1952) to distinguish the sense of harm from the subjective experience of pain that seems to accompany it.[35] Nociception takes place when free nerve endings in the skin, periosteum, joints, or some internal organs are exposed to intense chemical, mechanical, or thermal stimulation that threatens to produce tissue damage.

Electrophysiological studies of neuronal responses to tactile stimulation in primary sensory afferents, the dorsal column and trigeminal nuclei, and the ventral posterior nucleus of the thalamus are few in number, but they provide some useful information. Primary sensory afferents in the median nerve, that carries sensory signals from the hand to the spinal cord, can be classified according to the type of skin receptor they innervate. Skin receptors include slow-adapting Merkel cells, rapid-adapting Meissner corpuscles, and Pacinian corpuscles. They are specialized for the sensing of form and texture, microscopic slips between skin and object, and distant events through an object held in the hand, respectively.[36] Afferents from each type of receptor appear to cluster within the median nerve.[37] In studies with cats, this clustering appears to be maintained in cells of the cuneate and gracile nuclei. Within a receptor-specific region, each cell has a receptive field corresponding to a particular body area and the fields of cells within that region collectively represent the entire body.[38] Although there have been some studies of the response characteristics of cells of the ventroposterior lateral nucleus of the thalamus, results have been questioned and, at present, this remains to be resolved.[39]

Electrophysiological studies of neurons in the somatosensory cortex were inspired by the pioneering work of Vernon Mountcastle (1918–2015) at Johns Hopkins University in Baltimore, Maryland. In work that influenced Hubel and Wiesel and many others, Mountcastle discovered the columnar organization of the cortex.[40] Researchers from the Medical College of Pennsylvania in Philadelphia recorded the responses to touch of the skin of the palmer surface of the forepaw in neurons in the somatosensory cortex of raccoons. They discovered that many neurons showed maximal responding to a narrow, elongated touch stimulus in a particular orientation. Others fired maximally to a round stimulus applied anywhere within a receptive field.[41] The selectivity of these cells can be understood by the convergence of input from touch receptors from different areas of the raccoon's forepaw. They concluded that these neurons were somatosensory feature detectors analogous to the visual feature detectors found by Hubel and Wiesel, discussed earlier in this chapter.

Subsequent work revealed that neurons in the primary somatosensory cortex show a convergence of inputs from the different types of receptors that carry information about touch. A collaborative study involving researchers from the USA and Taiwan found that somatosensory cortical neurons of macaque monkeys respond during the duration of a skin indentation and at the offset of the touch stimulus. Primary sensory afferents in the ulnar and median nerves show *either* a sustained response (indicative of input from slow adapting receptors) *or* a response at stimulus offset (indicative of input from rapidly adapting receptors). The observation of both types of responses in the same neuron in the cortex was taken as strong evidence that somatosensory cortical neurons receive convergent input from different somatosensory receptor types. The researchers also found that these cells showed sensitivity to orientation of the skin indentation, replicating the earlier findings from studies with raccoons.[42] This orientation specificity and convergent input onto somatosensory cortical cells from different somatosensory receptor types would lead to cells that are activated by more specialized features of touch stimuli; for example, their maximum response may result from a combination of a particular form and texture along with a particular microslippage between the object and the skin. These cells are analogous to those found in the visual system, discussed earlier, that have complex fields specialized for specific features of visual stimuli and support the hierarchical model. However, because cells in somatosensory cortex receive convergent input that originates in different types of skin receptors, they are bimodal. The convergence of modalities represents another step in hierarchical processing.

Multimodal cortical cells

Many electrophysiological studies of the response characteristics of cortical neurons have found bi- or multimodal cells. Generally, primary sensory areas of the cortex project to adjacent cortical regions termed parasensory association cortex; neuronal cells in these areas are unimodal and respond to stimulus features as already discussed. Adjacent to parasensory association areas, at the junctions between two or more sensory modalities, multimodal cells are found. These multimodal areas include regions of the parietal, temporal, and frontal cortex.[43] Researchers recorded from one of these regions in cats, the anterior ectosylvian gyrus, where visual, auditory, and somatosensory information converges. They found cells that responded to visual and auditory stimulation, visual and somatosensory stimulation, auditory and somatosensory stimulation, or all three. They found that the receptive fields of these multisensory cells overlapped, that is, maximum responses were observed when the different sensory inputs originated in the same field.[44] These results provide further insight into how brain cells combine aspects of sensory information to become maximally responsive to particular stimuli in the environment.

In related studies, neurons that respond to auditory and somatosensory input were identified in the auditory cortex of macaque monkeys.[45] Similar multimodal cells were found in the parietotemporal cortical region of rats.[46] The responses of neurons in the gustatory cortex are modulated by somatosensory inputs and auditory inputs in rats.[29,34,47] Prefrontal cortical neurons in rhesus monkeys responded rapidly to vocalizations from other monkeys and to combined face-vocalization stimuli but more slowly to face stimuli, and the response was altered when the face-vocalization stimulus was made asynchronous.[48] All of these results support the idea that sensory/perceptual information is gleaned by the extraction of features within modalities and their eventual combination across modalities.

Many cells of the hippocampus, a limbic structure with strong interconnections with the entorhinal region of the cerebral cortex and that projects to the nucleus accumbens, respond to places in the environment and are therefore termed place cells. The 2014 Nobel Prize in Physiology or Medicine went to American-British neuroscientist John O'Keefe and to Norwegian neuroscientists May-Britt Moser and Edvard Moser for their discovery of place cells. In electrophysiological studies, O'Keefe and his co-workers found that individual cells of the hippocampus responded maximally when an animal was in a particular location within its environment.[49] They found that the timing of the place response changed with respect to an endogenous rhythm (theta) within the hippocampus as the rat moved through the part of the environment coded by the place cell.[51] They also found that the position and size of the fields of place cells changed when the borders of the test space were changed.[50] May-Britt Moser, Edvard Moser, and co-workers subsequently found that cells of the entorhinal cortex represent grids of place cells, defining the extended space of the environment.[52] This provides another example of the convergence of multiple inputs leading to cells that respond maximally to particular aspects of the environment.[53]

Some findings from human research corroborate the observation of multimodal brain regions that are activated maximally by concordant sensory/perceptual information from different modalities. A good example is the angular gyrus found at the junction of the occipital, temporal, and parietal lobes; this region is considered to be a cross-modal integrative hub.[54] Researchers from the UK used functional magnetic resonance imaging of the brain to identify regions with increased blood oxygenation level-dependent (BOLD) responses to audio and visual inputs presented either alone or in combination; the combinations were either semantically congruent or incongruent. They identified regions in the left superior temporal sulcus, including an area adjacent to the angular gyrus that were most activated when matched audiovisual inputs were presented.[55] This study did not have the resolution of electrophysiological studies that isolate single neurons, but results are consistent with the idea that there are brain regions that are maximally activated by multimodal input.

From the preceding discussion it is possible to get some idea of how information that is transformed into digital signals in bundles of axons coming from sensory regions can be combined through convergence at subsequent synaptic levels of the system until there are cells that collectively represent very complex environmental stimuli. *It must be the case that any stimulus we can discriminate activates a unique subset of cells in the brain.* If two stimuli activated exactly the same set of neurons in the brain, we would not be able to tell them apart.

The sophistication of our senses, vision for example, is astounding when we realize that all of the visual stimuli that are experienced by sighted people result from patterns of activity of neurons in the brain. Every person who we recognize, every animal or insect that we see, every word that we read has been realized because the light coming from those stimuli landed on our retinas where it altered the pattern of activity in our optic nerves. It is a wonder, and how the brain does it is still not fully understood.

Functional anatomy of motor systems

What is beyond these high-level subsets of cells that are uniquely activated by specific stimuli? Our sensory/perceptual abilities did not evolve to make us marvel at the world around us or to let us enjoy the beauty of a sunset. They evolved to improve our ability to operate effectively on the world to attain the things we need for survival. In just the same way that the primitive sensory abilities of *C. elegans* detect light, chemicals, osmotic gradients, and bodily contact, and use this input to steer the organism away from harmful stimuli and towards beneficial stimuli, our sophisticated sensory/perceptual systems allow us to navigate our physical environment. Thus, it might be expected that sensory/perceptual information will be transferred to response-output systems in the brain so that it can be used to control the musculature and therefore the behavior of the individual. This is a key point for understanding the anatomical organization of the nervous system.

As discussed, complex stimuli are detected through the convergence of synaptic inputs onto cells located along the pathways for that sensory modality and in multisensory areas, ending ultimately in the cerebral cortex at cells that respond to complex environmental stimuli, for example a face making a specific vocalization. *The cerebral cortex projects heavily upon the striatum consisting of the dorsally located caudate and putamen and the ventrally located nucleus accumbens and olfactory tubercle.* The striatum forms part of a larger complex of nuclei—collections of cell bodies—that are found, perhaps not surprisingly, just below the cortex in a region of the basal forebrain referred to as the basal ganglia. In anatomy textbooks, the basal ganglia are often described as parts of the extrapyramidal motor system.[56] The name "extrapyramidal" contrasts this system with the pyramidal system consisting of motor pathways that, in mammals, project from the cortex all the way to the spinal cord, forming eponymous pyramid-like protuberances on the ventral surface of the caudal brainstem on their way. Thus, all of that sophisticated sensory/perceptual information about our world that is so amazingly detected by our brains projects onto basal ganglia motor output systems.

Besides sensory/perceptual information that comes from the periphery of the body and projects from the cortex to the striatum, the striatum also receives information about the body's responses. Proprioceptive inputs from muscles and tendons project to the cortex and thence upon the striatum. Furthermore, copies of motor signals, termed "efference copies,"[57] are sent to the striatum. Thus, the striatum receives information about the body's posture and ongoing responses. These signals, like sensory/perceptual signals influence striatal output as discussed below.

The separation of motor output into pyramidal and extrapyramidal systems may be over simplistic. This is because effective corticospinal (pyramidal) neuronal function also depends on the basal ganglia. Cortical neurons activated by complex sensory/perceptual information project onto the striatum in mammals. From there signals are processed through the basal ganglia and then the axons of basal ganglia output structures (internal segment of the globus pallidus and zona reticulata of the substantia nigra) project onto the thalamus that, in turn, projects back to the cerebral cortex. The cortex then influences behavior through the corticospinal pathway. The cortex–basal ganglia–thalamus–cortex circuits are often referred to as loops.[58] Thus, the functioning of the pyramidal system relies on circuitry that includes the extrapyramidal system.

Motor control by the corticospinal system is of little relevance to most non-mammalian vertebrate species because they lack a corticospinal pathway.[59] Fish have a forebrain pallium, amphibians have some primordial cortical tissue, and reptiles and birds have a cerebral cortex; these areas receive projections from sensory systems and project to the striatal region of the basal ganglia.[60] In all these species that lack a corticospinal tract there are descending projections from the basal ganglia that can influence behavior. In fact, some of these descending projections are stronger in non-mammalian species than in mammals and may have weakened in mammals in parallel with the evolution of corticospinal projections.[61] Thus, regardless of whether or not a corticospinal tract is present, cortical sensory/perceptual information, including efference copy, projects upon the striatum and striatal output influences motor behavior; in mammals basal ganglia–thalamus–cortex loops may play a more prominent role (but see Note 62) and in non-mammalian species, descending projections from the basal ganglia may play a more prominent role.

Fish, amphibians, reptiles, and most birds do not have a corticospinal tract. In many non-primate mammals (e.g., cow, sheep, horse, rabbit) there is a corticospinal tract, but it only extends partway down the spinal cord, unlike the tract in primates that projects from the cerebral cortex all the way to the lumbar regions of the spinal cord.[63] Vertebrates that do not have a corticospinal tract generally have a smaller cortex and their motor capacities may not be as sophisticated as the complex digitation and tool use seen in primates; however, they still exhibit very complex behaviors that are effective in navigating and controlling their environments and they show incentive learning.

Because of its location within the spinal cord, the corticospinal tract is unlikely to be selectively damaged in an accident. However, it is possible to surgically sever the corticospinal tract in primates and such an experiment was carried out in rhesus monkeys in 1968 by Dutch neuroanatomist Hans Kuypers (1925–1989) and his colleague Donald Lawrence, working at the time at Case Western Reserve University in Cleveland, Ohio. Immediately following the surgery the monkeys held their heads up and were able to stand, walk, run, and climb. However, they were unable to use their limbs and hands independently of total body movement. Over the following eight weeks they regained independent use of their arms and hands, in reaching for food, for example, but even after five months they had not recovered the ability to use their fingers in the fine digitation (i.e., precision grip between thumb and forefinger) needed to pick up a morsel of food from a small food well. When they used their hand to grasp food, they had difficulty releasing the food.[64] These findings show that the corticospinal tract is important for fine motor control. Perhaps more importantly, they demonstrate the extent of motor control that is possible without the corticospinal tract.

Non-pyramidal motor control is effected by phylogenetically old descending pathways from the reticular region of the pons and medulla—the reticulospinal tracts—and the vestibulospinal tract. Projections to cranial motor nuclei, for example trigeminal and facial, are also involved. Striatal output nuclei including the internal segment of the globus pallidus and the substantia nigra zona reticulata, besides projecting to the thalamus, project caudally to midbrain/pontine regions, including the pedunculopontine tegmental nucleus.[65]

This nucleus also receives cerebellar input. It is part of the brainstem reticular formation and its descending output projects to the spinal cord as part of the reticulospinal pathway; it also projects to pontine and medullary reticular formation regions where it further influences locomotion and posture via the reticulospinal tract neurons originating from those regions.[66]

The tectospinal and rubrospinal tracts are phylogenetically newer non-pyramidal motor pathways. The tectospinal and rubrospinal tracts exert motor control from the midbrain. The red nucleus (Latin: *nucleus ruber*) is in the brainstem reticular formation and is the origin of the rubrospinal tract. It receives input from the cerebellum and its appearance in phylogeny is related to the presence of limbs or limb-like structures in many species.[67] It has undergone further modifications with the emergence of bipedalism and elaboration of the pyramidal/corticospinal system in some primates, including humans.[68] Elaboration of the tectospinal tract is correlated with the emergence of predatory behavior in mammals.[69] The origin of this tract in the midbrain tectum receives extensive visual, auditory, and somatosensory input. Outputs send motor commands via projections to the reticular formation and the direct tectrospinal pathway,[70] which control movements directed towards a specific location in space.[59]

A useful heuristic for thinking about the anatomy of the vertebrate brain is to begin with the primitive nervous system and then add further refinements of sensory/perceptual and motor capacities in a stepwise manner leading finally to the elaborate neuroanatomy of primates, including humans. This approach provides a rough outline for considering neuroanatomy but overlooks multiple sensory/perceptual and motor specializations found in various species that are themselves specialized for survival in particular environments. This approach begins with sensory-motor reflex circuits involving input from various sensory receptors that synapse in motor nuclei in the spinal cord and brainstem; an example is the withdrawal reflex that follows nociceptive input. Interconnections within the spinal cord and brainstem create central pattern generators. In the spinal cord, for example, these circuits "produce the synchronized, rhythmic patterns of motor-neuron excitation and inhibition that result in smooth propulsion through the water or to locomote across the land or fly through the air" (p. 102).[59] In the brainstem, similar circuits support the rhythmic motions of chewing, for example. The effective deployment of these reflex and pattern circuits is achieved by sensory input. Thus, sensory input, somatosensation from the body for example, projects onto motor nuclei in the spinal cord, brainstem reticular formation, and some cranial nerve nuclei. Other sensory modalities—vision, for example—via projections to the optic tectum, access the brainstem core (reticular formation) and cranial nerve nuclei where they control response circuitry. Descending outputs from the reticular formation, the reticulospinal pathway, carry motor commands that coordinate the activity of reflex and pattern circuitry. Somatosensory information is also relayed rostrally to the tectum, thalamus, and primitive cortex (pallium). Through phylogeny, the tectum receives progressively more elaborate multisensory input that allows for the detection of more complex features of the environment; its output projections to the brainstem reticular formation bring motor outputs under the control of these more complex features. The thalamus and pallium project to the striatum. Descending signals from the striatum to the pedunculopontine nucleus—part of the brainstem reticular formation—further modulate motor circuitry. As you can see later in this chapter and in Chapter 12, it is these circuits that are affected by dopamine and convey the effects of incentive learning to brainstem and spinal motor circuitry.

Further elaboration of motor capacities with the development of limbs and limb-like structures appears to lead to the appearance of the rubrospinal tract that brings cerebellar timing signals to reticular formation motor circuitry and also bypasses the brainstem and projects to the spinal cord. Neurons receiving multisensory signals in the tectum give rise to outputs that similarly project to the brainstem reticular formation but also bypass it and go directly to the spinal cord. Finally, with the elaboration of the cortex and its multisensory cell assemblies discussed earlier in this chapter comes the addition of the pyramidal corticospinal system, express lanes that carry cortical signals directly to motor circuits in the spinal cord. However, if motor nuclei received conflicting inputs from the cortex and other (non-pyramidal) sources, uncoordinated motor actions might result. To avoid this problem, cortical output also projects to the origins of the phylogenetically older motor pathways, the striatum, tectum, red nucleus, and brainstem reticular formation. This allows cortical output to spinal motor nuclei to coordinate its signals with those of other descending motor projections. Using this very brief heuristic, it is possible to understand some of the complex anatomy of the central nervous system by recognizing that it begins with a primitive sensory-motor core and adds the ability to better analyze sensory/perceptual input and to better operate on the environment with motor output in several phylogenetically newer layers.

It is useful to remember that the primitive sensory-motor core already contains striatal structures at its rostral end. All parts of the mammalian basal ganglia have been identified in lampreys, jawless (agnathan) fish-like animals that are phylogenetically the oldest group of living vertebrates. As is discussed shortly and in Chapter 12, the basal ganglia function in action selection through dopamine-mediated incentive learning. The observation of similar mechanisms in all vertebrates, including the oldest group, suggests that this mechanism has been conserved for over 560 million years of evolution.[71]

I was astounded recently to learn that the brains of members of another phylum, the Arthropoda, also have basal ganglia-like structures in part of their nervous system known as the central complex. Nicholas Strausfeld from the University of Arizona Tucson has identified what he termed the "deep homology of arthropod central complex and vertebrate basal ganglia."[72] He shows that a whole suite of homologous genes in insects and vertebrates is responsible for the derivation of analogous components of the central complex and basal ganglia. He describes how central complex structures (the fan-shaped body) in the insect (praying mantis in this case) are analogous to the vertebrate striatum; like striatal afferents, central complex inputs are activated by sensory stimuli, including visual and mechanosensory information. Strausfeld points out how information from different sensory modalities in the insect is processed through secondary neurons that are maximally activated by features of visual stimuli before projecting to the fan-shaped body; this is reminiscent of the processing of sensory/perceptual input in vertebrates as discussed earlier in this chapter. In insects, central complex outputs are critical for the selection of motor actions and the control of multijoint movement, again reminiscent of basal ganglia output to brainstem reticular formation and tectal regions that control movement in vertebrates. Finally, both the central complex of arthropods and the basal ganglia of vertebrates receive inputs from dopamine neurons.

I mentioned in Chapter 8 that dopamine may be implicated in incentive learning based on social stimuli in arthropods, including *Drosophila melanogaster*. It is perhaps worth noting in passing that members of other phyla also appear to show incentive learning based on dopamine. Thus, the nematode worm *C. elegans* learned a T-maze discrimination based on food, and genetically modified worms made dopamine-deficient by mutating the gene for tyrosine hydroxylase, the synthesizing enzyme for dopamine, were impaired in this task.[73] The Platyhelminthe flatworm *Dugesia japonica* showed a conditioned preference for a place associated with the dopamine-enhancing drug amphetamine and this preference was blocked by treatment with dopamine receptor-blocking drugs.[74] The marine mollusk *Aplysia* learned an operant biting response for electrical stimulation of the esophageal nerve,[75] which contains dopaminergic axons;[76] response-contingent iontophoretic application of dopamine to neurons post-synaptic to the esophageal nerve also served as an effective rewarding stimulus.[75] These studies add Nematoda, Platyhelminthes, and Molluska to Chordata and Arthropoda as phyla that appear to rely upon dopamine for incentive learning. In a review paper, Australian researchers Andrew Barron, Eirik Søvik, and Jennifer Cornish noted that dopamine has been implicated in the modulation of motor circuits in the five phyla mentioned above and also in Annelida and Cnidaria. Based on the observation that dopamine affects the amount of mouth opening to food stimuli in the cnidarian *Hydra japonica*, these authors speculate that "modulation of motor circuits in response to environmental stimuli could be one of the ancestral functions of dopamine" (p. 6).[77] These observations may push the evolutionary origin of mechanisms of dopamine-mediated incentive learning even earlier.

I have spent this time discussing the important role in motor control of the extrapyramidal motor system in vertebrates, with the striatum being one of the main output targets of the cortex, because it will help to emphasize the critical role played by dopamine in modulating the influence of stimuli on response output. The basal ganglia projections to the thalamus and back to the cortex and the addition of the corticospinal tract in the evolution of the central nervous system are elaborations of more primitive systems. It may be easier to understand the role of dopamine in the more primitive system and then to try to understand the implications of adding the basal ganglia–thalamus–cortex loops. Now it is time to add dopaminergic pathways to this anatomy.

Anatomy of dopamine systems and the basal ganglia

The ventral midbrain, also termed the ventral mesencephalon, is part of the brainstem, central neural tissue below the cortex, basal ganglia, and thalamus. In 1964, neuroanatomists Annica Dahlström and Kjell Fuxe, working at the Karolinska Institute in Stockholm, Sweden, reported the discovery, using the newly developed Falck-Hillarp formaldehyde histofluorescence technique,[78] of cell bodies of dopaminergic neurons located in the ventral midbrain in two major nuclei, the ventral tegmental area and the substantia nigra zona compacta.[79] The axons of these neurons project to the striatum: the ventral tegmental area largely to the ventrally located nucleus accumbens and olfactory tubercle, and the substantia nigra mainly to the more dorsally located caudate and putamen nuclei. The ventral tegmental area also has projections to limbic structures, including the hippocampus, amygdala, and medial prefrontal cortex. Because it receives strong projections from the hippocampus, one of the main structures of the limbic system, the nucleus accumbens is sometimes referred to as the limbic striatum.

The dopaminergic systems are named according to their region of origin and target structure. Thus, the system originating in the substantia nigra zona compacta and projecting to the striatum is termed the "nigrostriatal" dopaminergic system. The system originating in the ventral tegmental area, located in the midbrain or mesencephalon, and projecting to the nucleus accumbens, is sometimes referred to as the "mesoaccumbens" system. More commonly, the nucleus accumbens, hippocampus, and amygdala are lumped together as limbic structures and the projection from the ventral tegmental area of the mesencephalon to the nucleus accumbens, hippocampus, and amygdala is referred to as the "mesolimbic" dopaminergic system. Sometimes the projection from the ventral tegmental area to the medial prefrontal cortex is termed the "mesocortical" dopaminergic system. Finally, the limbic and cortical projections of the ventral tegmental area can be combined and so become the "mesolimbocortical" system.[80] Welcome to the fuzzy nomenclature of neuroanatomy.

Axons projecting into a structure have to end somewhere. Most commonly, they end at regions termed axon terminals or terminal "boutons" (from the French for "button") that are specialized for the release of neurotransmitters. Terminal boutons form one side of a synapse or synaptic gap between it and the target neuron on the other side. The target neuron has a specialized region termed the postsynaptic density where receptors for the neurotransmitter being released from the terminal bouton can affect the electrical and chemical activity of the postsynaptic cell.

The caudate, putamen, nucleus accumbens, and olfactory tubercle are made up primarily of projection neurons, a cell type termed "medium spiny neurons." Medium spiny caudate neurons number about 2.8 million per hemisphere in rats,[81] and constitute around 95 percent of the neurons of that structure. They are called "medium" because they are smaller than another more-scarce interneuron cell type of these nuclei termed "large aspiny neurons" and they are larger than glial cells.[82] They are termed "spiny" because their dendrites, the receptive zone of the neuron, are densely covered with little spines termed "dendritic spines;" anatomical studies with rats have estimated that, on average, a medium spiny neuron has about 10,000 spines.[83] It will probably come as no surprise that the dendrites of large aspiny neurons have very few dendritic spines.

The dendritic spines of medium spiny neurons are the site of contact between the thalamic and cortical neurons projecting into the striatum (including the nucleus accumbens and olfactory tubercle that receive hippocampal and olfactory cortical input) and the medium spiny neurons of the striatum.[84] Cortical neurons are those unimodal and multimodal cells that are activated by the features of stimuli and ongoing motor responses as discussed earlier in this chapter. They use glutamate as their neurotransmitter. Many, perhaps half of the same dendritic spines on medium spiny neurons that receive glutamatergic inputs from the cortex receive dopaminergic inputs from the ventral midbrain.[85] The structure of the spine as a tiny branch off the main dendritic shaft makes it possible for the glutamatergic and dopaminergic synapses that are common to that spine to produce interacting neurochemical effects in the cytoplasm of the spine that are somewhat isolated from the other spines and shaft of that dendrite.[86] The possible value of this arrangement is made clearer in Chapter 12.

The axons of cortical glutamatergic neurons projecting to the caudate (estimated to number 17 million per hemisphere in rats[87]) are highly branched. A single neuron may form, on average, in the order of 800 synapses.[87] Most of these synaptic contacts (about 95%) are made with dendritic spines of medium spiny neurons.[88] A single corticostriatal neuron does not form all of its synaptic contacts with a single medium spiny neuron. Instead, it contacts some (as many as 250 but probably many fewer; perhaps only about four) of the dendritic spines of each of many different medium spiny neurons.[87] Other corticostriatal neurons make contact with other dendritic spines on some of the same medium spiny neurons as the first corticostriatal neuron and with some different medium spiny neurons. And so on. In this way, individual medium spiny neurons receive synaptic contacts from multiple (estimated at around 134 at a minimum and over 5000 at a maximum) corticostriatal neurons with each medium spiny neuron receiving inputs from a somewhat different set of corticostriatal neurons.[84] A single corticostriatal neuron projects to a small region of the caudate (estimated to be, on average, 4% of the total caudate volume in a hemisphere of the rat[87]) so that specific cortical regions, for example visual regions or somatosensory regions, project to relatively specific striatal regions, preserving some of the regional specificity of the cortex in the dorsal striatum.[88]

The extent of branching of axons of mesolimbic and nigrostriatal dopaminergic neurons (estimated to number only about 20,000 per hemisphere of the mesencephalon in rats[89]) dwarfs that of corticostriatal neurons. Individual nigrostriatal dopaminergic neurons have been estimated to have as many as 400,000 synaptic regions,[90,91] at least two orders of magnitude more than corticostriatal neurons. The branches of axons of dopaminergic neurons form multiple synaptic contacts in series, referred to as *en passant* synapses. Like corticostriatal neurons, individual dopaminergic neurons make contact with the dendritic spines of many medium spiny neurons, but individual dopamine neurons make many more contacts with medium spiny neurons than individual corticostriatal neurons. In addition to synaptic contacts with the dendritic spines, shafts and perikarya of medium spiny neurons, the axons of dopaminergic neurons have varicosities where neurotransmitter is released but these varicosities are not in direct synaptic contact with a postsynaptic element. Dopamine release from varicosities is referred to as "volume transmission," suggesting influence at a distance. Neuroscientists Jonathan Moss and Paul

Bolam from Oxford University showed that dopaminergic axon varicosities are in close proximity (0.5–1.0 μm) to corticostriatal axospinous synapses and that dopamine released from varicosities is of sufficient concentration at those synapses to influence their function.[91] The modulating influence of dopamine on corticostriatal glutamatergic synapses is the central topic of Chapter 12.

As already mentioned, dopaminergic neurons are relatively few in number. This can be contrasted with the estimated 17 million glutamatergic neurons that project to the dorsal striatum in each hemisphere of the rat. This arrangement suggests that numerous corticostriatal projections carry relatively specific information to the medium spiny neurons; in fact, the information would be as specific as is made possible by the ability of cortical cells to discriminate individual details of stimuli. The relatively small number of dopaminergic neurons combined with their massive axonal branching and volume transmission, however, suggests that they may play a role in modulating the overall activity of the target region rather than carry specific detailed information.

Before considering the implications of this anatomical arrangement, I will mention two additional aspects of basal ganglia neuroanatomy because they have attracted a great deal of interest in recent years and because a complete description of the anatomical mechanisms of incentive learning will eventually need to incorporate them (see Chapter 12). The first is the direct and indirect pathway. Medium spiny projection neurons are of two subtypes characterized by the type of dopamine receptor they express and the neuropeptide molecule(s) that they appear to co-release with their inhibitory amino-acid neurotransmitter γ-aminobutyric acid (GABA). Some medium neurons express D1 dopamine receptors and co-release substance P, dynorphin, and GABA. These medium spiny neurons project from within the dorsal striatum directly to the output nuclei of the basal ganglia, the internal segment of the globus pallidus (entopeduncular nucleus in non-primates) and zona reticulata of the substantia nigra. This pathway is termed the "direct pathway." The "indirect pathway" in the dorsal striatum originates in medium spiny neurons that express D2 dopamine receptors and co-release enkephalin and GABA. They project to the external segment of the globus pallidus; it projects to the output nuclei of the basal ganglia and to the subthalamic nucleus. The subthalamic nucleus then projects to the output nuclei of the basal ganglia.[92]

The inputs to the spines of dorsal striatal medium spiny projection neurons of the direct and indirect pathways differ. Direct pathway medium spiny neurons receive input from cortical neurons that project within the telencephalon; indirect pathway medium spiny neurons receive input from neurons of the pyramidal tract that give rise to a collateral branch to the striatum.[93] The direct pathway promotes desired movements, whereas the indirect pathway inhibits undesired movements.[92] It might be the case that collaterals of pyramidal tract neurons that project to the indirect pathway serve to inhibit motor signals originating in the striatum and in this way prevent conflicting signals from the two motor regions, as discussed earlier in this chapter. However, one of the implications of this speculation about the function of the indirect pathway is that it might be less developed in mammals that have an incomplete corticospinal projection and perhaps absent in vertebrates that lack a corticospinal tract. Comparative anatomical studies show that the parcellation of pallidal neurons into two separate fields (external and internal segments) is absent in all non-mammalian tetrapods; however, separate striatal afferents containing substance P or enkephalin are present and separate neurons receiving their input have been identified throughout the pallidum in non-mammalian tetrapods.[94] Perhaps the appearance of a separated indirect pathway through the basal ganglia may correlate with the evolution of direct motor output from the cortex to the spinal cord, but more work is needed.

A direct and indirect pathway has been described in the nucleus accumbens, a ventral striatal structure.[95] Nucleus accumbens medium spiny neurons receive inputs from the thalamus, amygdala, hippocampus, and prefrontal cortex. Direct pathway neurons receive a stronger input from the hippocampus than indirect pathway neurons; both direct and indirect pathway neurons receive thalamic and prefrontal cortical input.[96] It is not known if some of the prefrontocortical–accumbens projections are from collaterals of pyramidal tract neurons. If they are it might be expected that they will project to the indirect pathway, paralleling the organization in the dorsal striatum. Further studies are needed to elucidate the connectivity of these circuits.

Some observations may not support the speculation that the indirect pathway inhibits unwanted movements when signals for movement are transmitted via the direct pathway. As discussed in Chapter 12, incentive learning may involve the strengthening of synaptic connections between striatally projecting cortical cells and medium spiny neurons. If the direct and indirect pathways work cooperatively it might be expected that when corticostriatal synapses onto medium spiny neurons of the direct pathway are strengthened, simultaneously activated corticostriatal synapses onto medium spiny neurons of the indirect pathway will also be strengthened. However, it appears that the opposite is the case, that is, when corticostriatal synapses onto medium spiny neurons of the direct pathway are strengthened, corticospinal synapses onto medium spiny neurons of the indirect pathway may be *weakened* (see Chapter 12). This result might suggest that the two pathways work in opposition to one another. The functional role of the direct and indirect pathways continues to be the topic of intense study.

The other aspect of striatal neuroanatomy that eventually needs to be incorporated into a complete understanding of the anatomical mechanisms of incentive learning has been referred to as ascending spiraling connections. In a seminal paper published in 2000, Suzanne Haber from the University of Rochester, New York, and colleagues analyzed intra-basal ganglia striatonigrostriatal circuits and identified interconnections of striatal regions with dopaminergic neurons that afforded an ascending spiraling of connectivity from the nucleus accumbens shell to the nucleus accumbens core, thence to the central striatal region and finally to the dorsolateral striatum, creating a hierarchy of information flow. The striatonigrostriatal circuits within the striatum both inhibit dopamine neurons via striatal projections to the substantia nigra zona compacta and excite dopamine neurons via striatal projections to the substantia nigra zona reticulata. Haber and colleagues suggested that afferents from the nucleus accumbens shell might not only inhibit dopamine neurons projecting there, a classic negative feedback function, but also facilitate excitation of dopamine neurons projecting to the nucleus accumbens core, facilitating feedforward of burst-firing signals associated with rewarding stimuli to the next striatonigrostriatal circuit that includes the nucleus accumbens core. This arrangement is reiterated for the forward facilitation of dopamine neuron signals to the central striatum and from there to the dorsolateral striatum.[97]

Recall that incentive learning involves the acquisition by neutral stimuli of an increased ability to elicit *approach* and *other* responses (Chapter 2). The specificity of stimuli that control responses increases from the ventral to the dorsal striatum in parallel with the sensory/perceptual cell assemblies found in the cortical regions that project there; the motor responses that send efference copies to the striatum are similarly more specific for inputs to dorsal than to ventral striatal regions, that is, efference copies for responses involving fine digitation and vocal control issue from cortical regions that project to the dorsal striatum. This suggests that spiraling circuits through the striatum may allow incentive learning about progressively finer sensory/perceptual details of the environment and the progressively more focused motor responses used to deal with them. Thus, ventral striatal regions may mediate the *approach* responses of incentive learning, responses that involve whole-body movement; the dorsal striatum, however, may mediate *other* responses of incentive learning, responses that involve the use of more specific musculature for manipulation, for example, that are instrumental in attaining a rewarding stimulus. Electrophysiological studies of the activity of striatal medium spiny neurons during incentive learning in monkeys have shown that the activity of more laterally located neurons is associated with the control of habitual actions.[98] Okihide Hikosaka and co-workers from the National Institute of Health in Bethesda, Maryland, have found that there is a further regionalization of control from the rostral to the caudal caudate nucleus in primates with more habitual responding being controlled by caudal regions.[62] Perhaps habitual responses are those that are more focused and under the control of relatively specific environmental stimuli. These studies support Haber's finding of spiraling control of responding through the striatum by striatonigrostriatal circuits.

Recall from the discussion in Chapter 5 that brain imaging studies have shown increased BOLD changes in the striatum or nucleus accumbens when participants are exposed to positive social stimuli such as a loved one or a cooperator. In the case of the cooperator, the social stimulus was a photo of a person whom the participant had met only once. When the photo of that person was followed by a cooperative outcome in a social game, an increased BOLD signal was detected in the region of the *nucleus accumbens*. When the photo of a passionately loved other was viewed, an increased BOLD signal was detected in the region of the *dorsal striatum*. The regional difference in the response observed in these two experiments might reflect the ascending spiraling connections described by Haber and others. When a stranger, a relatively novel social stimulus, is cooperative the strongest dopamine signal may be in the nucleus accumbens. In the case of a more familiar cooperative social stimulus such as a passionately loved other, the strongest dopamine signal may be in the striatum. This is, of course, speculative (and BOLD, not dopaminergic, responses were measured), but it maps these observations onto the spiraling connections described by Haber and her colleagues.

The following conceptualization is suggested by the processing of sensory/perceptual information that I have discussed in this chapter in the context of the neuronal structure and synaptic arrangement of the striatum, including the nucleus accumbens and olfactory tubercle. As an individual is moving through the environment, the efference copy and stimuli that are encountered, including other people, lead to activation of sensory/perceptual systems and subsets of cortical neurons. Those cortical neurons project to the striatum so there will be a subset of synapses on medium spiny neurons that is activated by any given stimulus. For example, striatal cells that respond to faces have been recorded in the macaque monkey.[99] As the stimuli change, the subset of activated corticostriatal synapses will change. From time to time, a rewarding stimulus will be encountered and this will lead to bursts of activity in dopaminergic neurons. Those stimuli that were encountered just before the rewarding stimulus occurred and that led to activation of a particular subset of corticostriatal synapses will become incentive stimuli with an increased ability to elicit approach and other responses. The action of a rewarding stimulus appears to be the strengthening of those synapses (Chapter 12). As a result of these putatively strengthened synapses, the stimuli encountered just before the rewarding stimulus occurred, when encountered again in the future, will have a stronger impact on response output systems, an increased ability to elicit approach and other responses.[100]

The synaptic arrangement of the dopaminergic neurons projecting to the striatum suggests that the dopamine signal is diffuse. The dopamine signal is produced by a small number of neurons that branch extensively. When a rewarding stimulus is encountered and dopamine neurons fire a burst of action potentials, the dopamine terminal zone, that is the interface of glutamatergic corticostriatal neurons and medium spiny striatal neurons, is awash in an increased concentration of dopamine. Dopamine putatively acts at those corticostriatal synapses that were most recently active to strengthen them. This means that there must be a mechanism for dopamine to be able to act selectively at a subset of synapses. A possible mechanism is the topic of Chapter 12.

As an individual moves through its environment and encounters various stimuli, those stimuli and the proprioceptive input and efference copy of their responses lead to activation of a subset of corticostriatal neurons and their synapses onto medium spiny neurons. When these synapses are activated they go into a putative transient *state of readiness* to be modified by dopamine. Theoretical neuroscientist Robert Miller, working at the time at Otago University in Dunedin, New Zealand, suggested the term "state of readiness" for this phenomenon.[101] If no rewarding stimulus is encountered and the individual moves on to other stimuli, those synapses previously activated will become silent and their state of readiness will dissipate. If, however, while a set of synapses is in a state of readiness, the dopamine signal arrives, it will alter the strength of those synapses. Timing is everything.

We know about the importance of timing for incentive learning from almost a century of behavioral experiments done primarily by psychologists. You will recall from Chapter 3 how incentive learning occurs in a lever-pressing task performed by a rat. The effects of a rewarding stimulus are to increase the incentive value of stimuli that were encountered just before the rewarding stimulus occurred. If the rewarding stimulus occurs just after the rat was close to the lever, the rat is more likely to return to the lever after eating the food pellet presumably because lever-related stimuli have acquired increased incentive value. The lever-related stimuli will lead to activation of a subset of corticostriatal neurons. If the synapses of those neurons are in a state of readiness when the rewarding stimulus occurs and dopamine neurons are activated, the synaptic strengthening that is incentive learning will take place. What will happen if the rewarding stimulus was not given immediately after the animal was close to the lever? The answer is that the synapses of the corticostriatal neurons activated by the lever and lever-related stimuli will no longer be in a state of readiness when the burst of activity in dopamine neurons produced by a rewarding stimulus takes place. Some corticostriatal neurons and their synapses will be in a state of readiness and dopamine putatively will strengthen those synapses but the goal of getting the lever and lever-related stimuli to control behavior will be thwarted. Numerous studies with animals have shown that the insertion of a delay between a to-be-conditioned stimulus and the rewarding stimulus leads to weaker conditioning. This was shown in lever-press acquisition experiments,[102] and in simpler experiments where the incentive value of a stimulus was measured using a reflexive response such as salivation.[103] In either case, lengthening the delay between the to-be-conditioned stimulus and the presentation of the rewarding stimulus led to weaker conditioning.

In the next chapter I discuss incentive learning at the neurochemical level. It is critical to identify the possible mechanism of the state of readiness produced by activity at corticostriatal synapses. The mechanism of the state of readiness will provide a means for dopamine to act selectively at a subset of synapses, even though it is released widely at many more synapses than those that it affects. The possible mechanism for how dopamine leads to synaptic strengthening at the selected synapses is also discussed. Results reveal that elegant neurochemical cascades lead to modifications of proteins that underlie synaptic strengthening. The process of incentive learning appears to involve protein synthesis, suggesting that it will be possible to begin to see how genetic variation can lead to differential sensitivity to dopamine-mediated learning. A consideration of these mechanisms may provide a means for understanding the contribution of genetic variations in dopamine-mediated learning to schizophrenia susceptibility.

Summary

The senses of vision, audition, olfaction, taste, and somatosensation each have specialized receptors for transducing environmental (or internal) stimuli into signals in the nervous system. In many cases those signals are directed towards motor nuclei for producing reflex responses such as withdrawing the hand from excessive heat. Those signals also ascend through the brain often via a series of nuclei and along the way axons detecting specific elements of a particular sense often converge onto higher-order neurons that then are activated by particular features of the stimulus. The convergence of features detected by different sensory modalities also occurs, leading to neurons that are activated by more complex multimodal stimuli. As a result, assemblies of cells in the cerebral cortex that respond to specific features detect complex environmental stimuli such as faces, conspecific vocalizations, or the bouquet of a particular wine. These sensory/perceptual capacities evolved to improve the ability of organisms to operate effectively on their environments to obtain fitness-enhancing biological needs such as food and cooperative social interactions, and to avoid danger. Operating on the environment means controlling behavioral responses and so it comes as no surprise that the heaviest projection area of the cerebral cortex is a motor region: the dorsal striatal nuclei, the caudate and putamen in primates, and ventral striatal nuclei, the nucleus accumbens, and olfactory tubercle. These are regions of the brain that project to brainstem motor nuclei that, in turn, control the musculature that underlies responses to environmental stimuli. Within the striatum, cortical projections frequently terminate on the dendritic spines of medium spiny neurons, the main efferents of these nuclei. Dopaminergic projection neurons from ventral mesencephalic nuclei also terminate on the same spines. Corticostriatal afferents branch so that their terminals contact a relatively small number of medium spiny neurons. By comparison, a small number of dopaminergic neurons branch far more extensively and each contacts a far larger number of medium spiny neurons. As a result of this arrangement, specific environmental (or internal) stimuli lead to activation of a specific subset of corticostriatal synapses; as the environmental stimuli change so does the activated subset of synapses. If a particular environmental stimulus is closely followed by a biologically important outcome, that is, a rewarding stimulus, dopaminergic neurons are activated and the burst of action potentials leads to a transient elevation in dopamine concentrations in striatal terminal areas. The combination of activity at the specific corticostriatal synapses most recently activated by particular environmental stimuli and, more generally, elevated dopamine concentrations produced by a rewarding stimulus leads to modifications of those specific corticostriatal synapses. As a result of the synaptic modifications, the stimuli that activated those specific corticostriatal synapses, through descending projections to motor areas, will acquire an increased ability to elicit approach and other responses in the future, that is, incentive learning.

Chapter 12

Mechanisms of dopamine-mediated incentive learning

As an animal moves through its environment it encounters different stimuli. The efference copy and proprioceptive signals generated by its movements (see Chapters 8 and 11) and each encountered stimulus leads to the activation of a set of cortical neurons that project to the striatum, including the nucleus accumbens and olfactory tubercle, where the synapses of those projections onto medium spiny neurons are activated. If a particular stimulus is followed by a rewarding stimulus, for example if a bird's nest yields tasty eggs for a fox, dopamine neurons will be activated. As a result, the scent of birds' nests and locations where they are found (e.g., marshy regions next to a lake or river) will become incentive stimuli for the fox, acquiring an enhanced ability to attract it in the future. Subsequently, when the fox is moving through its environment in search of food and encounters the scent of a bird's nest or a place where birds' nests have been found in the past, those stimuli will elicit approach and other responses. This is an example of dopamine-mediated incentive learning.[1]

Before embarking on a discussion of some of the molecular mechanisms of dopamine-mediated incentive learning, I need to state some caveats. Many of the molecular interactions that I describe in this chapter are thought to take place in the dendritic spines of medium spiny neurons of the striatum, including the nucleus accumbens and olfactory tubercle. However, as pointed out by researchers Wei-Dong Yao, Roger Spealman, and Jingping Zhang from Harvard Medical School in Southborough, Massachusetts, in a 2008 paper, "Direct assessment of [dopamine] signaling in spines ... is essentially lacking." They go on to say, "It is not known, for example, which second messenger systems are linked to [dopamine] receptors in spines and what signaling systems they engage" (p. 2060).[2] They point out some of the barriers to attaining this information: one is that direct electrophysiological approaches are prevented because dopaminergic neurotransmission is mediated "through a complex sequence of biochemical reactions involving second messengers, protein kinases, and protein phosphatases" (p. 2060);[2] another is that spines are generally not accessible by microscopic techniques (although newer techniques such as two-photon microscopy may overcome this limitation); additionally, validated methods are not available for isolating and purifying dendritic spines that could then be studied with conventional biochemical and pharmacological approaches. Notwithstanding these challenges, it is deemed highly likely that the dopamine–glutamate interactions described here take place in dendritic spines.[2] A further caveat is that some of the molecular events thought to be involved in dopamine-mediated incentive learning in the striatum, nucleus accumbens, and olfactory tubercle were originally described in non-striatal tissue such as the hippocampus and need to be confirmed in striatal tissue.[3] In the following I endeavor to identify where this is the case. These comments were made almost ten years ago (I am writing in February 2016), and enormous strides have been made in the intervening years towards confirming the molecular cascades that take place in dopaminoceptive striatal neurons; although differential involvement of some molecules in, for example, hippocampal versus striatal plasticity has been identified, many intracellular molecular events originally described in non-striatal tissue have been confirmed in the striatum. I am mindful of these caveats in the following.

The wave of phosphorylation

As discussed in Chapter 11, activity at corticostriatal synapses putatively will bring those synapses into a transient state of readiness for modification in case a rewarding stimulus occurs. If no rewarding stimulus occurs, the state of readiness rapidly dissipates, as suggested by the deleterious effects of delays between, on the one hand, to-be conditioned stimuli and the responses associated with them and, on the other, the presentation of a rewarding stimulus. The state of readiness may be coded by molecular events at the active synapses. The initial event includes the release of the neurotransmitter glutamate from the terminal boutons of corticostriatal neurons when electrical signals, action potentials, arrive there as a result of those neurons being activated by movement-related proprioceptive stimuli and stimuli in the environment. Glutamate diffuses across the synaptic gap where it occupies receptors for glutamate. There are several types of glutamate receptors that play different roles in synaptic plasticity; these include ionotropic and metabotropic receptors. For present purposes I will focus on the two ionotropic subtypes: N-methyl-D-aspartate (NMDA) receptors and α-amino-3-hydroxy-5-methyl-4-isoxazolepropionic acid (AMPA) receptors. A complete description of the molecular events underlying dopamine-mediated incentive learning eventually will include a role for metabotropic glutamate receptors.[4]

When NMDA receptors are sufficiently activated by glutamate, they allow calcium ions to enter the dendritic spine; calcium enters either through NMDA receptor channels or through voltage-sensitive calcium channels.[5] Neuroscientist Jeff Wickens, working at the time at the University of Otago in Dunedin, New Zealand, has suggested that this event initiates the state of readiness.[6] Calcium ion concentrations will be highest within the dendritic spines that receive active glutamatergic corticostriatal input and this elevated calcium concentration will produce a number of effects on molecules inside the dendritic spines; Wickens has suggested that spine morphology favors relative chemical (but not electrical) isolation of individual corticostriatal inputs from other corticostriatal inputs.[7] Some researchers have shown that activity at NMDA receptors and increased calcium concentrations within dendritic spines lead to a wave of transient phosphorylation events;[6,8] perhaps this can be seen as part of the state of readiness.

Stimulation of NMDA receptors and increased calcium concentrations in the dendritic spine may lead to phosphorylation and internalization of voltage-sensitive Kv4.2 potassium channels.[9] Potassium efflux normally begins the repolarization process that follows depolarization produced by an excitatory synaptic input. By internalizing Kv4.2 channels, repolarization is slowed thereby increasing the excitability of the dendritic spine. This may contribute to the state of readiness.

One of the molecules that is phosphorylated as a result of increased calcium concentrations in dendritic spines is calcium/calmodulin-dependent kinase II (CaMKII). Binding of calcium and calmodulin to the regulatory subunit of CaMKII changes its conformation allowing it to autophosphorylate at threonine 286, prolonging its action.[10] CaMKII, in turn, may promote the phosphorylation of a number of proteins. One example is the phosphorylation by CaMKII of serine 831 of the GluA1 subunit of AMPA receptors found in the postsynaptic density.[11] As a result, AMPA receptors have an increased conductance.[11,12] In this way phosphorylated AMPA receptors may serve to amplify the next corticostriatal signals at that dendritic spine. CaMKII may also promote the insertion (trafficking) of AMPA receptors into the postsynaptic membrane, further contributing to signal amplification.[12]

Increased intracellular calcium concentrations, activated calcium/diacylglycerol-activated protein kinase C (PKC) and CaMKII may promote the phosphorylation of mitogen-activated protein kinases, *viz.*, extracellular signal-regulated protein kinases 1 and 2 (ERK 1/2). PhosphoERK1/2 phosphorylates Kv4.2 channels, decreasing their open time and thereby increasing the excitability of the dendritic spine;[13] phosphoERK1/2 can also influence gene expression (see later) leading to long-term changes.[3],[14] These are some of the events that constitute the wave of phosphorylation that may be the state of readiness produced by stimulation of glutamate receptors.

NMDA receptor-induced increases in calcium concentration have another action that may contribute to the wave of phosphorylation. Neuroscientist Paul Greengard, who, as already discussed in Chapter 7, was co-recipient of the 2000 Nobel Prize in Physiology or Medicine for his pioneering work on signal transduction in neurons, and co-workers showed that increased calcium concentrations may lead to activation of protein phosphatase 2A (PP2A); PP2A, in turn, dephosphorylates *dopamine and cyclic adenosine 3, 5-monophosphate (cAMP)-regulated phosphoprotein-32* (DARPP-32) at threonine 75. Phosphothreonine-75 DARPP-32 is an inhibitor of cAMP-dependent protein kinase A (PKA).[15] Removal of this inhibition by dephosphorylating DARPP-32 at threonine 75 will promote the action of PKA if it is stimulated. As discussed in the following, PKA is activated by dopamine and can prevent a number of dephosphorylation events that normally follow the wave of phosphorylation. The dephosphorylation of DARPP-32 at threonine 75 may promote the wave of phosphorylation (Figure 12.1).

I sometimes find it hard to believe that all these neurochemical events are taking place from moment to moment during every minute of every day. As we navigate our environment encountering different sights, sounds, tastes, smells, and somatosensory inputs, the sensory/perceptual activations that those stimuli and our movements generate, as described in Chapter 11, lead to activation of unique assemblies of cortical neurons and therefore corticostriatal glutamatergic synapses. Each sufficiently strong synaptic activation by NMDA receptors leads to an increase in intracellular calcium, activation of CaMKII, and a wave of phosphorylation events, including those just described. Hot on the heels of the phosphorylation events is a wave of phosphatase activity to rapidly undo the wave of phosphorylation. Thus, synapses activated by briefly encountered environmental stimuli and motor actions remain in a state of readiness for only a short period, probably in the order of milliseconds or, at most, a few seconds, judging from the deleterious effects of imposing delays between to-be conditioned stimuli and unconditioned rewarding stimuli, as mentioned at the end of Chapter 11. I turn now to a consideration of the dephosphorylation stage.

The wave of phosphatase activity

Calcineurin (protein phosphatase 2B) is another calcium-dependent molecule. It has a higher affinity for calcium than PKC and CaMKII; high calcium

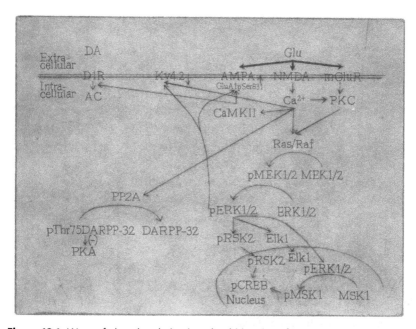

Figure 12.1 *Wave of phosphorylation in a dendritic spine of a striatal medium spiny neuron that receives a cortical glutamatergic input:* The release of glutamate (Glu) from the presynaptic cortical input stimulates α-amino-3-hydroxy-5-methyl-4-isoxazolepropionic acid (AMPA), N-methyl-D-aspartate (NMDA), and metabotropic glutamate receptors (mGluR). Sufficient stimulation of NMDA receptors results in elevated levels of intra-spinous calcium; this may lead to phosphorylation and internalization of voltage-sensitive potassium channels (Kv4.2↓), increasing excitability of the dendritic spine. Elevated Ca^{2+} may also lead to phosphorylation of calcium/calmodulin-dependent kinase II (CaMKII) that, in turn, phosphorylates serine 831 (pSer831) of the GluA1 subunit of AMPA receptors, increasing their conductance; CaMKII may also promote the insertion (↑) of AMPA receptors into the postsynaptic membrane, further contributing to signal amplification. Increased Ca^{2+} concentrations and activation of calcium/diacylglycerol-activated protein kinase C (PKC) may promote the phosphorylation of extracellular signal-regulated protein kinases 1 and 2 (pERK 1/2) through a chain of kinase activations that include Ras family and Raf family kinases that activate mitogen-activated protein kinase kinase (MEK)1/2. pERK1/2 phosphorylates Kv4.2 channels and influences the insertion of AMPA receptors into the membrane, further increasing excitability of the dendritic spine. pERK1/2 also phosphorylates p90 ribosomal S6 kinase2 (RSK2) that translocates to the nucleoplasm where it phosphorylates serine 133 of cyclic adenosine 3, 5-monophosphate (cAMP) response element-binding protein (CREB), possibly influencing gene transcription. In the nucleus, pERK1/2 activates mitogen- and stress-activated kinase-1 (pMSK1), which also phosphorylates CREB. pERK1/2 influences the transcription factor Elk 1. Increased calcium concentrations may lead to activation of protein phosphatase 2A (PP2A) that dephosphorylates *dopamine and cAMP-regulated phosphoprotein-32* (DARPP-32) at threonine 75 (Thr75). pThr75 DARPP-32 is an inhibitor of cAMP-dependent protein kinase A (PKA); removal of this inhibition may promote the action of PKA if it is stimulated. Finally, CaMKII enhances the coupling of D1 dopamine (DA) receptors (D1R) to adenylyl cyclase (AC), enhancing its action on cAMP formation from adenosine triphosphate (ATP) if the D1R is activated.

concentrations activate PKC and CaMKII, but as soon as calcium concentrations begin to drop, calcineurin activation will predominate.[16] Calcineurin is a protein phosphatase and its activation contributes to the undoing of the wave of phosphorylation described earlier. Rather than adding a phosphate group to a molecule and activating it (as is often, but not always, the case), calcineurin strips molecules of a phosphate group and thereby (usually) inhibits their action. One of the targets of calcineurin is Kv4.2, the voltage-sensitive potassium channel that is phosphorylated and internalized as a result of increased calcium concentrations, thereby increasing excitability of the dendritic spine (see earlier). By dephosphorylating Kv4.2, calcineurin stabilizes it in the membrane where it shortens the period of excitability of the dendrite.[17] This may diminish the state of readiness.

Calcineurin dephosphorylates the GluA1 subunit of AMPA receptors at serine 845. This decreases their open probability and conductance and reduces their insertion into the membrane.[18] This will decrease synaptic efficacy and may also diminish the state of readiness.

Another target of calcineurin is DARPP-32; it is dephosphorylated at threonine 34. Normally, phosphothreonine-34–DARPP-32 inhibits protein phosphatase 1 (PP1). By dephosphorylating DARPP-32 at threonine 34, calcineurin releases PP1 from inhibition and activates PP1.[15] Active PP1 continues the process of undoing some of the phosphorylation events that were started by the increased intracellular concentration of calcium. PP1 can dephosphorylate CaMKII decreasing its activity.[10] PP1 inhibits kinases upstream of ERK that normally lead to the phosphorylation of ERK1/2, thereby decreasing the effect of ERK1/2. By dephosphorylating striatal-enriched phosphatase (STEP), PP1 increases the affinity of STEP for phoshoERK1/2, promoting STEP's inhibition of phoshoERK1/2 (STEP provides an example in which dephosphorylation leads to activation).[19] Active ERK1/2 phosphorylates Kv4.2 potassium channels leading to their internalization and enhanced excitability of the membrane; inactivation of ERK1/2 reverses this process.[13] Active ERK1/2 also influences transcription (see the next section), an effect that will be reversed by PP1. In this way, even as calcium entry into the dendritic spine is activating proteins by phosphorylating them, it is activating a phosphatase to begin the work of dephosphorylating them again and thereby neutralizing the transient state of readiness putatively produced by the signal from a corticostriatal glutamatergic input (Figure 12.2). As I discuss later in this chapter, the dephosphorylation stage may do more than simply neutralizing the phosphorylation stage; it may result in long-lasting weakening of the synapse.

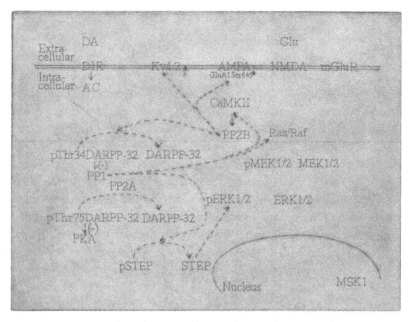

Figure 12.2 *Wave of phosphatase activity that follows the wave of phosphorylation in a dendritic spine of a striatal medium spiny neuron that receives a cortical glutamatergic input:* Intraspinous calcium concentrations may be increased by stimulation of *N*-methyl-D-aspartate (NMDA) receptors by glutamate (Glu). As Ca^{2+} concentrations begin to fall, stimulation of calcineurin (protein phosphatase 2B; PP2B) by calcium/calmodulin-dependent kinase II (CaMKII) begins to dominate. PP2B dephosphorylates voltage-sensitive potassium channels (Kv4.2) thereby stabilizing them (↑) in the membrane where they shorten the period of excitability of the dendrite. PP2B dephosphorylates the GluA1 subunit of α-amino-3-hydroxy-5-methyl-4-isoxazolepropionic acid (AMPA) receptors at serine (Ser) 845 reducing their insertion into the membrane (↓) and decreasing their conduction time. PP2B dephosphorylates *dopamine and cyclic adenosine 3, 5-monophosphate (cAMP)-regulated phosphoprotein-32* (DARPP-32) at threonine (Thr) 34, thereby releasing protein phosphatase 1 (PP1) from inhibition. PP1 decreases the activity of CaMKII. PP1 inhibits Ras and Raf family kinases, decreasing stimulation of the cascade that leads to phosphorylation of extracellular signal-regulated protein kinases 1 and 2 (pERK 1/2). PP1 dephosphorylates striatal-enriched phosphatase (STEP), increasing STEP's inhibition of pERK1/2. As activation of CaMKII drops, phosphorylation of protein phosphatase 2A (PP2A) will drop, shifting the balance of DARPP-32 back towards the form that is phosphorylated at threonine (Thr) 75, an inhibitor of cAMP-dependent protein kinase A (PKA). These events will serve to reverse the phosphorylation events that took place when Glu was first released. DA, dopamine; D1R, D1 dopamine receptor; AC, adenylyl cyclase; mGluR, metabotropic glutamate receptors; MSK1, mitogen- and-stress-activated kinase-1; (p)MEK, (phosphorylated) mitogen-actived protein kinase kinase.

Local enhancement of dopamine signaling

As already discussed, CaMKII will be phosphorylated and activated when calcium concentrations increase in the dendritic spine. Besides the phosphorylation events already mentioned, CaMKII may act on the enzyme adenylyl cyclase by increasing its coupling to dopamine D1 receptors (see Figure 12.1); adenylyl cyclase activates cAMP, part of the signaling cascade that follows dopaminergic stimulation of D1 receptors,[20] discussed later. Cooperative interactions of NMDA and D1 receptors have also been found in striatal membranes; stimulation of NMDA receptors by glutamate increases the number of D1 receptors on the plasma membrane surface and enhances D1 receptor-mediated cAMP formation.[2,21] As a result, when dopamine neurons are activated by a rewarding stimulus and dopamine is released at multiple terminal sites on multiple dendritic spines of many medium spiny neurons, it may have a greater impact on signaling in just those dendritic spines where there has been recent glutamatergic synaptic activity. This putative transient augmentation of dopamine receptor function may be part of the state of readiness that follows activity at glutamatergic synapses. If there is no signal at the dopamine receptor, the transiently enhanced ability of dopamine D1 receptors to stimulate cAMP formation will be ended.

Research from studies with the mollusk sea slug *Aplysia* provides convergent evidence for an influence of a sensory input on the ability of another receptor to activate adenylyl cyclase. In *Aplysia* the modulating input uses the monoamine neurotransmitter serotonin instead of dopamine and the terminals are found presynaptically on sensory neurons that contact motor output neurons. In part of his Nobel prize-winning research on the molecular mechanisms of learning and memory, neuroscientist Eric Kandel, co-recipient with Paul Greengard (and Arvid Carlsson, see Chapter 7) of the 2000 Prize in Physiology or Medicine, and his students and research associates, working at Columbia University in New York, showed how excitation at a sensory synapse transiently enhanced the ability of a serotonin synapse to activate adenylyl cyclase. No such enhancement took place at serotonin receptors located on other inactive sensory inputs. When serotonin synapses were activated leading to serotonin release at multiple synapses, this coupling resulted in a larger postsynaptic signal at serotonin synapses located on the recently active sensory input than those located on sensory neurons that had not been active. The larger postsynaptic signal led to modification of the recently active sensory synapse so that it was strengthened. No such modification took place at other sensory synapses that received serotonin inputs but that had not been augmented by the effects of recent activity.[22] Enhanced ability of serotonin receptors to stimulate adenylyl cyclase in the terminal of a recently active sensory input may contribute to a state of readiness.

The discovery by Kandel and associates of the influence of sensory inputs on the strength of serotonin signaling was made in classical conditioning experiments with *Aplysia*. They carried out differential classical conditioning. Two different sensory stimuli were produced by directly stimulating two different siphon sensory neurons. One of these sensory stimuli (conditioned stimulus) was paired with mild electrical shock to the tail (unconditioned stimulus). This mild aversive tail-shock stimulus causes the siphon-withdrawal reflex, a natural defensive reaction in *Aplysia*; instead of measuring the behavioral response, the researchers measured the postsynaptic potential in the motor neuron (unconditioned response) that receives input from the sensory neurons and projects to the siphon. As was expected from years of classical conditioning research with mammals, going all the way back to the iconic studies, carried out with dogs, by the Russian physiologist Ivan Pavlov (1849–1936), the sensory stimulus that was paired with tail shock gradually came to produce larger postsynaptic potentials in the motor neuron responsible for the siphon-withdrawal reflex (conditioned response); the other sensory stimulus, not paired with tail shock, did not acquire the ability to produce the conditioned response.[23] The terminals of the siphon sensory neurons receive serotonin input and both project to the same motor neuron. Previous work by Kandel and his group had discovered that activation of the serotonin input was necessary for producing the classical conditioning learning just described. The question was, how can a modulatory input, the serotonin input, selectively affect only one sensory synapse when that neuron contacts a number of sensory neurons? The answer turned out to be that serotonin,[24] although released at multiple sensory synapses that target the motor neuron, had a greater effect on neurotransmission by sensory neurons that were recently active, putatively because activity in the sensory neuron had enhanced the postsynaptic consequences of the serotonin input.

Returning to the dendritic spines of medium spiny neurons in the striatum, nucleus accumbens, and olfactory tubercle and recapitulating, some authors have described the events following activation of NMDA receptors as a wave of phosphorylation.[6,8] The phosphorylation events will take place in only the dendritic spines where the NMDA receptors had been strongly activated. These phosphorylation events will be transient because in very short order after the phosphorylation of a number of proteins, their dephosphorylation by phosphatases will take place. This transient wave of phosphorylation may be the state of readiness. If no phasic dopaminergic input occurs, the phosphorylation events may be quickly undone and the synapse may be no longer modifiable by a phasic dopaminergic input. If a phasic dopaminergic input occurs before the wave of phosphorylation has ended, the action of dopamine may lead to modifications that may be the neuromolecular substrate of incentive learning.

These considerations suggest the following. As an animal is moving through its environment it is constantly encountering stimuli. Those movements and stimuli activate sensory/perceptual pathways and assemblies of cortical neurons that are unique to each stimulus. The assemblies of cortical neurons project to the striatum, nucleus accumbens, and olfactory tubercle where their glutamatergic axon terminals are active, stimulating dendritic spines of medium spiny neurons. If the glutamatergic inputs are sufficiently strong, they activate NMDA (and AMPA) receptors leading to a transient wave of phosphorylation events. As the animal's behavior and the stimuli the animal encounters in its environment change, the activated set of cortical neurons changes and with it the activated set of corticostriatal synapses changes. Another wave of transient phosphorylation takes place in a new set of dendritic spines. And so on. This suggests that during waking there is always a subset of activated corticostriatal synapses and a corresponding wave of phosphorylation representing the transient state of readiness of those synapses for potential modification. If no rewarding stimulus occurs and therefore no burst of firing of dopaminergic neurons, the state of readiness quickly dissipates as the phosphatases undo the phosphorylation events and no incentive learning occurs. As I already mentioned earlier and discuss further in the next section, the dephosphorylation stage may do more than simply neutralize the phosphorylation stage; it may result in long-lasting weakening of the synapse.

Effects of the dopamine signal

What happens if a rewarding stimulus is encountered? As discussed in Chapter 5, a rewarding stimulus leads to phasic activation of dopaminergic neurons in the ventral midbrain and phasic increases in the synaptic concentration of dopamine in the dorsal striatum, nucleus accumbens, and olfactory tubercle. This will lead to the phasic stimulation of dopamine receptors located on the dendritic spines of many medium spiny neurons, especially because of the massively distributed dopamine signal, as described in Chapter 11. However, only a subset of those spines will be in a state of readiness, having experienced a glutamatergic input that produced a wave of phosphorylation. Those spines that are in a state of readiness will be those that were activated by the behavioral actions and environmental stimuli most recently produced and encountered by the animal, respectively. As mentioned in Chapter 7, phasic activation of dopaminergic neurons will increase synaptic concentrations of dopamine from the nanomolar to the micromolar range.[25] The affinity of D1- and D2-like receptors for dopamine differs, with D2-like receptors generally being stimulated by low dopamine concentrations (in the nanomolar range) and D1-like receptors generally being stimulated by higher dopamine concentrations (in the micromolar range).[26] Thus, rewarding stimulus-related phasic bursts of firing in dopaminergic neurons will result in the phasic stimulation of D1-lke receptors.

The dopaminergic input acting at D1-like dopamine receptors will lead to the stimulation of adenylyl cyclase and the activation of cAMP (see Chapter 7). Recall that one of the consequences of the glutamatergic input producing the state of readiness was an increase in the number of D1 receptors in the membrane and activation of CaMKII that putatively enhances the coupling of dopamine receptors to adenylyl cyclase. As a result, dopamine acting at dopamine receptors on dendritic spines that have recently received a glutamatergic input will have a greater impact on cAMP formation than dopamine acting at dopamine receptors at other dendritic spines that did not receive a glutamatergic input. Even from the first interaction of rewarding stimulus-related increases in synaptic dopamine with its receptors, the impact of the putative state of readiness on the postsynaptic effects of dopamine can be seen.

Dopamine-stimulated cAMP formation leads to activation of the well-known cAMP signaling pathway (Chapter 7). One of the targets of cAMP is cAMP-dependent PKA. PKA counteracts the effects of calcineurin on AMPA receptors in the striatum by phosphorylating the GluA1 subunit at serine 845.[27] This event may increase both activity and trafficking of AMPA receptors into the synapse.[28] This is one way that activation of dopamine receptors may oppose dephosphorylation and promote the wave of phosphorylation.

PKA phosphorylates threonine 34 of the phosphoprotein DARPP-32 and thereby activates its ability to inhibit PP1 by acting at its alpha catalytic subunit.[15] Recall that part of the wave of dephosphorylation that putatively undoes the state of readiness created by calcium influx at glutamatergic synapses is activation of the protein phosphatase calcineurin that dephosphorylates DARPP-32 at threonine 34 and thereby reduces its ability to inhibit PP1; this would promote the wave of dephosphorylation. Inhibiting PP1 makes PP1 unable to dephosphorylate and inactivate the phosphoproteins it normally targets (see later). Thus, stimulation of dopamine D1-like receptors and PKA activation counteracts the effect of calcineurin on DARPP-32 and the subsequent effects of PP1.

ERK1/2 is activated as a result of NMDA receptor-produced increases in calcium concentrations followed by a chain of kinase activations that include Ras family and Raf family kinases that activate mitogen-activated protein kinase kinase (MEK)1/2 leading to activated ERK1/2.[3,14] As already described, if no input occurs at dopamine receptors shortly following stimulation of NMDA receptors, PP1 inhibits kinases upstream of ERK1/2, interrupting the activation chain for ERK1/2 and dephosphorylates STEP, increasing its inhibition of ERK1/2. PKA, by allowing DARPP-32 to inhibit PP1, prevents the actions of PP1 on ERK1/2. ERK1/2 is then free to act on its various targets.[2,3,14] One is the Kv4.2 potassium channel that is inactivated by phosphoERK1/2, reducing potassium efflux from the dendritic spine and promoting its excitability. Another is insertion of AMPA receptors into the membrane, also promoting excitability by presynaptic inputs.[29] PhosphoERK1/2 may also promote translation of mRNAs and targeting of their proteins to the most recently active dendritic spines and it promotes the growth of new spines.[29,30]

Additional targets of ERK1/2 are transcription factors that influence gene expression in the nucleus. In the cytoplasm, phosphoERK1/2 phosphorylates p90 ribosomal S6 kinase2 (RSK2); phosphoRSK2 translocates to the nucleoplasm where it phosphorylates serine 133 of cAMP response element-binding protein (CREB), influencing gene transcription (see later).[29,31] In the nucleus, phosphoERK1/2 activates mitogen- and stress-activated kinase-1 (MSK1) that also phosphorylates CREB. PhosphoERK1/2 influences the transcription factor Elk 1 and the immediate early genes c-Fos and c-Jun.[29] MSK1 also acts on serine 10 of histone H3, influencing chromatin remodeling and subsequent gene expression.[29,32]

In their excellent paper on the role of ERK kinases in activity-dependent calcium signaling, neurobiologist Hilmar Bading from the University of Heidelberg in Germany and his student Simon Wiegert point out that "the magnitude of gene expression often depends on the combined activity of multiple signaling cascades. ..." For example, "nuclear ERK1/2-signaling is required but not sufficient to elicit robust, long-lasting CREB-dependent gene transcription" (p. 298).[29] As discussed in the next section, CREB is also activated by PKA. This suggests that if there is a glutamatergic NMDA receptor input and an increase in intracellular calcium concentration that leads to transient ERK1/2 activation, the level and/or duration of activation may *not* be sufficient to allow CREB to influence genes involved in the strengthening of synaptic connections. Similarly, if there is a dopamine input in the absence of a glutamatergic input, the action of dopamine–cAMP-stimulated PKA on CREB may *not* be sufficient to lead to the transcription of genes involved in the strengthening of synaptic connections. These considerations suggest that it may be the co-activation of a glutamate synapse followed by a dopamine synapse on a dendritic spine that is critical for the activation of genes that can lead to synaptic strengthening (see next section).[3,14,29] Gene activation could lead to long-term changes in the glutamate synapse that form part of the physiological substrate of incentive learning (Figure 12.3).

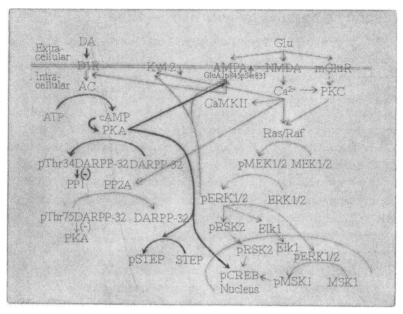

Figure 12.3 *Effects of the dopamine signal in a dendritic spine of a striatal medium spiny neuron that receives a cortical glutamatergic input:* Dopamine (DA) released when a rewarding stimulus is encountered will stimulate D1 receptors (D1R), activating adenylyl cyclase (AC), and leading to the formation of cyclic adenosine 3, 5-monophosphate (cAMP) from adenosine triphosphate (ATP). Note that the recent glutamate (Glu) input that activated N-methyl-D-aspartate (NMDA) receptors and led to an increase in intracellular Ca^{2+} will have activated calcium/calmodulin-dependent kinase II (CaMKII); one of the actions of CaMKII is to enhance the coupling of D1R to AC, increasing cAMP production. cAMP activates cAMP-dependent protein kinase A (PKA). Increased Ca^{2+} concentrations may lead to activation of protein phosphatase 2A (PP2A), which dephosphorylates *dopamine and cAMP-regulated phosphoprotein-32* (DARPP-32) at threonine 75 (Thr75). pThr75 DARPP-32 is an inhibitor of PKA; removal of this inhibition may promote the action of PKA if it is stimulated. PKA phosphorylates serine 845 (p845) of the GluA1 subunit of α-amino-3-hydroxy-5-methyl-4-isoxazolepropionic acid (AMPA) receptors and CaMKII phosphorylates serine 831 (pSer831), possibly increasing activity and trafficking (↑) of AMPA receptors into the synapse. PKA phosphorylates threonine 34 (pThr34) of DARPP-32 and thereby activates its ability to inhibit protein phosphatase 1 (PP1); this will prevent the inhibitory actions of PP1 associated with the wave of phosphatase activity described in Figure 12.2. PKA phosphorylates striatal-enriched phosphatase (pSTEP), decreasing its ability to inactivate phosphorylated extracellular signal regulated protein kinases 1 and 2 (pERK 1/2). Glu stimulation of NMDA receptors leading to elevated levels of intraspinous Ca^{2+} may lead to phosphorylation and internalization of voltage-sensitive potassium channels (Kv4.2⁻), increasing excitability of the dendritic spine. Stimulation of metabotropic glutamate receptors (mGluR) and increased Ca^{2+}

Signaling molecules in incentive learning

In 2004, Todor Gerdjikov, now at the University of Leicester in the UK, and I reviewed the evidence for a role for a number of signaling molecules in reward-related incentive learning.[33] At that time there was already good evidence for a role for PKA in the nucleus accumbens; results showed that disruption of PKA function produced a greater impairment of acquisition than of expression of incentive learning in conditioned approach, lever pressing for food, conditioned place preference based on amphetamine or cocaine, and conditioned activity studies (see later for a further discussion of testing acquisition vs expression). We also reviewed evidence that implicated nucleus accumbens PKC and ERK1/2 in the acquisition of conditioned place preference based on amphetamine. DARPP-32 knockout mice were impaired in the acquisition of a conditioned place preference based on cocaine implicating DARPP-32 in incentive learning. These results provide direct evidence for a role in incentive learning of some of the signaling molecules discussed in this chapter. Since publishing that paper, many additional studies have appeared that implicate one or more of the signaling molecules discussed earlier in incentive learning. I mention a few of those studies in the following two paragraphs.

In a recent paper, researchers from the University of Strasbourg, France, measured expression of the β catalytic subunit of PP1, PP1Cβ, in brain regions of rats trained to nose poke for food reward. They observed elevated levels of PP1Cβ in the striatum and nucleus accumbens 22 hours after a session of nose poking for food but not in yoked control rats that received food that was not contingent on responding.[34] Results show that PP1 activity is selectively altered in rats that have undergone operant conditioning for food reward. However, the correlational nature of the results and the long delay from behavioral testing to harvesting of brain tissue make it difficult to link the results to the precise timing

---

concentrations may activate calcium/diacylglycerol-activated protein kinase C (PKC) and promote the phosphorylation of ERK 1/2 through a chain of kinase activations that include Ras family and Raf family kinases that activate mitogen-activated protein kinase kinase (MEK)1/2. pERK1/2 phosphorylates Kv4.2 channels and influences the insertion of AMPA receptors into the membrane, further increasing excitability of the dendritic spine. pERK1/2 also phosphorylates p90 ribosomal S6 kinase2 (RSK2), which translocates to the nucleoplasm where it phosphorylates serine 133 of cAMP response element-binding protein (pCREB). In the nucleus, pERK1/2 activates mitogen-and-stress-activated kinase-1 (pMSK1), which also phosphorylates CREB. pERK1/2 influences the transcription factor Elk 1. PKA activates CREB and it may be the combined effects of signaling at Glu synapses and DA synapses that leads to the transcription of genes involved in the strengthening of synaptic connections.

of the putative incentive learning-related neuromolecular events described earlier. In related work by Cornell Medical College, New York, researcher Barry Kosofsky and colleagues, levels of serine 133-phosphorylated CREB were elevated in the nucleus accumbens of mice re-exposed to conditioned incentive stimuli based on cocaine in the conditioned place preference apparatus; increased levels of DARPP-32 phosphorylated at threonine 34, making it a potent inhibitor of PP1, were also observed.[35] These results are consistent with a role for CREB, DARPP-32, and PP1 in the mechanisms of incentive learning. Researchers from the University of Pittsburgh directly tested the effects of glutamate NMDA receptor blockade or ERK1/2 blockade in the nucleus accumbens on CREB phosphorylation following exposure to a food-related conditioned incentive stimulus; they observed a significant reduction. They also showed that ERK1/2 phosphorylation following exposure to the conditioned stimulus depended on stimulation of NMDA and dopamine D1-like receptors.[36] A conditioned incentive stimulus that has been established by pairings with food can itself produce phasic dopamine release and new incentive learning (Chapter 5; also see later). This excellent work shows that during incentive learning ERK1/2 and CREB activation depend on both NMDA and D1-like receptor stimulation, supporting the mechanism described earlier.

A recent study from Bharathidasan University in Tiruchirappalli, India, reported increased levels of ERK1/2 and CREB phosphorylation in the telencephalon of goldfish (*Carassius auratus*) that were killed 30 or 60 minutes after performing a food-related color discrimination incentive learning task; a treatment that inhibited the CREB pathway impaired learning.[37] These results support a role for CREB in incentive learning and suggest that the signaling pathways involved in incentive learning may be conserved throughout vertebrate phylogeny.

As mentioned in Chapter 11, studies with arthropods implicate dopamine in incentive learning in invertebrates and in many cases some of the signaling molecules already discussed have been shown to be involved. In the fruit fly *Drosophila melanogaster*, a genetic mutant termed *dumb* that lacks D1 dopamine receptors was impaired in incentive learning to a cue previously paired with food when tested in a discrimination task in a T-maze and the deficit was rescued by reinstating dopamine D1 receptor expression.[38] Other genetic mutants have been tested in a food-rewarded place conditioning task or in a conditioned avoidance version of the task that also assesses incentive learning (see Chapter 3), and a number of additional incentive learning-impaired animals have been identified. Among the mutants identified are the amusingly named *dunce, rutabaga, amnesiac, radish, turnip*, and *leonardo* mutants.[39] In the *dunce* mutant, the deficient gene encodes a calcium/calmodulin-stimulated adenylyl cyclase. In the *rutabaga* mutant, the deficient gene codes for a cAMP phospho-diesterase, an enzyme that degrades cAMP. The *amnesiac* gene encodes a peptide that activates adenylyl cyclase. In *radish* mutants the affected protein is a target of PKA.[40] Finally, the *turnip* and *leonardo* mutations may affect PKC.[39] This is only a small subset of the large number of mutants now identified.[41] Thus, a number of *Drosophila* mutants that show impaired incentive learning have altered function of molecules implicated in the mechanism of incentive learning in vertebrates, as discussed earlier in this chapter.

As discussed in Chapter 11, dopamine has been implicated in food reward-related learning in the mollusk *Aplysia*. Response-contingent, but not random, activation of the esophageal nerve branch led to patterned ingestion-related biting activity. This effect depended on dopamine,[42] and was shown also to depend on cAMP and PKA; evidence of an associative convergence of PKC activity and dopamine signaling also was found, possibly supporting the importance of timing of different inputs for the putative plasticity mediated by dopamine.[43] It will be of interest eventually to identify environmental stimuli (e.g., odors, tastes) that, by the action of dopamine, become incentive stimuli, controlling food-seeking movements in *Aplysia*.

To recap briefly, the scenario is as follows. Environmental stimuli lead to activation of a subset of corticostriatal glutamatergic synapses. At those synapses the increase in calcium concentration may create a state of readiness characterized by the phosphorylation and activation of a number of proteins. At the same time, phosphatases, including calcineurin and PP1, are activated that begin to undo some of the phosphorylation events that putatively characterize the state of readiness and in short order activity returns to baseline (or synaptic weakening takes place as discussed in the next section). However, if there is a dopaminergic input immediately following the glutamatergic input, signaling molecules activated by the dopamine input, including PKA, prevent the effects of PP1 and other phosphatases thereby prolonging the phosphorylation events begun by the glutamatergic input and they also more directly augment some of the same phosphorylation pathways that glutamate impacts (Figures 12.1–12.3). This may lead to strengthening of the corticostriatal synapse so that in the future the environmental stimuli that activated that synapse have an increased ability to elicit approach and other responses. These intracellular molecular events may be the mechanism of dopamine-mediated incentive learning.

Short-term and long-term incentive learning

Incentive learning might have short-term and long-term components and those putative components might be mediated by different mechanisms.

Regarding the putative short-term component, recall that one of the consequences of increased calcium concentrations in the dendritic spine is activation of CaMKII and phosphorylation of AMPA receptors at serine 831 of the GluA1 subunit, and that phosphorylated AMPA receptors have an increased conductance and increased trafficking to the membrane surface.[11,12] As a result, stimulation of AMPA receptors in that synapse can have an increased impact on the postsynaptic cell, producing a larger excitatory postsynaptic potential that is more likely to affect the firing rate of the medium spiny neuron. Recall further that another consequence of the calcium input and activation of CaMKII was to activate calcineurin that dephosphorylates AMPA receptors at serine 845 of the GluA1 subunit reducing conductance and trafficking to the membrane surface.[18] Thus, activating and competing deactivating events occur close together in time. The case with Kv4.2 is similar; these potassium channels are phosphorylated and internalized by increased calcium concentrations but then dephosphorylated and externalized by the actions of calcineurin.[9,16] However, if a dopamine input occurs while this is going on (i.e., putatively while the dendritic spine is in a state of readiness), activation of PKA has at least two effects that will promote excitability of the glutamate synapse: (1) PKA will lead to phosphorylation of the GluA1 subunit of AMPA receptors at serine 845 promoting their conductance and trafficking to the membrane surface;[27] and (2) PKA will phosphorylate DARPP-32 at threonine 34,[15] reversing the inactivating effects of calcineurin, allowing DARPP-32 to inhibit PP1, removing the inhibitory effect of PP1 on ERK1/2 and thereby promoting the influence of ERK1/2 on the internalization of Kv4.2 channels (Figure 12.3).[29] As a result, the increased conductance and trafficking to the membrane surface of AMPA receptors and the internalization and deactivation of Kv4.2 channels will persist, leading to increased excitability of the glutamatergic synapse. This might be the mechanism of a short-term form of incentive learning.

Support for this idea again comes from the work of Eric Kandel and his many students and colleagues. They carried out studies of the possible molecular mechanisms of learning, employing slices of brain tissue from the hippocampus of rats. Using a combination of electrical stimulation and recording techniques, they found that the postsynaptic consequences of activating an input were strengthened following a strong stimulation of that input. This phenomenon is termed "long-term potentiation." Its discovery in the hippocampus of anaesthetized rabbits is attributed to Timothy Bliss from the National Institute of Medical Research, at the time located in the Mill Hill district of London, UK, and Terje Lømo from the University of Oslo, Norway.[44] What Kandel and his co-workers found was that long-term potentiation had at least two components, a genuinely long-term component that relied on protein synthesis and a more transient short-term component lasting one to three hours that was protein synthesis independent.[45] It may be that the short-term component was mediated, in part, by phosphorylated AMPA receptors and Kv4.2 potassium channels. Their phosphorylation does not depend on protein synthesis, resulting instead from covalent modifications of existing proteins, as described earlier. It is at present unclear what maintains the short-term modifications of existing proteins. One possibility is that CaMKII, once activated, autophosphorylates at threonine 286 and thereby becomes independent of calcium concentrations; it can then putatively maintain synaptic strength in the short term, perhaps by interacting with AMPA or NMDA receptors.[46] However, the molecular mechanisms of short-term synaptic strengthening remain to be fully worked out.

Long-term synaptic strengthening requires protein synthesis. PKA activated by the dopamine input has downstream targets that may lead to long-term strengthening of the corticostriatal synapse. One of them is CREB. This molecule is constitutively bound to CREB binding sites in the promoter region of many genes. When activated, CREB influences gene transcription and the synthesis of new proteins. Those proteins can then participate in strengthening the glutamatergic synapse that started this whole process by going into a state of readiness just before a rewarding stimulus occurred and dopaminergic neurons were activated. There are a number of important questions about how CREB signaling is regulated. One is that dopaminergic input to any dendritic spine, whether it has a state of readiness or not, will activate dopamine D1-like receptor signaling, including PKA activation and CREB phosphorylation. How does the mechanism act selectively so that CREB-initiated transcription events modify the most recently active corticostriatal glutamatergic synapse? One answer that should immediately come to mind is that the PKA signal may be amplified at dendritic spines in a state of readiness because the glutamatergic input may have led to enhanced coupling of dopamine D1-like receptors to adenylyl cyclase through the action of CaMKII.[20] This would lead to a larger CREB signal from the dendritic spines that most recently had a glutamatergic input than those that did not (see earlier).

Another way to selectively affect the CREB signal in dendritic spines that most recently had a glutamatergic input would be for the glutamatergic input to produce a molecular event that augmented the effect of PKA on CREB. As already discussed, the ERK1/2 signal provides a possible candidate. When there has been a glutamatergic input followed quickly by a dopaminergic input, the combined influence of ERK1/2-activated RSK2 and MSK1 and dopamine–PKA-activated CREB in the nucleus may be necessary for CREB-mediated gene transcription.[29,32,47] These events may lead to new protein synthesis that forms the basis of long-term synaptic strengthening. A recent paper reported that six- to eight-day-old larval zebrafish showed a conditioned place preference 36 hours after the place was paired with social reward; a protein synthesis inhibitor blocked this effect.[48] These results remind us of the conservation of reward-related learning across species, that social stimuli can be powerful rewards (Chapter 8), and emphasize the role of dopamine-dependent protein synthesis in incentive learning.

Once the actions of CREB produce messenger RNA (mRNA) and new proteins that can contribute to the strengthening of recently active corticostriatal glutamatergic synapses on the dendritic spines of medium spiny neurons, how do those gene products find their way to the right synapses? The new mRNA transcripts may be converted to the proteins they code for at ribosomes in the cell body. Now the proteins have to find their way back to the dendritic spines where the glutamate and dopamine inputs acted in concert to initiate the whole process to begin with. An alternative is that the mRNA itself travels back to the relevant dendritic spines where it is converted to the protein it codes for. In either case, the problem remains of finding the right place. How does newly synthesized protein or mRNA find its way to the small subset of dendritic spines that were in a state of readiness when the dopamine signal arrived?

The general answer to this question is that there is a tag, some sort of biochemical marker that signals the right place. The tag may last for about 30 minutes.[47] This putative marker might be set up as a result of the conjunction of glutamatergic NMDA and dopaminergic D1-like receptor activity in the dendritic spine. We might expect that when a corticostriatal glutamatergic NMDA input is active and initiates the wave of phosphorylation events that putatively represents the state of readiness, it also sets up a potential signaling molecule (tag), perhaps by phosphorylating it. If no rewarding stimulus occurs and therefore no dopaminergic input takes place, the state of readiness is quickly lost as phosphatases undo the phosphorylation events, including the phosphorylation of the putative tag. However, if a rewarding stimulus occurs and the dopaminergic input is activated while the dendritic spine is in a state of readiness, the action of dopamine D1-like receptor signaling might sustain the phosphorylation of the tag. This signal would now be set up only in the dendritic spines that were in a state of readiness when a rewarding stimulus occurred and dopaminergic neurons were activated.[49] An alternative to setting up the signal when the wave of phosphorylation occurs to create the state of readiness would be to have some molecular event that occurs only as a result of the conjunction of glutamatergic NMDA and dopaminergic D1-like receptor inputs to serve as the signal. For example, just as ERK1/2 activated by the glutamatergic input and PKA activated by the dopaminergic input work in concert to influence the effect of CREB on transcription, two molecular events, one resulting from signaling at the glutamatergic input and the other resulting from signaling at the dopaminergic input, may act on a molecule that then serves as the tag for that dendritic spine. There is some evidence for both of these mechanisms from studies of long-term synaptic plasticity in the hippocampus.[49]

The new proteins that are thought to contribute to changes in synaptic effectiveness include the protein products (in brackets) of the immediate early genes *FOSB* (FosB and its splice variant ΔFosB),[50] *c-Fos* (c-fos), and *EGR1* (Zif268) that are transcription factors.[51] Proteins that may contribute to long-term remodeling of recently active synapses, including postsynaptic density 95, homer, filamentous actin,[52] and cyclin-dependent kinase 5,[53] are among perhaps several dozen proteins that are regulated by CREB or immediate early gene signaling;[54] however, studies are needed that look at gene expression resulting from conjoint activity at glutamate and dopamine synapses. The mechanisms that link the synthesis of new proteins to eventual synaptic strengthening remain to be worked out. Neuroscientists Terry Robinson from the University of Michigan in Ann Arbor and Bryan Kolb from the University of Lethbridge in Alberta, Canada, review studies identifying increases in dendritic spine density and branching of the distal dendrites of medium spiny neurons in the nucleus accumbens of animals that were treated with the dopamine-enhancing drugs amphetamine or cocaine; small effects were seen even after a single injection.[55] These changes may be the end result of the expression of new proteins that follows a conjunction of activity at a particular subset of corticostriatal synapses and rewarding stimulus-related phasic activation of dopaminergic neurons.

The results of a recent paper from Japanese researchers are of interest at this point for several reasons. They used optogenetic techniques (see later) to separately stimulate dopamine D1 receptor and glutamate inputs to medium spiny projection neurons of the striatum of mice. Their main dependent variable was spine morphology detected with two-photon microscopy. Dendritic spine morphology is correlated with spine function and dendritic spines enlarge during long-term potentiation of synapses onto them. They found that activation of glutamatergic inputs led to spine enlargement when dopamine inputs were activated within a time window of 0.3–2 seconds following the glutamate input; the enlargement lasted at least 50 minutes, the longest they tested after paired stimulus presentation. They showed further that the glutamate input required NMDA receptors, increased intracellular calcium concentrations, induction of CaMKII, and protein synthesis. The effect of the dopamine input on glutamate-induced changes in spines depended on cAMP, PKA, DARPP-32, and inhibition of PP1. They linked glutamate input and CaMKII activation to potentiation of dopamine signaling and showed that this was necessary for the dopamine input to produce activation of PKA of sufficient strength to lead to spine enlargement.[56] Results clearly show the importance of timing of the glutamate and dopamine inputs for modifications of the effect of the glutamate input to take place. They additionally suggest the importance of protein synthesis and changes in spine morphology for incentive learning.

The dopamine D3 receptor may be involved in incentive learning. Recall from Chapter 7 that behavioral experiments, for example using conditioned activity, show that D3 receptor antagonists are more effective at blocking the expression of incentive conditioning than they are at blocking establishment. The study of Bernard Le Foll et al. showed further that the paired group (that received cocaine injections immediately prior to placement into the test environment) had increased expression of D3 receptors and D3 receptor mRNA in the nucleus accumbens compared with an unpaired group (that received cocaine in a different environment).[57] Results suggested that D3 receptors may be synthesized and added to the membrane in paired animals. Little is known about the mechanism by which D3 receptors might influence incentive learning. Pierre Sokoloff from the Pierre Fabre Research Center in Castres and colleagues from France reported electron microscopy findings showing D3 receptor immunoreactivity in presumed *glutamatergic* synapses on the heads of dendritic spines of medium spiny neurons in the nucleus accumbens of rats. They suggested a direct interaction between D3 receptors and NMDA or AMPA receptors.[58] This observation raises the intriguing possibility that D3 receptors contribute to changes in corticostriatal glutamate synaptic effectiveness thought to underlie incentive learning. Further studies of the mechanisms by which D3 receptors are expressed and how they possibly interact with glutamate receptors are needed.

AMPA receptors are thought to be involved in long-term synaptic strengthening. Some years ago, Todor Gerdjikov and I reviewed the possible contribution of NMDA and AMPA receptors to reward-related incentive learning.[59] Behavioral tests that we covered included conditioned approach, lever pressing for food, brain stimulation, or drug reward, and conditioned place preference based on amphetamine, cocaine, morphine, or food. Results generally revealed that NMDA receptor antagonists disrupted the acquisition of learning in these behavioral tests but had little effect when given in the expression phase after the incentive learning had been acquired. This differential effect was seen with systemic injections or intra-nucleus accumbens injections of NMDA receptor antagonist drugs. Although fewer data were available for the effects of AMPA receptor antagonists in these behavioral tests, the available data showed conversely that AMPA receptor antagonists more consistently disrupted the expression of incentive learning than its acquisition. Results are consistent with a critical role for NMDA receptors in the acquisition of reward-related incentive learning and a more central role for AMPA receptors in its expression.

As discussed earlier, one of the components of the putative state of readiness is phosphorylation of AMPA receptors at serine 831 of the GluA1 subunit; this leads to increased trafficking of AMPA receptors to the membrane surface and an increase in their conductance, both events that will enhance synaptic transmission at that dendritic spine if another glutamatergic input occurs there. The nuclear events, *viz.* gene expression and new protein synthesis, that take place when a glutamatergic input is followed by phasic firing of dopamine neurons may lead to structural changes in the dendritic spine that underlie a more stable and long-term incentive learning. The details of such a mechanism need to be worked out.

Role of the indirect pathway in incentive learning

All of the discussion up to this point in this chapter has focused on incentive learning-associated molecular changes that may take place in medium spiny projection neurons of the striatum that express dopamine D1 receptors. Recall from Chapter 11 that these are neurons of the direct pathway in the basal ganglia. About half of the medium spiny neurons express D2 receptors and form the indirect pathway. What happens in D2 receptor-expressing medium spiny projections neurons when reward-related learning occurs? As discussed in the following paragraphs, data suggest that *when incentive learning is taking place and corticostriatal glutamatergic synapses onto neurons of the direct pathway are being strengthened, corticostriatal glutamatergic synapses onto neurons of the indirect pathway are being weakened.*

New molecular tools have made it possible to independently activate or inhibit neurons of the direct or indirect pathway. Optogenetics uses viral vectors to express light-sensitive molecules, for example channelrhodopsins or halorhodopsins; these can be expressed specifically within genetically defined neurons such as those of the direct or indirect pathway.[60] Channelrhodopsins and halorhodopsins are similar to the light-sensitive molecules of the retina. When a particular frequency of light is shone upon neurons expressing a particular channelrhodopsin or halorhodopsin, those neurons are, respectively, activated or inhibited. Optogenetic techniques can be used in awake, behaving animals. Researchers at the Gladstone Institute, University of California San Francisco and Stanford University showed that optogenetic activation of direct pathway neurons through chronically implanted optical fibers led to motor activation and optogenetic activation of indirect pathway neurons led to motor inhibition in mice.[61]

Incentive learning involves the acquisition by stimuli of an increased ability to elicit approach and other responses. The molecular mechanisms discussed in this chapter suggest a strengthening of cortical connections to the D1 receptor-expressing pathway; the implication by optogenetic studies of this pathway in motor activation is consistent with this strengthening. A simultaneous weakening of cortical glutamatergic synapses onto D2 receptor-expressing neurons of the indirect pathway would further promote the activating effects of incentive stimuli (see Cui et al. in Note 61). Electrophysiological studies provide some evidence that D2 receptor stimulation contributes to the weakening of glutamatergic corticostriatal synapses. Paolo Calabresi and co-workers in Rome, Italy, reported long-term synaptic depression in the striatum following tetanic stimulation of the cortex. This effect depended on D2 and metabotropic glutamate receptor stimulation (for excellent reviews see Note 63).[62] It also depended on endocannabinoid signaling that was stimulated by the synergistic action of dopamine, glutamate and calcium;[63] perhaps glutamate signaling (including increased intracellular calcium concentrations) produces a state of readiness in dendritic spines of D2 receptor-expressing medium spiny projection neurons of the indirect pathway like that described earlier for the D1 receptor-expressing neurons of the direct pathway. If a phasic dopamine signal arrives during this putative state of readiness, stimulation of the synthesis of the endocannabinoids anandamide and 2-arachidonyl glycerol may lead to a decrease in the probability of glutamate release from presynaptic terminals resulting from the action of endocannabinoids on cannabinoid receptors located there.[64] This may form part of a mechanism for weakening the influence of environmental stimuli on the indirect pathway, thereby reducing motor inhibition produced by those stimuli. Recall from Chapter 7 that antagonists acting at D1- or D2-like receptors were able to block incentive learning; recent results from studies using optogenetic activation of dopaminergic neurons in place conditioning and self-stimulation experiments similarly show the necessity of both D1 and D2 receptors for reward-related learning.[65] These results support the suggestion that incentive learning may involve both strengthening of cortical synapses onto direct pathway neurons and weakening of cortical synapses onto indirect pathway neurons.

Sophisticated molecular technologies were used recently by psychiatrist and neuroscientist Eric Nestler and colleagues at Icahn School of Medicine at Mount Sinai, New York, to shed further light on the role of D2 receptor-expressing medium spiny neurons in incentive learning. Fiber photometry calcium imaging allowed them to record from genetically distinct subpopulations of striatal neurons in awake, behaving mice. Mice underwent place preference conditioning with cocaine and recordings were then taken during the drug-free test day when the mice had access to both sides of the apparatus. As expected, mice showed a conditioned place preference, spending more time in the cocaine-paired compartment. Entry into the drug-paired compartment during test simultaneously increased the activity of D1 receptor-expressing medium spiny neurons and decreased the activity of D2 receptor-expressing medium spiny neurons.[66] Like the electrophysiological results reviewed earlier, these results support the suggestion that incentive learning may involve both strengthening of cortical synapses onto direct pathway neurons and weakening of cortical synapses onto indirect pathway neurons. The high temporal resolution of the calcium imaging provided further detail. D1 receptor-expressing medium spiny neurons showed their peak activation in the approximately one second immediately prior to entering the drug-paired side; by comparison, D2 receptor-expressing neurons showed their peak reduction in activation during the 1–2 seconds immediately following entry into the drug-paired side. The authors made the intriguing speculation that "D1 activity drives the motivation to enter a paired compartment, with the reduced activity of D2 cells after entry driving the motivation to remain in that compartment" (p. 2727).[66] Further studies are needed with non-drug, natural rewards such as food to evaluate the generality of this observation.

Downstream signaling following stimulation of D2 receptors in D2 receptor-expressing medium spiny projection neurons has not been studied to the same extent as that associated with stimulation of D1 receptors. One signaling molecule that is activated by stimulation of D2 receptors is glycogen synthase kinase-3 (GSK-3).[67] Ellen Unterwald and associates from Temple University in Philadelphia, Pennsylvania, showed that blockade of GSK-3 during conditioning sessions prevented the establishment of a conditioned place preference based on cocaine in mice.[68] Rebekah Wickens and Susan Quartarone, working in my laboratory, have recently shown that a GSK-3 inhibitor injected systemically or directly into the nucleus accumbens similarly blocked conditioned place preference based on amphetamine. We found that the dose of the GSK-3 inhibitor needed to block acquisition was lower than the dose needed to block expression. Thus, in separate groups several doses were tested by injecting them each day prior to conditioning sessions and in other groups conditioned with amphetamine, the GSK-3 inhibitor was given prior to the test session.[69] Findings implicate GSK-3 in both acquisition and expression of conditioned place preference based on amphetamine, but the finding that acquisition is more sensitive to disruption than expression further implicates GSK-3 more strongly in acquisition. One study has implicated GSK-3 in long-term depression of synaptic strength in the hippocampus,[70] but, to date, no studies have investigated the possible role of GSK-3 in the striatum in long-term depression.

Activation of GSK-3 leads to inhibition of the transcription factor β-catenin.[71] The canonical Wnt signaling pathway activates β-catenin.[72] Wnt signaling plays a critical role in development of the nervous system,[73] and a few recent studies have implicated Wnt in memory in the hippocampus.[74] Farhana Islam and Kathleen Xu, working in my laboratory, found that nucleus accumbens Wnt signaling plays a role in incentive learning. In conditioned place preference studies, they injected a Wnt palmitoylation inhibitor either before conditioning sessions with amphetamine or before test sessions. A dose-dependent blockade of preference for the drug-paired side was found in both phases, but a lower dose was effective at blocking acquisition than expression, suggesting that Wnt signaling may be more important for the establishment of incentive learning than its expression.[75] Whether the Wnt signaling that appears to be involved in incentive learning takes place in D1 or D2 receptor-expressing medium spiny neurons or in other neurons of the striatum remains to be determined.

From the discussion of the importance of timing for incentive learning in the D1 receptor-expressing direct pathway, it would follow that timing is similarly important for incentive learning in the D2 receptor-expressing pathway. Environmental stimuli and stimuli produced by ongoing muscular activity putatively would lead to activity at a subset of corticostriatal glutamatergic synapses onto D2 receptor-expressing medium spiny projection neurons, bringing them into a state of readiness. If a phasic activation of dopaminergic neurons produced by rewarding stimuli takes place, those synapses in a putative state of readiness may be weakened by the action of dopamine acting at D2 receptors and possibly signaling through endocannabinoids and GSK-3. Jean-Martin Beaulieu of Laval University in Quebec City, Canada, and colleagues have studied D2 receptor signaling extensively and provide many details of the molecular events that may be involved in D2 receptor-mediated plasticity.[67] Further studies of the molecular events underlying modification of cortical connections to indirect pathway neurons are eagerly awaited.

As discussed in Chapter 7, the early discoveries of D1- and D2-like receptors in the late 1970s characterized them, respectively, as activating and inhibiting the adenylyl cyclase–cAMP cascade. At the time, the direct and indirect pathways had not been described and general thinking was that D1- and D2-like receptors were co-localized on the same neurons. This led to some confusion because, on the one hand, D1- and D2-like receptors seemed to act antagonistically towards one another when their action on the adenylyl cyclase–cAMP cascade was considered but, on the other, they seemed to act in a complementary manner when their contribution to the stimulation of motor activity or reward-related incentive learning was considered (see Chapter 7). The identification of the direct and indirect pathways and their independent, respective, location of D1 and D2 receptors (for the most part; a small proportion of striatal medium spiny projection neurons co-express D1 and D2 receptors) has helped to resolve this confusion. D1 and D2 receptors appear to work cooperatively in their control of incentive learning; D1 receptor stimulation resulting from phasic bursts of activity in dopamine neurons activates adenylyl cyclase and a cascade of intracellular events that result in strengthening of recently active corticostriatal synapses and D2 receptor stimulation simultaneously appears to weaken cortical synapses onto D2-expressing medium spiny projection neurons by an adenylyl cyclase–cAMP-independent mechanism.

Possible mechanism of inverse incentive learning

It remains the case that D2 receptor stimulation inhibits adenylyl cyclase in medium spiny neurons of the indirect pathway. However, *in indirect pathway neurons, the adenylyl cyclase–cAMP cascade is not activated by D1 receptors but instead by adenosine 2A (A2A) receptors.*[76] Under conditions when dopamine neurons are producing tonic activity and synaptic concentrations of dopamine are maintained perhaps in the nanomolar range,[77] dopamine acting at D2 receptors inhibits adenylyl cyclase and prevents downstream signaling through A2A receptors. However, when dopamine neuron activity is transiently inhibited and synaptic concentrations of dopamine drop, perhaps, for example when an expected rewarding stimulus fails to occur (termed "negative prediction error" by Wolfram Schultz and colleagues[78]), D2 receptor-mediated dopaminergic inhibition of adenylyl cyclase will be removed and cAMP-mediated downstream signaling will be able to take place.[79] Results suggest that this signaling can lead to synaptic strengthening (see below). Because the indirect pathway has inhibitory effects on motor activity, strengthening of cortical connections to medium spiny projection neurons of this pathway should lead to a *reduced* ability of the stimuli and efference copy that activate those cortical synapses to elicit approach and other responses. This is, of course, inverse incentive learning.

You will recall from Chapter 6 that inverse incentive learning takes place when stimuli are associated with a decrease in dopaminergic neurotransmission. Inverse incentive learning is the loss by stimuli of their ability to elicit approach and other responses. I suggested in Chapter 6 that the brief inhibition of dopamine neuron firing that takes place when an expected rewarding stimulus fails to appear—negative prediction error—might produce inverse incentive learning. *Inverse incentive learning might be associated with the strengthening of corticostriatal glutamatergic projections onto the indirect pathway and the weakening of related connections onto direct pathway neurons.* Both potentiation of cortical synapses onto indirect pathway neurons and depression of cortical synapses onto direct pathway neurons have been reported in electrophysiological experiments and recent behavioral data are in the early stages of unraveling these mechanisms.

Like the strengthening of connections onto D1 receptor-expressing medium spiny neurons that appears to depend on activation of the cAMP–PKA pathway, the strengthening of connections onto D2 receptor-expressing medium spiny neurons appears to depend on the cAMP–PKA pathway. However, whereas dopamine stimulates this cascade in D1 receptor-expressing neurons of the direct pathway, the cAMP–PKA cascade is stimulated by A2A receptors in D2 receptor-expressing neurons of the indirect pathway. Under normal conditions, when dopamine neurons are firing in a tonic manner, the concentration of dopamine at synapses expressing D2 receptors may be high enough that stimulation of dopamine receptors inhibits adenylyl cyclase preventing adenosine from acting through A2A receptors to initiate the cascade of molecular signals that appears to be necessary for strengthening of glutamatergic connections onto the dendritic spine. However, when dopamine neurons are inhibited, for example as the result of failure of a predicted rewarding stimulus to occur, the D2 receptor-mediated inhibition of adenylyl cyclase is removed and the cascade can be activated by adenosine, possibly leading to inverse incentive learning.

Electrophysiological studies have shown long-term potentiation of corticostriatal synapses onto D2 receptor-expressing neurons of the indirect pathway; this long-term potentiation is dependent on *low* dopamine, NMDA receptor stimulation, and requires stimulation of A2A receptors.[80] Studies have implicated adenylyl cyclase, cAMP, PKA, DARPP-32, CREB, and ERK, but more studies are needed.[63] It may be that stimulation of A2A receptors leads to strengthening of glutamatergic synapses onto indirect pathway neurons via many of the same signaling molecules that have been implicated in D1 receptor-mediated strengthening of glutamatergic synapses onto direct pathway neurons. It may also be the case that glutamatergic inputs onto indirect pathway neurons produce a state of readiness for A2A receptor-mediated plasticity. However, as was the case for long-term depression of these synapses, further studies are needed to work out the molecular details of long-term potentiation of the indirect pathway and the relevance of long-term potentiation results for understanding the mechanisms of synaptic plasticity that takes place under physiological conditions.

In inverse incentive learning studies we, and others, have observed increases in descent latencies in the bar test following pairings of placement on the bar with low-dose haloperidol-induced decreases in D2 receptor stimulation and we have observed conditioned increases in descent latencies when paired animals are tested following an injection of saline (Chapter 6). In very recent as-yet-unpublished studies my doctoral student, Jeffery Rocca, has found that pretreatment with the adenosine receptor antagonist theophylline prior to injections of haloperidol dose-dependently reduced increased descent latencies over days. These results support a role for adenosine in producing the putative synaptic strengthening of glutamatergic synapses onto D2 receptor-expressing medium spiny neurons that may underlie inverse incentive learning. In additional studies, we did not observe significant sensitization following pairings of placement on the bar with low-dose treatment with the D1-like receptor antagonist SCH23390. Neither did we observe conditioned increases in descent latency in a saline test.[81] These results suggest that it is a decrease in synaptic transmission at D2 or D2 and D1 receptors, not at D1 receptors alone that leads to inverse incentive learning. Much remains to be done.

In the same way that incentive learning seems to involve strengthening of glutamatergic corticostriatal connections onto D1 receptor-expressing medium spiny projection neurons *and* weakening of glutamatergic corticostriatal connections onto D2 receptor-expressing medium spiny projection neurons, inverse incentive learning may involve strengthening of glutamatergic corticostriatal connections onto D2 receptor-expressing medium spiny projection neurons, as just discussed, *and* weakening of glutamatergic contrcostriatal connections onto D1 receptor-expressing medium spiny projection neurons (Table 12.1). In electrophysiological studies, long-term depression of cortical synapses onto direct pathway neurons has been reported but only in the presence of low dopamine.[63] Like long-term depression of corticostriatal synapses of the indirect pathway, this effect involves the endogenous cannabinoids anandamide and 2-arichydonyl glycerol in rats and mice.[82,83]

Some results implicate D2 receptors and muscarinic cholinergic receptors in long-term depression of glutamatergic synapses onto direct pathway neurons. Cholinergic synapses originate from large aspiny neurons of the striatum that connect with medium spiny neurons.[84] D2 receptors may act to lower acetylcholine release by inhibiting cholinergic interneurons.[82] This putative inhibition may then reduce the inhibitory effect of acetylcholine on endocannabinoid synthesis in direct pathway neurons and subsequent increases in endocannabinoid synthesis may reduce glutamate release from presynaptic terminals, contributing to long-term depression.[63] The mechanisms underlying weakening of cortical connections onto direct pathway neurons are a work in progress.

The possible role of striatal cholinergic interneurons in the putative mechanisms and circuitry of incentive learning and inverse incentive learning provides a specific example of what may be a more general case concerning striatal

Table 12.1 Possible role of the direct and indirect pathway in incentive and inverse incentive learning.

	Glutarnate synapses onto direct (D1) pathway neurons	Glutamate synapses onto indirect (D2) pathway neurons
Incentive learning	Strengthening via D1 receptor, cAMP, PKA, DARPP-32, CREB/ERK	Weakening via endocannabinoids?
Inverse incentive learning	Weakening via endocannabinoids?	Strengthening via A2A receptor, cAMP, PKA, DARPP-32, CREB/ERK

Incentive learning may involve strengthening of glutamatergic synapses onto D1 receptor-expressing medium spiny neurons (MSNs) of the direct pathway and weakening of glutamatergic synapses onto D2 receptor-expressing MSNs of the indirect pathway. The strengthening mechanism may involve the D1 receptor, cyclic adenosine 3, 5-monophosphate (cAMP), c-AMP-dependent protein kinase A (PKA), *dopamine and cAMP-regulated phosphoprotein-32* (DARPP-32), and the combined influences of cAMP response element binding protein (CREB) and extracellular signal regulated kinase 1/2 (ERK) on gene expression; the weakening mechanism might involve endocannabinoids. Inverse inventive learning may involve strengthening of glutamatergic synapses onto MSNs of the indirect pathway and weakening of synapses onto MSNs of the direct pathway. Strengthening may involve adenosine 2A (A2A) receptors, cAMP, PKA, DARPP-32, and CREB/ERK; weakening may involve endocannabinoids.

interneurons. As I pointed out in Chapter 11, the other approximately five percent of neurons in the striatum include not only large aspiny cholinergic interneurons, but also five subtypes of interneurons that use γ-aminobutyric acid (GABA) as their neurotransmitter. These GABAergic interneurons include parvalbumin-expressing fast-spiking interneurons; neurons that co-express neuropeptide Y, somatostatin, and nitric oxide synthase along with GABA, and are termed low-threshold spiking interneurons; GABA and neuropeptide Y-only expressing neurogliaform interneurons; tyrosine hydroxylase-expressing interneurons; and calretinin-expressing interneurons.[84] Charles Gerfen from the National Institute of Mental Health in Bethesda, Maryland, and D. James Surmeier from Northwestern University in Chicago, Illinois, have worked extensively on the neuroanatomical circuitry and mechanisms of neuroplasticity in the striatum; they and colleagues have reviewed in detail some of the connections of interneurons with medium spiny projection neurons of the striatum.[85]

An example of interneurons in the striatum is the parvalbumin-expressing fast-spiking interneurons that receive cortical glutamatergic input and GABAergic input from neurons of the external segment of the globus pallidus. They synapse onto direct and indirect pathway medium spiny projection neurons; however, their connections onto direct pathway neurons may be stronger. Stimulation of D2 receptors of the indirect pathway leads to a reduction of GABAergic input to fast-spiking interneurons, reducing inhibition of direct pathway neurons. This connectivity provides a means for communication between direct and indirect pathway outputs.[86] Another example is inter-neurons co-expressing neuropeptide Y, somatostatin, and nitric oxide synthase along with GABA; their function is poorly understood. They express D1-like D5 receptors and connect to distal dendrites in the striatum; perhaps they provide a means for the direct pathway to influence the indirect pathway, but further studies are needed.[85] Some years ago, neuroscientist Sheena Josselyn, now at the Hospital for Sick Children and the University of Toronto, while working in my laboratory discovered that stimulation of neuropeptide Y receptors in the nucleus accumbens produced incentive learning using the conditioned place preference procedure; she showed further that a dopamine receptor antagonist blocked this effect.[87] These results implicate striatal interneurons that release neuropeptide Y in incentive learning. A complete description of the mechanisms of incentive learning will eventually include striatal interneurons and their interactions with medium spiny projection neurons and their cortical inputs. It will also be necessary to better understand the functional relationship between astrocytes and neurons in the basal ganglia; recent work has shown that different subpopulations of astrocytes selectively respond to D1 or D2 receptor-expressing medium spiny projection neurons.[88]

Novel stimuli are unconditioned incentive stimuli insofar as they can elicit approach and other responses. How do striatal circuits respond to novel stimuli and how do those circuits change their responses to novel stimuli when novel stimuli turn out not to be predictors of biologically important outcomes such as rewarding stimuli? Recall from Chapter 6 that novel stimuli lead to increased dopamine neuronal activity and increased dopamine release in the nucleus accumbens. These increases are generally short-lived, only being seen upon the first few presentations of novel stimuli after which the dopamine response is no longer seen. These neurochemical responses parallel behavioral observations that animals initially orient to, and sometimes approach and interact with, novel stimuli, but these responses quickly subside upon repeated exposures to the novel stimulus; this pattern is often referred to as "habituation."[89] Recall further the electrophysiological observation of Jon Horvitz and colleagues, discussed in Chapter 6; they found that dopamine neuron responses to novel stimuli, by contrast to dopamine neuron responses to rewarding stimuli, are followed by a brief period of inhibition (similar to negative prediction error). Perhaps novelty-induced dopamine activity produces an exploration bonus, increasing the chances that the individual will find a rewarding stimulus in a novel environment.[90] Horvitz et al. suggested that novel stimuli may produce a rapid initial excitation in dopamine neurons that takes place before the rewarding or non-rewarding status of the event can be processed and that the post-excitation inhibition serves to counteract the initial burst in cases where a rewarding stimulus fails to occur.[91]

The mechanisms of habituation are not fully understood.[92] Recent work in my laboratory has revealed that inverse incentive learning is augmented by pre-exposure to the environmental stimuli subsequently paired with decreased dopamine neurotransmission.[93] This finding raises the possibility that habituation may be mediated by mechanisms similar to those involved in inverse incentive learning. Only speculation is possible at this point. Increased synaptic concentrations of dopamine produced by novel stimuli might be expected to produce incentive learning by the mechanisms described earlier in this chapter. Perhaps a period of inhibition of dopamine neurons immediately following a period of excitation is sufficient to reverse the molecular cascades normally leading to incentive learning, as implied by Horvitz et al.[91] Besides putatively arresting the incentive learning mechanism in both D1 and D2 receptor-expressing medium spiny projection neurons, the inhibition of dopamine neuron firing may lead to activation of the putative inverse incentive learning mechanism, strengthening the indirect pathway and weakening the direct pathway. Such a mechanism might lead to the observed loss of dopaminergic neuronal and behavioral activation observed to follow repeated presentations of novel stimuli as habituation takes place.

Incentive stimuli and dopamine release

The mechanisms of incentive learning discussed in this chapter involve modifications of corticostriatal synapses. Extensive data, many reviewed in Chapter 5, reveal that conditioned incentive stimuli acquire the ability to activate dopamine neurons and produce dopamine release. Thus, there may be two distinct aspects of incentive learning: (i) modifications of corticostriatal glutamatergic synapses; and (ii) acquisition by previously neutral stimuli of the ability to activate dopamine neurons and produce dopamine release. Recall that once incentive learning has taken place, conditioned incentive stimuli for a time retain the ability to elicit approach and other responses, even when dopamine receptors are blocked (Chapters 2 and 9). For example, untrained rats treated with a dopamine receptor blocker fail to learn to lever press for food.[94] or to make avoidance responses,[95] but trained rats similarly treated continue to respond for food,[96] and to make avoidance responses,[97] showing a gradual, extinction-like decline in responding. Recall from Chapter 9 that these observations are consistent with the well-documented delayed response to antipsychotic medications in schizophrenia. If conditioned incentive stimuli in trained animals rely on dopamine release for their ability to control responding, treatment with dopamine receptor blocking drugs should have immediate effect at blocking the behavioral effects of those stimuli. However, if conditioned incentive stimuli rely instead on modified corticostriatal glutamatergic connections for their ability to control responding, as discussed in this chapter, responding might be expected to continue, at least for a while, in the presence of dopamine receptor-blocking drugs. As discussed extensively in this book, this has been observed frequently. The observations suggest that, with use in the absence of dopamine, modified corticostriatal glutamatergic connections gradually return to baseline strength.

The question then arises as to how conditioned incentive stimuli acquire the ability to produce dopamine release and what is the function of this plastic change. One possibility is that dopamine-mediated modifications of corticostriatal synapses (as discussed earlier) lead to this ability; if this is the case, the mechanism remains to be elucidated. Alternatively, a number of findings suggest that there is plasticity of glutamatergic connections onto dopaminergic neurons in their nucleus of origin, the ventral tegmental area.

The mechanisms underlying the ability of reward-related stimuli to activate ventral tegmental area dopaminergic neurons have been reviewed in an excellent paper by behavioral neuroscientist Robert Ranaldi from the City University of New York in Flushing.[98] It is a remarkable story in the present context. The dendrites of ventral tegmental area dopaminergic neurons receive glutamatergic inputs from a number of brain regions, including the periaqueductal gray, pedunculopontine tegmental nucleus, nuclei of the amygdala, bed nucleus of the stria terminalis, and medial prefrontal cortex. The dendrites of the same dopaminergic neurons receive cholinergic inputs from neurons of the pedunculopotine and lateral dorsal tegmental nuclei. Instead of dopamine modifying glutamatergic synapses in an activity-dependent manner when reward-related learning takes place, as described in this chapter, it appears that acetylcholine plays this role in modifying glutamatergic synapses onto dopamine neurons in the ventral tegmental area. This organization suggests that environmental stimuli activate glutamatergic inputs; the precise role played by the various brain regions from which these inputs arise remains to be worked out.[99] Rewarding stimuli activate the cholinergic inputs.[98]

Just as the specific subset of cortical glutamatergic neurons and their corresponding synapses onto medium spiny neurons of the striatum changes as environmental stimuli change, so it may be that the specific subset of glutamatergic synapses onto dopaminergic neurons of the ventral tegmental area changes as environmental stimuli change. Stimulation of glutamate receptors may create a state of readiness in ventral tegmental area dopaminergic neurons like that created in medium spiny projection neurons. When a rewarding stimulus is encountered, cholinergic input neurons are activated. Acetylcholine, acting on muscarinic cholinergic receptors, may depolarize ventral tegmental area dopamine neurons leading to burst firing, producing the reward signal already discussed extensively. The muscarinic cholinergic input may also activate a molecular signaling cascade involving adenylyl cyclase, cAMP, and PKA within dopaminergic neurons that may interact with glutamatergic inputs that are in a putative state of readiness to produce synaptic strengthening. ERK has also been implicated in plasticity in the ventral tegmental area.[100] As a result of these putative molecular events, in the future, environmental stimuli that activate those synapses may acquire the ability themselves to activate dopamine neurons.

Ranaldi reviews much of what is known about the mechanisms of reward-related learning in the ventral tegmental area.[98] NMDA glutamatergic receptor stimulation and muscarinic cholinergic receptor stimulation are both necessary for plastic changes to occur. NMDA receptor stimulation will lead to increases in intracellular calcium concentrations and other downstream molecular changes that may contribute to synaptic modification. Once a stimulus has acquired the ability to activate dopamine neurons, that ability appears to be mediated by AMPA glutamatergic receptors; this is parallel to the findings discussed earlier in this chapter that NMDA receptors are more important for the establishment of incentive learning at corticostriatal synapses and that AMPA receptors are more important for its expression. Just as dopamine appears to produce plastic changes by modifying non-dopaminergic (glutamatergic) synapses in the striatum, so it is that acetylcholine appears to produce plastic changes by modifying non-cholinergic (also glutamatergic) synapses in the ventral tegmental area. The results of a recent study by Ranaldi and his students support the idea that cholinergic inputs are more important for establishment than expression of incentive learning. They show that the anticholinergic drug, scopolamine, given systemically during pairing of a light and food stimulus reduced the ability of the light to act as a conditioned reward in subsequent drug-free testing; giving the same doses of the anticholinergic prior to testing in animals that had received the light-food pairings while in an un-drugged state failed to affect the expression of learning.[101] Further studies are needed to work out the details of the mechanisms mediating synaptic plasticity in the ventral tegmental area, but initial observations suggest striking similarities to the mechanisms of incentive learning thought to operate in the striatum.

The findings discussed in this chapter and those reviewed by Ranaldi suggest that incentive learning has at least two separate components. Rewarding stimuli have an unconditioned ability to produce burst firing in ventral tegmental area dopamine neurons, possibly mediated by cholinergic inputs. Environmental and proprioceptive stimuli that are present just prior to rewarding stimuli will produce a putative state of readiness at their synaptic contacts with medium spiny projection neurons of the striatum and possibly in dopaminergic neurons of the ventral tegmental area. In the striatum, the conjunction of molecular events produced by glutamate and by activation of the cAMP–PKA cascade and associated intracellular signaling molecules by dopamine appears to lead to enhanced glutamate synaptic strength onto D1 receptor-expressing neurons, endocannabinoid mechanisms may lead to decreased glutamate synaptic strength onto D2 receptor-expressing neurons and, in the ventral tegmental area, it is possible that similar signaling events to those observed in D1 receptor-expressing neurons, produced by the action of glutamate and acetylcholine may lead to modification of glutamatergic synapses onto dopamine neurons. Thus, incentive learning may involve synaptic changes in at least two separate regions through independent but similar molecular mechanisms. In discussing the work of Ann Graybiel and colleagues in Chapter 5, I provide some suggestions for how conditioned dopamine release may operate to produce a gradient of incentive value in any particular environment.

Before ending this chapter, it is important to point out that dopamine appears to play a role in synaptic plasticity in other brain regions, including the prefrontal cortex and the hippocampus. Work by Eric Kandel and many others has shown that glutamate acting at NMDA receptors and dopamine acting at D1 receptors is necessary in the hippocampus for the late phase of long-term potentiation. This effect of dopamine appears to involve cAMP, PKA, CREB, ERK, and transcription and translation events leading to new protein synthesis.[102] Similarly, work by Thérèse Jay from the Université Paris Descartes and others has shown that dopamine–glutamate interactions appear to be necessary for long-term potentiation and working memory in the prefrontal cortex; many of the same signaling molecules have been implicated.[103] How these functions of dopamine are related to its action in the striatum in incentive learning remains to be explained.

Summary

As an animal moves through its environment, the internal sensory events that result from its movement and the stimuli that it encounters in its environment activate assemblies of cortical glutamatergic neurons that project to the striatum where they make synaptic contact with dendritic spines of medium spiny efferent neurons. As the incoming stimuli change, the uniquely activated subset of corticostriatal synapses changes. When corticostriatal synapses are sufficiently activated, calcium enters postsynaptic dendritic spines and initiates a wave of phosphorylation events that may constitute a state of readiness for modification. If a rewarding stimulus is not encountered, a subsequent wave of phosphatase activity quickly undoes the putative state of readiness. If a rewarding stimulus is encountered, increased concentrations of dopamine produced by bursting activity in striatal dopamine afferents initiates a cascade of intraspinous events in D1 receptor-expressing medium spiny neurons that may prevent the phosphatases from undoing the wave of phosphorylation produced by the cortical input. Additionally, some intracellular signaling molecules activated by the dopamine input may work synergistically with signaling events produced by the glutamatergic cortical input. The end result may be that corticostriatal synapses on D1 receptor-expressing medium spiny neurons active just prior to encountering a rewarding stimulus are altered so that they have a greater impact on response output systems in the future; this may be part of the mechanism of dopamine-mediated incentive learning. Putative synaptic changes may have both short-term and long-term components mediated by different mechanisms with the long-term modification relying on protein synthesis. In the presence of high dopamine concentrations, signaling at D2 receptors on dendritic spines of D2 receptor-expressing medium spiny neurons may prevent synaptic strengthening by inhibiting adenosine signaling through receptors that activate the cAMP–PKA cascade; these synapses may actually be weakened through other mechanisms involving endocannabinoids.

When extracellular concentrations of dopamine drop, for example during negative prediction errors, the opposite may occur, that is, corticospinous glutamatergic synapses onto D2 receptor-expressing medium spiny neurons may be strengthened and those onto D1 receptor-expressing medium spiny neurons may be weakened. This may be part of the mechanism of inverse incentive learning. Less is known about the mechanisms of these putative modifications. Synaptic strengthening may involve the effect of constitutively active adenosine acting at A2A receptors leading to activation of cAMP–PKA signaling that synergizes with signaling initiated by glutamate released at the corticospinous synapse of D2 receptor-expressing medium spiny neurons. Weakening at corticospinous glutamatergic synapses onto D1 receptor-expressing neurons may involve endocannabiinoids.

When incentive learning occurs, environmental stimuli that are encountered just prior to receiving a rewarding stimulus acquire the ability themselves to activate dopaminergic neurons. The underlying mechanisms for this modification may be similar to those for modifications of corticostriatal glutamatergic synapses. Thus, glutamatergic neurons from a number of brain regions including the cortex project into the ventral tegmental area where they synapse with dopaminergic cells located there. Dopamine cells also receive cholinergic inputs that are activated when a rewarding stimulus is encountered. Some findings suggest that cholinergic inputs may modify the strength of glutamatergic inputs, providing another area where synaptic modifications may contribute to incentive learning.

Chapter 13

Dopamine and mental experience

The relationship between the brain and the mind continues to be a topic of considerable interest to philosophers and neuroscientists. The mind can be studied with little or no reference to the brain. For over a century, psychologists have asked people about their perceptual experiences and memories of events that the researcher controls and presents to the participant. These studies have provided a rich corpus of knowledge about how various stimulus configurations affect perceptual experiences, for example in the case of visual illusions, and about how information is stored and retrieved from memory.[1] However, these psychological studies, like anatomical studies of the brain, provide little insight into the relationship between the brain and the mind.

Evidence linking brain and mind

There is ample evidence that mental experiences are changed by alterations of the brain. Certain kinds of localized brain damage, for example, lead to alterations in the perceptions and/or memories of affected individuals. One example comes from the studies of Roger Sperry (1913–1994), who worked at the California Institute of Technology and elsewhere. Sperry received the Nobel Prize in Physiology or Medicine in 1981 for his studies of the perceptual experiences of individuals who had had their corpus callosum transected as a (successful) treatment for epilepsy.[2] The corpus callosum (great commissure) is the large fiber bundle that connects the two cerebral hemispheres of the brain. Sperry and co-workers found that a patient with a transected corpus callosum could indicate, by showing the appropriate number of fingers with his left hand, how many times that hand had been touched by the experimenter; however, when asked to *state* how many touches he had experienced, the patient, apparently relying on language-producing circuitry located predominantly in the left side of the brain (the sensory input from the left hand would go to the right side of the brain), was unable to accurately specify the number. He (the language-expressing left hemisphere) apparently was not aware that he (the non-language-expressing right hemisphere) had felt the stimuli or made the response.[3] Sperry and his co-workers concluded that "the split brain behaves in many respects like two separate brains" (p. 1749).[4]

By presenting brief stimuli to one side of the visual field at a time, Sperry and colleagues were able to evaluate the relatively independent perceptual abilities of the two hemispheres in patients with a transected corpus callosum. This was made possible because of the anatomical organization of the connections of the two hemiretinae in each eye to the brain. They found that the patient could select correctly (better than chance) with his left hand, from a set of five pictures, the one that had been presented to the left visual field and, similarly, he could select correctly with his right hand the image presented to the right visual field. However, he could not use his left hand to correctly select the picture matching the image delivered to the right visual field. When a stimulus was presented to the left visual field and the patient was asked to use his right hand (controlled by the left—verbal—hemisphere) to select the matching picture, the patient "would commonly deny having seen anything and often seemed puzzled that he should be asked to pick up a card" (p. 225).[5] Sperry summarized the general picture that has come out of studies of "split-brain" patients:

> [they have] an apparent doubling in most of the realms of conscious awareness. Instead of the normal unified stream of consciousness, these patients behave in many ways as if they have two independent streams of conscious awareness, one in each hemisphere, each of which is cut off from and out of contact with the mental experiences of the other. In other words, each hemisphere seems to have its own separate and private sensations; its own perceptions; its own concepts; and its own impulses to act, with related volitional, cognitive, and learning experiences (p. 724).[6]

These observations provide compelling evidence that mental experiences are changed by alterations of the brain.

There are extensive examples from studies of people with brain damage that show that mental experiences are altered in affected individuals. An interesting example is provided by the influential work of neuroscientists Melvyn Goodale, David Milner, respectively from Western University in London, Ontario, and University of St. Andrews in Scotland, and colleagues. They reported on a patient who, at the age of 34, as a result of accidental exposure to carbon monoxide, suffered permanent bilateral localized loss of cortical tissue (ventrolateral occipital cortex and cortex in the parasagittal occipitoparietal region). The patient was able to talk normally and to communicate effectively after the accident. Among a range of observations, these researchers found that the patient was unable to perceive the orientation of a slot into which a card could be inserted. She apparently had little or no mental experience of the slot's orientation when shown the slot and asked about it. In spite of this, she was able to insert a card into the slot by rotating the card appropriately in her hand as she moved it towards the slot.[7] This result showed that this type of brain damage altered the mental experience of visual stimuli. It further showed dissociation between brain regions that contribute to the mental experience of visual stimuli, such as the slot, and brain regions that control neural projections to musculature responsible for the posture of the hand when inserting a card into the slot at various orientations. Other researchers showed opposite dissociation in patients with damage to the parietal lobe; these patients are able to judge the orientation of a slot, that is, they have mental experience of the slot, but are unable to effectively perform the motor task of insetting something into the slot.[8] These intriguing results show that mental experience is altered following brain damage and further that some brain regions are more involved than others in producing mental experiences.[9]

Wilder Penfield (1891–1976), working at the Montreal Neurological Institute and Hospital that he founded in 1934, carried out some of the most influential work relating brain and mind. Penfield was a neurosurgeon and one of his challenges was the treatment of severely epileptic individuals whose seizures could not be controlled with medication. Previous neurosurgeons, for example Englishman Victor Horsley (1857–1916), had found that epileptic seizures could be reduced or eliminated by removing the region of the brain where the seizures were generated, know as the epileptic focus.[10] In later years an epileptic focus could be indicated with the aid of electroencephalographic techniques with surface recording electrodes, a technique pioneered at the Institute by Penfield's close colleague Herbert Jasper (1906–1999).[11] Once the suspected region of the focus was identified, the operation could be carried out under local anesthesia while the patient was sedated but awake because the brain does not have pain sensors like other organs of the body. Thus, under local anesthesia, the scalp and the bone overlying the region of the focus would be removed. Penfield then used a metal probe to gently stimulate various regions of the brain and asked the awake patient to report on his or her experiences. This was done to map the region of the focus so that when the tissue removal was finally carried out, Penfield could be careful not to remove regions that were vital for speech, for example. What is most intriguing is what Penfield observed during his mapping procedure. In his words:

> [What the stimulations produced] were electrical activations of the sequential record of consciousness, a record that had been laid down during the patient's earlier experience. The patient "re-lived" all that he had been aware of in that earlier period of time as in a moving-picture "flashback."
>
> On the first occasion, when one of these "flashbacks" was reported to me by a conscious patient (1933), I was incredulous. On each subsequent occasion, I marveled" (p. 21).[12]

Penfield found that patients sometimes reported memories when he mildly stimulated regions of the temporal lobe. In his book, *The Mystery of the Mind*, published in 1975, Penfield quotes some of his patients describing vivid experiences from their past when he mildly stimulated a particular area of the brain. If he stimulated another area, a different experience would be reported. Stimulation of some areas did not produce memory experiences. From these studies it seems very clear that when particular neurons are activated in the brain, mental experiences result.[13]

In his informative book *Brain Control: A Critical Examination of Brain Stimulation and Psychosurgery*, University of Michigan Ann Arbor psychologist and neuroscientist Elliot Valenstein provides a thoughtful consideration of possible threats and therapeutic advances that may arise from studies of the brain. In his chapter on the effects of brain manipulations on the control of specific behaviors, he includes a section on human responses to brain stimulation. He says that "Considerable light can be shed on the effects of brain stimulation by examining the human evidence, since it is only in these cases that we can obtain verbal reports" (p. 104).[14] He provides a richly referenced review of studies reporting patients' mental experiences when particular regions of their brains are stimulated. By the time he wrote the book, tens of thousands of patients had been examined in operations designed to mitigate various symptoms, including emotional or behavioral disturbances such as aggression; chronic pain; motor abnormalities such as chorea; or epilepsy, as already discussed in the case of Penfield's work. Valenstein points out the nature of reports of mental experiences by patients when their brains are stimulated, emphasizing the unpredictability, generality, and situational dependence of these responses. Stimulation of the same area within the same individual may produce reports of different experiences at different times and stimulation of the same area from individual to individual does not produce the same experiences. Valenstein provides valuable insight into the underlying mechanisms contributing to these differences and discusses often-misunderstood implications of brain manipulations. For present purposes, his work reviews extensive evidence that changes in the brain lead to changes in mental experience.

The relationship between brain and mind is informed by the experiences of Henry Molaison (1926–2008), discussed in Chapter 4. After undergoing a bilateral medial temporal lobectomy as a radical treatment for intractable epilepsy, HM's memory abilities were permanently altered. You will recall that the operation resulted in severe anterograde amnesia, with some retrograde memory loss, but memories that were stored from his earlier life were apparently intact. Thus, HM could remember his family, where he went to school, and events of World War Two that he lived through before his operation. He could not, however, remember new facts and events from after the time of the operation. In support of the concept of multiple memory systems, HM showed evidence of learning and memory on a number of tasks, including mirror-drawing and the pursuit rotor (see Chapter 4). However, he showed no declarative knowledge of having done the tasks when re-introduced to them. The rich spectrum of memories for facts and events encountered each day that we all have as part of our mental experience was lost to HM as a result of the surgery that was done to treat his epilepsy. By changing HM's brain, the surgery changed his mind.

The effects of psychoactive drugs on mental experience provide another link between brain and mind. Alcohol is a drug that is widely used by humans. Among other things, alcohol alters neurotransmission mediated by γ-aminobutyric acid in the brain,[15] and, as discussed in Chapter 10, influences dopaminergic neurotransmission.[16] The acute effects of alcohol on mental experience are probably familiar to many of the readers of this chapter and are often alluded to in literature and film. They include, for example, feelings of elevated mood, arousal, talkativeness, and excitement while blood alcohol levels are rising followed by feelings of depressed mood, difficulty concentrating, and fatigue when blood alcohol levels are falling.[17] Mood refers to a mental state that a person is experiencing at a particular time. The observation that the consumption of alcohol alters brain neurotransmission and mood provides evidence that mood itself results from the action of neurotransmitters in the brain.

LSD refers to "lysergic acid diethylamide," an ergot-derived compound synthesized by Swiss chemist Albert Hofmann (1906–2008) in 1938 while working at Sandoz Laboratories.[18] Hofmann presagingly describes how in 1943 while synthesizing a new batch of LSD, "I was interrupted in my work by unusual sensations" (p. 57)![19] Hofmann experienced slight dizziness and went home early. The next day he dutifully provided his superior with a written report of what had happened: "In a dream-like state, with eyes closed ... an uninterrupted stream of fantastic pictures of extraordinary plasticity with intense, kaleidoscope-like play of colors surged in on me" (p. 58).[19] Wanting to further explore this interesting phenomenon, Hofmann carried out additional "self-experiments" and reported further on his mental experiences. He commented, "It was particularly remarkable how every acoustic perception, such as the sound of a door handle or a passing automobile, became transformed into optical perceptions. Every sound generated a vividly changing image, corresponding in form and color" (p. 59);[19] this phenomenon is known as "synesthesia." Thus began the modern era of mind-altering experiences produced by psychedelic drugs, including related compounds such as psilocybin and mescaline.[20-22] This era saw the rise of advocates of these mind-expanding agents, including Timothy Leary (1920–1996), Richard Alpert (Ram Dass), and others.[23] LSD, psilocybin, and mescaline affect serotonergic neurotransmission in the brain.[22] The effects of these agents provide another example of how changes in neurotransmission in the brain lead to changes in the mental experiences reported by people.

Evidence linking dopamine and mental experience

The examples reviewed in the previous section leave little doubt that changes in the brain can produce changes in mental experience. It then becomes reasonable to ask: Do alterations in dopaminergic neurotransmission affect mental experience and, if so, how? Among the approaches to exploring this question are imaging studies of the correlation between mental experiences and indices of dopaminergic neurotransmission, and the verbal reports of unmedicated patients with schizophrenia and Parkinson's disease. I next discuss some examples.

Psychiatrist and Director of the National Institute of Drug Abuse in the United States, Nora Volkow, and her many colleagues have carried out a number of imaging studies using positron emission tomography (PET) to identify changes in dopaminergic neurotransmission produced by cocaine. In the same studies, she and her colleagues evaluated, using rating scales, the mental experience of cocaine. They found a positive correlation between cocaine's ability to block the dopamine transporter and reports of mental experiences such as feeling "high" or experiencing a "rush" in human volunteers. The dopamine transporter normally clears dopamine from synapses terminating its action; by blocking the transporter, cocaine prolongs the action of dopamine. They also observed that the time course of the "high" paralleled the time course of cocaine concentrations within the striatum.[24] These results suggest that the mental experience of getting "high" on cocaine and related drugs may be associated with enhanced dopaminergic neurotransmission in the striatum.

It is not necessary to use a drug of abuse like cocaine to produce correlated increases in dopaminergic neurotransmission and desirable mental experiences. Neurologist Alain Dagher and colleagues from McGill University in Montreal showed the same relationship using food reward. Participants fasted for 16 hours on two occasions. After one of the fasts their brains were scanned using PET with the dopamine receptor ligand [^{11}C]raclopride; after the other fast, they ate one of their favorite meals and then were similarly scanned. Results showed that after the meal, the binding of [^{11}C]raclopride in the dorsal striatum (caudate and putamen) was significantly decreased, indicating that more endogenous dopamine was present to compete with the [^{11}C]raclopride (see

Chapter 5). They had the participants rate the meal for "pleasantness" and found a significant positive relationship between those ratings and dopamine increases in the caudate and putamen.[25] This result shows that the mental experience of "enjoyment" of a meal is correlated with the level of dopamine released in the dorsal striatum as a result of eating a meal.

In PET studies with human participants addicted to cocaine, Volkow and co-workers showed that drug-associated cues (e.g., places where drugs are taken, people with whom drugs are taken, paraphernalia used to administer drugs) produce strong evidence of increases in striatal dopamine and that these increases are associated with mental experiences of "craving" (e.g., desire to use the drug, anticipation of positive outcome, etc.).[26] In similar studies with healthy participants, Volkow et al. showed that food-related cues also appear to increase striatal dopamine that is associated with reports of the "desire" for food.[27] The finding that drug or food reward-related cues can lead to increases in striatal dopamine release in human participants is consistent with many findings from animal research reviewed in Chapter 5 showing that conditioned incentive stimuli produce increased firing of dopaminergic neurons and increased concentrations of dopamine in the striatum. The mental experiences of "craving" or "desire" appear to be associated with conditioned increases in striatal dopamine release produced by drug- or food-related stimuli;[28] however, as discussed in the next paragraph, it is also possible that other neuronal events associated with incentive learning affect these mental experiences.

As discussed near the end of Chapter 12, conditioned incentive stimuli appear to activate previously modified (by dopamine) corticostriatal glutamatergic synapses *and* dopaminergic neurons. When drug- or food-related conditioned incentive stimuli are encountered, both of these events are thought to occur. As discussed in Chapter 2, it appears that conditioned incentive stimuli initially retain their increased ability to elicit approach and other responses even when dopaminergic neurotransmission is blocked. This finding suggests that putatively modified corticostriatal glutamatergic synapses can control responding in the absence of increased dopaminergic neurotransmission. It may be that these synapses also play a key role in producing the mental experience of "craving." Thus, Volkow and colleagues found that drug-induced increases in striatal dopamine concentrations elicit "craving" in cocaine abusers in the presence but not in the absence of drug-related cues.[29] Perhaps craving can occur even when dopaminergic neurotransmission is blocked. Some researchers have found that dopamine receptor antagonist drugs *fail* to block the ability of cocaine-related cues to elicit "desire" in cocaine abusers.[30] In this latter case, dopamine receptor antagonist drugs will block the postsynaptic actions of dopamine in the striatum but will not immediately alter the strength of previously modified corticostriatal glutamatergic synapses that are activated by cues associated with drug taking. These observations support a possible link between cue-induced activation of corticostriatal synapses and the mental experience of "craving." From the excellent work of Nora Volkow, her colleagues and other research groups, it is clear that the mental experience of being "high" and those of "craving" or "desire" are associated with striatal neuronal responses to drug-associated cues.

Changes in dopaminergic neurotransmission appear to affect mental experiences. Another way to learn more about the nature of this possible relationship might be from reports of their mental experiences by unmedicated people in a psychotic state. For the relationship between decreased dopaminergic neurotransmission and mental experience, the reports of non-medicated people with Parkinson's disease or of those who have been treated with a dopamine receptor-blocking drug may provide some insight. Fortunately, such reports exist. Although many of these reports are anecdotal, they are consistent with a brain–mind link and may enrich understanding of that link.

People in a psychotic state often have a diagnosis of schizophrenia and are treated with dopamine receptor-blocking drugs that may affect their reported mental experiences. To discover mental experiences that are unaltered by antipsychotic drugs in people with schizophrenia, it will be important to interview unmedicated patients. Fortunately, relevant reports can be found and they are a valuable resource. Prior to the discovery of chlorpromazine and the dawning of the era of relatively effective pharmacological treatment for psychoses (see Chapters 7 and 9), there were many hospitalized patients with schizophrenia who were not treated with dopamine receptor-blocking medications. Some of these patients were interviewed and their descriptions of their mental experiences were recorded by researchers interested in the nature of the mental changes associated with schizophrenia. The reports of the mental experiences of these patients provide a candid look into the possible relationship between increased dopaminergic neurotransmission (and its putative effects, e.g., altered corticostriatal glutamatergic neurotransmission) and mental experience.

If dopaminergic neurotransmission is overactive in people with schizophrenia and if increased dopamine concentrations in the striatum produce mental experiences such as "high" or "rush," as reported by Volkow and colleagues (see earlier), patients with schizophrenia might be expected to have relatively constant mental experiences of an elevated mood state. The reports of patients (see later) reveal that this is clearly not the case. Fortunately, experimental results provide an explanation. Volkow and colleagues showed that methylphenidate, a drug that, like cocaine, blocks the dopamine transporter leading to increased synaptic concentrations of dopamine, produces different effects on mental experience depending on its route of administration. When taken intravenously, methylphenidate, like cocaine, produces the mental experience of "high;" however, when given orally, methylphenidate fails to produce a "high." At appropriate doses, intravenous and oral methylphenidate lead to a similar blockade of the dopamine transporter and increases in synaptic dopamine, but the time course is different: intravenous administration leads to peak effects within ten minutes, whereas the effects of oral administration do not peak until about 60 minutes after ingestion. These results show that it is the *rate* at which methylphenidate and cocaine enter the brain and block the transporter that determines the elevated mental experience described as "high."[31]

If patients with schizophrenia have relatively chronically elevated levels of dopaminergic neurotransmission (see Chapter 9), they may not experience elevated mental states like those that result from a sudden rise in synaptic concentrations of dopamine. However, elevated levels of dopamine may engage the incentive learning mechanisms described in Chapter 12, leading to an enhanced ability of stimuli associated with elevated dopamine to elicit approach and other responses. Thus, the mental experiences of non-medicated people with schizophrenia might be more related to excessive incentive learning than to sudden increases in synaptic dopamine.

Researchers working in the middle of the twentieth century at what was then the Dundee Royal Mental Hospital in Scotland were interested in the psychological nature of the deficit in people in the early stages of psychosis. They included Scotsman Andrew McGhie (1926–1988), who emigrated to Canada in 1968 to take up a post at Queen's University in Kingston, Ontario, where he became Head of the Department of Psychology in 1981. McGhie developed a theory of psychosis in schizophrenia that posited faulty mechanisms of attention, resulting in sensory overload. He based this on the reports of patients recorded in informal talking sessions and *inter alia* on empirical observations of the impaired ability of the patients to find a target in a visual array of stimuli.[32] McGhie and his colleagues provide many examples of patients' reports of their mental experiences; these patients were in the early stages of the disease and the subsequent course of the illness confirmed the diagnosis of schizophrenia. One patient said,

> It's as if I am too wide awake—very, very alert. I can't relax at all. Everything seems to go through me. I just can't shut things out (p. 104).[33]

Another said:

> Things are coming in too fast. I lose my grip of it and get lost. I am attending to everything at once and as a result I do not really attend to anything (p. 104).[33]

In 1960, Norma MacDonald, who was living with schizophrenia, published a brief biography in which she describes some of her mental experiences. Many of her comments clearly reflect the enhanced responsiveness or sensitivity to stimuli described by McGhie. Here is one example:

> I … want to explain … the exaggerated state of awareness in which I lived before, during, and after my acute illness. At first it was as if parts of my brain "awoke" which had been dormant, and I became interested in a wide assortment of people, events, places, and ideas which normally would make no impression on me (p. 218).[34]

In another part of her article she said:

> Every face in the windows of a passing streetcar would be engraved on my mind, all of them concentrating on me and trying to pass me some sort of message (p. 218).[34]

German psychiatrist Emil Kraepelin (1856–1926) reported similar mental experiences of patients in his 1913 book, translated into English in 1919, entitled *Dementia Praecox and Paraphrenia*.[35] Patients comment "everything is as though accentuated … " (p. 14); Kraepelin stated that a patient "cannot bring order into the jumble of his thoughts, there is an 'entanglement in his mind' " (p. 23).[35] Kraepelin linked some of the common behaviors observed in patients with schizophrenia to this overwhelming sensory/perceptual input:

> Many patients close their eyes, cover their faces with their hands, cover themselves up, draw the bedcover over their head, and convulsively hold it fast; "This position is pleasant for the eyes and more restful for the inner life," explained a patient (p. 49).[35]

McGhie concluded that individuals find themselves less able to direct their attention. He suggested that attentional control is increasingly determined by changes in the environment.[32] Perhaps it is possible to understand these experiences as manifestations of excessive incentive learning. As I discussed with Andy McGhie many years ago, we both had the same idea about the nature of the deficit in schizophrenia, it being an inability to ignore irrelevant stimuli. The faulty filter described by McGhie can be understood as the manifestation of excessive dopamine-mediated incentive learning. The mental experiences described by patients and associated with this putatively excessive dopamine-mediated incentive learning may be the compelling importance of stimuli that should normally be ignored.

People who chronically abuse large doses of amphetamine or cocaine often report mental experiences that are apparently delusions and sometimes hallucinations. Psychiatrist Robert Post, at the time at the National Institute of Mental Health in Bethesda, Maryland, describes how chronic users do not appear to be intoxicated, confused, or disoriented. Delusions can be characterized by suspiciousness, misinterpretation of events, or groundless jealousies.[36] Others describe how the perceptual distortions induced by an excess of cocaine are usually related to increased perceptual sensitivity. For example, faraway voices sound nearby or random street noises organize into the sound of marching feet.[37] These observations and those described by patients with schizophrenia suggest that increases in dopaminergic neurotransmission create a mental experience of intense clarity or importance of stimuli that normally do not have that effect.

Following from the putative illuminating mental effects of elevated dopamine, it might be expected that the decrease in dopaminergic neurotransmission in Parkinson's disease or following treatment with dopamine receptor-blocking drugs will have an opposite effect on mental experience, dulling the mental impact of stimuli that normally might be of some interest. This appears to be what has been found. As was the case with schizophrenia, where an examination of the possible mental effects of the disorder uncontaminated by antidopaminergic medication was possible in patient reports recorded prior to the advent of antipsychotic medications, the self-reports of post-encephalic patients with Parkinson's-like symptoms who lived without dopamine-replacement therapy prior to the advent of L-3,4-dihydroxyphenylalanine (L-DOPA) therapy (see Chapter 9) may provide a relatively uncontaminated glimpse into the mental effects of decreased dopaminergic neurotransmission. In this regard, the scientific community owes a great debt to the neurologist and prolific writer Oliver Sacks (1933–2015). In his widely acclaimed bestseller, *Awakenings*, first published in 1973, Sacks provides an unparalleled compendium of the comments of post-encephalic patients with Parkinson's-like symptoms who languished in the back wards or hospitals, some for over 40 years, about their mental experiences while in a dopamine depletion-related incapacitated state.

I read *Awakenings* during the summer of 2010 while on vacation in Nova Scotia. I had picked up the book from the public library before leaving. When I borrowed the book, I was unaware that it had been published over the years in several editions, some containing Sacks' copious footnotes and some without the notes. It was my very good fortune that the copy I had was an edition with all of the original notes,[38] because I found much of the material I was looking for in the notes. I read *Awakenings* with the explicit goal of finding descriptions of the mental experiences of patients about what it was like being Parkinsonian without medication. Sacks' book chronicles the course of the lives of a number of patients who were given L-DOPA. With this medication, patients "woke up," hence the title of the book, and their personalities again emerged; it is a fascinating and recommended read. It became possible for patients, some who had been mute for years, to talk about their mental experiences while in an unmedicated Parkinson's-like state.

I wondered, would the unmedicated Parkinson's-like individual have a rich mental life filled with the recollections, plans, dreams, and fears normally experienced but be unable to convert any intention into action? Some of Sacks' comments bear on this question, but the answer is not immediately clear. When discussing the meaning of "akinesia," Sacks speaks of a retardation or resistance that slows or eliminates movement, speech, and even thought. Patients may will an action but then a "counter-will" (Sacks' term) or "resistance" prevents it. On the one hand, it sounds like movements might be willed but then arrested by a counter-will. On the other, the definition makes it sound like even thought may be greatly slowed or arrested. So do unmedicated Parkinson's-like patients have mental experience?

Sacks quotes a patient's comment when she was given L-DOPA therapy: "Parkinsonism is gravity, L-DOPA is levity" (p. 8, footnote 11).[38] He continues:

> (T)here is … in many akinetic patients, a corresponding "stickiness" of mind and bradyphrenia, the thought stream as slow and sluggish as the motor stream. The thought stream, the stream of consciousness, speeds up in these patients with L-DOPA… (pp. 8–9, footnote 12).[38]

These comments strongly suggest that the motor slowing experienced in Parkinson's-like disease has associated with it a mental slowing. This suggests that individuals with Parkinson's disease may not have the rich mental life that is experienced by people with intact dopaminergic neurotransmission.

It appears that as decreases in dopamine levels progress with the disease, motor slowing and mental slowing proceed in parallel. The will is not lost immediately but gradually weakens as thoughts slow. Thus, Sacks describes French neurologist Jean-Martin Charcot's (1825–1893) observations of patients who would sit for hours not only motionless, but also with no impulse to move, apparently lacking will to engage in any activity. Before L-DOPA, patients apparently registered what was happening around them but with a lack of attention and a profound indifference. Aspects of being and behavior, including thoughts, appetites, and feelings, no less than movements, were greatly diminished. One patient, after receiving L-DOPA, reported "It is so long since I had any feelings" (pp. 101–102).[38] This suggests that unmedicated patients with Parkinson's disease do not think or feel, or, perhaps, that the thought that does occur takes place very slowly. Apparently, without dopamine there is not only a loss of movement, but also a diminution or loss of attention, thought, and feeling.

An unmedicated Parkinson's-like individual does perceive. One patient, after receiving L-DOPA, described her experience while in a Parkinson's-like state:

> I ceased to have any moods ... I ceased to care about anything. Nothing *moved* me—not even the death of my parents. I forgot what it felt like to be happy or unhappy. Was it good or bad? It was neither. It was nothing (p. 71, Sacks' italics).[38]

Another patient who was unresponsive for 43 years, upon awakening with L-DOPA reported:

> I can give you the date of Pearl Harbor ... I can give you the date of Kennedy's assassination. I've registered it all—but none of it seems real ... I've been a spectator for the last forty-three years (p. 83, footnote 58).[38]

Yet another patient described her experience as being aware of what was happening around her and of what the date was but that she had "*no feeling of happening*" (p. 167, Sacks' italics),[38] only the feeling that time had stopped. These comments suggest that there was mental experience, as already described, but no feeling. The Parkinson's-like patient does perceive events but she does not have any feeling about them. It would appear that dopamine is not necessary for mental experience per se. Stimuli that are associated with low dopamine may undergo inverse incentive learning. By definition, such stimuli lose their ability to elicit approach and other responses. These stimuli also appear to lose their ability to produce emotional mental experiences.

Some patients who responded to L-DOPA subsequently entered a state of enhanced dopaminergic neurotransmission. This may have been associated with hyperkinesia, the opposite of the bradykinesia, seen before L-DOPA was introduced. There are often comments about mental experiences while in this state that are opposite and complementary to those described earlier for decreased dopamine. For example, one patient in a state of enhanced dopaminergic neurotransmission reported being *forced* to think things, the opposite of the reduction or absence of thought before L-DOPA. In his usual eloquent way, Sacks describes the art, a drawing of a tree, of one patient before L-DOPA:

> ... a small, meager thing, stunted, impoverished, a bare winter tree with no foliage at all,

on L-DOPA:

> ... the tree acquires vigor, life, imagination—and foliage

and during L-DOPA-induced dopaminergic hyperfunctioning:

> ... the tree may acquire a fantastic ornateness and exuberance, exploding with a florescence of new branches and foliage with little arabesques, curlicues, and whatnots, until finally its original form is completely lost beneath this enormous, this baroque, elaboration (p. 155, footnote 80).[38]

One patient described her experience on L-DOPA as:

> So tingly, like my blood is champagne. I am bubbling and bubbling and bubbling inside (p. 156).[38]

Increased dopaminergic neurotransmission led to mental experiences of elation or lightness.

It seems that even when dopaminergic neurotransmission is low and producing a Parkinson's-like state, signals in cortical circuits can "break through" to produce motor acts. For example, Sacks described the apparent lifting of Parkinson's disease by interesting or activating situations (I discuss *kinesia paradoxa* in Chapter 9). Immobile patients can walk if another person accompanies them. One patient described it this way:

> When you walk with me, I feel in myself your own power of walking. I *partake* of the power and freedom you have. I *share* your walking powers, your perceptions, your feelings, your existence (p. 282, Sacks' italics).[38]

People with Parkinson's disease can similarly be activated by music. These observations suggest that some stimuli may be able to activate a hypofunctioning dopamine system or corticostriatal glutamatergic synapses to the level needed for motor control to be engaged. In recent years it has been found that social cooperation can activate regions of the brain that contain dopaminergic cell bodies or that receive dopaminergic input (see Chapter 8). Findings from functional magnetic resonance imaging (fMRI) studies may provide independent support for the observation that stimuli provided by socially cooperative others can produce motor activation in patients with Parkinson's disease.

Two additional observations from Sacks' book caught my attention. One was that a patient who received L-DOPA declared, "I feel like a man in love" (p. 209).[38] fMRI studies have shown that being in the early stages of romantic love leads to indirect evidence of increased dopaminergic activity (see Chapter 8). Perhaps it follows that L-DOPA-enhanced dopaminergic activity can lead to feeling like being in love. The other was the idea of latent Parkinson's disease. The idea was that there may be people with low dopamine levels but not levels low enough to cause symptoms. However, when these people experience life events that may lead to lowering of dopaminergic neurotransmission, for example depression, the symptoms of Parkinson's disease may suddenly emerge (p. 238, footnote 115).[38]

The stories of post-encephalic patients with Parkinson's-like disease who were treated with L-DOPA provide a unique opportunity to learn about the mental experiences of people who live in a state of low dopamine. Now that L-DOPA and related drugs are available it is rare to find people in this state. Thus, *Awakenings* is a valuable resource for students of dopamine and behavior, in particular, and neurotransmitters and behavior, in general. Dr. Sacks has provided a treasure trove of clinical observations. The state of dopamine hypofunction found in Parkinson's disease is associated with mental experiences characterized by a loss of interest in stimuli, inattention, and muted feelings about facts and events that normally are associated with feelings described, for example, as "happy" or "sad."

Another source of information about the mental experiences of being in a state of altered dopaminergic neurotransmission is the reports of people who have been given dopamine receptor-antagonist drugs for the treatment of psychotic or manic symptoms. In this regard, I found the book *A Gift of Stories: Discovering How to Deal with Mental Illness*, edited by Julie Leibrich of Dunedin, New Zealand, and published in 1999, of particular interest.[39] This book contains the brief personal stories of 21 people who suffer from or have suffered from mental illness, including that of the author herself in the final chapter. Some of the stories may reflect the effects on mental experience of a continuum of levels of activity of brain dopamine systems. As already discussed, excessive activity can lead to psychoses and insufficient activity is associated with Parkinson's disease (Chapter 9). The level of dopamine activity in most people is normally between these two extremes, but even within this "normal" range, there may be a continuum from low normal to high normal. At the high end, people are creative, witty, excited about and interested in things, and energetic. At the low end they are generally less interested in things, less witty, and not very energetic. Often as a person moves towards psychoses, they pass through a period of high energy and creativity. This is often described as a desirable state characterized by intense energy. Treatments for psychosis decrease dopaminergic neurotransmission; the patient may experience Parkinson's-like motoric side effects if the dose of the drug is too high. Even if the dose is not too high, the person may be shifted along that normal continuum towards the lower end where they have less creativity, interest, and energy. The comments of some of the people who relate their experiences in *A Gift of Stories* reflect this dynamic.

The effects of decreased dopamine function were reflected in the comments of a bipolar poet taking antipsychotic medication:

> The medication I take suppresses my illness and keeps it under control but it also suppresses the creativity and I feel that the two are intertwined together (p. 43).[39]

He says that when he is on medication he writes very little. Another patient with bipolar disorder says his fantasy world can be very pleasurable; experiencing mania or psychosis is like taking cocaine. (Cocaine is a drug that elevates dopaminergic neurotransmission (see earlier)). A third patient with bipolar disorder talking about the highs said "the colours were just amazing" (p. 131).[39] These comments provide some clues to the close relationship between level of dopaminergic neurotransmission and mental experience of the world.

In another of his books, *The Man Who Mistook His Wife for a Hat and Other Clinical Tales*, published in 1985, Oliver Sacks recounts the story of a patient with Tourette's syndrome, Witty Ticcy Ray, who was treated with the dopamine receptor antagonist haloperidol (Haldol). Under the influence of the drug:

> He is slow and deliberate in his movements and judgments, with none of the impatience, the impetuosity, he showed before Haldol, but equally, none of the wild improvisations and inspirations. Even his dreams are different in quality: "straight wish-fulfillment," he says, "with none of the elaborations, the extravaganzas, of Tourette's". He is less sharp, less quick in repartee, no longer bubbling with witty tics or ticcy wit. He no longer enjoys or excels at ping-pong or other games; he no longer feels "that urgent killer instinct, the instinct to win, to beat the other man"; he is less competitive, then, and also less playful; and he has lost the impulse, or the knack, of sudden "frivolous" moves which take everyone by surprise. He has lost his obscenities, his coarse chutzpah, his spunk. He has come to feel, increasingly, that something is missing" (p. 100).[40]

Haloperidol blocks dopamine receptors in the brain thereby reducing dopaminergic neurotransmission. The mental changes described by Sacks in this patient suggest a strong link between dopaminergic brain systems and mental experience.

Do non-human animals have mental experiences?

So far in this chapter I have reviewed evidence that changes in the brain are associated with changes in mental experience. This provided the basis for assessing the relationship between changes in dopaminergic neurotransmission and mental experience. Evidence suggests that rapid elevations in synaptic concentrations of dopamine are associated with mental experiences such as feeling "high" or getting a "rush." Chronically elevated dopamine can lead to mental experiences of increased awareness of people and things in the environment and enhanced energy; chronically depressed dopamine leads to mental experiences of loss of interest in people and things, and low energy. Following from these observations, one might ask if animals other than humans have mental experiences associated with changes in their brains, in general, and associated with changes in dopaminergic neurotransmission, in particular. If so, how could we find out?

One approach is to use inductive logic, arguing that since changes in the brain lead to changes in mental experience in humans, related changes in the brains of other animals have a high probability of leading to changes in their mental experience. The question remains, how would we know?

The most direct way to answer the question would be to ask. Although animals are unable to speak to us, they can respond differentially to communicate information that might suggest they have mental experiences. For example, in a procedure termed "drug discrimination," animals can learn to reliably press one of two levers when they are in a drug state (e.g., following an injection of cocaine) versus when they are in a non-drug state (e.g., following an injection of saline). If the discrimination is trained with a cocaine dose of ten milligrams per kilogram of body weight (mg/kg) and the animal is then tested periodically with a lower dose, for example 1.25 mg/kg, it will choose the cocaine lever less often. If it is tested with 0.63 mg/kg, it chooses the cocaine lever even less often but still more often than the saline lever. Results from several doses generate a generalization curve.[41] These data show that an animal can respond differentially depending on the drug state the animal is in. The drug state can be referred to as "interoceptive" cues produced by the drug. These cues are inside the animal with no corresponding external stimulus. Some experiments compared a compound (chlorpromazine) that has effects outside the brain and also on the brain versus a similar compound (quaternary chlorpromazine) that has the same effects outside the brain but does not act on the brain (i.e., does not cross the blood–brain barrier) at moderate doses; rats learned to discriminate chlorpromazine from saline, and quaternary chlorpromazine did not substitute for chlorpromazine.[42] This suggests that to respond differentially animals rely on cues produced by the action of the drug on their brains.

Drug discrimination studies led European neuropharmacologist Francis Colpaert (1950–2010) to suggest that drug-induced states in animals are analogous to the subjective states produced by drugs in humans. Colpaert suggested that drug discrimination "carries the exciting promise of rendering amenable to experimental analysis animals (*sic*) experiences, which, by their nature, have been considered as out of the range of scientific inquiry" (p. 338).[43] In drug discrimination experiments with cocaine, for example, placing a trained animal into the operant chamber is like asking the question "Do you feel like you have been injected with the training dose of cocaine?" The animal's lever-press responses provide an answer to the question. This is analogous to asking a human if they feel the effect of a drug and we have to rely on the response of the human as the only source of this information. Perhaps drug discrimination provides a peek into the possible mental experiences of non-human animals, but, by comparison to the richness of human communication, it appears to provide rather limited access.

If we have such limited access to the possible mental experiences of other animals, perhaps the best approach is to avoid talking about them altogether or, alternatively, to very explicitly separate discussions of brain mechanisms from discussions of possible mental experiences associated with the operation of brain mechanisms. It is clearly feasible to talk about reward-related learning without reference to possible mental states associated with rewarding stimuli; I have written this book in that way. In this chapter, I have discussed some of the work relating changes in dopaminergic neurotransmission to human mental experience. With the development of neuroimaging methodologies, this area of research is proliferating rapidly. However, notwithstanding the possible exception of drug discrimination, there is no parallel line of enquiry in non-human animals. It may be unnecessary and possibly misleading to use language that refers to mental experiences when discussing the brain mechanisms of reward-related learning and other psychological phenomena, especially when trying to generalize those mechanisms across species.

In this regard, I have found the position recently articulated by New York University neuroscientist Joseph LeDoux, a prominent researcher and author, to provide valuable guidance. LeDoux has spent much of his career studying the neurobiology of fear conditioning. His work has provided great insight into the brain mechanisms underlying the learning, detection and response to threats. He points out that, in humans, there is dissociation between the brain mechanisms associated with threat and those associated with the mental experience of "fear." It is therefore desirable to adopt "terms that distinguish processes that give rise to conscious feelings of fear from processes that operate nonconsciously in detecting and responding to threats" (p. 2873).[44] This makes the case for humans but perhaps an equally compelling argument can be made for avoiding terms that refer to mental experiences in non-human animals because we have little or not access to those putative mental experiences.

LeDoux and others point out that the circuits and cellular and molecular mechanisms involved in reward-related learning may not be the same as the mechanisms that give rise to mental experiences such as "pleasure."[44,45] This makes the case for avoiding the use of terms that reflect mental experience when studying those circuits and cellular and molecular mechanisms of reward-related learning. We do not know if non-human animals even have mental experiences of reward-related learning. In spite of the concerns expressed by LeDoux and others, the terms used to describe the effects of rewarding stimuli on behavior continue to contribute to the confusion between empirically derived mechanisms and mental experiences.

The now classic 1978 study by Roy Wise and colleagues showing that a dopamine receptor-blocking drug led to a gradual decline in responding for food reward was entitled "Neuroleptic-induced 'anhedonia' in rats: pimozide blocks reward quality of food."[46] This paper has been cited nearly 500 times. It strongly influenced research into the role of dopamine in reward-related learning, as discussed in this book, but it conflated the neural mechanism with possible mental experiences arising from the operation of the mechanism. This conflation has continued to dog research in the area of reward-related learning.

The excellent empirical work of neuroscientist Kent Berridge from the University of Michigan Ann Arbor and colleagues has identified elements of reward-related learning that have brought the field to a new level of understanding of the mechanisms. In parallel, however, they have perpetuated the conflation of neural mechanism and possible mental experience by referring to these elements using terms that refer to mental experience. Berridge and colleagues studied the rhythmic midline tongue protrusions, lateral tongue protrusions, and paw licking, constituting the orofacial expressions normally seen in rats when they taste a sucrose solution; these behaviors serve to maximize ingestion of this highly calorific food. They found that decreases in dopaminergic neurotransmission did not affect these responses to sucrose. However, decreases in dopaminergic neurotransmission interfered with incentive learning as expected; thus, dopamine receptor blockers decreased the acquisition of approach responses to sucrose-associated cues but did not affect the pattern of orofacial expressions when sucrose was encountered.[47] This is an important distinction that informs our understanding of the organization of the nervous system with sweet gustatory sensory inputs activating reflex circuitry leading to orofacial expressions quite independent of the dopamine-mediated learning associated with those inputs.

Berridge and colleagues conveniently referred to the orofacial and incentive learning components of reward-related behaviors as "liking" and "wanting," respectively: dopamine plays a critical role in "wanting," whereas "liking" appears to be independent of dopamine. "Liking" referred to the "objective affective reaction" that corresponds to the mental experience of "pleasure."[47] In their 1978 paper, Wise et al. refer to the effects of dopamine receptor blockade on behavior using the term "anhedonia," meaning "lack of pleasure," taken from the Greek word for "pleasure" and the combining term for its negation.[46] Berridge and others showed that Wise et al. were incorrect in their assertion that dopamine receptor blockade induced an "anhedonic" state since clearly the objectively defined orofacial movements that constituted the dependent variable for "pleasure" were unaffected by dopamine receptor blockade. Berridge et al. have no quarrel with the finding of Wise et al. that dopamine receptor blockade leads to the gradual loss of incentive learning about stimuli that control lever-press responding.

The concern of LeDoux about the use of the term "fear conditioning" is that it blurs the distinction between neural mechanisms for learning about threatening stimuli and the possible mental experiences associated with the operation of those mechanisms. The same concern applies to the use of the terms "pleasure," "liking," and "wanting." These terms can be defined by objective measures as, for example, "liking," defined by Berridge and colleagues as a particular type of orofacial movements. The definition may be convenient shorthand for an objective measure, but it also refers to a subjective state and the two may be easily confused. Especially when speaking about non-human animals, the use of language that conflates objective behavioral observations and their underlying neural mechanisms, on the one hand, and the possible mental experiences associated with them, on the other, runs the risk of inferring mental experiences that we may have no way of objectively verifying.

A marvel of dopamine-mediated reward-related incentive learning is its apparent presence throughout vertebrate species and its possible presence in other phyla.[48] As I discuss in Chapter 12, similar neurochemical mechanisms may operate across multiple species to produce this type of learning. One of the perils of using language that conflates neural mechanisms and behavioral observations with possible mental experience is that discussions of incentive learning in multiple species may imply that those species have mental experiences associated with rewarding stimuli. A 2012 review paper entitled "Neural mechanisms of reward in insects" provides an example. This paper includes excellent coverage of relevant insect work and concludes that the elements of reward-related learning in insects include both "wanting" and "liking."[49] At present we have no means to scientifically investigate the possibility that insects, for example, have mental experiences.[50] In the absence of this ability, it behooves our science to strive for terminology that minimizes the conflation of neural mechanisms and their associated behavioral observations with possible mental experience that may accompany them. An alternative to "liking" might be "orofacial behaviors associated with sweet tastes" and an alternative to "wanting" might be "incentive learning."

It may be possible to argue that the use of the term "reward" suffers from the same problems as terms such as "fear," "liking," "wanting," and "pleasure," conflating objectively observables with mental experiences. As I discuss in Chapter 2, Skinner tried to circumvent this possible problem by using the term "reinforcer" to refer to a rewarding stimulus and "reinforcement" to refer to its presentation. I could have used those terms throughout this book, but, as I explain in Chapter 2, the terms "reinforcer" and "reinforcement" are strongly associated with radical behaviorism that has been shown to have a number of limitations. As I explain in Chapter 2, I have used the term "reward" to avoid the somewhat rigid framework implied by behaviorism's "reinforce." I do not think that the term "reward" has strong implications of mental experiences compared with, for example, the term "pleasure." However, it continues to be important that psychologists and neuroscientists acknowledge the difference between neural and behavioral mechanisms, on the one hand, and mental experience, on the other, and strive to use language that minimizes confusion between the two.

Summary

There is very strong evidence that mental experience arises from the activity of the brain. For example, various forms of brain damage lead to alterations in mental experience. Psychoactive drugs that alter neurotransmitter function alter mental experience in parallel, sometimes with spectacular mental consequences for the individual. PET studies show that the mental experience of feeling "high" or having a "rush" following cocaine is strongly correlated with the level of dopamine receptor occupancy in the striatum, and the ratings of "pleasantness" of a meal are similarly correlated with dopamine receptor occupancy in the dorsal striatum. These findings suggest that the mental experiences of people who are suffering from diseases that affect dopaminergic neurotransmission may be altered and observations from unmedicated patients provide evidence that they are. People with schizophrenia who are thought to suffer from hyperdopaminergia report that stimuli encountered in their environment, including sounds or the faces of others, take on added importance—appear interesting—becoming difficult to shut out. Parkinson's-like patients who suffer from a loss of dopaminergic neurons report that nothing moves them, that they cease to feel happy or sad; they are disinterested, passive spectators. When people with schizophrenia are treated with antipsychotic dopamine receptor-blocking drugs, they report a gradual loss of interest in things that previously interested them; when patients with Parkinson's disease are treated with medications that elevate brain dopamine, they again become interested in things that are happening around them. These and many related findings show that mental experience arises from activity of the brain.

Do non-human animals have mental experience? How would we know? In humans we learn about the mental experiences of others by communication using language, but this option is absent or very limited with other species. Rats can learn to make a discrimination based on a drug state, for example the state associated with a particular dose of cocaine. Through discriminated responding, a well-trained rat can communicate if and by how much the dose has changed and the rat can communicate how similar or dissimilar a different drug is to the original one. These results suggest that drugs produce discriminable effects on the brain of animals that might be like mental experiences in humans, but we have no further information about those putative experiences. In the absence of reliable means for evaluating the possible mental experiences of other animals, it may be advisable, when discussing the behavioral neuroscience of non-human animals, to avoid the use of language that implies mental experience. The terms "reward-related learning" or "incentive learning" may be preferable over terms such as "pleasure" or "wanting" to describe the effects of increased synaptic concentrations of dopamine on the behavior of animals.

References and notes

Chapter 1

1. When I was an undergraduate student at the University of Western Ontario in the early 1970s, while I was reading for an essay I read a paper that used the analogy of reinforcement acting like the moon on the tides:

   Hildum DC, Brown RW (1956) Verbal reinforcement and interviewer bias. *Journal of Abnormal and Social Psychology* 53: 108–111.

   Although they used the analogy somewhat differently than I am using it here, the idea always stuck with me that there are natural phenomena all around us and whether or not we understand them, they unfold before us and influence our lives. The effect of rewarding stimuli on behavior is a particularly interesting example because it steers us through life even though we may be blissfully unaware of it.

Chapter 2

1. There was extensive work done in the twentieth century on the so-called laws of learning. Edward Thorndike (1874–1949) is often cited as the originator of the law of effect, stating the relationship between reward and behavior. Many others followed, including B.F. Skinner (1904–1990) with his *The Behavior of Organisms* in 1938. For an overview of work on animal behavior and the putative laws of learning, see Nicholas Mackintosh's (1935–2015) excellent 1974 book.

   Mackintosh NJ (1974) *Psychology of Animal Learning*. Academic Press: New York.

   Skinner BF (1938) *The Behavior of Organisms: An Experimental Analysis*. B.F. Skinner Foundation: Cambridge, MA.

   Thorndike EL (1898) Some experiments on animal intelligence. *Science* 7: 818–824.

   Thorndike EL (1911) *Animal Intelligence: Experimental Studies*. Macmillan Company: New York.

2. Beninger RJ, Kendall SB (1975) Behavioral contrast in rats with different reinforcers and different response topographies. *Journal of the Experimental Analysis of Behavior* 24: 267–280.

3. Williams BA (2002) Behavioral contrast redux. *Animal Learning & Behavior* 30: 1–20.

4. One example of the implications of behavioral contrast in a clinical setting is that the frequency of misbehavior may increase in a non-clinical setting if reinforcement for that behavior in a clinical setting is reduced or removed as part of a behavioral training program. See:

   Murphy ES, McSweeney FK, Smith RG, McComas JJ (2003) Dynamic changes in reinforcer effectiveness: theoretical, methodological and practical implications for applied research. *Journal of Applied Behavior Analysis* 36: 421–438.

5. Cooper JO, Heron TE. Heward WL (2007) *Applied Behavior Analysis* (2nd ed.). Prentice Hall: Upper Saddle River, NJ.

    Davidson JR (2013) *Sink into Sleep: A Step-by-Step Workbook for Reversing Insomnia.* Demos Health: New York.

6. Garcia J, Koelling RA (1966) Relation of cue to consequence in avoidance learning. *Psychonomic Science* 4: 123–124

    Garcia J, McGowan BK, Ervin FR, Koelling RA. (1968) Cues: their relative effectiveness as a function of the reinforcer. *Science* 160: 794–795.

7. Breland K, Breland M (1961) The misbehavior of organisms. *American Psychologist* 16: 681–684.

    Breland K, Breland M (1966) *Animal Behavior.* The Macmillan Company: New York.

8. Jenkins HM, Moore BR (1973) The form of the auto-shaped response with food or water reinforcers. *Journal of the Experimental Analysis of Behavior* 20: 163–181

9. Many of the findings that challenged the putative laws of learning are discussed in the following volumes:

    Hinde RA, Stevenson-Hinde J, eds. (1973) *Constraints on Learning: Limitations and Predispositions.* Academic Press: New York.

    Klein SB, Mowrer RR, eds. (1989) *Contemporary Learning Theories: Pavlovian Conditioning and the Status of Traditional Learning Theory.* Lawrence Erlbaum Associates: Hillsdale, NJ.

    Klein SB, Mowrer RR, eds. (1989) *Contemporary Learning Theories: Instrumental Conditioning Theory and the Impact of Biological Constraints on Learning.* Lawrence Erlbaum Associates: Hillsdale, NJ.

    Seligman MEP, Hager JL, eds. (1972) *Biological Boundaries of Learning.* Appleton Century Crofts: New York.

10. Lorenz K (1950) Innate behaviour patterns. In: *Symposium of the Society for Experimental Biology, No. 4, Physiological Mechanisms in Animal Behaviour.* Academic Press: New York.

    Tinbergen N (1951) *The Study of Instinct.* Oxford: Clarendon.

    For a recent history of ethology and the work of Lorenz and Tinbergen see:

    Burkhardt RW, Jr. (2005) *Patterns of Behavior: Konrad Lorenz, Niko Tinbergen, and the Founding of Ethology.* University of Chicago Press: Chicago, IL.

11. Garcia J, McGowan BK, Green KF (1972) Biological constraints on conditioning. In: Black AH, Prokasy WF, eds., *Classical Conditioning II: Current Research and Theory.* Appleton Century Crofts: New York, pp. 3–27.

    Wilcoxon HC, Dragoin WB, Kral PA (1971) Illness-induced aversions in rat and quail: Relative salience of visual and gustatory cues. *Science* 171: 826–828.

12. Evans S (1936) The role of kinaesthesis in the establishment and control of the maze habit. *Pedagogical Seminary and Journal of Genetic Psychology* 48: 177–198.

    Macfarlane DA (1930) The role of kinaesthesis in maze learning. *University of California Publications in Psychology* 4: 277–305.

13. Dalbir Bindra (1922–1980), working at McGill University in the 1970s, explained that incentive-motivational theories appeared in the 1930s but had little influence until the

1950s when they began to appear in the accounts of learning and performance of a number of prominent psychologists. In parallel, Robert Bolles (1928–1994), working at Hollins College in Virginia and then at the University of Washington in Seattle, was an influential incentive-learning theorist. The writings of both men have had an enduring influence on the field of animal learning:

Bindra D (1974) A motivational view of learning, performance, and behavior modification. *Psychological Review* 81: 199–213.

Bindra D (1976) *A Theory of Intelligent Behavior.* John Wiley & Sons: New York.

Bolles RC (1967) *Theory of Motivation.* Harper & Row: New York.

Bolles RC (1972) Reinforcement, expectancy, and learning. *Psychological Review* 79: 394–409

14. This was the definition I used in my writing about incentive learning, for example in my 1983 paper. For this definition, I cited Dalbir Bindra, who described reinforcing stimuli as having "'incentive-motivational' properties which influence the response-energizing capabilities of the stimuli that contribute to the occurrence of the response" (Bindra 1974, p. 199, see Note 13 for full reference). See also:

Beninger RJ (1983) The role of dopamine in locomotor activity and learning. *Brain Research Reviews* 6: 173–196.

Bindra D (1978). How adaptive behavior is produced: a perceptual-motivational alternative to response-reinforcement. *Behavioral and Brain Sciences* 1: 41–91.

15. In addition to my 1983 paper cited in Note 14, there have been many reviews of the role of dopamine in behavioral processes including reward-related learning:

Beninger RJ, Miller R (1998) Dopamine D-1 like receptors and reward-related incentive learning. *Neuroscience and Biobehavioral Reviews* 22: 335–345.

Berridge KC, Robinson KE (1998) What is the role of dopamine in reward: hedonic impact, reward learning, or incentive salience? *Brain Research Reviews* 28: 309–369.

Crow TJ (1979) Catecholamine reward pathways and schizophrenia: the mechanism of the antipsychotic effect and the site of the primary disturbance. *Federation Proceedings* 38: 2462–2467.

Di Chiara G (2005) Dopamine, motivation and reward. In: Dunnett SB, Bentivoglio M, Bjorklund A, Hokfelt T, eds., *Handbook of Chemical Neuroanatomy Volume 21: Dopamine.* Elsevier: New York, pp. 309–394.

Fibiger HC. Phillips AG (1988) Mesocorticolimbic dopamine systems and reward. *Annals of the New York Academy of Sciences* 537: 206–215.

Horvitz JC, Choi WY, Morvan C, Eyny Y, Balsam PD (2007) A "good-parent" function of dopamine: transient modulation of learning and performance during stages of training. *Annals of the New York Academy of Sciences* 1104: 270–288.

Ikemoto S (2010) Brain reward circuitry beyond the mesolimbic dopamine system: a neurobiological theory. *Neuroscience and Biobehavioral Reviews* 35: 129–150.

Miller R, Wickens JR, Beninger RJ (1990) Dopamine D-1 and D-2 receptors in relation to reward and performance: a case for the D-1 receptor as the primary site of action of neuroleptic drugs. *Progress in Neurobiology* 34: 143–189.

Robbins TW, Everitt BJ (1982) Functional studies of the central catecholamines. *International Review of Neurobiology* 23: 303–365.

Robbins TW, Everitt BJ (1996) Neurobehavioural mechanisms of reward and motivation. *Current Opinions in Neurobiology* 6: 228–236.

Salamone JD, Correa M (2012) Mysterious motivational functions of mesolimbic dopamine. *Neuron* 76: 470–485.

White NM (1989) A functional hypothesis concerning the striatal matrix and patches: mediation of S-R memory and reward. *Life Sciences* 45: 1943–1957.

Wise RA (1978) Catecholamine theories of reward: a critical review. *Brain Research* 152: 215–247.

Wise RA (1982) Neuroleptics and operant behavior: the anhedonia hypothesis. *Behavioral and Brain Sciences* 5: 39–87.

16. Olds J, Milner P (1954) Positive reinforcement produced by electrical stimulation of the septal area and other regions of rat brain. *Journal of Comparative and Physiological Psychology* 47: 419–427.

17. Brown RE, Milner PM (2003) The legacy of Donald O Hebb: more than the Hebb synapse. *Nature Reviews: Neuroscience* 4: 1013–1019.

18. Ball GG, Micco DJ Jr, Berntson GG (1974) Cerebellar stimulation in the rat: complex stimulation-bound oral behaviors and self-stimulation. *Physiology and Behavior* 13: 123–127.

Carter DA, Phillips AG (1975) Intracranial self-stimulation at sites in the dorsal medulla oblongata. *Brain Research* 94: 155–160.

Huang GH, Routttenberg A (1971) Lateral hypothalamic self-stimulation pathways in *Rattus norvegicus*. *Physiology and Behavior* 7: 419–432.

Olds J (1956) A preliminary mapping of electrical reinforcing effects in the rat brain. *Journal of Comparative and Physiological Psychology* 49: 281–285.

Routtenberg A, Sloan M (1972) Self-stimulation in the frontal cortex of *Rattus norvegicus*. *Behavioral Biology* 7: 567–572.

Simon H, Le Moal M, Cardo B (1975) Self stimulation in the dorsal pontine tegmentum in the rat. *Behavioral Biology* 13: 339–347.

19. Dahlström A, Fuxe K (1964) Evidence for the existence of monoamine-containing neurons in the central nervous system. I. Demonstration of monoamines in the cell bodies of brain stem neurons. *Acta Physiologica Scandinavica* 232(Suppl.): 1–55.

20. German DC, Bowden DM (1974) Catecholamine systems as the neural substrate for intracranial self-stimulation: a hypothesis. *Brain Research* 73: 381–419.

21. Zarevics P, Settler PE (1979) Simultaneous rate-independent and rate-dependent assessment of intracranial self-stimulation: evidence for the direct involvement of dopamine in brain reinforcement mechanisms. *Brain Research* 169: 499–512.

22. Franklin KBJ, McCoy SN (1979) Pimozide-induced extinction in rats: stimulus control rules out motor deficit. *Pharmacology, Biochemistry and Behavior* 11: 71–75.

23. Beninger RJ, Freedman NL (1982) The use of two operants to examine the nature of pimozide induced decreases in responding for brain stimulation. *Physiological Psychology* 10: 409–412.

24. Wise, RA Spindler J, de Wit H, Gerber GJ (1978) Neuroleptic-induced "anhedonia" in rats: pimozide blocks reward quality of food. *Science* 201: 262–264.

25. I, in fact, was co-author on one of the papers that appeared soon after the classic study of Wise et al. (Note 24) and that took issue with their conclusions. The paper was:

Mason ST, Beninger RJ, Fibiger HC, Phillips AG (1980) Pimozide-induced suppression of responding: evidence against a block of food reward. *Pharmacology, Biochemistry and Behavior* 12: 917–923.

This was my first publication on which I was not the first author. What I realized at the time was that one of the things junior authorship meant was not being able to have the final word on the content of the paper. In retrospect, I could have withdrawn my name from the paper if I did not agree with its conclusions, but I was an ambitious postdoctoral fellow at the time and felt that I needed the publication to enhance my chances of getting a job. In this paper, we tested rats in the same conditions as those used by Wise et al. Among other things, we found that after being trained to lever press for food, a group tested with non-reward responded at a higher rate than a similarly trained group tested with non-reward after injection of the dopamine receptor antagonist pimozide. We concluded that pimozide and extinction could not have an identity of action because of the apparent additive effects of the two manipulations. If Wise et al. (Note 24) had not claimed equivalence of pimozide plus reward compared with non-reward, but instead had said that the two manipulations produced similar effects, our data were in general agreement.

I still remember receiving a phone call from Roy Wise shortly after this paper appeared. Like him, I was one of the proponents of the hypothesis that dopamine played a major role in reward-related learning. I was somewhat abashed as he queried me about the paper I had co-authored with Mason, Fibiger, and Phillips. I remember telling him the same thing I wrote above, that I felt I needed the publication and that I did not have senior authorship on the paper so did not have final say on its conclusions. I do not remember his response except that he chuckled and I am happy to say he never held this paper against me.

Other papers that appeared around the same time and that challenged the conclusion of Wise et al. that a history of responding for food reward while being treated with a dopamine receptor-blocking drug was equivalent to responding for non-reward include:

Ettenberg A, Cinsavich SA, White N (1979) Performance effects with repeated-response measures during pimozide-produced dopamine receptor blockade. *Pharmacology Biochemistry and Behavior* 11: 557–561.

Faustman WO, Fowler SC (1981) Use of operant response duration to distinguish the effects of haloperidol from nonreward. *Pharmacology Biochemistry and Behavior* 15: 327–329.

Greenshaw AJ, Sanger DJ, Blackman DE (1981) The effects of pimozide and of reward omission on fixed-interval behavior of rats maintained by food and electrical brain stimulation. *Pharmacology Biochemistry and Behavior* 15: 227–233.

Phillips AG, Fibiger HC (1979) Decreased resistance to extinction after haloperidol: implications for the role of dopamine in reinforcement. *Pharmacology, Biochemistry and Behavior* 10: 751–760.

Tombaugh T (1981) Effects of pimozide on nondiscriminated and discriminated performance in the pigeon. *Psychopharmacology* 73: 137–141.

Tombaugh T, Anisman H, Tombaugh J (1980) Extinction and dopamine receptor blockade after intermittent reinforcement training: failure to observe functional equivalence. *Psychopharmacology* 70: 19–28.

Tombaugh TN, Szostak C, Voorneveld P, Tombaugh JW (1982) Failure to obtain functional equivalence between dopamine receptor blockade and extinction: Evidence supporting a sensory-motor conditioning hypothesis. *Pharmacology, Biochemistry and Behavior* 16: 67–72.

Tomabugh TN, Tomabugh J, Anisman H (1979) Effects of dopamine receptor blockade on alimentary behaviors—home cage food-consumption, magazine training, operant acquisition, and performance. *Psychopharmacology* 66: 219–225.

26. Threat conditioning is a common approach to the study of aversive conditioning; it involves pairing a neutral stimulus such as a tone or a particular place with aversive foot shock and then subsequently evaluating the response to threat, i.e., freezing behavior, when the animal is re-exposed to the stimulus. Often such studies do not include the opportunity to make avoidance responses and are more concerned with the learning of the stimulus-shock association than with the reward-related learning associated with shock offset. Some studies use operant avoidance tasks where an animal is trained to press a lever to delay the onset of foot shock. See:

    Sidman M (1953) Avoidance conditioning with brief shocks and no exteroceptive warning stimulus. *Science* 118: 157–158.

27. The electric shock typically used in these experiments is considered mild and normally does not exceed 0.5 mA. There are ethical considerations about delivering noxious stimuli to animals that would emphasize the use of mild shock stimuli. There are, in addition, practical reasons insofar as more intense shock may disrupt the behavior of the animal to an extent that obviates conduct of the experiment. See:

    Sagvolden T (1976) Free-operant avoidance behavior in rats with lateral septal lesions: effect of shock intensity. *Brain Research* 110: 559–574.

28. Although a tone or light signal can be and often is used to signal the impending shock, it is not necessary in the one-way version of the avoidance task. The stimuli associated with the shock side, including its visual appearance and spatial location, provide reliable information signaling the impending shock. Sometimes a two-way version of the task is used where an audio or visual signal comes on in the "safe" side, signaling the coming shock that can be avoided by the rat if it shuttles back to the original side. As you might imagine, some rats find it difficult to return to a place where they were previously shocked; this is discussed in the main text in the coming pages of Chapter 2.

29. Mowrer OH (1947) On the dual nature of learning—a re-interpretation of "conditioning" and "problem-solving." *Harvard Educational Review* 17: 102–148.

30. Dinsmoor JA (2001) Stimuli inevitably generated by behavior that avoids electric shock are inherently reinforcing. *Journal of the Experimental Analysis of Behavior* 75: 311–333.

31. Norton PJ, Price EC (2007) A meta-analytic review of adult cognitive-behavioral treatment outcomes across anxiety disorders. *Journal of Nervous and Mental Diseases* 195: 521–531.

    Recent findings suggest that pharmacological treatments in conjunction with exposure to conditioned aversive stimuli may affect memory reconsolidation and accelerate extinction of aversive conditioning underlying phobias; see:

Kindt M, Soeter M, Vervliet B (2009) Beyond extinction: erasing human fear responses and preventing the return of fear. *Nature Neuroscience* 12: 256–258.

32. Bolles RC (1970) Species-specific defense reactions and avoidance learning. *Psychological Review* 77: 32–48.

33. Fogel SM, Smith CT, Beninger RJ (2009) Evidence for 2-stage models of sleep and memory: learning-dependent changes in spindles and theta in rats. *Brain Research Bulletin* 79: 445–451.

    Fogel SM, Smith CT, Beninger RJ (2010) Too much of a good thing? Elevated baseline sleep spindles predict poor avoidance performance in rats. *Brain Research* 1319: 112–117.

    Fogel SM, Smith CT, Higginson CD, Beninger RJ (2010) Different types of avoidance behavior in rats produce dissociable post-training changes in sleep. *Physiology and Behavior* 102: 170–174.

34. Reynolds GS (1961) Attention in the pigeon. *Journal of the Experimental Analysis of Behavior* 4: 203–208.

35. Cooper BR, Breese GR, Grant LD, Howard JL (1973) Effects of 6-hydroxydopamine treatments on active avoidance responding: evidence for involvement of brain dopamine. *Journal of Pharmacology and Experimental Therapeutics* 185: 358–370.

36. In the introduction to their paper reporting the results of studies of possible mechanisms underlying avoidance learning, Davis et al. (1961) stated "The CAR (conditioned avoidance response) test had been widely used for the characterization of potential new 'psychoactive agents' in spite of differences among psychologists in their interpretation of the events involved in avoidance conditioning and in spite of uncertainty of the mechanisms of drug effects on the CAR" (p. 268).

    Davis WM Capehart J, Llewellin WL (1961) Mediated acquisition of a fear-motivated response and inhibitory effects of chlorpromazine. *Psychopharmacologia* 2: 268–276.

37. Courvoisier S (1956) Pharmacodynamic basis for the use of chlorpromazine in psychiatry. *Journal of Clinical and Experimental Psychopathology* 17: 25–37.

38. Carlsson A, Lindqvist M (1963) Effects of chlorpromazine or haloperidol on formation of 3-methoxytyramine and normetanephrine in mouse brain. *Acta Pharmacologica et Toxicologica* 20: 140–144.

Chapter 3

1. Tolman EC (1948) Cognitive maps in rats and men. *Psychological Review* 55: 189–208.

2. Gail Patterson from the University of Minnesota, Twin Cities, provides a scholarly and fascinating account of Skinner's (re)-discovery of the method of successive approximations, termed "response shaping," while working for the war effort in 1943 at a secret location (at the time) in downtown Minneapolis:

    Patterson GB (2004) A day of great illumination: B. F. Skinner's *discovery* of shaping. *Journal of the Experimental Analysis of Behavior* 82: 317–328.

3. Kimble GA (1961) *Hilgard and Marquis Conditioning and Learning*. Methuen & Co. Ltd: London, p. 74.

4. Skinner BF (1987) *Upon further reflection*. Prentice-Hall: Englewood Cliffs, NJ.

5. Darwin C (1859) *On the Origin of Species by Means of Natural Selection on the Preservation of Favoured Races in the Struggle for Life.* John Murray: London.

6. Griffiths AJF, Miller JH, Suzuki DT, Lewontin RC, Gelbart WM (2000) *An Introduction to Genetic Analysis* (7th ed.). Freeman: New York.

7. Dawkins R (1986) *The Blind Watchmaker.* Norton & Company: New York.

8. The configuration of stimuli in the two sides of a place conditioning apparatus that results in rats spending about an equal amount of time in each side can be found in:

   Brockwell NT, Ferguson DS, Beninger RJ (1996) A computerized system for the simultaneous monitoring of place conditioning and locomotor activity in rats. *Journal of Neuroscience Methods* 64: 227–232.

9. Hoffman DC, Beninger RJ (1989) The effects of selective dopamine D1 and D2 receptor antagonists on the establishment of agonist-induced place conditioning. *Pharmacology, Biochemistry and Behavior* 33:273–279

   Spyraki C, Fibiger HC, Phillips AG (1982) Dopaminergic substrates of amphetamine-induced place preference conditioning. *Brain Research* 253: 185–193.

10. Abrahams BS, Rutherford JD, Mallet PE, Beninger RJ (1998) Place conditioning with the dopamine D1-like agonist SKF 82958 but not SKF 81297 or SKF 77434. *European Journal of Pharmacology* 343: 111–118.

    Hoffman DC, Beninger RJ (1988) Selective D1 and D2 dopamine agonists produce opposing effects in place conditioning but not in conditioned taste aversion learning. *Pharmacology, Biochemistry and Behavior* 31: 1–8.

    Morency MA, Beninger RJ (1986) Dopaminergic substrates of cocaine-induced place conditioning. *Brain Research* 399: 33–41.

    Thomas Tzschentke from the University of Tübingen, then Grunenthal GbH in Aachen, Germany has comprehensively reviewed the extensive literature on the effects of different classes of drugs on incentive learning in conditioned place preference tasks:

    Tzschentke TM (1998) Measuring reward with the conditioned place preference paradigm: a comprehensive review of drug effects, recent progress and new issues. *Progress in Neurobiology* 56: 613–672.

    Tzschentke TM (2007) Measuring reward with the conditioned place preference (CPP) paradigm: update of the last decade. *Addiction Biology* 12: 227–462.

11. Di Chiara G (1995) The role of dopamine in drug abuse viewed from the perspective of its role in motivation. *Drug and Alcohol Dependence* 38: 95–137.

12. Beninger RJ, Olmstead MC (2000) The role of dopamine in the control of locomotor activity and reward-related incentive learning. In: Miller R, Wickens J, eds., *Brain Dynamics and the Striatal Complex.* Harwood Academic Press: Chur, pp. 29–50.

13. Beninger RJ, Cooper TA, Mazurski EJ (1985) Automating the measurement of locomotor activity. *Neurobehavioral Toxicology and Teratology* 7:79–85.

14. See Skinner and Mackintosh in Note 1 of Chapter 2.

15. Pickens RW, Crowder WF (1967) Effects of CS-US interval on conditioning of drug response, with assessment of speed of conditioning. *Psychopharmacologia* 11: 88–94.

16. Beninger RJ, Herz RS (1986) Pimozide blocks establishment but not expression of cocaine-produced environment-specific conditioning. *Life Sciences* 38: 1425–1431.

17. Beninger RJ, Hahn BL (1983) Pimozide blocks establishment but not expression of amphetamine-produced environment-specific conditioning. *Science* 220: 1304–1306.

18. Post RM (1980) Intermittent versus continuous stimulation: effect of time interval on the development of sensitization or tolerance. *Life Sciences* 26: 1275–1282.

19. Post RM, Lockfeld A, Squillace KM, Contel NR (1981) Drug-environment interaction: context dependency of cocaine-induced behavioral sensitization. *Life Sciences* 28: 755–760.

20. See Note 27 in Chapter 2.

21. Beninger RJ, Mason ST, Phillips AG, Fibiger HC (1980) The use of conditioned suppression to evaluate the nature of neuroleptic-induced avoidance deficits. *Journal of Pharmacology and Experimental Therapeutics* 213: 623–627.

22. Beninger RJ, Phillips AG, Fibiger HC (1983) Prior training and intermittent retraining attenuate pimozide-induced avoidance deficits. *Pharmacology, Biochemistry and Behavior* 18:619–624.

Chapter 4

1. Squire LR (1987) *Memory and Brain*. Oxford University Press: New York.

   Squire LR (2004) Memory systems of the brain: a brief history and current perspectives. *Neurobiology of Learning and Memory* 82: 171–177.

   Squire LR, Clark RE, Bayley PJ (2004) Medial temporal lobe function and memory. In: Gazzaniga MS, ed., *The Cognitive Neurosciences III*. MIT Press: Cambridge, MA, pp. 691–708.

   Squire LR, Knowlton BJ (1995) Memory, hippocampus and brain systems. In: Gazzaniga MS, ed., *The Cognitive Neurosciences*. MIT Press: Cambridge, MA, pp. 825–837.

   Squire LR, Knowlton BJ (2000) The medial temporal lobe, the hippocampus, and the memory systems of the brain. In: Gazzaniga MS, ed., *The New Cognitive Neurosciences*. MIT Press: Cambridge, MA, pp. 765–779.

2. Corkin S (2013) *Permanent Present Tense: The Unforgettable Life of the Amnesic Patient, H.M.* Basic Books: New York.

3. Scoville WB, Milner B (1957) Loss of recent memory after bilateral hippocampal lesions. *Journal of Neurology, Neurosurgery and Psychiatry* 20: 11–21.

4. Milner B (1962) Les troubles de la mémoire accompagnant des lésions hippocampiques bilatérales. In: *Physiologie de l'Hippocampe*. Centre National de la Recherche Scientifique: Paris, pp. 257–272 [English translation in Milner PM, Glickman S, eds., (1965) *Cognitive Processes and the Brain*. Van Nostrand: Princeton, NJ, pp. 97–111].

5. Corkin S (1968) Acquisition of motor skill after medial temporal-lobe excision. *Neuropsychologia* 6: 255–265.

6. Warrington EK, Weiskrantz L (1970) The amnesic syndrome: consolidation or retrieval? *Nature* 228: 628–630.

   Warrington EK, Weiskrantz L (1974) The effect of prior learning on subsequent retention in amnesic patients. *Neuropsychologia* 12: 419–428.

   Warrington EK, Weiskrantz L (1978) Further analysis of the prior learning effect in amnesic patients. *Neuropsychologia* 16: 169–177.

For a review see:

Shimamura P (1986) Priming effects in amnesia: evidence for a dissociable memory function. *The Quarterly Journal of Experimental Psychology Section A: Human Experimental Psychology* 38: 619–644.

7. Gluck MA, Bower GH (1988) From conditioning to category learning: an adaptive network model. *Journal of Experimental Psychology: General* 117: 227–247.

8. The groundbreaking report of Ehringer and Hornykiewicz showing the depletion of dopamine in the brains of Parkinson's patients was published in German:

    Ehringer H, Hornykiewicz O (1960) Verteilung von Noradrenalin und Dopmmin (3-Hydroxytyramin) im Gehirn des Menschen und ihr Verhalten bei Erkrankungen des extrapyramidalen Systems. *Klinische Wochenschrift* 38: 1236–1239.

    See:

    Hornykiewicz O (2010) A brief history of levodopa. *Journal of Neurology* 257 (Suppl. 2): S249–S252.

9. Knowlton BJ, Mangles JA, Squire LR (1996) A neostriatal habit learning system in humans. *Science* 273: 1399–1402.

10. Perretta J, Pari G, Beninger RJ (2005) Effects of Parkinson's disease on two putative nondeclarative memory tasks: probabilistic classification and gambling. *Cognitive and Behavioral Neurology* 18: 185–192.

11. Charbonneau D, Riopelle RJ, Beninger RJ (1996) Impaired incentive learning in treated Parkinson's disease. *Canadian Journal of Neurological Sciences* 23: 271–278.

12. Bechara A, Damasio H, Tranek D, Damasio AR (1997) Deciding advantageously before knowing the advantageous strategy. *Science* 275: 1293–1295.

13. Fukui H, Murai T, Fukuyama H, Hayashi T, Hanakawa T (2005) Functional activity related to risk anticipation during performance of the Iowa Gambling Task. *Neuroimage* 24: 253–259.

14. Bechara A, Damasio AR, Damasio H, Anderson SW (1994) Insensitivity to future consequences following damage to human prefrontal cortex. *Cognition* 50: 7–15.

15. Bechara A, Tranel D, Damasio H, Damasio AR (1996) Failure to respond automatically to anticipated future outcomes following damage to prefrontal cortex. *Cerebral Cortex* 6: 215–225.

    Bechara A, Damasio H, Tranel D, Anderson SW (1998) Dissociation of working memory from decision making within the human prefrontal cortex. *Journal of Neuroscience* 4: 428–437.

    Clark J, Manes F, Antoun N, Sahakian BJ, Robins TW (2003) The contributions of lesion laterality and lesion volume to decision-making impairments following frontal lobe damage. *Neuropsychologia* 41: 1474–1483.

    Manes F, Sahakian B, Clark L, Rogers R, Antoun N, Aitken M, Robbins T (2002) Decision-making processes following damage to the prefrontal cortex. *Brain* 125: 624–639.

16. Tulving E (1983) *Elements of Episodic Memory.* Clarendon Press: Oxford.

17. Clayton NS, Dickinson A (1998) Episodic-like memory during cache recovery by scrub jays. *Nature* 395: 272–274.

Clayton NS, Dickinson A (1999) Scrub jays (*Aphelocoma coerulescens*) remember the relative time of caching as well as the location and content of their caches. *Journal of Comparative Psychology* 113: 403–416.

Clayton NS, Griffiths DP, Emery NJ, Dickinson A (2001) Elements of episodic-like memory in animals. *Philosophical Transactions of the Royal Society of London B* 356: 1483–1491.

Clayton NS, Yu KS, Dickinson A (2001) Scrub jays (*Aphelocoma coerulenscens*) form integrated memories of the multiple features of caching episodes. *Journal of Experimental Psychology Animal Behavior Processes* 27: 17–29.

18. Babb SJ, Crystal JD (2005) Discrimination of what, when, and where: implications for episodic-like memory in rats. *Learning and Motivation* 36: 177–189.

Babb SJ, Crystal JD (2006) Discrimination of what, when, and where is not based on time of day. *Learning & Behavior* 34: 124–130.

Babb SJ, Crystal JD (2006) Episodic-like memory in the rat. *Current Biology* 16: 1317–1321.

19. McDonald RJ, White NM (1993) A triple dissociation of memory systems: hippocampus, amygdala and dorsal striatum. *Behavioral Neuroscience* 107: 3–22

See also:

Packard MG, Hirsh R, White NM (1989) Differential effects of fornix and caudate nucleus lesions on two radial maze tasks: evidence for multiple memory systems. *Journal of Neuroscience* 9: 1465–1472.

20. Beatty WW, Rush JR (1983) Spatial working memory in rats: effects of monoaminergic antagonists. *Pharmacology, Biochemistry and Behavior* 18: 7–12

See also:

Levin ED, Galen DM, Ellison GD (1987) Chronic haloperidol effects on oral movements and radial-arm maze performance in rats. *Pharmacology, Biochemistry and Behavior* 26: 1–6.

McGurk SR, Levin ED, Butcher LL (1988) Cholinergic-dopaminergic interactions in radial-arm maze performance. *Behavioral and Neural Biology* 49: 234–239.

21. Beninger RJ, Phillips AG (1980) The effect of pimozide on the establishment of conditioned reinforcement. *Psychopharmacology* 68: 147–153.

22. O'Keefe J, Dostrovsky J (1971) The hippocampus as a spatial map. Preliminary evidence from unit activity in the freely-moving rat. *Brain Research* 34: 171–175.

O'Keefe J, Nadel L (1978) *The Hippocampus as a Cognitive Map*. Oxford University Press: Oxford.

23. LeDoux J (2007) The amygdala. *Current Biology* 17: R868–R874.

24. Alexander GE, DeLong MR, Strick PL (1986) Parallel organization of functionally segregated circuits linking basal ganglia and cortex. *Annual Review of Neuroscience* 9: 357–381.

25. If the dorsal striatal lesion was made by electrocoagulation it would also damage the dopaminergic axons and terminals in that area eliminating, in that area, the dopamine release associated with reward. McDonald and White (Note 19 above) carried out an additional experiment where they made the lesions using the excitotoxin kainic acid. Excitotoxic lesions damage cell bodies but generally leave fibers of passage intact. They observed similar

results in their rats that received excitotoxic lesions of the dorsal striatum to those that received electrolytic lesions of that area. This result shows that even when dopaminergic axons and terminals are putatively intact in the dorsal striatum, lesion animals are impaired on the stimulus–response task but not the spatial learning or cue preference tasks.

26. Sherry DF, Schacter DL (1987) The evolution of multiple memory systems. *Psychological Review* 94: 439–454.

27. Baudry M, Zhu G, Liu Y, Want Y, Briz V, Bi X (2015) Multiple cellular cascades participate in long-term potentiation and in hippocampus-dependent learning. *Brain Research* 1621: 73–81.

    Goodman J, Packard MG (2015) The influence of cannabinoids on learning and memory processes of the dorsal striatum. *Neurobiology of Learning and Memory* 125: 1–14.

28. Ahlenius S, Engel J, Zöller M (1977) Effects of apomorphine and haloperidol on exploratory behavior and latent learning in mice. *Physiological Psychology* 5: 290–294.

29. Tolman EC, Honzik CH (1930) Introduction and removal of reward, and maze performance in rats. *University of California Publications in Psychology* 4: 257–275.

30. Blodgett HC (1929) The effect of the introduction of reward upon the maze performance or rats. *University of California Publications in Psychology* 4: 113–134.

31. Ichihara K, Nabeshima T, Kameyama T (1989) Differential effects of pimozide and SCH 23390 on acquisition of learning in mice. *European Journal of Pharmacology* 164: 189–195.

32. Recall from Chapter 2 the 1978 publication by Wise et al. (*Science* 201: 262–264) reporting that treatment with the dopamine receptor blocker pimozide was equivalent to drug-free testing without reward. In Note 25 of Chapter 2, I described how a number of researchers challenged this conclusion of Wise et al. by showing that in some situations treatment with a dopamine receptor-blocking drug and non-reward were not equivalent. I argued that the *pattern* of responding in animals treated with dopamine receptor blockers was similar (not equivalent) to that seen in animals responding for non-reward. Perhaps ironically, the paper by Ahlenius et al. (Note 28 above), although its publication antedated the report of Wise et al. by a year, contributed to the side of the argument that opposed a role for dopamine in learning. At the time there was little attention being paid to the possibility that there were multiple memory systems in animals and that dopamine might be more importantly involved in one of them.

33. Poldrack RA, Clark J, Paré-Blagoev EJ, Shohamy D, Creso Moyano J, Myers C, Gluck MA (2001) Interactive memory systems in the human brain. *Nature* 414: 546–550.

34. Brown RM, Robertson EM (2007) Off-line processing: reciprocal interactions between declarative and procedural memories. *Journal of Neuroscience* 27: 10468–10475.

    Cho SS, Yoon EJ, Lee J-M, Kim SE (2012) Repetitive transcranial magnetic stimulation of the left dorsolateral prefrontal cortex improves probabilistic category learning. *Brain Topography* 25: 443–449.

    Foerde K, Knowlton BJ, Poldrack RA (2006) Modulation of competing memory systems by distraction. *Proceedings of the National Academy of Sciences of the United States of America* 103: 11778–11783.

Lee AS, Duman RS, Pittenger C (2008) A double dissociation revealing bidirectional competition between striatum and hippocampus during learning. *Proceedings of the National Academy of Sciences of the United States of America* 105: 17163–17168.

Poldrack RA, Rodriguez P (2004) How do memory systems interact? Evidence from human classification learning. *Neurobiology of Learning and Memory* 82: 324–332.

Seger CA, Cincotta M (2006) Dynamics of frontal, striatal and hippocampal systems during rule learning. *Cerebral Cortex* 16: 1546–1555.

Shohamy D, Myers CE, Kalanithi J, Gluck MA (2008) Basal ganglia and dopamine contributions to probabilistic category learning. *Neuroscience and Biobehavioral Reviews* 32: 219–236.

35. Klimkowicz-Mrowiec A, Slowik A, Krzywoszanski L, Herzog-Krzywoszanski R, Szczudlik A (2008) Severity of explicit memory impairment due to Alzheimer's disease improves effectiveness of implicit learning. *Journal of Neurology* 255: 502–509.

36. Corkin S (1982) Some relationships between global amnesias and the memory impairment in Alzheimer's disease. In: Corkin S, Davis KL, Growdon JH, Usdin E, Wrutman RJ, eds., *Aging Volume 19, Alzheimer's Disease: A Report of Progress and Research*. Raven Press: New York, pp. 149–164.

37. Voermans NC, Petersson KM, Daudey L, Weber B, van Spaendonck KP, Kremer HPH, Fernández G (2004) Interaction between the human hippocampus and the caudate nucleus during route recognition. *Neuron* 43: 427–435.

See associated commentary:

Hartley T, Burgess N (2005) Complementary memory systems: competition, cooperation and compensation. *Trends in Neurosciences* 28: 169–170.

38. Vonsattel JPG, Keller C, Corets Ramirez EP (2011) Huntington's disease—neuropathology. In: Weiner WJ, Tolosa E, eds., *Handbook of Chemical Neurology, Volume 100, Hyperkinetic Movement Disorders*. Elsevier: Amsterdam, pp. 83–100.

39. Richardson MP, Strange BA, Dolan RJ (2004) Encoding of emotional memories depends on amygdala and hippocampus and their interactions. *Nature Neuroscience* 7: 278–285.

40. Kubikova L, Košťál L (2010) Dopaminergic system in birdsong learning and maintenance. *Journal of Chemical Neuroanatomy* 39: 112–123.

Smulders TV (2006) A multi-disciplinary approach to understanding hippocampal function in food-hoarding birds. *Reviews in the Neurosciences* 17: 53–69.

Chapter 5

1. Milner PM (1970) *Physiological Psychology*. Holt, Rinehart & Winston: New York.

2. Bobiller P, Mouret JR (1971) The alterations of the diurnal variations of brain tryptophan, biogenic amines and 5-hydroxyindole acetic acid in the rat under limited time feeding. *International Journal of Neuroscience* 2: 271–282.

3. Glick S (2011) Rosalyn Sussman Yallow (1921–2011) *Nature* 474: 580.

4. Heffner TG, Hartman JA, Seiden LS (1980) Feeding increases dopamine metabolism in the rat brain. *Science* 208: 1168–1170.

5. Blackburn JR, Phillips AG, Jakubovic A, Fibiger HC (1986) Increased dopamine metabolism in the nucleus accumbens and striatum following consumption of a nutritive meal

but not a palatable non-nutritive saccharine solution. *Pharmacology, Biochemistry and Behavior* 25: 1095–1100.

In this paper the authors also included a group that was fed with the non-nutritive sweetener, saccharine. This group showed no significant changes in DOPAC:dopamine or HVA:dopamine ratios after one hour of access to saccharine. This was surprising because saccharine has been shown in some studies to produce reward-related learning. It has been shown in more recent studies carried out at the University of Chicago, using more sensitive in vivo voltammetric methods that both sucrose and saccharine increase dopamine release in the nucleus accumbens core and that the dopamine signal produced by sucrose is longer lasting than that produced by saccharine. Cues predictive of reward also acquire the ability to activate dopamine neurons (see the following paragraph in the text); this paper showed that saccharine-predictive cues evoke less dopamine release than sucrose-predictive cues:

McCutcheon JE, Beeler JA, Roitman MF (2012) Sucrose-predictive cues evoke greater phasic dopamine release than saccharine-predictive cues. *Synapse* 66: 346–351.

6. A further paper from Lew Seiden's lab in Chicago reported that a significant rise in DOPAC following feeding in food-restricted rats was not seen until the second hour after access to food. This finding added time-dependency as another consideration when using postmortem biochemical techniques to assess the effects of stimuli such as food on dopamine. Subsequent use of in vivo microdialysis and in vivo voltammetry provided superior temporal resolution. See:

Heffner TG, Vosmer GA, Seiden LS (1984) Time-dependent changes in hypothalamic dopamine metabolism during feeding in the rat. *Pharmacology, Biochemistry and Behavior* 20: 947–949.

7. Simansky KJ, Bourbonais KA, Smith GP (1985) Food-related stimuli increase the ratio of 3,4-dihydroxyphenylacetic acid to dopamine in the hypothalamus. *Pharmacology, Biochemistry and Behavior* 23: 253–258.

8. Schiff SR (1982) Conditioned dopaminergic activity. *Biological Psychiatry* 17: 135–154.

9. Blackburn JR, Phillips AG, Jakubovic A, Fibiger HC (1989) Dopamine and preparatory behavior: II. A neurochemical analysis. *Behavioral Neuroscience* 103: 15–23.

10. Bermant G (1961) Response latencies of female rats during sexual intercourse. *Science* 133: 1771–1773.

Everitt BJ, Fray P, Kostarczyk E, Taylor S, Stacey P (1987) Studies of instrumental behavior with sexual reinforcement in male rats (*Rattus norvegicus*): I, Control by brief visual stimuli paired with a receptive female. *Journal of Comparative Psychology* 101: 395–406.

11. Lanuza E, Novejarque A, Marínez-Ricós J, Martínez-Hernández J, Agustín-Pavón C, Martínez-García F (2008) Sexual pheromones and the evolution of the reward system of the brain: the chemosensory function of the amygdala. *Brain Research Bulletin* 75: 460–466.

12. Mas M, del Castillo AR, Guerra M, Davidson JM, Battaner E (1987) Neurochemical correlates of male sexual behavior. *Physiology and Behavior* 41: 341–345.

13. Ahlenius S, Carlsson A, Hillegaart V, Hjorth S, Larsson K (1987) Region-selective activation of brain monoamine synthesis by sexual activity in male rats. *European Journal of Pharmacology* 144: 77–82.

See also:

Ahlenius S, Hillegaart V, Hjorth S, Larsson K (1991) Effects of sexual interactions on the in vivo rate of monoamine synthesis in forebrain regions of the male rat. *Behavioural Brain Research* 46: 117–122.

14. Vega-Matuszczuk J, Hillegaart V, Larsson K, Ahlenius S (1993) Effects of exposure to an estrous female on forebrain monoaminergic neurotransmission in the non-copulating male rat. *Brain Research* 630: 82–87.

15. Pepeu G (1973) The release of acetylcholine from the brain: an approach to the study of central cholinergic mechanisms. *Progress in Neurobiology* 2: 259–288.

16. Beninger RJ, Tighe SA, Jhamandas K (1984) Effects of chronic manipulations of dietary choline on locomotor activity, discrimination learning and cortical acetylcholine release in aging adult Fisher 344 rats. *Neurobiology of Aging* 5: 29–34.

17. Gaddum JH (1961) Push-pull cannulae. *Journal of Physiology* 155: P1–P2.

18. Myers R (1972) Methods for perfusing different brain structures. In: Myers R, ed., *Methods in Psychobiology Volume 2.* Academic Press: London, pp. 169–211.

19. Martin GE, Myers RD (1976) Dopamine efflux from the brain stem of the rat during feeding, drinking and lever-pressing for food. *Physiology and Behavior* 4: 551–560.

20. Brito L, Davson H, Levin E, Murray M, Snider N (1966) The concentration of free amino acids and other electrolytes in cerebrospinal fluid: in vivo dialysis of brain and blood plasma of the dog. *Journal of Neurochemistry* 13: 1057–1067.

21. Jose Manuel Rodriguez Delgado (1915–2011) was a Spanish physiologist who studied at Yale University. He developed technologies for stimulating the brain, including electrodes and the chemitrode, and was involved in the development of an early version of the cardiac pacemaker.

    Delgado JMR, DeFeudis FV, Roth RH, Ryugo DK, Mitruka BK (1972) Dialytrode for long term intracerebral perfusion in awake monkeys. *Archives Internationales de Pharmacodyamie et de Thérapie* 198: 9–21.

22. Ungerstedt U, Pycock C (1974) Functional correlates of dopamine neurotransmission. *Bulletin der Schweizerischen Akademie der Medizinischen Wissenschaften* 1278: 1–13.

23. For reviews see:

    Bourne JA (2003) Intracerebral microdialysis: 30 years as a tool for the neuroscientist. *Clinical and Experimental Pharmacology and Physiology* 30: 16–24.

    Chefer VI, Thompson AC, Zapata A, Shippenberg TS (2009) Overview of brain microdialysis. *Current Protocols in Neuroscience* Supplement 47 Unit 7.1.

    Salamone JD (1996) The behavioral neurochemistry of motivation: methodological and conceptual issues in studies of the dynamic activity of nucleus accumbens dopamine. *Journal of Neuroscience Methods* 64: 137–149.

    Westerink BHC (1995) Brain microdialysis and its application for the study of animal behaviour. *Behavioural Brain Research* 70: 103–124.

24. Church WH, Justice JB Jr, Neill DB (1987) Detecting behaviorally relevant changes in extracellular dopamine with microdialysis. *Brain Research* 412: 397–399.

25. Ahn S, Phillips AG (2007) Dopamine efflux in the nucleus accumbens during within-session extinction, outcome-dependent, and habit-based instrumental responding for reward. *Psychopharmacology* 191: 641–651.

Hajnal A, Norgren R (2001) Accumbens dopamine mechanisms in sucrose intake. *Brain Research* 904: 76–84.

Hernandez L, Hoebel BG (1988) Feeding and hypothalamic stimulation increase dopamine turnover in the nucleus accumbens. *Physiology and Behavior* 44: 599–606.

Hernandez L, Hoebel BG (1988) Food reward and cocaine increase extracellular dopamine in the nucleus accumbens as measured by microdialysis. *Life Sciences* 42: 1705–1712.

Martel P, Fantino M (1996) Mesolimbic dopaminergic system activity as a function of food reward: a microdialysis study. *Pharmacology, Biochemistry and Behavior* 53: 221–226.

McCullough LD, Cousins MS, Salamone JD (1993) A role of nucleus accumbens dopamine in responding on a continuous reinforcement operant schedule: a neurochemical and behavioral study. *Pharmacology, Biochemistry and Behavior* 46: 581–586.

Ostund SB, Wassum KM, Murphy NP, Balleine BW, Maidment NT (2011) Extracellular dopamine levels in striatal subregions track shifts in motivation and response cost during instrumental conditioning. *Journal of Neuroscience* 31: 200–207.

Radhakishun FS, van Ree JM, Westerink BHC (1988) Scheduled eating increases dopamine release in the nucleus accumbens of food-deprived rats as assessed with on-line brain dialysis. *Neuroscience Letters* 85: 351–356.

Segovia KN, Correa M, Salamone JD (2011) Slow phasic changes in nucleus accumbens dopamine release during fixed ratio acquisition: a microdialysis study. *Neuroscience* 196: 178–188.

26. Beaufour CC, Le Bihan C, Hamon M, Thiébot M-H (2001) Extracellular dopamine in the rat prefrontal cortex during reward-, punishment- and novelty-associated behaviour. Effects of diazepam. *Pharmacology, Biochemistry and Behavior* 69: 133–142.

Hernandez L, Hoebel BG (1990) Feeding can enhance dopamine turnover in the prefrontal cortex. *Brain Research Bulletin* 25: 975–979.

27. Yoshida M, Yokoo H, Mizoguchi K, Kawahara H, Tsuda A, Nishikawa T, Tanaka M (1992) Eating and drinking cause increased dopamine release in the nucleus accumbens and ventral tegmental area in the rat: measurement by in vivo microdialysis. *Neuroscience Letters* 139: 73–76.

28. Hajnal A, Smith GP, Norgren R (2004) Oral sucrose stimulation increases accumbens dopamine in the rat. *American Journal of Physiology—Regulatory, Integrative and Comparative Physiology* 286: R31–R37.

29. Bassareo V, De Luca MA, Di Chiara G (2002) Differential expression of motivational stimulus properties by dopamine in nucleus accumbens shell versus core and prefrontal cortex. *Journal of Neuroscience* 22: 4709–4719.

Bassareo V, Di Chiara G (1997) Differential influence of associative and nonassociative learning mechanisms on the responsiveness of prefrontal and accumbal dopamine transmission to food stimuli in rats fed *ad libitum*. *Journal of Neuroscience* 17: 851–861.

See also:

Cenci MA, Kalén P, Mandel RJ, Björklund A (1992) Regional differences in the regulation of dopamine and noradrenaline release in the medial frontal cortex, nucleus accumbens and caudate-putamen: a microdialysis study in the rat. *Brain Research* 581: 217–228.

30. Bassareo V, Di Chiara G (1999) Differential responsiveness of dopamine transmission to food-stimuli in nucleus accumbens shell/core compartments. *Neuroscience* 89: 637–641.

    Bassareo V, Musio P, Di Chiara G (2011) Reciprocal responsiveness of nucleus accumbens shell and core dopamine to food- and drug-conditioned stimuli. *Psychopharmacology* 214: 687–697.

31. Datla KP, Young AMJ, Gray JA, Joseph MH (2002) Conditioned appetitive stimulus increases dopamine in the nucleus accumbens of the rat. *European Journal of Neuroscience* 16: 1987–1993.

    See also:

    Phillips AG, Cacca G, Ahn S (2008) A top-down perspective on dopamine, motivation and memory. *Pharmacology, Biochemistry and Behavior* 90: 236–249.

32. Fiorino DF, Coury A, Fibiger HC, Phillips AG (1993) Electrical stimulation of reward sites in the ventral tegmental area increases dopamine transmission in the nucleus accumbens of the rat. *Behavioural Brain Research* 55: 131–141.

    Miliaressis E, Emond C, Merali Z (1991) Re-evaluation of the role of dopamine in intracranial self-stimulation using *in vivo* microdialysis. *Behavioural Brain Research* 46: 43–48.

    Nakahara D, Ozaki N, Kapoor V, Nagatsu T (1989) The effects of uptake inhibition on dopamine release from nucleus accumbens of the rat during self- or forced stimulation of the medial forebrain bundle: a microdialysis study. *Neuroscience Letters* 104: 136–140.

    Nakahara D, Ozaki N, Miura Y, Miura H, Nagatsu T (1989) Increased dopamine and serotonin metabolism in rat nucleus accumbens produced by intracranial self-stimulation of the medial forebrain bundle by *in vivo* microdialysis. *Brain Research* 495: 178–181.

    Rada PV, Mark GP, Hoebel BG (1998) Dopamine release in the nucleus accumbens by hypothalamic stimulation-escape behavior. *Brain Research* 782: 228–234.

    You, Z-B, Chen Y-Q, Wise RA (2001) Dopamine and glutamate release in the nucleus accumbens and ventral tegmental area of rat following lateral hypothalamic self-stimulation. *Neuroscience* 107: 629–639.

33. Ranaldi R, Pocock D, Zereik R, Wise RA (1999) Dopamine fluctuations in the nucleus accumbens during maintenance, extinction, and reinstatement of intravenous D-amphetamine self-administration. *Journal of Neuroscience* 19: 4102–4109.

    Wise RA, Newton P, Leeb K, Burnette B, Pocock D, Justice JB Jr (1995) Fluctuations in nucleus accumbens dopamine concentration during intravenous cocaine self-administration in rats. *Psychopharmacology* 120: 10–20.

    See also:

    Hembly SE, Co C, Kroves TR, Smith JE, Dworkin SI (1997) Differences in extracellular dopamine concentrations in the nucleus accumbens during response-dependent and response-independent cocaine administration in the rat. *Psychopharmacology* 133: 7–16.

34. Bassareo V, De Luca MA, Di Chiara G (2007) Differential impact of pavlovian drug conditioned stimuli on in vivo dopamine transmission in the rat accumbens shell and core and in the prefrontal cortex. *Psychopharmacology* 191: 689–703.

    Duvauchelle CL, Ikegami A, Asami S, Robens J, Kressin K, Castaneda E (2000) Effects of cocaine context on NAcc dopamine and behavioral activity after repeated intravenous cocaine administration. *Brain Research* 862: 49–58.

    Fontana DJ, Post RM, Pert A (1993) Conditioned increases in mesolimbic dopamine overflow by stimuli associated with cocaine. *Brain Research* 629: 31–39.

    Gonzales RA, Weiss F (1998) Suppression of ethanol-reinforced behavior by naltrexone is associated with attenuation of the ethanol-induced increase in dialysate dopamine levels in the nucleus accumbens. *Journal of Neuroscience* 18: 10663–10671.

    Ito R, Dalley JW, Howes SR, Robbins TW, Everitt BJ (2000) Dissociation in conditioned dopamine release in the nucleus accumbens core and shell in response to cocaine cues and during cocaine-seeking behavior in rats. *Journal of Neuroscience* 20: 7489–7495.

    Katner SN, Kerr TM, Weiss F (1996) Ethanol anticipation enhances dopamine efflux in the nucleus accumbens of alcohol-preferring (P) but not Wistar rats. *Behavioural Pharmacology* 7: 669–674.

    Weiss F, Lorang MT, Bloom FE, Koob GF (1993) Oral alcohol self-administration stimulates dopamine release in the rat nucleus accumbens: genetic and motivational determinants. *Journal of Pharmacology and Experimental Therapeutics* 267: 250–258.

    Weiss F, Maldonado-Vlaar CS, Parsons LH, Kerr KM, Smith DL, Ben-Shahar O (2000) Control of cocaine-seeking behavior by drug-associated stimuli in rats: effects on recovery of extinguished operant-responding and extracellular dopamine levels in amygdala and nucleus accumbens. *Proceedings of the National Academy of Sciences of the United States of America* 97: 4321–4336.

    Not all authors have found that conditioned stimuli that signal a drug of abuse increase extracellular dopamine:

    Bradberry CW, Barrett-Larimore RL, Jatlow P, Rubina SR (2000) Impact of self-administered cocaine and cocaine cues on extracellular dopamine in mesolimbic and sensorimotor striatum in rhesus monkeys. *Journal of Neuroscience* 20: 3874–3883.

35. Pfaus JG, Damsma G, Nomikos GG, Wenkstern DG, Blaha CD, Phillips AG, Fibiger HC (1990) Sexual behavior enhances central dopamine transmission in male rat. *Brain Research* 530: 345–348.

36. Damsma G, Pfaus JG, Wenkstern D, Phillips AG, Fibiger HC (1992) Sexual behavior increases dopamine transmission in the nucleus accumbens and striatum of male rats: comparison with novelty and locomotion. *Behavioral Neuroscience* 106: 181–191.

    Dominguez J, Riolo JV, Xu Z, Hull EM (2001) Regulation by the medial amygdala of copulation and medial preoptic dopamine release. *Journal of Neuroscience* 21: 349–355.

    Fiorino DF, Coury A, Phillips AG (1997) Dynamic changes in nucleus accumbens dopamine efflux during the Coolidge effect in male rats. *Journal of Neuroscience* 17: 4849–4855.

    Fumero B, Fernandez-Vera JR, Gonzalez-Mora JL, Mas M (1994) Changes in monoamine turnover in forebrain areas associated with masculine sexual behavior: a microdialysis study. *Brain Research* 662: 233–239.

Hull EM, Eaton RC, Moses J, Lorrain D (1993) Copulation increases dopamine activity in the medial preoptic area of male rats. *Life Sciences* 52: 935–940.

Mas M, Fumero B, Fernandez-Vera JR, Gonzalez-Mora JL (1995) Neurochemical correlates of sexual exhaustion and recovery as assessed by in vivo microdialysis. *Brain Research* 675: 13–19.

Melis MR, Succu S, Mascia MS, Cortis L, Argiolas A (2003) Extra-cellular dopamine increased in the paraventricular nucleus of male rats during sexual activity. *European Journal of Neuroscience* 17: 1266–1272.

Pleim ET, Matochik JA, Barfield RJ, Auerbach SB (1990) Correlation of dopamine release in nucleus accumbens with masculine sexual behavior in rats. *Brain Research* 524: 160–163.

Putnam SK, Du J, Sato S, Hull EM (2001) Testosterone restoration of copulatory behavior correlates with medial preoptic dopamine release in castrated male rats. *Hormones and Behavior* 39: 216–224.

Sato Y, Wada H, Horita H, Suzuki N, Shibuya A, Adachi H, et al. (1995) Dopamine release in the medial preoptic area during male copulatory behavior in rats. *Brain Research* 692: 66–70.

Wenkstern D, Pfaus JG, Fibiger HC (1993) Dopamine transmission increase in the nucleus accumbens of male rats during their first exposure to sexually receptive female rats. *Brain Research* 618: 41–46.

37. Kleitz-Nelson HK, Dominguez JM, Ball GF (2010) Dopamine release in the medial preoptic area is related to hormonal action and sexual motivation. *Behavioral Neuroscience* 124: 773–779.

Kleitz-Nelson HK, Dominquez JM, Cornil CA, Ball GF (2010) Is sexual motivational state linked to dopamine release in the medial preoptic area? *Behavioral Neuroscience* 124: 300–304.

38. Becker JB, Rudnick CN, Jenkins WJ (2001) The role of dopamine in the nucleus accumbens and striatum during sexual behavior in the female rat. *Journal of Neuroscience* 21: 3236–3241.

Jenkins WJ, Becker JB (2003) Dynamic increase in dopamine during paced copulation in the female rat. *European Journal of Neuroscience* 18: 1997–2001.

Mermelstein PG, Becker JB (1995) Increased extracellular dopamine in the nucleus accumbens and striatum of female rat during paced copulatory behavior. *Behavioral Neuroscience* 109: 354–365.

Pfaus JG, Damsma G, Wenkstern D, Fibiger HC (1995) Sexual activity increases dopamine transmission in the nucleus accumbens and striatum of female rats. *Brain Research* 693: 21–30.

39. Kohlert JG, Meisel RL (1999) Sexual experience sensitizes mating-related nucleus accumbens dopamine responses of female Syrian hamsters. *Behavioural Brain Research* 99: 45–52.

Kohlert JG, Rowe RK Meisel RL (1997) Intromissive stimulation from the male increases extracellular dopamine release from fluoro-gold-identified neurons within the medbrain of female hamsters. *Hormones and Behavior* 32: 143–154.

Meisel RL, Camp DM, Robinson TE (1993) A microdialysis study of ventral striatal dopamine during sexual behavior in female Syrian hamsters. *Behavioural Brain Research* 55: 151–157.

40. Curtis JT, Stowe JR, Wang Z (2003) Differential effects of intraspecific interactions on the striatal dopamine system in social and non-social voles. *Neuroscience* 118: 1165–1173.

41. Studies cited in Note 36 that also showed that conditioned sexual stimuli produced increased dopamine release in male rats include: Damsma et al. (1992), Dominguez et al. (2001), Hull et al. (1993), Melis et al. (2003), and Putnam et al. (2001). The studies cited in Note 36 reported that sexually experienced male Japanese quail showed increased dopamine release in the medial preoptic area when exposed to receptive but inaccessible females.

42. Studies cited in Note 38 that also showed that conditioned sexual stimuli produced increased dopamine release in female rats include: Jenkins and Becker (2003) and Pfaus et al. (1995).

43. Kettermann H (1997) Alexander von Humboldt and the concept of animal electricity. *Trends in Neurosciences* 20: 239–242.

44. Matteuchi C (1838) Sur le courant électrique ou proper de la grénouille. *Annales de Chemie et de Physique* 67: 93–106.

45. Meltzer SJ (1897) Emil du Bois-Reymond. *Science* 5: 217–219.

    Pearce JMS (2001) Emile Heinrich du Bois-Reymond (1818-1896). *Journal of Neurology, Neurosurgery and Psychiatry* 71: 620.

46. De Palma A, Pareti G (2011) Bernstein's long path to membrane theory: radical change and conservation in nineteenth-century German electrophysiology. *Journal of the History of the Neurosciences* 20: 306–337.

47. Hodgkin A (1979) Edgar Douglas Adrian, Baron Adrian of Cambridge: 30 November 1889-4 August 1977. *Biographical Memoires of Fellows of the Royal Society* 25: 1–73.

48. Hodgkin AL, Huxley AF, Katz B (1952) Measurement of current-voltage relations in the membrane of the giant axon of *Loligo. Journal of Physiology* 116: 424–448.

    Hodgkin AL, Huxley AF (1952) Currents carried by sodium and potassium ions through the membrane of the giant axon of *Loligo. Journal of Physiology* 116: 449–472.

    Hodgkin AL, Huxley AF (1952) The components of membrane conductance in the giant axon of *Loligo. Journal of Physiology* 116: 473–496.

    Hodgkin AL, Huxley AF (1952) The dual effect of membrane potential on sodium conductance in the giant axon of *Loligo. Journal of Physiology* 116: 497–506.

    Hodgkin AL, Huxley AF (1952) A quantitative description of membrane current and its application to conduction and excitation in nerve. *Journal of Physiology* 117: 500–544.

    Schwiening CJ (2012) A brief historical perspective: Hodgkin and Huxley. *Journal of Physiology* 590: 2571–2575.

49. Stuart DG, Brownstone RM (2011) The beginning of intracellular recording in spinal neurons: facts, reflections and speculations. *Brain Research* 1409: 62–93.

50. Bunney BS, Aghajanian GK, Roth RH (1973) Comparison of effects of L-dopa, amphetamine and apomorphine on firing rate of rat dopaminergic neurons. *Nature New Biology* 245: 123–125.

Bunney BS, Walters JR, Roth RH, Aghajanian GK (1973) Dopaminergic neurons: effect of antipsychotic drugs and amphetamine on single cell activity. *Journal of Pharmacology and Experimental Therapeutics* 185: 560–571.

See also:

Grace AA, Bunney BS (1980) Nigral dopamine neurons: intracellular recording and identification with L-dopa injection and histoflorescence. *Science* 210: 654–656.

Grace AA, Bunney BS (1983) Intracellular and extracellular electrophysiology of nigral dopaminergic neurons—1. Identification and characterization. *Neuroscience* 10: 301–315.

Mogenson GJ, Jones DL, Yim CY (1980) From motivation to action: functional interface between the limbic system and the motor system. *Progress in Neurobiology* 14: 69–97.

51. Shi W-X (2009) Electrophysiological characteristics of dopamine neurons: a 35-year update. *Journal of Neural Transmission* Supplementa 73: 103–119.

52. Miller JD, Sanghera MK, German DC (1981) Mesencephalic dopaminergic unit activity in the behaviorally conditioned rat. *Life Sciences* 29: 1255–1263.

53. Ljungberg T, Apicella P, Schultz W (1992) Responses of monkey dopamine neurons during learning of behavioral reactions. *Journal of Neurophysiology* 67: 145–163.

54. Schultz W (1986) Responses of midbrain dopamine neurons to behavioral trigger stimuli in the monkey. *Journal of Neurophysiology* 56: 1439–1462.

Schultz W, Romo R (1990) Dopamine neurons of the monkey midbrain: contingencies of responses to stimuli eliciting immediate behavioral reactions. *Journal of Neurophysiology* 63: 607–624.

55. See Note 24, Chapter 2.

56. This ability of conditioned incentive stimuli to themselves produce incentive learning is seen in conditioned reward tasks where a new response is learned based on a conditioned stimulus previously paired with reward. See Note 21 in Chapter 4 and pages 235–237 in Mackintosh (1974) in Note 1 of Chapter 2.

57. Zaghloul KA, Blanco JA, Weidemann CT, McGill K, Jaggi JL, Baltuch GH, Kahana MJ (2009) Human substantia nigra neurons encode unexpected financial rewards. *Science* 323: 1496–1499.

58. Pan W-X, Schmidt R, Wickens JR, Hyland BI (2008) Tripartite mechanism of excitation suggested by dopamine neuron activity and temporal difference model. *Journal of Neuroscience* 24: 9619–9631.

59. Pan W-X, Schmidt R, Wickens JR, Hyland BI (2005) Dopamine cells respond to predicted events during classical conditioning: evidence for eligibility traces in the reward-learning network. *Journal of Neuroscience* 25: 6235–6242.

60. Schultz W (1998) Predictive reward signal of dopamine neurons. *Journal of Neurophysiology* 80: 1–27.

See also:

Schultz W (2007) Behavioral dopamine signals. *Trends in Neuroscience* 30: 203–210.

Schultz W (2013) Updating dopamine reward signals. *Current Opinions in Neurobiology* 23: 229–238.

Tobler PN, Dickinson A, Schultz W (2003) Coding of predicted reward omission by dopamine neurons in the conditioned inhibition paradigm. *Journal of Neuroscience* 23: 10402–10410.

Waelti P, Dickenson A, Schultz W (2001) Dopamine responses comply with basic assumptions of formal learning theory. *Nature* 412: 43–48.

61. Hollerman JR, Schultz W (1998) Dopamine neurons report an error in the temporal prediction of reward during learning. *Nature Neuroscience* 1: 304–309.

    Ljungberg T, Apicella P, Schultz W (1991) Responses of monkey midbrain dopamine neurons during delayed alternation performance. *Brain Research* 586: 337–341.

    Schultz W, Apicella P, Ljungberg T (1993) Responses of monkey dopamine neurons to reward and conditioned stimuli during successive steps of learning a delayed response task. *Journal of Neuroscience* 13: 900–913.

62. Gerstner W, Sprekeler H, Deco D (2012) Theory and simulation in neuroscience. *Science* 338: 60–65.

    Schultz W, Dayan P, Montague PR (1997) A neural substrate of prediction of reward. *Science* 275: 1593–1599.

    Sutton RS (1988) Learning to predict by the methods of temporal differences. *Machine Learning* 3: 9–44.

    Sutton RS, Barto AG (1990) Time derivative models of Pavlovian reinforcement. In: Gabriel M, Moore J, eds., *Foundations of Adaptive Networks*. MIT Press: Cambridge, MA, pp. 497–537.

63. Berridge KC (2007) The debate over dopamine's role in reward: the case for incentive salience. *Psychopharmacology* 191: 391–431.

    Glimcher PW (2011) Understanding dopamine and reinforcement learning: the dopamine reward prediction error hypothesis. *Proceedings of the National Academy of Sciences of the United States of America* 108(Suppl. 3): 15647–15654.

64. Heyrovsky J (1924) The processes at the mercury dropping cathode. II. The hydrogen overpotential. *Transactions of the Faraday Society* 19: 785–788.

65. Borland LM, Michael AC (2007) An introduction to electrochemical methods in neuroscience. In: Michael AC, Borland LM, eds., *Electrochemical Methods for Neuroscience*. CRC Press: Boca Raton, FL, pp 1–17.

    Stamford JA (1985) In vivo voltammetry: promise and perspective. *Brain Research Reviews* 10: 119–135.

66. Kissinger PT, Hart JB, Adams RN (1973) Voltammetry in brain tissue—a new neurophysiological measurement. *Brain Research* 55: 209–213.

67. Gonon F, Buda A, Cespuglio R, Jouvet M, Pujol JF (1980) In vivo electrochemical detection of catechols in the neostriatum of anaesthetized rats: dopamine and DOPAC? *Nature* 286: 902–904.

    Gonon FG, Fombarlet CM, Buda MJ, Pujol JF (1981) Electrochemical treatment of pyrolytic carbon fiber electrodes. *Analytic Chemistry* 53: 1386–1389.

    Gonon FG, Navarre F, Buda MJ (1984) In vivo monitoring of dopamine release in the rat brain with differential pulse voltammetry. *Analytic Chemistry* 56: 573–575.

Ponchon JL, Cespuglio R, Gonon F, Jouvet M, Pujol JF (1979) Normal pulse polarography with carbon fiber electrodes for in vitro and in vivo determination of catecholamines. *Analytical Chemistry* 51: 1483–1486.

68. Keller RW, Stricker EM, Zigmond MJ (1983) Environmental stimuli but not homeostatic challenges produce apparent increase in dopaminergic activity in the striatum: an analysis by in vivo voltammetry. *Brain Research* 279: 159–170.

69. D'Angio M, Scatton B (1989) Feeding or exposure to food odors increases extracellular DOPAC (as measured by in vivo voltammetry) in the prefrontal cortex of food-deprived rats. *Neuroscience Letters* 96: 223–228.

70. Joseph MH, Hodges H, Gray JA (1989) Lever pressing for food reward and in vivo voltammetry: evidence for increase in extracellular homovanillic acid, the dopamine metabolite, and uric acid in the rat caudate nucleus. *Neuroscience* 32: 195–201.

71. Joseph MH, Hodges H (1990) Lever pressing for food reward and changes in dopamine turnover and uric acid in rat caudate and nucleus accumbens studied chronically by in vivo voltammetry. *Journal of Neuroscience Methods* 34: 143–149.

72. Richardson NR, Gratton A (1996) Behavior-relevant changes in nucleus accumbens dopamine transmission elicited by food reinforcement: an electrochemical study in rat. *Journal of Neuroscience* 16: 8160–8169.

    Richardson NR, Gratton A (1998) Changes in medial prefrontal cortical dopamine levels associated with response-contingent food reward: an electrochemical study in rat. *Journal of Neuroscience* 18: 9130–9138.

73. Wightman RM, Robinson DL (2002) Transient changes in mesolimbic dopamine and their association with "reward." *Journal of Neurochemistry* 82: 721–735.

74. Wilson GS, Johnson MA (2008) In-vivo electrochemistry: what can we learn about living systems? *Chemical Reviews* 108: 2462–2481.

75. Day JJ, Roitman MF, Wightman RM, Carelli RM (2007) Associative learning mediates dynamic shifts in dopamine signaling in the nucleus accumbens. *Nature Neuroscience* 10: 1020–1028.

76. Roitman MF, Stuber GD, Phillips PEM, Wightman RM, Carelli RM (2004) Dopamine operates as a subsecond modulator of food seeking. *Journal of Neuroscience* 24: 1265–1271.

77. Cacciapaglia F, Saddoris MP, Wightman RM, Carelli RM (2012) Differential dopamine release dynamics in the nucleus accumbens core and shell track distinct aspects of goal-directed behavior for sucrose. *Neuropharmacology* 62: 2050–2056.

78. Richardson NR, Gratton A (2008) Changes in nucleus accumbens dopamine transmission associated with fixed- and variable-interval schedule-induced feeding. *European Journal of Neuroscience* 27: 2714–2723.

79. Oliveira-Maia AJ, Roberts CD, Walker QD, Luo B, Kuhn C, Simon SA, Nicolelis MAL (2011) Intravascular food reward. *PLOS ONE* 6: e24992.

80. Nakazato T (2005) Striatal dopamine release in the rat during a cued lever-press for food reward and the development of changes over time measured using high-speed voltammetry. *Experimental Brain Research* 166: 137–146.

81. Brown HD, McCutcheon JE, Cone JJ, Ragozzino ME, Roitman MF (2011) Primary food reward and reward-predictive stimuli evoke different patterns of phasic

dopamine signaling throughout the striatum. *European Journal of Neuroscience* 34: 1997–2006.

This paper appeared about the same time as that of Cacciapaglia et al. (Note 77) and there was a conflicting finding in the two papers. Studying well-trained rats, Cacciapaglia et al. reported increased dopamine release in the nucleus accumbens core and shell following the conditioned stimulus associated with food and increased dopamine release in only the shell region following food. Brown et al. found increased dopamine release in the nucleus accumbens core to both the conditioned stimulus and food and no change in the shell. One possibility is that the level of training differed in the two experiments. Untrained animals show an increase in dopamine release in the nucleus accumbens core to food presentation but not to a cue that precedes the food. As training progressed, the dopamine signal in the nucleus accumbens core began to occur during the cue and began to subside during food itself. If the rats in the Brown et al. study were less extensively trained than those in the Cacciapaglia et al. study, the former study might have been observing changes in dopamine release associated with an earlier stage of training when the nucleus accumbens core dopamine signal was still seen to both the cue and food itself. Another difference between the studies was that Cacciapaglia et al. used a cue-signaled lever pressing operant task whereas Brown et al. used an operant discrimination task involving the presentation of two different cues, one that signaled that lever presses would produce reward and the other, non-reward. The use of an operant discrimination task may result in different dopamine dynamics in the nucleus accumbens core and shell than the use of a simpler cue-signaled task. Further studies are eagerly awaited.

82. Natori S, Yoshimi K, Takahashi T, Kagohashi M, Oyama G, Shimo Y, Hattori N, Kitazawa S (2009) Subsecond reward-related dopamine release in the mouse dorsal striatum. *Neuroscience Research* 63: 267–272.

83. Yoshimi K, Naya Y, Mitani N, Kato T, Inoue M, Natori S, et al. (2011) Phasic reward responses in monkey striatum as detected by voltammetry with diamond microelectrodes. *Neuroscience Research* 71: 49–62.

84. Shang C-F, Li X-Q, Yin C, Liu B, Wang Y-F, Zhou Z, Du J-L (2015) Amperometric monitoring of sensory-evoked dopamine release in awake larval zebrafish. *Journal of Neuroscience* 35: 15291–15294.

85. Howe MW, Tierney PL, Sandberg TG, Phillips PEM, Graybiel AM (2013) Prolonged dopamine signaling in striatum signals proximity and value of distant rewards. *Nature* 500: 575–579.

86. For a discussion of Hull and Spence's use of the fractional anticipatory goal response see:

Hull CL (1943) *Principles of Behavior*. Appleton-Century-Crofts: New York.

Kimble GA (1961) *Hilgard and Marquis Conditioning and Learning*. Methuen & Co Ltd: London, pp. 146–150, 173, and elsewhere.

Marx MH, Hillix WA (1963) *Systems and Theories in Psychology*. McGraw-Hill: New York, pp 241–256, and elsewhere.

Spence KW (1956) *Behavior Theory and Conditioning*. Yale University Press: New Haven, CT.

87. Heien MLAV, Khan AS, Ariansen JL, Cheer JE, Phllips PEM, Wassum KM, Wightman RM (2005) Real-time measurement of dopamine fluctuations after cocaine in the brain of behaving rats. *Proceedings of the National Academy of Sciences of the United States of America* 102: 10023–10028.

88. Aragona BJ, Day JJ, Roitman MF, Cleaveland NA, Wightman RM, Carelli RM (2009) Regional specificity in the real-time development of phasic dopamine transmission patterns during acquisition of a cue-cocaine association in rats. *European Journal of Neuroscience* 30: 1889–1899.

Wheeler RA, Aragona BJ, Fuhrmann KA, Jones JL, Day JJ, Cacciapaglia F, et al. (2011) Cocaine cues drive opposing context-dependent shifts in reward processing and emotional state. *Biological Psychiatry* 69: 1067–1074.

89. Blaha CD, Phillips AG (1990) Application of in vivo electrochemistry to the measurement of changes in dopamine release during intracranial self-stimulation. *Journal of Neuroscience Methods* 34: 125–133.

90. Kilpatrick MR, Rooney MB, Michael DJ, Wightman RM (2000) Extracellular dopamine dynamics in the rat caudate-putamen during experimenter-delivered and intracranial self-stimulation. *Neuroscience* 96: 697–706.

91. Beyene M, Carelli RM, Wightman RM (2010) Cue-evoked dopamine release in the nucleus accumbens shell tracks reinforcer magnitude during intracranial self-stimulation. *Neuroscience* 169: 1682–1688.

Cheer JF, Aragona BJ, Heien MLAV, Seipel AT, Carelli RM, Wightman RM (2007) Coordinated accumbal dopamine release and neural activity drive goal-directed behavior. *Neuron* 54: 237–244.

Owesson-White CA, Cheer JF, Beyene M, Carelli RM, Wightman RM (2008) Dynamic changes in accumbens dopamine correlate with learning during intracranial self-stimulation. *Proceedings of the National Academy of Sciences of the United States of America* 105: 11957–11962.

92. Mas M, Gonzalez-Mora JL, Louilot A, Solé C, Guadalupe T (1990) Increased dopamine release in the nucleus accumbens of copulating male rats as evidenced by in vivo voltammetry. *Neuroscience Letters* 110: 303–308.

93. Louilot A, Gonzalez-Mora JL, Guadalupe T, Mas M (1991) Sex-related olfactory stimuli induce a selective increase in dopamine release in the nucleus accumbens of male rats. A voltammetric study. *Brain Research* 553: 313–317.

Mitchell JB, Gratton A (1991) Opioid modulation and sensitization of dopamine release elicited by sexually relevant stimuli: a high speed chronoamperometric study in freely behaving rats. *Brain Research* 551: 20–27.

Robinson DL, Heien MLAV, Wightman MR (2002) Frequency of dopamine concentration transients increases in dorsal and ventral striatum of male rats during introduction of conspecifics. *Journal of Neuroscience* 22: 10477–10486.

Robinson DL, Phillips REM, Budygin EA, Trafton BJ, Garris PA, Wightman RM (2001) Sub-second changes in accumbal dopamine during sexual behavior in male rats. *NeuroReport* 12: 2549–2552.

94. Flagel SB, Clark JJ, Robinson TE, Mayo L, Czuj A, Willuhn I, et al. (2011) A selective role for dopamine in stimulus-reward learning. *Nature* 469: 53–57.
See also:

Flagel SB, Cameron SM, Pickup KN, Watson SJ, Akil H, Robinson TE (2011) A food predictive cue must be attributed with incentive salience for it to induce c-fos mRNA expression in cortico-striatal-thalamic brain regions. *Neuroscience* 196: 80–96.

95. See Mackintosh (1974) in Note 1 of Chapter 2, pp. 233 ff.

96. Bugelski BR (1938) Extinction with and without sub-goal reinforcement. *Journal of Comparative Psychology* 26: 121–134.

97. Bradley WG (2008) History of medical imaging. *Proceedings of the American Philosophical Society* 152: 349–361.

98. Bonte FJ (1976) Nuclear medicine pioneer prize, 1976: David E. Kuhl, M.D. *Journal of Nuclear Medicine* 17: 518–519.

    Kuhl DE, Edwards RQ (1963) Image separation radioisotope scanning. *Radiology* 80: 653–662.

99. Luciagnani G, Bastianello S (2006) Neuroimaging: a story of physicians and basic scientists. *Functional Neurology* 21: 133–136.

100. The discoveries of the Joliot-Curies followed from those of Irène's parents, Marie Skłodowska-Curie (1867–1934) and Pierre Curie (1859–1906), who shared the Nobel Prize in Physics in 1903 for their studies of radioactivity. Marie won an unprecedented second Nobel Prize in 1911, this time in Chemistry, for her discovery and characterization of the radioactive elements radium and polonium.

101. Ter-Pogossian MM (1992) The origins of positron emission tomography. *Seminars in Nuclear Medicine* 22: 140–149.

102. Raichle ME (1998) Behind the scenes of functional brain imaging: a historical and physiological perspective. *Proceedings of the National Academy of Sciences of the United States of America* 95: 765–772.

103. Kety SS (1951) The theory and applications of the exchange of inert gas at the lungs and tissues. *Pharmacological Reviews* 3: 1–41.

    Landau WM, Freygang WH Jr, Roland LP, Sokoloff L, Kety SS (1955) The local circulation of the living brain; values in the unanesthetized and anesthetized cat. *Transactions of the American Neurological Association* 1955-1956 (80th Meeting): 125–129.

104. Ingvar GH, Risberg J (1965) Influence of mental activity on regional cerebral blood flow in man. *Acta Neurologica Scandinavica* 41(Suppl. 14): 183–186s.

105. Lassen N, Ingvar D, Skinhøj E (1978) Brain function and blood flow. *Scientific American* 239: 62–71.

106. Holzman PS (2000) Seymour S Kety 1915–2000. *Nature Medicine* 6: 727.

107. Phelps ME (1977) Emission computed tomography. *Seminars in Nuclear Medicine* 7: 337–365.

    Phelps ME (2004) In tribute of Edward J. Hoffman, PhD (1942–2004) *Molecular Imaging and Biology* 6: 271–274.

108. Raichle ME (2008) A brief history of human brain mapping. *Trends in Neuroscience* 32: 118–128.

109. Belliveau JW, Kennedy DN, McKinstry RC, Buchbinder BR, Weisskoff RM, Cohen MS, et al. (1991) Functional mapping of the human visual cortex by magnetic resonance imaging. *Science* 254: 716–719.

110. Small DM, Jones-Gotman M, Dagher A (2003) Feeding-induced dopamine release in dorsal striatum correlates with meal pleasantness ratings in healthy human volunteers. *NeuroImage* 19: 1709–1715.

111. Koepp MJ, Gunn RN, Lawrence AD, Cunningham VJ, Dagher A, Jones T, et al. (1998) Evidence for striatal dopamine release during a video game. *Nature* 393: 266–268.

112. Pappata S, Dehaene S, Poline JB, Gregoire MC, Jobert A, Delforge J, et al. (2002) *In vivo* detection of striatal dopamine release during reward: a PET study with [¹¹C]raclopride and a single dynamic scan approach. *NeruoImage* 16: 1015–1027.

113. Martin-Soelch C, Szczepanik J, Nugent A, Barhaghi K, Rallis D, Herscovitch P, et al. (2011) Lateralization and gender differences in the dopaminergic response to unpredictable reward in the human ventral striatum. *European Journal of Neuroscience* 33: 1706–1715.

   Schott BH, Minuzzi L, Krebs RM, Elmenhorst D, Lang M, Winz OH, et al. (2008) Mesolimbic functional magnetic resonance imaging activations during reward anticipation correlate with reward-related ventral striatal dopamine release. *Journal of Neuroscience* 28: 14311–14319.

114. Zald DH, Boilear I, El-Dearedy W, Gunn R, McGlone F, Dichter GS, Dagher A (2004) Dopamine transmission in the human striatum during monetary reward tasks. *Journal of Neuroscience* 24: 4105–4112.

115. Boilieu I, Dagher A, Leyton M, Welfeld K, Booij L, Diksic M, Benkelfat C (2007) Conditioned dopamine release in humans: a positron emission tomography [¹¹C] raclopride study with amphetamine. *Journal of Neuroscience* 27: 3998–4003.

116. Francis S, Rolls ET, Bowtell R, McGlone F, O'Doherty J, Browning A, et al. (1999) The representation of pleasant touch in the brain and its relationship with taste and olfactory areas. *NeuroReport* 10: 453–459.

   O'Doherty J, Rolls ET, Francis S, Bowtell R, McGlone F (2001) Representation of pleasant and aversive taste in human brain. *Journal of Neurophysiology* 85: 1315–1321.

117. O'Doherty J, Rolls ET, Francis S, Bowtell R, McGlone F, Kobal G, et al. (2000) Sensory-specific satiety-related olfactory activation of the human orbitofrontal cortex. *NeuroReport* 11: 893–897.

118. Berns GS, McClure SM, Pagnoni G, Montague PR (2001) Predictability modulates human brain response to reward. *Journal of Neuroscience* 21: 2793–2798.

119. O'Doherty JP, Deichmann R, Critchley HD, Dolan RJ (2002) Neural responses during anticipation of a primary taste reward. *Neuron* 38: 815–826.

120. Pagoni G, Zink CF, Montague R, Berns GS (2002) Activity in human ventral striatum locked to errors of reward prediction. *Nature Neuroscience* 5: 97–98.

121. McClure SM, Berns GS, Montague PR (2003) Temporal prediction errors in a passive learning task activate human striatum. *Neuron* 38: 339–346.

   McClure SM, Ericson KM, Laibson DI, Loewenstein G, Cohen JD (2007) Time discounting for primary rewards. *Journal of Neuroscience* 27: 5796–5804.

   O'Doherty JP, Buchanan TW, Seymour B, Dolan RJ (2006) Predictable neural coding of reward preference involves dissociable responses in human ventral midbrain and ventral striatum. *Neuron* 49: 157–166.

   O'Doherty JP, Dayan P, Friston K, Critchley H, Dolan RJ (2003) Temporal difference models and reward-related learning in the human brain. *Neuron* 38: 329–337.

O'Doherty J, Dayan P, Schultz J, Deichmann R, Friston K, Dolan RJ (2004) Dissociable roles of ventral and dorsal striatum in instrumental conditioning. *Science* 304: 452–454.

Vallentin VV, O'Doherty JP (2009) Overlapping prediction errors in dorsal striatum during instrumental learning with juice and money reward in the human brain. *Journal of Neurophysiology* 102: 3384–3391.

122. D'Ardenne K, McClure SM, Nystrom, Cohen JD (2008) BOLD responses reflecting dopaminergic signals in human ventral tegmental area. *Science* 319: 1264–1267.

123. Park K, Kang HK, Seo JJ, Kim HJ, Ryu SB, Jeong GW (2001) Blood-oxygenation-level-dependent functional magnetic resonance imaging for evaluating cerebral regions of female sexual arousal response. *Urology* 57: 1189–1194.

Park K, Seo JJ, Kang HK, Ryu SB, Kim HJ, Jeong GW (2001) A new potential of blood oxygenation level dependent (BOLD) functional MRI for evaluating cerebral centers of penile erection. *International Journal of Impotence Research* 13: 73–81.

124. Arnow BA, Desmond JE, Banner LL, Glover GH, Solomon A, Polan ML, et al. (2002) Brain activation and sexual arousal in healthy, heterosexual males. *Brain* 125: 1014–1023.

Karama S, Lecours AR, Leroux J-M, Bourgouin P, Beaudoin G, Joubert S, Bearuregard M (2002) Areas of brain activation in males and females during viewing of erotic film excerpts. *Human Brain Mapping* 16: 1–13.

125. Ahron I, Etcoff N, Ariely D, Chabris CF, O'Connor E, Breiter HC (2001) Beautiful faces have variable reward value: fMRI and behavioral evidence. *Neuron* 32: 537–551.

126. Kranz F, Ishai A (2006) Face perception is modulated by sexual preference. *Current Biology* 16: 63–68.

O'Doherty J, Winston J, Critchley H, Perrett D, Burt DM, Dolan RJ (2003) Beauty in a smile: the role of medial orbitofrontal cortex in facial attractiveness. *Neuropsychologia* 41: 147–155.

127. Kampe KKW, Frith CD, Dolan RJ, Frith U (2001) Reward value of attractiveness and gaze. *Nature* 413: 589.

128. Bray S, O'Doherty J (2007) Neural coding of reward-prediction error signals during classical conditioning with attractive faces. *Journal of Neurophysiology* 97: 3036–3045.

129. Thut G, Schultz W, Roelcke U, Nienhusmeier M, Missimer J, Maguire RP, Leenders KL (1997) Activation of the human brain by monetary reward. *NeuroReport* 8: 1225–1228.

130. Rogers RD, Owen AM, Middleton HC, Williams EJ, Pickard JD, Sahakian BJ, Robbins TW (1999) Choosing between small, likely rewards and large, unlikely rewards activated inferior and orbital prefrontal cortex. *Journal of Neuroscience* 20: 9029–9038.

131. Delgado MR, Nystrom LE, Fissel C, Noll DC, Fiez JA (2000) Tracking the hemodynamic response to reward and punishment in the striatum. *Journal of Neurophysiology* 84: 3072–3077.

Dreher J-C, Kohn P, Berman KF (2006) Neural coding of distinct statistical properties of reward information in humans. *Cerebral Cortex* 16: 561–573.

Elliott R, Friston KJ, Dolan RJ (2000) Dissociable neural responses in human reward systems. *Journal of Neuroscience* 20: 6159–6165.

Elliott R, Newman JL, Longe OA, Deakin JFW (2003) Differential response patterns in the striatum and orbitofrontal cortex to financial reward in humans: a parametric functional magnetic resonance imaging study. *Journal of Neuroscience* 23: 303–307.

Elliott R, Newman JL, Longe OA, Deakin JFW (2004) Instrumental responding for rewards is associated with enhanced neuronal response in subcortical reward systems. *NeuroImage* 21: 984–990.

Ino T, Nakai R, Azuma T, Kimura T, Fukuyama H (2010) Differential activation of the striatum for decision making and outcomes in a monetary task with gain and loss. *Cortex* 46: 2–14.

Klein-Flügge MC, Hunt LT, Bach DR, Dolan RJ, Behrens TEJ (2011) Dissociable reward and timing signals in human midbrain and ventral striatum. *Neuron* 72: 654–664.

Knutson B, Adams CM, Fong GW, Hommer D (2001) Anticipation of increasing monetary reward selectively recruits nucleus accumbens. *Journal of Neuroscience* 21: RC 159 1–5.

Knutson B, Fong GW, Adams CM, Varner JL, Hommer D (2001) Dissociation of reward anticipation and outcome with event-related fMRI. *NeuroReport* 12: 3683–3687.

Knutson B, Westdrop A, Kaiser E, Hommer D (2000) FMRI visualization of brain activity during a monetary incentive delay task. *NeuroImage* 12: 20–27.

Nieuwenhuis S, Heslenfeld DJ, von Geusau NJA, Mars RB, Holroyd CB, Yeung N (2005) Activity in human reward-sensitive brain areas is strongly context dependent. *NeuroImage* 25: 1302–1309.

Small DM, Gitelman D, Simmons K, Bloise SM, Parrish T, Mesulam M-M (2005) Monetary incentives enhance processing in brain regions mediating top-down control of attention. *Cerebral Cortex* 15: 1855–1865.

Smith DV, Hayden BY, Truong T-K, Song AW, Platt ML, Huettel SA (2010) Distinct value signals in anterior and posterior ventromedial prefrontal cortex. *Journal of Neuroscience* 30: 2490–2495.

Tanaka SC, Balleine BW, O'Doherty P (2008) Calculating consequences: brain systems that encode the causal effects of actions. *Journal of Neuroscience* 28: 6750–6755.

Zink CF, Pagnoni G, Martin-Skurski ME, Chappelow JC, Berns GS (2004) Human striatal responses to monetary reward depend on saliency. *Neuron* 42: 509–517.

For reviews see:

Chau DT, Roth RA, Green AI (2004) The neural circuitry of reward and its relevance to psychiatric disorders. *Current Psychiatry Reports* 6: 391–399.

Egerton A, Mehta MA, Montgomery AJ, Lappin JM, Howes OD, Reeves SJ, et al. (2009) The dopaminergic basis of human behaviors: a review of molecular imaging studies. *Neuroscience and Biobehavioral Reviews* 33: 1109–1132.

Knutson B, Cooper JC (2005) Functional magnetic resonance imaging of reward prediction. *Current Opinion in Neurology* 18: 411–417.

132. Breiter HC, Aharon I, Kahneman D, Dale A, Shizgal P (2001) Functional imaging of neural responses to expectancy and experience of monetary gains and losses. *Neuron* 30: 619–639.

Chritchley HD, Mathias CJ, Dolan RJ (2001) Neural activity in the human brain relating to uncertainty and arousal during anticipation. *Neuron* 29: 537–545.

Delgado MR, Locke HM, Stenger VA, Fiez JA (2003) Dorsal striatal responses to reward and punishment: effects of valence and magnitude manipulations. *Cognitive, Affective, & Behavioural Neuroscience* 3: 27–38.

Miyapuram KP, Tobler P, Gregorios-Pippas L, Schultz W (2012) BOLD responses in reward regions to hypothetical and imaginary monetary rewards. *NeuroImage* 59: 1692–1699.

O'Doherty J, Kringelbach ML, Rolls ET, Hornak J, Andrews C (2001) Abstract reward and punishment representations in the human orbitofrontal cortex. *Nature Neuroscience* 4: 95–102.

133. Scott DJ, Stohler CS, Egnatuk CM, Wang H, Koeppe RA, Zubieta J-K (2007) Individual difference in reward responding explain placebo-induced expectations and effects. *Neuron* 55: 325–336.

134. Dreher J-C, Meyer-Lindenberg A, Kohn P, Berman KF (2008) Age-related changes in midbrain dopaminergic regulation of the human reward system. *Proceedings of the National Academy of Sciences of the Unites States of America* 105: 15106–15111.

Urban NBL, Slifstein M, Meda S, Xu X, Ayoub R, Medina O, et al. (2012) Imaging human reward processing with positron emission tomography and functional magnetic resonance imaging. *Psychopharmacology* 221: 67–77.

Also see Schott et al. in Note 113.

135. Breiter HC, Gollob RL, Weisskoff RM, Kennedy DN, Makris N, Berke JD, et al. (1997) Acute effects of cocaine on human brain activity and emotion. *Neuron* 19: 591–611.

136. Jenkins BG (2012) Pharmacologic magnetic resonance imaging (phMRI): imaging drug action in the brain. *NeuroImage* 62: 1072–1085.

137. For a review see:

Knutson B, Gibbs SEB (2007) Linking nucleus accumbens dopamine and blood oxygenation. *Psychopharmacology* 191: 813–822.

Chapter 6

1. Chiodo LA, Antelman SM, Caggiula AR, Lineberry CG (1980) Sensory stimuli alter the discharge rate of dopamine (DA) neurons: evidence for two functional types of DA cells in the substantia nigra. *Brain Research* 189: 455–549.

2. See Note 53 in Chapter 5.

3. Rebec GV, Christensen JRC, Guerra C, Bardo MT (1997) Regional and temporal differences in real-time dopamine efflux in the nucleus accumbens during free-choice novelty. *Brain Research* 776: 61–67.

4. Legault M, Wise RA (2001) Novelty-evoked elevations of nucleus accumbens dopamine: dependence on impulse flow from the ventral striatum and glutamatergic neurotransmission in the ventral tegmental area. *European Journal of Neuroscience* 13: 819–828.

5. Bunzeck N, Düzel E (2006) Absolute coding of stimulus novelty in the human substantia nigra/VTA. *Neuron* 51: 369–379.

6. Horvitz JC, Stewart T, Jacobs BL (1997) Burst activity of ventral tegmental dopamine neurons is elicited by sensory stimuli in the awake cat. *Brain Research* 759: 251–258.

7. Horvitz *et al.* (2007): see Note 15 in Chapter 2.

8. Steinfels GF, Heym J, Strecker RE, Jacobs BL (1983) Behavioral correlates of dopaminergic unit activity in freely moving cats. *Brain Research* 258: 217–228.

   Steinfels GF, Heym J, Strecker RE, Jacobs BL (1983) Response of dopaminergic neurons in cats to auditory stimuli presented across the sleep-waking cycle. *Brain Research* 277: 150–154.

9. Fiorillo CD, Yun SR, Song MR (2013) Diversity and homogeneity in responses of midbrain dopamine neurons. *Journal of Neuroscience* 33: 4693–4709.

   Fiorillo CD, Yun SR, Song MR (2013) Multiphasic temporal dynamics in responses of midbrain dopamine neurons to appetitive and aversive stimuli. *Journal of Neuroscience* 33: 4710–4725.

   Fiorillo CD (2013) Two dimensions of value: dopamine neurons represent reward but not aversiveness. *Science* 341: 546–549.

10. Cabib S, Puglisi-Allegro S (1994) Opposite responses of mesolimbic dopamine system to controllable and uncontrollable aversive experience. *Journal of Neuroscience* 14: 3333–3340.

    Puglisi-Allegra S, Imperato A, Angelucci L, Cabib S (1991) Acute stress induces time-dependent responses in dopamine mesolimbic system. *Brain Research* 554: 217–222.

    Thierry AM, Tassin JP, Blanc G, Glowinski J (1976) Selective activation of the mesocortial DA system by stress. *Nature* 263: 242–244.

11. Abercrombie ED, Keefe KA, DiFrischia DS, Zigmond MJ (1989) Differential effect of stress on in vivo dopamine release in the striatum, nucleus accumbens, and medial frontal cortex. *Journal of Neurochemistry* 52: 1655–1658.

    Bassareo V, De Luca MA, Di Chiara G (2002) Differential expression of motivational stimulus properties by dopamine in nucleus accumbens shell versus core and prefrontal cortex. *Journal of Neuroscience* 22: 4709–4719.

    Cenci MA, Kalén P, Mandel RJ, Björklund A (1992) Regional differences in the regulation of dopamine and noradrenaline release in medial frontal cortex, nucleus accumbens and caudate-putamen: a microdialysis study in the rat. *Brain Research* 581: 217–228.

    Keef KA, Sved AF, Zigmond MJ, Abercrombie ED (1993) Stress-induced dopamine release in the neostriatum: evaluation of the role of action potentials in nigrostriatal dopamine neurons or local initiation by endogenous excitatory amino acids. *Journal of Neurochemistry* 61: 1943–1952.

    Rada PV, Mark GP, Hoebel BG (1998) Dopamine release in the nucleus accumbens by hypothalamic stimulation-escape behavior. *Brain Research* 782: 228–234.

    Saulskaya N, Marsden CA (1995) Conditioned dopamine release: dependence upon N-methyl-D-aspartate receptors. *Neuroscience* 67: 57–63.

    Sorg BA, Kalivas PW (1991) Effects of cocaine and footshock stress on extracellular dopamine levels in the ventral striatum. *Brain Research* 559: 26–39.

Taber MT, Fibiger HC (1997) Activation of the mesocortical dopamine system by feeding: lack of a selective response to stress. *Neuroscience* 77: 295–298.

Wilkinson LS, Humby T, Killcross AS, Torres EM, Everitt BJ, Robbins TW (1998) Dissociations in dopamine release in medial prefrontal cortex and ventral striatum during the acquisition and extinction of classical aversive conditioning in the rat. *European Journal of Neuroscience* 10: 1019–1026.

Young AMJ (2004) Increased extracellular dopamine in nucleus accumbens in response to unconditioned and conditioned aversive stimuli: studies using 1 min microdialysis in rats. *Journal of Neuroscience Methods* 138: 57–63.

Young AMJ, Ahier RG, Upton RL, Joseph MH, Gray JA (1998) Increased extracellular dopamine in nucleus accumbens of the rat during associative learning of neutral stimuli. *Neuroscience* 83: 1175–1183.

Young AMJ, Joseph MH, Gray JA (1993) Latent inhibition of conditioned dopamine release in the rat nucleus accumbens. *Neuroscience* 54: 5–9.

12. Imperato A, Puglisi-Allegra S, Casolini P, Angelucci L (1991) Changes in brain dopamine and acetylcholine release during and following stress are independent of the pituitary-adrenocortical axis. *Brain Research* 538: 111–117.

13. Weiss F, Imperato A, Casu MA, Mascia MS, Gessa GL (1997) Opposite effects of stress on dopamine release in the limbic system of drug-naïve and chronically amphetamine-treated rats. *European Journal of Pharmacology* 337: 219–222.

14. Puglisi-Allegra, Imperato, Angelucci L, Cabib S (1991) Acute stress induces time-dependent responses in dopamine mesolimbic system. *Brain Research* 554: 217–222.

15. Imperato A, Angeluci L, Casolini P, Zocchi A, Puglisi-Allegra S (1992) Repeated stressful experiences differently affect limbic dopamine release during and following stress. *Brain Research* 577: 194–199.

16. McCullough LD, Sokolowski JD, Salamone JD (1993) A neurochemical and behavioral investigation of the involvement of nucleus accumbens dopamine in instrumental avoidance. *Neuroscience* 52: 919–925.

17. See Note 68 in Chapter 5.

18. Bertolucci-D'Angio A, Serrano A, Scatton B (1990) Differential effects of forced loco-motion, tail-pinch, immobilization, and methyl-β-carboline carboxylate on extracellular 3,4-dihydroxyphenylacetic acid levels in the rat striatum, nucleus accumbens, and prefrontal cortex: an in vivo voltammetric study. *Journal of Neurochemistry* 55: 1208–1215.

Doherty MS, Gratton A (1997) NMDA receptors in nucleus accumbens modulate stress-induced dopamine release in nucleus accumbens and ventral tegmental area. *Synapse* 26: 225–234.

Louilot A, Le Moal M, Simon H (1986) Differential reactivity of dopaminergic neurons in the nucleus accumbens in response to different behavioral situations. An in vivo voltammetric study in freely moving rats. *Brain Research* 397: 395–400.

19. Oleson EB, Gentry RN, Chioma VC, Cheer JF (2012) Subsecond dopamine release in the nucleus accumbens predicts conditioned punishment and its successful avoidance. *Journal of Neuroscience* 32: 14804–14808.

20. Anstrom KK, Woodward DJ (2005) Restraint increases dopaminergic burst firing in awake rats. *Neuropsychopharmacology* 30: 1832–1840.

Chiodo LA, Antelman SM, Caggiula AR, Lineberry CG (1980) Sensory stimuli after the discharge of dopamine (DA) neurons: evidence for two functional types of DA cells in the substantia nigra. *Brain Research* 189: 544–549.

21. Strecker RE, Jacobs BL (1985) Substantia nigra dopaminergic unit activity in behaving cats: effect of arousal on spontaneous discharge and sensory evoked activity. *Brain Research* 361: 339–350.

22. Kiaytkin EA (1988) Functional properties of presumed dopamine-containing and other ventral tegmental area neurons in conscious rats. *International Journal of Neuroscience* 42: 21–43.

23. Joshua M, Adler A, Mitelman, R, Vaadia E, Bergman H (2008) Midbrain dopaminergic neurons and striatal cholinergic interneurons encode the difference between reward and aversive events at different epochs of probabilistic classical conditioning trials. *Journal of Neuroscience* 28: 11673–11684.

24. Brischoux R, Chakraborty S, Beierley DI, Ungless MA (2009) Phasic excitation of dopamine neurons in the ventral VTA by noxious stimuli. *Proceedings of the National Academy of Sciences of the United States of America* 106: 4894–4899.

    Ungless MA, Argilli E, Bonci A (2010) Effects of stress and aversion on dopamine neurons: implications for addiction. *Neuroscience and Biobehavioral Reviews* 35: 151–156.

25. Mirenowicz J, Schultz W (1996) Preferential activation of midbrain dopamine neurons by appetitive rather than aversive stimuli. *Nature* 379: 449–451.

    See also:

    Schultz W (2007) Multiple dopamine functions at different time courses. *Annual Review of Neuroscience* 30: 259–288.

    Schultz (2007): see Note 60 in Chapter 5.

26. Schultz W (2010) Dopamine signals for reward value and risk: basic and recent data. *Behavioral and Brain Functions* 6: 24.

27. Blomberg-Martin E, Matsumoto M, Hikosaka O (2010) Dopamine in motivational control: rewarding, aversion, and alerting. *Neuron* 68: 815–834.

28. Ungless MA, Magill PJ, Bolam JP (2004) Uniform inhibition of dopamine neurons in the ventral tegmental area by aversive stimuli. *Science* 303: 2040–2042.

    See also Brischoux et al., Note 25.

29. Matsumoto M, Hikosaka O (2009) Two types of dopamine neurons distinctly convey positive and negative motivational signals. *Nature* 459: 837–841.

    This paper makes a strong case for a subset of dopamine cells that is fired by aversive stimuli. However, Christopher Fiorillo et al. (2013 *Journal of Neuroscience* 33: p 4693; see Note 9) comment extensively on the methodology. They argue that the air-puff stimulus that was used as an aversive stimulus was, in fact, very mild and close to neutral; it may even have produced dopamine neuron activation because it was signaled and could have been associated with the opportunity to avoid the air puff to the eye. Fiorillo et al. point out that the apparent regional difference in dopamine neurons that respond to reward and aversion reported by Matsumoto and Hikosaka was confounded with direction of electrode penetration, with apparent aversion-activated cells found earlier in the day when penetration were more dorsolateral and the air puff was relatively novel. Matsumoto and Hikosaka observed that a conditioned stimulus associated with an air puff produced dopamine neuron activation. They identified dopamine neuron activation by comparing the response to that produced by a stimulus that putatively predicted no outcome; however, that stimulus may have been producing negative prediction error because it was also presented in the context of a highly valued reward (juice). In other words, the apparent activation of dopamine neurons by an aversive conditioned stimulus may have been a result of comparing the response to that produced by a conditioned stimulus that resulted in inhibition of dopamine neuron firing. Further studies are needed to resolve these concerns.

In a subsequent paper, Matsumoto and colleagues showed that in mice, optogenetically identified dopamine neurons are inhibited by an aversive air puff. They showed further that conditioned olfactory stimuli that reliably signal aversive air puffs themselves produce decreases in dopamine neuron activity. See:

Matsumoto H, Tian J, Uchida N, Watabe-Uchida M (2016) Midbrain dopamine neurons signal aversion in a reward-context-dependent manner. *eLIFE* 5: e17328.

30. Costall B, Naylor RJ (1975) Detection of the neuroleptic properties of clozapine, sulpiride and thioridazine. *Psychopharmacologia* 43: 69–74.

31. Sanberg PR, Bunsey MD, Giordano M, Norman AB (1988) The catalepsy test: its ups and downs. *Behavioral Neuroscience* 102: 748–759.

32. Amtage J, Schmidt WJ (2003) Context-dependent catalepsy intensification is due to classical conditioning and sensitization. *Behavioural Pharmacology* 14: 563–567.

    Lanis A, Schmidt WJ (2001) NMDA receptor antagonists do not block the development of sensitization of catalepsy, but make its expression state-dependent. *Behavioural Pharmacology* 12: 143–149.

    Riedinger K, Kulak A, Schmidt WJ, von Ameln-Mayerhofer A (2011) The role of NMDA and AMPA/kainite receptors in the consolidation of catalepsy sensitization. *Behavioural Brain Research* 218: 194–199.

    Schmidt WJ, Beninger RJ (2006) Behavioural sensitization in addiction, schizophrenia, Parkinson's disease and dyskinesia. *Behavioural Pharmacology* 10: 161–166.

    Schmidt WJ, Tzschentke T, Kretschmer BD (1999) State-dependent blockade of haloperidol-induced sensitization of catalepsy by MK-801. *European Journal of Neuroscience* 11: 3365–3368.

    Srinivasan J, Schmidt, WJ (2004) Intensification of cataleptic response in 6-hydroxydopamine-induced neurodegeneration of substantia nigra is not dependent on the degree of dopamine depletion. *Synapse* 51: 213–218.

33. Klein A, Schmidt WJ (2003) Catalepsy intensifies context-dependently irrespective of whether it is induced by intermittent or chronic dopamine deficiency. *Behavioral Pharmacology* 14: 49–53.

34. Antelman SM, Kocan D, Edwards DJ, Knopf S, Perel JM, Stiller R (1986) Behavioral effects of a single neuroleptic treatment grow with the passage of time. *Brain Research* 385: 58–67.

    Banasikowski TJ, Beninger RJ (2012) Haloperidol conditioned catalepsy in rats: a possible role for D1-like receptors. *International Journal of Neuropsychopharmacology* 15: 1525–1534.

Banasikowski TJ, Beninger RJ (2012) Reduced expression of haloperidol conditioned catalepsy in rats by the dopamine D3 receptor antagonists nafadotride and NGB 2904. *European Neuropsychopharmacology* 22: 761–768.

Carey RJ (1987) Conditioning and the delayed onset of a haloperidol-induced behavioral effect. *Biological Psychiatry* 22: 269–277.

35. Rocca JF, Lister JG, Beninger RJ (2016) Spiroperidol, but not eticlopride or aripiprazole, produces gradual increases in descent latencies in the bar test in rats. *Behavioural Pharmacology* 28: 30–36.

36. Schimmel LNP, Banasikowski TJ, Hawken ER, Dumont EC, Beninger RJ (2015) Brain regions associated with inverse incentive learning: c-Fos immunohistochemistry after haloperidol sensitization on the bar test in rats. *Behavioural Brain Research* 293: 81–88.

37. Banasikowski T (2012) Dopamine D1-like, D2 and D3 receptor subtypes in catalepsy sensitization and conditioning in rats: implications for motor function, motivation and learning. PhD thesis, Queen's University, Kingston, ON, Canada.

38. Mackintosh N (1974). See Note 1 in Chapter 2.

39. This study was originally done by Banasikowski (see Note 37); Kathleen Xu, working in my laboratory, replicated the effect in the groups reported here.

40. Key BJ (1961) Effects of chlorpromazine and lysergic acid diethylamide on the rate of habituation of the arousal response. *Nature* 190: 275–277.

41. See Beninger (1983) in Note 14 in Chapter 2 and:

Beeler JA, Daw N, Frazier CR, Zhuang X (2010) Tonic dopamine modulates exploitation of reward learning. *Frontiers in Behavioral Neuroscience* 4: Article 170.

42. The concept of an inverse agonist arose as a result of observations of the effects of drugs affecting γ-aminobutyric acid (GABA) neurotransmission. The $GABA_A$ receptor has a site on it that is termed the "benzodiazepine site" because benzodiazepine compounds (e.g., the anxiolytic drug diazepam, marketed as Valium) acts at that site to *increase* GABAergic neurotransmission. The drug flumazenil (Ro 15-1788) was discovered to be an antagonist at the benzodiazepine site that could effectively block the effects of benzodiazepines and could be used, for example, to treat benzodiazepine overdose. Together benzodiazepines and flumazenil covered the usual pharmacological actions of drugs at receptors, agonist and antagonist, respectively. Subsequently, the β-carbolines were discovered, endogenous agents that act at the benzodiazepine site to *decrease* GABAergic neurotransmission. Since the standard terms "agonist" and "antagonist" were already used to describe classes of drugs that affected the benzodiazepine site, a new term was needed. "Inverse agonist" was the term chosen to describe an agent that acts at the same receptor site as an agonist but produces an effect opposite in direction to that produced by the agonist. Researchers at Hoffman-La Roche & Co. in Basel, Switzerland, were perhaps the first to use the term in the following paper:

Polc P, Bonetti ER, Schaffner R, Haefely W (1982) A three-state model of the benzodiazepine receptor explains the interactions between benzodiazepine antagonist Ro 15-1788, benzodiazepine tranquilizers, β-carbolines, and phenobarbitone. *Naunyn-Schmiedeberg's Archives of Pharmacology* 321: 260–264.

43. See Note 10 of Chapter 2.

44. Lubow RE (1989) *Latent Inhibition and Conditioned Attention Theory*. Cambridge University Press: Cambridge.

45. Bethus I, Muscat R, Goodall G (2006) Dopamine manipulations limited to preexposure are sufficient to modulate latent inhibition. *Behavioral Neuroscience* 120: 554–563.

   Young AMJ, Moran PM, Joseph MH (2005) The role of dopamine in conditioning and latent inhibition: what, when, where and how? *Neuroscience and Biobehavioral Reviews* 29: 963–976.

46. See Schultz et al. (1997), Hollerman and Schultz (1998) and Waelti et al. (2001) in Notes 60–62 of Chapter 5 and:

   Schultz W (2013) Updating dopamine reward signals. *Current Opinion in Neurobiology* 23: 229–238.

47. D'Souza MS, Duvauchelle CL (2008) Certain and uncertain cocaine expectations influence accumbens dopamine responses to self-administered cocaine and non-rewarded operant behavior. *European Neuropsychopharmacology* 18: 628–638.

48. Mangiavacchi S, Masi F, Scheggi S, Leggio B, De Montis MG, Gamvrana C (2001) Long-term behavioral and neurochemical effects of chronic stress exposure in rats. *Journal of Neurochemistry* 79: 1113–1121.

49. Seligman MEP, Maier SF (1967) Failure to escape traumatic shock. *Journal of Experimental Psychology* 74: 1–9.

   Overmier JB, Seligman MEP (1967) Effects of inescapable shock upon subsequent escape and avoidance responding. *Journal of Comparative and Physiological Psychology* 63: 28–33.

   Overmier JB (1996) Richard L. Solomon and learned helplessness. *Integrative Physiological and Behavioral Science* 31: 331–337.

Chapter 7

1. Rang HP (2006) The receptor concept: pharmacology's big idea. *British Journal of Pharmacology* 147: S9–S16.

2. Sutherland EW, Rall TW (1958) Fractionation and characterization of a cyclic adenine ribonucleotide formed by tissue particles. *Journal of Biological Chemistry* 232: 1077–1091.

3. Walsh DA, Perkins JP, Krebs EG (1968) An adenosine 3′,5′-monophosphate-dependant protein kinase from rabbit skeletal muscle. *Journal of Biological Chemistry* 243: 3763–3765.

   This discovery formed part of the body of work that led Krebs and his colleague Edmond Fischer to receive the Nobel Prize in Physiology or Medicine in 1992.

4. Miyamoto E, Kuo JF, Greengard P (1969) Adenosine 3′,5′-monophosphate-dependent protein kinase from brain. *Science* 165: 63–65.

5. Kebabian JW, Greengard P (1971) Dopamine-sensitive adenyl cyclase: possible role in synaptic transmission. *Science* 174: 1346–1349.

   Kebabian JW, Petzold GL, Greengard P (1972) Dopamine-sensitive adenylate cyclase in caudate nucleus of rat brain, and its similarity to the "dopamine receptor." *Proceedings of the National Academy of Science of the United States of America* 69: 2145–2149.

6. Snyder SH (2011) What dopamine does in the brain. *Proceedings of the National Academy of Science of the United States of America* 108: 18869–18871.

7. Arvid Carlsson's studies of dopamine and its relationship to Parkinson's disease led to him receiving the Nobel Prize in Physiology or Medicine in 2000; Carlsson was a co-recipient of the Prize with Eric Kandel and Paul Greengard, whose work is discussed in this chapter, as well as Chapters 9 and 12.

 Carlsson A, Lindqvist M, Magnusson T, Waldeck B (1958) On the presence of 3-hydroxytyramine in brain. *Science* 127: 471.

8. See Note 8, Chapter 4

9. Laverty R, Sharman DF (1965) The estimation of small quantities of 3,4-hydroxyphenylethylamine in tissues. *British Journal of Pharmacology* 24: 538–548.

10. McAfee DA, Schorderet M, Greengard P (1971) Adenosine 3',5'-monophosphate in nervous tissue: increase associated with synaptic transmission. *Science* 171: 1156–1158.

11. Ungerstedt U, Butcher LL Butcher SG, Andén N-E, Fuxe K (1969) Direct chemical stimulation of dopaminergic mechanisms in the neostriatum of the rat. *Brain Research* 14: 461–471.

12. Andén N-E, Butcher SG, Corrodi H, Fuxe K, Ungerstedt U (1970) Receptor activity and turnover of dopamine and noradrenaline after neuroleptics. *European Journal of Pharmacology* 11: 303–314.

 Andén N-E, Corrodi H, Fuxe K, Ungerstedt U (1971) Importance of nervous impulse flow for the neuroleptic induced increase in amine turnover in central dopamine neurons. *European Journal of Pharmacology* 15: 193–199.

 Andén N-E, Roos B-E, Werdinius B (1964) Effects of chlorpromazine, haloperidol and reserpine on the levels of phenolic acids in rabbit corpus striatum. *Life Sciences* 3: 149–158.

 Corrodi H, Fuxe K, Hökfelt T (1967) The effects of neuroleptics on the activity of central catecholamine neurones. *Life Sciences* 6: 767–774.

 Nybäck H, Sedvall G (1968) Effect of chlorpromazine on accumulation and disappearance of catecholamines formed from tyrosine-c14 in brain. *Journal of Pharmacology and Experimental Therapeutics* 162: 294–301.

 See also Note 38 in Chapter 2.

13. Van Rossum JM (1966) The significance of dopamine-receptor blockade for the mechanism of action of neuroleptic drugs. *Archives Internationales de Pharmacodynamie et de Therapie* 160: 92–94.

 Van Rossum JM (1967) The significance of dopamine-receptor blockade for the action of neuroleptic drugs. In: Brill H, Cole JO, Deniker P, Hippius H, Bradley PB, eds., *Neuro-Psycho-Pharmacology, Proceedings of the Fifth International Congress of the Collegium Internationale Neuro-Psychopharmacologicum, March 1966*. Excerpta Medica Foundation: Amsterdam, pp. 321–329.

14. Clement-Cormier YC, Kebabian JW, Petzold GL, Greengard P (1974) Dopamine-sensitive adelylate cyclase in mammalian brain: a possible site of action of antipsychotic drugs. *Proceedings of the National Academy of Sciences of the United States of America* 71: 1113–1117.

 See also:

 Miller RJ, Horn A, Iverson LL (1974) The action of neuroleptic drugs on dopamine-stimulated adenosine 3'5'-monophosphate production in rat neostriatum and limbic forebrain. *Molecular Pharmacology* 10: 759–766.

15. Seeman P (1981) Brain dopamine receptors. *Pharmacological Reviews* 32: 229–313.

    Zingales IA (1971) A gas chromatographic method for the determination of haloperidol in human plasma. *Journal of Chromatography* 54: 15–24.

16. Paton WDM, Rang HP (1965) The uptake of atropine and related drugs by intestinal smooth muscle of the guinea-pig in relation to acetylcholine receptors. *Proceedings of the Royal Society of London Series B, Containing Papers of a Biological Nature* 163: 1–44.

17. Snyder SH (1984) Drug and neurotransmitter receptors in the brain. *Science* 224: 22–31.

18. Pert CB, Snyder SH (1973) Opiate receptor: demonstration in nervous tissue. *Science* 179: 1011–1014.

    Corroborative reports appeared later in the same year:

    Simon EJ, Hiller JM, Edelman I (1973) Stereospecific binding of the potent narcotic analgesic (3H) etorphine to rat-brain homogenate. *Proceedings of the National Academy of Sciences of the United States of America* 70: 1947–1949.

    Terenius L (1973) Characteristics of the "receptor" for narcotic analgesics in synaptic plasma membrane fraction from rat brain. *Acta Pharmacologica et Toxicologica* 33: 377–384.

19. Seeman P, Chau-Wong M, Tedesco J, Wong K (1975) Brain receptors for antipsychotic drugs and dopamine: direct binding assays. *Proceedings of the National Academy of Sciences of the United States of America* 72: 4376–4380.

    See also:

    Seeman P, Lee T, Chau-Wong M, Wong K (1976) Antipsychotic drug doses and neuroleptic/dopamine receptors. *Nature* 261: 717–719.

20. Madras B (2013) History of the discovery of the antipsychotic dopamine D2 receptor: a basis for the dopamine hypothesis of schizophrenia. *Journal of the History of the Neurosciences* 22: 62–78.

21. Burt DR, Creese I, Snyder SH (1976) Properties of [^{3}H]haloperidol and [^{3}H]dopamine binding associated with dopamine receptors in calf brain membranes. *Molecular Pharmacology* 12: 800–812.

    Snyder SH, Creese I, Burt DR (1975) The brain's dopamine receptor: labeling with [^{3}H] dopamine and [^{3}H]haloperidol. *Psychopharmacology Communications* 1: 663–673.

22. Spano PF, Govoni S, Trabucci M (1978) Studies of the pharmacological properties of dopamine receptors in various areas of the central nervous system. In: Roberts PJ, Woodruff GN, Iversen LL, eds., *Advances in Biochemical Psychopharmacology, Volume 19: Dopamine.* Raven Press: New York, pp. 155–165.

23. Kebabian JW, Calne DB (1979) Multiple receptors for dopamine. *Nature* 277: 93–96.

    See also:

    Kebabian JW, Tsuruta K, Cote TE, Grewe CW (1982) The activity of substituted benzamides in biochemical models of dopamine receptors. In: Stanley M, Rotrosen J, eds., *Advances in Biochemical Psychopharmacology, Volume 35: The Benzamides: Pharmacology, Neurobiology, and Clinical Aspects.* Raven Press: New York, pp. 17–49.

24. Cote TE, Frey EA, Grewe CW, Kebabian JW (1983) Evidence that the D-2 dopamine receptor in the intermediate lobe of the rat pituitary gland is associated with an

inhibitory guanyl nucleotide component. *Journal of Neural Transmission* Supplementum 18: 139–147.

25. Mukherjee C, Caron MG, Coverstone M, Lefkowitz RJ (1975) Identification of β-adrenergic receptors in frog erythrocyte membranes with (-)-[³H]alprenolol. *Journal of Biological Chemistry* 250: 4869–4875.

    Williams LT, Lefkowitz RJ (1976) Identification of α-adrenergic receptors by [³H] dihydroergocryptine binding. *Science* 192: 791–793.

26. The G protein was discovered by Martin Rodbell (1925–1998) and Al Gilman, work that earned them the 1994 Nobel Prize in Physiology or Medicine. See:

    Lefkowitz RJ (1994) Rodbell and Gilman win 1994 Nobel Prize for Physiology and Medicine. *Trends in Pharmacological Sciences* 15: 442–444.

27. Dixon RAF, Kobilka BK, Strader DJ, Benovic JL, Dohlman HG, Frielle T, et al. (1986) Cloning of the gene and cDNA for mammalian β-adrenergic receptor and homology with rhodopsin. *Nature* 321: 75–79.

28. Lefkowitz RJ (2013) A brief history of G-protein coupled receptors (Nobel lecture) *Angewandte Chemie International Edition* 52: 6367–6378.

29. Polymerase chain reaction (PCR) is a technique for amplifying a small number of copies of DNA by orders of magnitude, providing an alternative to slow and labor-intensive purification techniques. Kary Mullis, working at Cetus Corporation in Emeryville, California, developed PCR technology in 1983. Mullis was the co-recipient of the 1993 Nobel Prize in Chemistry for this discovery. See:

    Mullis KB (1990) The unusual origin of the polymerase chain reaction. *Scientific American* 262: 56–65.

30. Bunzow JR, Van Tol HHM, Grandy DK, Albert P, Salon J, Christie M, et al. (1988) Cloning and expression of a rat D₂ dopamine receptor cDNA. *Nature* 336: 783–787.

31. Dearry A, Gingrich JA, Falardeau P, Fremeau RT, Bates MD, Caron MG (1990) Molecular cloning and expression of the gene for a human D₁ dopamine receptor. *Nature* 347: 72–76.

    Monsma FJ Jr., Mahan LC, McVittie LD, Gerfen CR, Sibley DR (1990) Molecular cloning and expression of a D1 dopamine receptor linked to adenylyl cyclase activation. *Proceedings of the National Academy of Sciences of the United States of America* 87: 6723–6727.

    Sunahara RK, Niznik HB, Weiner DM, Stormann TM, Brann MR, Kennedy JL, et al. (1990) Human dopamine D₁ receptor encoded by an intronless gene on chromosome 5. *Nature* 347: 80–83.

    Zhou Q-Y, Grandy DK, Thambi L, Kushner JA, Van Tol HHM, Cone R, et al. (1990) Cloning and expression of human and rat D₁ dopamine receptors. *Nature* 347: 76–80.

32. Sokoloff P, Giros B, Martes M-P, Bouthenet M-L, Schwartz J-C (1990) Molecular cloning and characterization of a novel dopamine receptor (D₃) as a target for neuroleptics. *Nature* 347: 146–151.

33. Van Tol HHM, Bunzow JR, Guan H-C, Sunahara RK, Seeman P, Niznik HB, Civelli O (1991) Cloning of the gene for a human dopamine D₄ receptor with high affinity for the antipsychotic clozapine. *Nature* 350: 610–614.

34. Sunahara RK, Guan H-C, O'Dowd BF, Seeman P, Laurier LG, Ng G, et al. (1991) Cloning of the gene for a human dopamine D$_5$ receptor with higher affinity for dopamine than D1. *Nature* 350: 614–619.

35. Beninger RJ (1991) Receptor subtype-specific dopamine agonists and antagonists and conditioned behaviour. In: Willner P, Scheel-Krüger J, eds., *The Mesolimbic Dopamine System: From Motivation to Action.* Chichester: John Wiley and Sons, pp. 273–299.

    Beninger RJ (1992) D1 receptor involvement in reward-related learning. *Journal of Psychopharmacology* 6: 34–42.

    Beninger RJ (1993) Role of D1 and D2 receptors in learning. In: Waddington J, ed., *D$_1$: D$_2$ Dopamine Receptor Interactions: Neuroscience and Psychopharmacology.* London: Academic Press, pp. 115–157.

    Beninger RJ, Hoffman DC, Mazurski EJ (1989) Receptor subtype-specific dopaminergic agents and conditioned behavior. *Neuroscience and Biobehavioral Reviews* 13: 122–133.

    Beninger RJ, Mazurski EJ, Hoffman DC (1991) Receptor subtype-specific dopaminergic agents and unconditioned behaviour. *Polish Journal of Pharmacology and Pharmacy* 43: 507–528.

    Beninger RJ, Nakonechny PL (1996) Dopamine D1-like receptors and molecular mechanisms of incentive learning. In: Beninger RJ, Palomo T, Archer T, eds., *Dopamine Disease States.* Madrid: CYM Press, pp. 407–431.

    See also Beninger and Miller (1998) and Miller et al. (1990) in Note 15, Chapter 2.

36. Ungerstedt U, Ljundberg T, Ranje C (1977) Dopamine neurotransmission and the control of behaviour. In Cools AR, Lohman AHM, van den Bercken JHL, eds., *Psychobiology of the Striatum.* North-Holland Publishing Company: Amsterdam, pp. 85–97.

37. See Beninger (1983) in Note 14 in Chapter 2.

38. Setler PE, Sarau HM, Zirkle CL, Saunders HL (1978) The central effects of a novel dopamine agonist. *European Journal of Pharmacology* 50: 419–430.

39. See Beninger et al. (1991) in Note 35.

40. Fletcher GH, Starr MS (1985) SKF 38393 and apomorphine modify locomotion and exploration in rats placed in a holeboard by separate actions at D-1 and D-2 receptors. *European Journal of Pharmacology* 117: 381–385.

41. Hahn RA, MacDonald BR (1984) Primate cardiovascular responses mediated by dopamine receptors: effects of N,N-di-*n*-propyldopamine and LY171555. *Journal of Pharmacology and Experimental Therapeutics* 229: 132–138.

42. Braun AR, Chase TN (1986) Obligatory D-1/D-2 receptor interaction in the generation of dopamine agonist related behaviors. *European Journal of Pharmacology* 131: 301–306.

    McDevitt JT, Setler PE (1981) Differential effects of dopamine agonists in mature and immature rats. *European Journal of Pharmacology* 72: 69–75.

43. Lyons M, Robbins T (1975) The action of central nervous system stimulant drugs: a general theory concerning amphetamine effects. In: Essman W, Valzelli L, eds., *Current Developments in Psychopharmacology, Volume 2.* Spectrum Publications: New York, pp. 80–163.

44. Jackson DM, Hashizume M (1987) Bromocriptine-induced locomotor stimulation in mice is modulated by dopamine D-1 receptors. *Journal of Neural Transmission* 69: 131–145.

Walters JR, Bergstrom DA, Carlson JH, Chase TN, Braun AR (1987) D1 dopamine receptor activation required for postsynaptic expression of D2 agonist effects. *Science* 236: 719–722.

For further references see Beninger et al. (1991) in Note 35 and:

Waddington JL, Dally SA (1993) Regulation of unconditioned motor behaviour by D_1:D_2 interactions. In: Waddington J, ed., D_1:D_2 *Dopamine Receptor Interactions: Neuroscience and Psychopharmacology*. Academic Press: London, pp. 51–78.

45. Hyttel J (1983) Functional evidence for selective dopamine D-1 receptor blockade by SCH 23390. *Neuropharmacology* 23: 15951401.

46. O'Boyle KM, Waddington JL (1984) Identification of the enantiomers of SK&F 83566 as specific and stereoselective antagonists at the striatal D-1 dopamine receptor: comparisons with the D-2 enantioselectivity of Ro 22-1319. *European Journal of Pharmacology* 106: 219–220.

    O'Boyle KM, Waddington JL (1984) Selective and stereospecific interactions of R-SK&F 38393 with [³H]piflutixol but not [³H]spiperone binding to striatal D_1 and D_2 dopamine receptors: comparisons with SCH 23390. *European Journal of Pharmacology* 98: 433–436.

47. Christensen AV, Arnt J, Hyttel J, Larsen J-J, Svendsen O (1984) Pharmacological effects of a specific dopamine D-1 antagonist SCH 23390 in comparison with neuroleptics. *Life Sciences* 34: 1529–1540.

48. See Beninger et al. (1991) in Note 35.

49. Blume E (1983) Street drugs yield primate Parkinson's model. *JAMA* 250: 13–14.

    Langston JW, Ballard P, Tetrud JW, Irwin I (1983) Chronic Parkinsonism in humans due to a product of meperidine-analog synthesis. *Science* 219: 979–980.

50. Arnt J (1985) Hyperactivity induced by stimulation of separate dopamine D-1 and D-2 receptors in rats with bilateral 6-OHDA lesions. *Life Sciences* 37: 717–723.

    Breese GR, Duncan GE, Napier C, Bondy SC, Iorio LC, Mueller RA (1987) 6-Hydroxydopamine treatments enhance behavioral responses to intracerebral microinjections of D1 and D2 dopamine agonists into nucleus accumbens and striatum without changing dopamine antagonist binding. *Journal of Pharmacology and Experimental Therapeutics* 240: 167–176.

    Breese GR, Mueller RA (1985) SCH-23390 antagonism of a D-2 dopamine agonist depends upon catecholamine neurons. *European Journal of Pharmacology* 113: 109–114.

51. Barone P, Bankiewicz KS, Corsini GU, Kopin IJ, Chase TN (1987) Dopaminergic mechanisms in hemiparkinsonian monkeys. *Neurology* 37: 1592–1595.

    Close SP, Marriott AS, Pay S (1985) Failure of SKF 38393-A to relieve Parkinsonian symptoms induced by 1-methyl-4-phenyl-1,2,3,6-tetrahydropyridine in the marmoset. *British Journal of Pharmacology* 85: 320–322.

    Falardeau P, Bouchard S, Bédard PJ, Boucher R, Di Paolo T (1988) Behavioral and biochemical effect of chronic treatment with D-1 and/or D-2 dopamine agonists in MPTP monkeys. *European Journal of Pharmacology* 150: 59–66.

    Nomoto M, Jenner P, Marsden CD (1985) The dopamine D2 agonist LY 141865, but not the D1 agonist SKF 38393, reverses Parkinsonism induced by

1-methyl-4-phenyl-1,2,3,6-tetrahydropyridine (MPTP) in the common marmoset. *Neuroscience Letters* 57: 37–41.

Nomoto M, Jenner P, Marsden CD (1988) The D1 agonist SKF 38393 inhibits the antiparkinsonian activity of the D2 agonist LY 171555 in the MPTP-treated marmoset. *Neuroscience Letters* 93: 275–280.

52. Braun AR, Fabbrini G, Mouradian MM, Serrati C, Baron P, Chase TN (1987) Selective D-1 dopamine receptor agonist treatment of Parkinson's disease. *Journal of Neural Transmission* 68: 41–50.

Lieberman AN, Goldstein M (1985) Bromocriptine in Parkinson disease. *Pharmacological Reviews* 37: 217–227.

53. For a review see:

Hurley MJ, Jenner P (2006) What has been learnt from study of dopamine receptors in Parkinson's disease? *Pharmacology and Therapeutics* 111: 715–728.

54. Fowler SC, Liou J-R (1994) Microcatalepsy and disruption of forelimb usage during operant behavior: differences between dopamine D_1 (SCH-23390) and D_2 (raclopride) antagonists. *Psychopharmacology* 115: 24–30.

Fowler SC, Liou J-R (1998) Haloperidol, raclopride, and eticlopride induce microcatalepsy during operant performance in rats, but clozapine and SCH 23390 do not. *Psychopharmacology* 140: 81–90.

55. See Note 15 in Chapter 2, Note 6 in Chapter 6, Note 60 in Chapter 9, and Note 56 in this chapter.

56. Choi WY, Morvan C, Balsam PD, Horvitz JC (2009) Dopamine D1 and D2 antagonist effects on response likelihood and duration. *Behavioral Neuroscience* 123: 1279–1287.

See also:

Horvitz JC (2001) The effects of D1 and D2 receptor blockade on the acquisition and expression of a conditioned appetitive response. *Appetite* 37: 119–120.

57. Azzara AV, Bodanr RJ, Delamater AR, Sclafani A (2001) D_1 but not D_2 dopamine receptor antagonism blocks the acquisition of a flavor preference conditioned by intragastric carbohydrate infusions. *Pharmacology, Biochemistry and Behavior* 68: 709–720.

58. Kraft TT, Yakubov Y, Huang D, Fitzgerald G, Acosta V, Natanova E, et al. (2013) Dopamine D1 and opioid receptor antagonism effects on the acquisition and expression of fat-conditioned flavor preferences in BALD/c and SWR mice. *Pharmacology, Biochemistry and Behavior* 110: 127–136.

59. Touzani K, Bodnar RJ, Sclafani A (2013) Glucose-conditioned flavor preference learning requires co-activation of NMDA and dopamine D1-like receptors within the amygdala. *Neurobiology of Learning and Memory* 106: 95–101.

See also:

Andrzejewski ME, Spencer RC, Kelley AC (2005) Instrumental learning, but not performance, requires dopamine D1-receptor activation in the amygdala. *Neuroscience* 135: 335–345.

60. Intermittent pairing in used because it produces a more durable conditioned reward effect. See:

Knott PD, Clayton KN (1966) Durable secondary reinforcement using brain stimulation as the primary reinforcer. *Journal of Comparative and Physiological Psychology* 61: 151–153.

Zimmerman DW (1959) Sustained performance in rats based on secondary reinforcement. *Journal of Comparative and Physiological Psychology* 52: 353–358.

Zimmerman DW (1963) Influence of three stimulus conditions upon the strength of a secondary reinforcement effect. *Psychological Reports* 13: 135–139.

61. See Note 95 in Chapter 5.

62. Beninger RJ, Phillips AG (1980) The effect of pimozide on the establishment of conditioned reinforcement. *Psychopharmacology* 68: 147–153.

63. Fletcher PJ, Higgins GA (1997) Differential effects of ondansetron and α-flupenthixol on responding for conditioned reward. *Psychopharmacology* 134: 64–72.

    Killcross AS, Everitt BJ, Robbins TW (1997) Symmetrical effects of amphetamine and alpha-flupenthixol on conditioned punishment and conditioned reinforcement: contrasts with midazolam. *Psychopharmacology* 129: 141–152.

    Robbins TW, Watson BA, Gaskin M, Ennis C (1983) Contrasting interactions of pipradrol, *d*-amphetamine, cocaine, cocaine analogues, apomorphine and other drugs with conditioned reinforcement. *Psychopharmacology* 80: 113–119.

    For a review see:

    Sutton MA, Beninger RJ (1999) Psychopharmacology of conditioned reward: evidence for a rewarding signal at D_1-like dopamine receptors. *Psychopharmacology* 144: 95–110.

64. Beninger RJ, Ranaldi R (1992) The effects of amphetamine, apomorphine, SKF 38393, quinpirole and bromocriptine on responding for conditioned reward in rats. *Behavioural Pharmacology* 3: 155–163.

65. Colpaert FC, van Bever WFM, Leyson JEMP (1976) Apomorphine: chemistry, pharmacology, biochemistry. *International Review of Neurobiology* 19: 225–268.

66. Scheel-Krüger J (1971) Comparative studies of various amphetamine analogues demonstrating different interaction with the metabolism of the catecholamines in the brain. *European Journal of Pharmacology* 14: 47–59.

    Westerink BHC (1979) The effects of drugs on dopamine biosynthesis and metabolism in the brain. In: Horn AS, Korf J, Westerink BHC, eds., *The Neurobiology of Dopamine*. Academic Press: London, pp. 255–291.

67. Robbins TW (1975) The potentiation of conditioned reinforcement by psychomotor stimulant drugs: a test of Hill's hypothesis. *Psychopharmacology* 45: 103–114.

    Robbins TW (1976) Relationship between reward-enhancing and stereotypical effects of psychomotor stimulant drugs. *Nature* 264: 57–59.

    Robbins TW (1978) The acquisition of responding with conditioned reinforcement: effects of pipradrol, methylphenidate, *d*-amphetamine, and nomifensine. *Psychopharmacology* 58: 79–87.

    Robbins TW, Koob GF (1978) Pipradrol enhances reinforcing properties of stimuli paired with brain stimulation. *Pharmacology, Biochemistry and Behavior* 8: 219–222.

    See also: Robbins et al. (1983) in Note 63.

68. Beninger RJ, Rolfe NG (1995) Dopamine D1-like receptor agonists impair responding for conditioned reward in rats. *Behavioural Pharmacology* 6: 1–9.

    Ranaldi R, Pantalony D, Beninger RJ (1995) The D1 agonist SKF 38393 attenuates amphetamine-produced enhancement of responding for conditioned reward. *Pharmacology, Biochemistry and Behavior* 52: 131–137.

69. See the discussion in Beninger and Miller in Note 15, Chapter 2. Also:

    Abrahams BS, Rutherford JD, Mallet PE, Beninger RJ (1998) Place conditioning with the dopamine D1-like agonist SKF 82958 but not SKF 81297 or SKF 77434. *European Journal of Pharmacology* 343: 111–118.

    Hoffman DC, Beninger RJ (1988) Selective D1 and D2 dopamine agonists produce opposing effects in place conditioning but not in conditioned taste aversion learning. *Pharmacology, Biochemistry and Behavior* 31: 1–8.

    Hoffman DC, Beninger RJ (1989) The effects of selective dopamine D1 and D2 receptor antagonists on the establishment of agonist-induced place conditioning. *Pharmacology, Biochemistry and Behavior* 33: 273–279.

    Hoffman DC, Dickson PR, Beninger RJ (1988) The dopamine D2 receptor agonists, quinpirole and bromocriptine produce conditioned place preferences. *Progress in Neuro-Psychopharmacology and Biological Psychiatry* 12: 315–322.

    White NM, Packard MG, Hiroi N (1991) Place conditioning with dopamine-D1 and D2 agonists induced peripherally or into nucleus accumbens. *Psychopharmacology* 103: 271–276.

    See also Morency and Beninger in Note 10.

70. See Note 12 in Chapter 3.

71. Smithies O, Gregg RG, Boggs SS, Koralewski MA, Kucherlapati RS (1985) Insertion of DNA sequences into the human chromosomal beta-globin locus by homologous recombination. *Nature* 317: 230–234.

    Wong EA, Capecchi MR (1986) Analysis of homologous recombination in cultured mammalian cells in transient expression and stable transformation assays. *Somatic Cell and Molecular Genetics* 12: 63–72.

72. Evans MJ, Kaufman MH (1981) Establishment in culture of pluripotential cells from mouse embryos. *Nature* 292: 154–156.

73. Bradley A, Evans M, Kaufman MH, Robertson E (1984) Formation of germ-line chimaeras from embryo-derived teratocarcinoma cell lines. *Nature* 309: 255–256.

74. Artzt K (2012) Mammalian developmental genetics in the twentieth century. *Genetics* 192: 1151–1163.

    Gondo Y (2008) Trends in large-scale mouse mutagenesis: from genetics to functional genomics. *Nature Reviews Genetics* 9: 803–810.

    Hall B, Limaye A, Kulkarni AB (2009) Overview: generation of gene knockout mice. *Current Protocols in Cell Biology* 44: Unit 19.

    Manis JP (2007) Knock out, knock in, knock down—genetically manipulated mice and the Nobel Prize. *New England Journal of Medicine* 357: 2426–2429.

    Vogel G (2007) A knockout award in medicine. *Science* 318: 178–179.

75. Evettts KD, Uretsky NJ, Iversen LL, Iversen SD (1970) Effects of 6-hydroxydopamine on CNS catecholamines, spontaneous motor activity and amphetamine induced hyper-activity in rats. *Nature* 225: 961–962.

76. Breese GR, Traylor TD (1971) Depletion of brain noradrenaline and dopamine by 6-hydroxydopamine. *British Journal of Pharmacology* 42: 88–99.

77. Marshall JF, Richardson JS, Teitelbaum P (1974) Nigrostriatal bundle damage and the lateral hypothalamic syndrome. *Journal of Comparative and Physiological Psychology* 87: 808–830.

Ungerstedt U (1971) Adipsia and aphagia after 6-hydroxydopamine-induced degeneration of the nigrostriatal dopamine system. *Acta Physiologica Scandinavica* 367(Suppl.): 95–122.

Zigmond MJ, Stricker EM (1973) Recovery of feeding and drinking by rats after intraventricular 6-hydroxydopamine or lateral hypothalamic lesions. *Science* 182: 717–720.

78. Marshall JF (1984) Behavioral consequences of neuronal plasticity following injury to nigrostriatal dopaminergic neurons. In: Scheff SW, ed., *Aging and Recovery of Function in the Central Nervous System*. Plenum Press: New York, pp. 102–127.

Stricker EM, Zigmond MJ (1976) Recovery of function following damage to central catecholaminergic neurons: a neurochemical model for the lateral hypothalamic syndrome. In: Sprague JM, Epstein AN, eds., *Progress in Neurobiology and Physiological Psychology*. Academic Press: New York, pp. 121–189.

79. Zigmond MJ, Stricker EM (1985) Adaptive properties of monoaminergic neurons and their functional implications. In: Lajtha A, ed., *Handbook of Neurochemistry Volume 9*. Plenum Press: New York, pp. 87–102.

Zigmond MJ, Stricker EM, Berger TW (1987) Parkinsonism: insights from animal models utilizing neurotoxic agents. In: Coyle JT, ed., *Experimental Models of Dementing Disorders: A Synaptic Neurochemical Perspective*. Alan R. Liss: New York, pp. 1–38.

80. Bruno JP, Snyder AM, Stricker EM (1984) Effect of dopamine-depleting brain lesions on suckling and weaning in rats. *Behavioral Neuroscience* 98: 151–161.

Porter BM, Bruno JP (1989) Food intake of rats depleted of dopamine as neonates is impaired by inhibition of catecholamine biosynthesis. *Neuroscience Letters* 107: 295–300.

Weihmuller FB, Bruno JP (1989) Drinking behavior and motor function in rat pups depleted of brain dopamine during development. *Developmental Psychobiology* 22: 101–114.

81. Erinoff L, MacPhail RC, Heller A, Seiden LS (1979) Age-dependent effects of 6-hydroxydopamine on locomotor activity in the rat. *Brain Research* 164: 195–205.

Pappas BA, Gallivan JV, Dugas T, Saari M, Ings R (1980) Intraventricular 6-hydroxydopamine in the newborn rat and locomotor responses to drugs in infancy: no support for the dopamine depletion model of minimal brain dysfunction. *Psychopharmacology* 70: 41–46.

Shaywitz BA, Teicher MH, Cohen DJ, Anderson GM, Young JG (1984) Dopaminergic but not adrenergic mediation of hyperactivity and performance deficits in developing rat pup. *Psychopharmacology* 17: 386–396.

Shaywitz BA, Yager RD, Klopper JH (1976) Selective brain dopamine depletion in developing rats: an experimental model of minimal brain dysfunction. *Science* 191: 305–308.

82. Heffner TG, Seiden LS (1983) Impaired acquisition of an operant response in young rats depleted of brain dopamine in neonatal life. *Psychopharmacology* 79: 115–119.

Stellar JR, Waraczynski M, Bruno JP (1988) Neonatal dopamine depletions spare lateral hypothalamic stimulation reward in adult rats. *Pharmacology, Biochemistry and Behavior* 30: 365–370.

Takeichi T, Kurumiya S, Umemoto M, Olds ME (1986) Roles of catecholamine terminals and intrinsic neurons of the ventral tegmentum in self-stimulation investigated in neonatally dopamine-depleted rats. *Pharmacology, Biochemistry and Behavior* 241: 1101–1109.

See also Shaywitz et al. (1976) in Note 81.

83. Breese GR, Baumeister AA, McCown TJ, Emerick SG, Frye GD, Crotty K, Mueller RA (1984) Behavioral differences between neonatal and adult 6-hydroxydopamine-treated rats to dopamine agonists: relevance to neurological symptoms in clinical syndromes with reduced brain dopamine. *Journal of Pharmacology and Experimental Therapeutics* 231: 343–354.

Breese GR, Baumeister AA, McCown TJ, Emerick SG, Frye GD, Crotty K, Mueller RA (1984) Neonatal-6-hydroxydopamine treatment: model of susceptibility for self-mutilation in the Lesch-Nyan syndrome. *Pharmacology, Biochemistry and Behavior* 21: 459–461.

Breese GR, Baumeister A, Napier TC, Frye GD, Mueller RA (1985) Evidence that D-1 dopamine receptors contribute to the supersensitive behavioral responses induced by L-dihydroxydopamine. *Journal of Pharmacology and Experimental Therapeutics* 235: 287–295.

84. Joyce JN, Frohna PA, Neal-Beliveau BS (1996) Functional and molecular differentiation of the dopamine system induced by neonatal denervation. *Neuroscience and Biobehavioral Reviews* 20: 453–486.

85. Kolb, B, Teskey GC (2010) Age, experience, injury and the changing brain. *Developmental Psychobiology* 54: 311–325.

86. Gore BB, Zweifel LS (2013) Genetic reconstruction of dopamine D1 receptor signaling in the nucleus accumbens facilitates natural and drug reward responses. *Journal of Neuroscience* 33: 8640–8649.

87. El-Ghundi M, O'Dowd BF, Erclik M, George SR (2003) Attenuation of sucrose reinforcement in dopamine D_1 receptor deficient mice. *European Journal of Neuroscience* 17: 851–862.

88. Tran AH, Tamura R, Uwano T, Kobayashi T, Katsuki M, Ono T (2005) Dopamine D1 receptors involved in locomotor activity and accumbens neural responses to prediction of reward associated with place. *Proceedings of the National Academy of Sciences of the United States of America* 102: 2117–2122.

89. Karasinska JM, George SR, Cheng R, O'Dowd BF (2005) Deletion of dopamine D1 and D3 receptors differentially affects spontaneous behaviour and cocaine-induced locomotor activity, reward and CREB phosphorylation. *European Journal of Neuroscience* 22: 1741–1750.

Miner Ll, Drago J, Chamberlain PM, Donovan D, Uh GR (1995) Retained cocaine conditioned place preference in D1 receptor deficient mice. *NeuroReport* 6: 2314–2316.

90. Caine SB, Thomsen M, Gavriel KI, Berkowitz JS, Gold LH, Koob GF, et al. (2007) Lack of self-administration of cocaine in dopamine D_1 receptor knock-out mice. *Journal of Neuroscience* 28: 13140–13150.

91. El-Ghundi M, George SR, Drago J Fletcher PJ, Fan T, Nguyen T, et al. (1998) Disruption of dopamine D1 receptor gene expression attenuates alcohol-seeking behavior. *European Journal of Pharmacology* 353: 149–158.

Short JL, Ledent C, Drago J, Lawrence AJ (2006) Receptor crosstalk: characterization of mice deficient in dopamine D_1 and adenosine A_{2A} receptors. *Neuropsychopharmacology* 31: 525–534.

92. Nitz DA, Kargo WJ, Fleischer J (2007) Dopamine signaling and the distal reward problem. *NeuroReport* 18: 1833–1836.

93. El-Ghundi M, Fletcher PJ, Drago J, Sibley DR, O'Dowd BF, George SR (1999) Spatial learning deficit in dopamine D1 receptor knockout mice. *European Journal of Pharmacology* 383: 95–106.

94. Ortiz O, Delgado-García JM, Espadas I, Bahí A, Tullas R, Dreyer J-L, et al. (2010) Associative learning and CA3-CA1 synaptic plasticity are impaired in D_1 R null, *Drd1a*–/– mice and in hippocampal siRNA silenced *Drd1a* mice. *Journal of Neuroscience* 30: 12288–12300.

95. Caine SB, Negus SS, Mello NK, Patel S, Bristow L, Kulagowski J, et al. (2002) Role of dopamine D2-like receptors in cocaine self-administration: studies with D2 receptor mutant mice and novel D2 receptor antagonists. *Journal of Neuroscience* 22: 2977–2988.

96. Elmer GI, Pieper JO, Rubinstein M, Low MJ, Grandy DK, Wise RA (2002) Failure of intravenous morphine to serve as an effective instrumental reinforer in dopamine D2 receptor knock-out mice. *Journal of Neuroscience* 22: RC224 1–6.

97. Elmer GI, Pieper JO, Levy J, Rubenstein M, Low MJ, Grandy DK, Wise RA (2005) Brain stimulation and morphine reward deficits in dopamine D2 receptor-deficient mice. *Psychopharmacology* 182: 33–44.

98. Dockstader CL, Rubinstein M, Grandy DK, Low MJ, van der Kooy D (2001) The D_2 receptor is critical in mediating opiate motivation only in opiate-dependent and withdrawn mice. *European Journal of Neurosicence* 13: 995–1011. Note: there is some disagreement about the possible interactive effects of opiate dependency and dopamine D2 receptor knockout on place preference based on morphine.

Maldonado R, Saiardi A, Velverde O, Samad TA, Roques BP, Borrelli E (1997) Absence of opiate rewarding effects in mice lacking dopamine D2 receptors. *Nature* 388: 586–589.

99. Tran AH, Tamura R, Uwano T, Kobayashi T, Katsuki M, Matsumoto G, Ono T (2002) Altered accumbens neural responses to prediction of reward associated with place in dopamine D2 receptor knockout mice. *Proceedings of the National Academy of Sciences of the United States of America* 99: 8986–8991.

100. Yan Y, Kong H, Wu EJ, Newman AH, Xu M (2013) Dopamine D3 receptors modulate reconsolidation of cocaine memory. *Neuroscience* 241: 32–40.

101. Kong H, Kuang W, Xu M (2011) Activation of dopamine D3 receptors inhibits reward-related learning induced by cocaine. *Neuroscience* 176: 152–161 But see Karasinska et al. in Note 89.

102. Narita Mi, Mizuo K, Mizoguchi H, Sakata M, Narita Ma, Tseng LF, Suzuki T (2003) Molecular evidence for the functional role of dopamine D_3 receptor in morphine-induced rewarding effect and hyperlocomotion. *Journal of Neuroscience* 23: 1006–1012.

103. Dulawa SC, Grandy DK, Low MJ, Paulus MP, Geyer MA (1999) Dopamine D4 receptor-knock-out mice exhibit reduced exploration of novel stimuli. *Journal of Neuroscience* 19: 9550–9556.

104. Helms CM, Gubner NR, Wilhelm CJ, Mitchell SH, Grandy DK (2008) D_4 receptor deficiency in mice has limited effects on impulsivity and novelty seeking. *Pharmacology, Biochemistry and Behavior* 90: 387–393.

105. Nemirovsky SI, Avale ME, Drunner D, Rubinstein M (2009) Reward-seeking and discrimination deficits displayed by hypodopaminergic mice are prevented in mice lacking dopamine D4 receptors. *Synapse* 63: 991–997.

    Young JW, Powell SB, Scott CN, Zhou X, Geyer MA (2011) The effect of reduced dopamine D4 receptor expression in the 5-choice continuous performance task: separating response inhibition from premature responding. *Behavioural Brain Research* 222: 183–192.

106. Thanos PK, Bermeo C, Rubinstein M, Suchland KL, Wang GJ, Grady DK, Volkow ND (2010) Conditioned place preference and locomotor activity in response to methylphenidate, amphetamine and cocaine in mice lacking dopamine D_4 receptors. *Journal of Psychopharmacology* 24: 897–904.

107. Thanos PK, Habibi R, Michaelides M, Patel UB, Suchland K, Anderson BJ, et al. (2010) Dopamine D4 receptor (D4R) deletion in mice does not affect operant responding for food and cocaine. *Behavioural Brain Research* 207: 508–511.

108. Ebstein RP, Novick O, Umansky R, Priel B, Osher Y, Blaine D, et al. (1996) Dopamine D4 receptor (*D4DR*) exon III polymorphism associated with the human personality trait of novelty seeking. *Nature Genetics* 12: 78–80.

109. LaHoste GJ, Swanson JM, Wigal SB, Glabe C, Wigal T, King N, Kennedy JL (1996) Dopamine D4 receptor gene polymorphism is associated with attention deficit hyperactivity disorder. *Molecular Psychiatry* 1: 121–124.

110. Karlsson R-M, Hefner KR, Sibley DR, Holmes A (2008) Comparison of dopamine D1 and D5 receptor knockout mice for cocaine locomotor sensitization. *Psychopharmacology* 200: 117–127.

111. Beninger RJ, Banasikowski TJ (2008) Dopaminergic mechanisms of reward-related incentive learning: focus on the dopamine D_3 receptor. *Neurotoxicity Research* 14: 57–70.

112. Higley AE, Kiefer SW, Li X, Gaál J, Xi Z-X, Gardner EL (2011) Dopamine D_3 receptor antagonist SB-277011A inhibits methamphetamine self-administration and methamphetamine-induced reinstatement of drug-seeking in rats. *European Journal of Pharmacology* 659: 187–192.

    Higley AE, Spiller K, Grundt P, Newman AH, Kiefer SW, Xi Z-X, Gardner EL (2011) PG01037, a novel dopamine D_3 receptor antagonist, inhibits the effects of methamphetamine in rats. *Journal or Psychopharmacology* 25: 263–273.

113. Peng X-Q, Ashby CR, Jr., Spiller K, Li X, Li J, Thomasson N, et al. (2009) The preferential dopamine D3 antagonist S33138 inhibits cocaine reward and cocaine-triggered relapse to drug-seeking behavior in rats. *Neuropharmacology* 56: 752–760.

114. Song R, Yang R-F, Wu N, Su R-B, Li J, Peng X-Q, et al. (2011) YQA14: a novel dopamine D_3 receptor antagonist that inhibits cocaine self-administration in rats and mice, but not in D_3 receptor-knockout mice. *Addiction Biology* 17: 259–273.

115. Di Ciano P (2008) Drug seeking under a second-order schedule of reinforcement depends on dopamine D_3 receptors in the basolateral amygdala. *Behavioral Neuroscience* 122: 129–139.

116. Achat-Mendes C, Grundt P, Cao J, Platt DM, Newman AH, Spealman RD (2010) Dopamine D3 and D2 receptor mechanisms in the abuse-related behavioral effects of cocaine: studies with preferential antagonists in squirrel monkeys. *Journal of Pharmacology and Experimental Therapeutics* 334: 556–565.

117. Cheung THC, Loriaux AL, Weber SM, Chandler KN, Lenz JD, Schaan RF, et al. (2013) Reduction of cocaine self-administration and D3 receptor-mediated behavior by two novel dopamine D3 receptor-selective partial agonists, OS-3-106 and WW-III-55. *Journal of Pharmacology and Experimental Therapeutics* 347: 410–423.

118. Cheung THC, Nolan BC, Hammerslag LR, Weber SM, Durbin JP, Peartree NA, et al. (2012) Phenylpiperazine derivatives with selectivity for dopamine D3 receptors modulate cocaine self-administration in rats. *Neuropharmacology* 63: 1346–1359.

119. See the Higley et al. reference in Note 112.

120. Song R, Bi G-H, Zhang H-Y, Yang R-F, Gardner EL, Li J, Xi Z-X (2014) Blockade of D3 receptors by YQA14 inhibits cocaine's rewarding effects and relapse to drug-seeking behavior in rats. *Neuropharmacology* 77: 398–405.

121. Khaled MATM, Araki KF, Li B, Coen KM, Marinelli PW, Varga J, et al. (2010) The selective dopamine D_3 receptor antagonist SB-277-11-A, but not the partial agonist BP 897, blocks cue-induced reinstatement of nicotine-seeking. *International Journal of Neuropsychopharmacology* 13: 181–190.

122. Spiller K, Xi Z-X, Peng X-Q, Newman AH, Ashby CR, Jr., Heidbreder C, et al. (2008) The selective dopamine D_3 receptor antagonists SB-277011A and NGB 2904 and the putative partial D_3 receptor agonist BP-897 attenuate methamphetamine-enhanced brain stimulation reward in rats. *Psychopharmacology* 196: 533–542.

123. Koffarnus MN, Collins GT, Rice KC, Chen J, Woods JH, Winger G (2011) Self-administration of agonists selective for dopamine D_2, D_3 and D_4 receptors by rhesus monkeys. *Behavioural Pharmacology* 23: 331–338.

124. Hu R, Song R, Yang R, Su R, Li J (2013) The dopamine D_3 receptor antagonist YQA14 that inhibits the expression and drug-primed reactivation of morphine-induced conditioned place preference. *European Journal of Pharmacology* 720: 212–217.

125. Banasikowski TJ, Bespalov A, Drescher K, Behl B, Unger L, Haupt A, et al. (2010) Double dissociation of the effects of haloperidol and the dopamine D3 receptor antagonist AB-127 on acquisition vs. expression of cocaine conditioned activity in rats. *Journal of Pharmacology and Experimental Therapeutics* 335: 506–515.

126. Stewart J (1992) Conditioned stimulus control of the expression of sensitization of the behavioral activating effects of opiate and stimulant drugs. In: Gormezano I, Wasserman

EA, eds., *Learning and Memory: Behavioral and Biological Substrates*. Lawrence Erlbaum Publishers: Hillsdale, NJ, pp. 129–159.

Steward J, Vezina P (1988) Conditioning and behavioral sensitization. In: Kalivas PW, Barnes CD, eds., *Sensitization in the Nervous System*. Telford Press: Caldwell, NJ, pp. 207–224.

See also Note 18 in Chapter 3.

127. Liang J, Zheng X, Chen J, Li Y, Xing X, Bai Y, Li Y (2011) Roles of BDNF, dopamine D$_3$ receptors, and their interactions in the expression of morphine-induced context-specific locomotor sensitization. *European Neuropsychopharmacology* 21: 825–834.

128. Banasikowski T, Beninger RJ (2012) Reduced expression of haloperidol conditioned catalepsy in rats by the dopamine D3 receptor antagonists nafadotride and NGB 2904. *European Neuropsychopharmacology* 22: 761–768.

129. Mogg K, Bradey BP, O'Neill B, Bani M, Merlo-Pich E, Koch A, et al. (2012) Effect of dopamine D$_3$ receptor antagonism on approach responses to cues in overweight and obese individuals. *Behavioural Pharmacology* 23: 603–608.

130. Le Foll B, Frances H, Diaz J, Schwartz JC, Sokoloff P (2002) Role of the dopamine D$_3$ receptor in reactivity to cocaine-associated cues in mice. *European Journal of Neuroscience* 15: 2016–2026.

131. Yan Y, Pushparaj A, Le Strat Y, Gamaleddin I, Barnes C, Justinova Z, et al. (2012) Blockade of dopamine D4 receptors attenuates reinstatement of extinguished nicotine-seeking behavior in rats. *Neuropsychopharmacology* 37: 685–696.

132. Woolley ML, Waters KA, Reavill C, Bull S, Lacroix LP, Martyn AJ, et al. (2008) Selective dopamine D$_4$ receptor agonist A-412997 improves cognitive performance and stimulates motor activity without influencing reward-related behaviour in rat. *Behavioural Pharmacology* 19: 765–776.

133. Ebstein RP, Novick O, Umansky R, Priel B, Osher Y, Blaine D, et al. (1996) Dopamine D4 receptor (*D4DR*) exon III polymorphism associated with human personality trait of novelty seeking. *Nature Genetics* 12: 78–80.

134. St Onge JR, Floresco SB (2009) Dopaminergic modulation of risk-based decision making. *Neuropsychopharmacology* 34: 681–697.

135. Koffanus MN, Hewman AH, Grundt P, Rice KC, Woods JH (2011) Effects of selective dopaminergic compounds on a delay-discounting task. *Behavioural Pharmacology* 22: 300–311.

136. Ferré S, Baler R, Bouvier M, Caron MG, Devi LA, Durroux T, et al. (2009) Building a new conceptual framework for receptor heteromers. *Nature Chemical Biology* 5: 131–134.

137. Jordan BA, Devi LA (1999) G-protein-coupled receptor heterodimerization modulates receptor function. *Nature* 399: 697–700.

138. Chun LS, Free RB, Doyle TB, Huang X-P, Rankin ML, Sibley DR (2013) D$_1$-D$_2$ dopamine receptor synergy promotes calcium signaling via multiple mechanisms. *Molecular Pharmacology* 84: 190–200.

Hasbi A, O'Dowd BF, George SR (2010) Heteromerization of dopamine D2 receptor with dopamine D1 or D5 receptors generates intracellular calcium signaling by different mechanisms. *Current Opinion in Pharmacology* 10: 93–99.

Lee SP, So CH, Rashid AJ, Varghese G, Cheng R, Lança AJ, et al. (2004) Dopamine D1 and D2 receptor co-activation generates a novel phospholipase C-mediated calcium signal. *Journal of Biological Chemistry* 279: 35671–35678.

Perreault ML, Hasbi A, Alijaniaram M, Fan T, Varghese G, Fletcher PJ, et al. (2010) The dopamine D1-D2 receptor heteromer localizes in dynorhphin/enkephalin neurons. *Journal of Biological Chemistry* 285: 36625–36634.

Perreault ML, Hasbi A, O'Dowd BF, George SR (2011) The dopamine D1-D2 receptor heteromer in striatal medium spiny neurons: evidence for a third distinct neuronal pathway in basal ganglia. *Frontiers in Neuroanatomy* 5: article 31.

Some recent opposition to the existence of D1–D2 receptor heteromers has also appeared:

Frederick AL, Yano H, Trifilieff P, Vishwasrao HD, Biezonski D, Mészáros J, et al. (2015) Evidence against dopamine D1/D2 receptor heteromeres. *Molecular Psychiatry* 20: 1373–1385.

139. Personal communication with Susan R. George, Pharmacology Department, University of Toronto.

140. Ferré S, Agnati LF, Ciruela F, Lluis C, Woods AS, Fuxe K, Franco R (2007) Neurotransmitter receptor heteromers and their integrative role in "local modules": the striatal spine module. *Brain Research Reviews* 55: 55–67.

Ferré S, Ciruela R, Woods AS, Lluis C, Franco R (2007) Functional relevance of neurotransmitter receptor heteromers in the central nervous system. *Trends in Neurosciences* 30: 440–446.

Ferré S, Goldberg SR, LLuis C, Franco R (2009) Looking for the role of cannabinoid receptor heteromers in striatal function. *Neuropharmacology* 56(Suppl. 1): 226–234.

Prinster SC, Hague C, Hall RA (2005) Heterodimerization of G protein-coupled receptors: specificity and functional significance. *Pharmacological Reviews* 57: 289–298.

141. Fiorentini C, Busi C, Gorruso E, Gotti C, Spano PF, Missale C (2008) Reciprocal regulation of dopamine D1 and D3 receptor function and trafficking by heterodimerization. *Molecular Pharmacology* 74: 59–69.

Marcellino D, Ferré S, Casadó V, Cortés A, Le Foll B, Mazzola C, et al. (2008) Identification of dopamine D1–D3 receptor heteromers: indications for a role of synergistic D1–D3 receptor interactions in the striatum. *Journal of Biological Chemistry* 283: 26016–26025.

142. Scott L, Aperia A (2009) Interaction between *N*-methyl-D-aspartate acid receptors and D2 dopamine receptors: an important mechanism for brain plasticity. *Neuroscience* 158: 62–66.

143. Ferré S (2008) An update on the mechanisms of the psychostimulant effects of caffeine. *Journal of Neurochemistry* 105: 1067–1079

Ferré S, Borycz J, Goldberg SR, Hope BT, Morales M, Lluis C, et al. (2005) Role of adenosine in the control of homosynaptic plasticity in striatal excitatory synapses. *Journal of Integrative Neuroscience* 4: 445–464.

Ferré S, Quiroz C, Woods AS, Cunha R, Popoli P, Lluis C, et al. (2008) An update on adenosine A_{2A}-dopamine D_2 receptor interactions: implications for the function of G protein-coupled receptors. *Current Pharmaceutical Design* 14: 1468–1474.

144. Soria G, Castañe A, Ledent C, Parmentier M, Maldonado R, Valverde O (2006) The lack of A_{2A} adenosine receptors diminishes the reinforcing efficacy of cocaine. *Neuropsychopharmacology* 31: 978–987.

145. Kern, A, Albarran-Zeckler R, Walsh HE, Smith RG (2012) Apo-ghrelin receptor forms heteromers with DRD2 in hypothalamic neurons and is essential for anorexigenic effects of DRD2 agonism. *Neuron* 73: 317–332.

Chapter 8

1. Rilling JK, Sanfey AG, Aronson JA, Nystrom LE, Cohen JD (2004) Opposing BOLD responses to reciprocated and unreciprocated altruism in putative reward pathways. *NeuroReport* 15: 2539–2543.

See also:

Sun P, Zheng L, Li L, Guo X, Zhang W, Zheng V (2016) The neural responses to social cooperation in gain and loss contexts. *PLOS ONE* 11: e0160503.

2. Rilling JK, Gutman DA, Zeh, TR, Pagnoni G, Berns GS, Kitts CD (2002) A neural basis for social cooperation. *Neuron* 35: 395–405.

3. See Notes 135 and 136 in Chapter 5.

4. King-Casas B, Tomlin D, Anen C, Cramerer CF, Quartz SR, Montague PR (2005) Getting to know you: recognition and trust in a two-person economic exchange. *Science* 308: 78–83.

See also:

Kishida KT, Montague PR (2012) Imaging models of valuation during social interaction in humans. *Biological Psychiatry* 72: 93–100.

5. Aron A, Fisher H, Mashek DJ, Strong G, Li H, Brown LL (2005) Reward, motivation, and emotion systems associated with early-stage intense romantic love. *Journal of Neurophysiology* 94: 327–337.

See also:

Bartels A, Zeki S (2000) The neural basis of romantic love. *NeuroReport* 11: 3829–3834.

Ortigue S, Bianchi-Demicheli R, Hamilton AF, Grafton ST (2007) The neural basis of love as a subliminal prime: an event-related functional magnetic resonance imaging study. *Journal of Cognitive Neuroscience* 19: 1218–1230.

Ortigue S, Bianchi-Demicheli, Pastel N, Frum C, Lewis JW (2010) Neuroimaging of love: fMRI meta-analysis evidence toward new perspectives in sexual medicine. *Journal of Sexual Medicine* 7: 3541–3552.

Xu X, Aron A, Brown L, Cao G, Feng T, Wang X (2010) Reward and motivation systems: a brain mapping study of early-stage intense romantic love in Chinese participants. *Human Brain Mapping* 32: 249–257.

6. Acevedo BP, Aron A, Fisher HE, Brown LL (2012) Neural correlates of long-term intense romantic love. *Social, Cognitive and Affective Neuroscience* 7: 145–159.

7. Bartels A, Zeki S (2004) The neural correlates of maternal and romantic love. *NeuroImage* 21: 1155–1166.

See also:

Noriuchi M, Kikuchi Y, Senoo A (2008) The functional neuroanatomy of maternal love: mother's response to infant's attachment behaviors. *Biological Psychiatry* 63: 415–423.

8. Klucharev V, Smidts A, Fernández G (2008) Brain mechanisms of persuasion: how "expert power" modulates memory and attitudes. *Social, Cognitive and Affective Neuroscience* 3: 353–366.

9. Walter NT, Markettt SA, Montag C, Reuter M (2011) A genetic contribution to cooperation: dopamine-relevant genes are associated with social facilitation. *Social Neuroscience* 6: 289–301.

10. O'Connell LA, Hofmann HA (2011) The vertebrate mesolimbic reward system and social behavior network: a comparative synthesis. *Journal of Comparative Neurology* 519: 3599–3639.

    See also:

    Stoesz BM, Hare JF, Snow WM (2013) Neurophysiological mechanisms underlying affiliative social behavior: insight from comparative research. *Neuroscience and Biobehavioral Reviews* 37: 123–132.

11. Sofroniew MV (1983) Morphology of vasopressin and oxytocin neurons and their central and vascular projections. *Progress in Brain Research* 60: 101–114.

12. Lim MM, Young LJ (2006) Neuropeptidergic regulation of affiliative behavior and social bonding in animals. *Hormones and Behavior* 50: 506–517.

13. Pedersen CA, Ascher JA, Monroe YL, Prange AJ Jr (1982) Oxytocin induces maternal behavior in virgin female rats. *Science* 216: 648–650.

    Pedersen CA, Caldwell JD, Walker C, Ayers G, Mason GA (1994) Oxytocin activates the postpartum onset of maternal behavior in the ventral tegmental and medial preoptic areas. *Behavioral Neuroscience* 108: 1163–1171.

14. Strathearn L (2011) Maternal neglect: oxytocin, dopamine and the neurobiology of attachment. *Journal of Neuroendocrinology* 23: 1054–1065.

15. Williams JR, Carter CS, Insel T (1992) Partner preference development in female prairie voles is facilitated by mating or the central infusion of oxytocin. *Annals of the New York Academy of Sciences* 652: 487–489.

16. Donaldson ZR, Young LJ (2008) Oxytocin, vasopressin, and the neurogenetics of sociality. *Science* 322: 900–904.

17. Numan M, Stolzenberg DS (2009) Medial preoptic area interactions with dopamine neural systems in the control of the onset and maintenance of maternal behavior in rats. *Frontiers in Neuroendocrinology* 30: 46–64.

18. Love TM, Enoch M-A, Hodgkinson CA, Peciña M, Mickey B, Koeppe RA, et al. (2012) Oxytocin gene polymorphisms influence human dopaminergic function in a sex-dependent manner. *Biological Psychiatry* 72: 198–206.

19. Winslow JR, Hastings N, Carter CS, Harbaugh CR, Insel TR (1993) A role for central vasopressin in pair bonding in monogamous prairie voles. *Nature* 365: 545–548.

20. Lim MM, Wang Z, Olazabal DE, Rem X, Terwilliger EF, Young LJ (2004) Enhanced partner preference in a promiscuous species by manipulating the expression of a single gene. *Nature* 429: 754–757.

21. Skuse DH, Gallagher L (2011) Genetic influences on social cognition. *Pediatric Research* 69: 85R–91R.

22. Fisher HE, Aron A, Brown LL (2006) Romantic love: a mammalian brain system for mate choice. *Philosophical Transactions of the Royal Society B Biological Sciences* 361: 2173–2186.

23. Grant KA, Shively CA, Nader MA, Ehrenkaufer RL, Line SW, Morton TE, et al. (1998) Effect of social status on striatal dopamine D_2 receptor binding characteristics in cynomolgus monkeys assessed with positron emission tomography. *Synapse* 29: 80–83.

24. Stolzenberg DS, McKenna JB, Keough S, Hancock R, Numan MJ, Numan M (2007) Dopamine D_1 receptor stimulation of the nucleus accumbens or the medial preoptic area promotes the onset of maternal behavior in pregnancy-terminated rats. *Behavioral Neuroscience* 121: 907–919.

    Stolzenberg DS, Zhang KY, Luskin K, Ranker L, Bress J, Numan M (2010) Dopamine D_1 receptor activation of adenylyl cyclase, not phospholipase C, in the nucleus accumbens promotes maternal behavior in rats. *Hormones and Behavior* 57: 96–104.

    See also Note 17.

    See review by:

    Rilling JK, Young LJ (2014) The biology of mammalian parenting and its effect on offspring social development. *Science* 345: 771–776.

25. Champagne FA, Chretien P, Stevenson CW, Zhang TY, Gratton A, Meaney MJ (2004) Variations in nucleus accumbens dopamine associated with individual differences in maternal behavior in the rat. *Journal of Neuroscience* 24: 4113–4123.

26. Hansen S (1994) Maternal behavior of female rats with 6-OHDA lesions of the ventral striatum: characterization of the pup retrieval deficit. *Physiology and Behavior* 55: 615–620.

    Hansen S, Harthon C, Willin E, Lofberg L, Svensson K (1991) The effects of 6-OHDA-induced dopamine depletions in the ventral or dorsal striatum on maternal and sexual behavior in the female rat. *Pharmacology, Biochemistry and Behavior* 39: 71–77.

27. Giordano B, Johnson AE, Rosenblatt JS (1990) Haloperidol-induced disruption of retrieval behavior and reversal with apomorphine in lactating rats. *Physiology and Behavior* 48: 211–214.

    Keer SE, Stern JM (1999) Dopamine receptor blockade in the nucleus accumbens inhibits maternal retrieval and licking, but enhances nursing in lactating rats. *Physiology and Behavior* 67: 659–669.

    Numan M, Numan MJ, Pliakou N, Stolzenberg DS, Mullins OJ, Murphy JM, Smith CD (2005) The effects of D1 and D2 dopamine receptor antagonism in the medial preoptic area, ventral pallidum, or nucleus accumbens on the maternal retrieval response and other aspects of maternal behavior in rats. *Behavioral Neuroscience* 119: 1588–1604.

    Stern JM, Taylor LA (1991) Haloperidol inhibits maternal retrieval and licking, but facilitates nursing behavior and milk ejection in lactating rats. *Journal of Neuroendocrinology* 3: 591–596.

28. Alfonso VM, King S, Chatterjee D, Fleming A (2009) Hormones that increase maternal responsiveness affect accumbal dopaminergic responses to pup- and food-stimuli in the female rat. *Hormones and Behavior* 56: 11–23.

    Hansen S, Bergvall AH, Nyiredi S (1993) Interaction with pups enhances dopamine release in the ventral striatum of maternal rats: a microdialysis study. *Pharmacology, Biochemistry and Behavior* 45: 673–676.

29. Fleming AS, Kosmit M, Deller M (1994) Rats pups are potent reinforcers to the maternal animal: effects of experience, parity, hormones and dopamine function. *Psychobiology* 22: 44–53.

    Lee A, Clancy S, Fleming AS (1999) Mother rats bar-press for pups: effects of lesions of the mpoa and limbic sites on maternal behavior and operant responding for pup-reinforcement. *Behavioural Brain Research* 100: 15–31.

30. Thiel KJ, Okum AC, Neisewander JL (2008) Social reward-conditioned place preference: a model revealing an interaction between cocaine and social context rewards in rats. *Drug and Alcohol Dependence* 96: 202–212.

    See also:

    Fritz M, El Rawas R, Salti A, Klement S, Bardo MT, Kemmler G, et al. (2011) Reversal of cocaine-conditioned place preference and mesocorticolimbic Zif268 expression by social interaction in rats. *Addiction Biology* 16: 273–284.

    El Rawas R, Klement S, Kummer KK, Fritz M, Dechant G, Saria A, Zemig G (2012) Brain regions associated with the acquisition of conditioned place preference for cocaine vs. social interaction. *Frontiers in Behavioral Neuroscience* 6: article 63.

31. Gunaydin LA, Grosenick L, Finkelstein JC, Kauvar IV, Fenno LE, Adhikari A, et al. (2014) Natural neural projection dynamics underlying social behavior. *Cell* 157: 1535–1551.

32. Bartal IB-A, Decety J, Mason P (2011) Empathy and pro-social behavior in rats. *Science* 334: 1427–1430.

33. Brudzynski SM (2013) Ethotransmission: communication of emotional states through ultrasonic vocalizations in rats. *Current Opinions in Neurobiology* 23: 310–317.

34. Burgdorf J, Kroes RA, Moskal JR, Pfaus JG, Brudzynski SM, Panksepp J (2008) Ultrasonic vocalizations of rats (*Rattus norvegicus*) during mating, play, and aggression: behavioral concomitants, relationship to reward, and self-administration of playback. *Journal of Comparative Psychology* 122: 357–367.

35. Anstrom KK, Miczek KA, Budygin EA (2009) Increased phasic dopamine signaling in the mesolimbic pathway during social defeat in rats. *Neuroscience* 161: 3–12.

    Tidey JW, Miczek KA (1996) Social defeat stress selectively alters mesocorticolimbic dopamine release: an in vivo microdialysis study. *Brain Research* 721: 140–149.

36. Miczek KA, Nikulina EM, Shimamoto A, Covington HE III (2011) Escalated or suppressed cocaine reward, tegmental BDNF, and accumbal dopamine caused by episodic versus continuous social stress in rats. *Journal of Neuroscience* 31: 9848–9857.

    Shimamoto A, DeBold JF, Holly EN, Miczek KA (2011) Blunted accumbal dopamine response to cocaine following chronic social stress in female rats: exploring a link between depression and drug abuse. *Psychopharmacology* 218: 271–279.

    See also:

    Tanaka K, Furuyashiki T, Kitaoka S, Senzai Y, Imoto Y, Segi-Nishida E, et al. (2012) Prostaglandin E_2-mediated attenuation of mesocortical dopaminergic pathway is critical to susceptibility to repeated social defeat stress in mice. *Journal of Neuroscience* 32: 4319–4329.

37. Aragona BJ, Liu Y, Yu YJ, Curtis JT, Detwiler JM, Insel TR, Wang Z (2006) Nucleus accumbens dopamine differentially mediates the formation and maintenance of monogamous pair bonds. *Nature Neuroscience* 9: 133–139s.

Aragona BJ, Wang Z (2004) The prairie vole (*Microtus ochrogaster*): an animal model of behavioral neuroendocrine research on pair bonding. *ILAR Journal* 45: 35–45.

Aragona BJ, Wang Z (2009) Dopamine regulation of social choice in a monogamous rodent species. *Frontiers in Behavioral Neuroscience* 3: article 15.

Burkett JP, Young LJ (2012) The behavioral, anatomical and pharmacological parallels between social attachment, love and addiction. *Psychopharmacology* 224: 1–26.

Curtis JT, Liu Y, Aragona BJ, Wang Z (2006) Dopamine and monogamy. *Brain Research* 1126: 76–90.

38. Aragona BJ, Liu Y, Curtis JT, Stephan FK, Wang Z (2003) A critical role for nucleus accumbens dopamine in partner-preference formation in male prairie voles. *Journal of Neuroscience* 23: 3483–3490.

Wang Z, Yu G, Cascio C, Liu Y, Gingrich B, Insel TR (1999) Dopamine D2 receptor-mediated regulation of partner preference in female prairie voles (*Microtus ochrogaster*): a mechanism for pair bonding? *Behavioral Neuroscience* 113: 602–611.

39. Gingrich B, Liu Y, Cascio C, Wang Z, Insel TR (2000) Dopamine D2 receptors in the nucleus accumbens are important for social attachment in female prairie voles (*Microtus ochrogaster*). *Behavioral Neuroscience* 114: 173–183.

40. Bell MR, Meerts SH, Sisk CL (2010) Male Syrian hamsters demonstrate a conditioned place preference for sexual behavior and female chemosensory stimuli. *Hormones and Behavior* 58: 410–414.

Bell MR, Sisk CL (2013) Dopamine mediates testosterone-induced social reward in male Syrian hamsters. *Endocrinology* 154: 1225–1234.

41. Schulz KM, Richardson HN, Romeo RD, Morris JA, Lookingland KJ, Sisk CL (2003) Medial preoptic area dopaminergic responses to female pheromones develop during puberty in the male Syrian hamster. *Brain Research* 988: 139–145.

42. Meisel RL, Joppa MA, Rowe RK (1996) Dopamine receptor antagonists attenuate conditioned place preference following sexual behavior in female Syrian hamsters. *European Journal of Pharmacology* 309: 21–24.

43. Schwartzer JJ, Ricci LA, Kelloni RH Jr (2013) Prior fighting experience increases aggression in Syrian hamsters: implications for a role of dopamine in the winner effect. *Aggressive Behavior* 39: 290–300.

44. Fish EW, DeBold JF, Miczek KA (2005) Escalated aggression as a reward: corticosterone and GABA$_A$ receptor positive modulators in mice. *Psychopharmacology* 182: 116–127.

May ME, Kennedy CH (2009) Aggression as positive reinforcement in mice under various ratio- and time-based reinforcement schedules. *Journal of the Experimental Analysis of Behavior* 91: 185–196.

45. Couppis MH, Kennedy CH (2008) The rewarding effect of aggression is reduced by nucleus accumbens dopamine receptor antagonism in mice. *Psychopharmacology* 197: 449–456.

46. van Erp AM, Miczek KA (2000) Aggressive behavior, increased accumbal dopamine, and decreased cortical serotonin in rats. *Journal of Neuroscience* 20: 9320–9335.

47. von Holst E (1954) Relations between the central nervous system and the peripheral organs. *British Journal of Animal Behavior* 2: 89–94.

48. Riters LV (2011) Pleasure seeking and birdsong. *Neuroscience and Biobehavioral Reviews* 35: 1837–1845.

49. Heimovics SA, Riters LV (2008) Evidence that dopamine within motivation and song control brain regions regulates birdsong context-dependently. *Physiology and Behavior* 95: 258–266.

50. Alger SJ, Juang C, Riters LV (2011) Social affiliation relates to tyrosine hydroxylase immunolabeling in male and female zebra finches (*Taeniopygia guttata*). *Journal of Chemical Neuroanatomy* 42: 45–55.

51. Sasaki A, Sotnikova TD, Gainetdinov RP, Jarvis ED (2006) Social context-dependent singing-related dopamine. *Journal of Neuroscience* 26: 9010–9014.

52. Huang Y-C, Hessler NA (2008) Social modulation during songbird courtship potentiates midbrain dopaminergic neurons. *PLOS ONE* 3(10): e3281.

53. Goodson JL, Kabelik D, Kelly AM, Rinaldi J, Klatt JD (2009) Midbrain dopamine neurons reflect affiliation phenotypes in finches and are tightly coupled to courtship. *Proceedings of the National Academy of Sciences of the United States of America* 106: 8737–8742.

54. Harding CF (2004) Brief alteration in dopaminergic function during development causes deficits in adult reproductive behavior. *Journal of Neurobiology* 61: 301–308.

55. Rauceo S, Harding CF, Maldonado A, Gaysinkaya L, Tulloch I, Rodriguez E (2008) Dopaminergic modulation of reproductive behavior and activity in male zebra finches. *Behavioural Brain Research* 187: 133–139.

56. Pawlisch BA, Riters LV (2010) Selective behavioral responses to male song are affected by the dopamine agonist GBR-12909 in female European starlings (*Sturnus vulgaris*). *Brain Research* 1353: 113–124.

57. Leblois A (2013) Social modulation of learned behavior by dopamine in the basal ganglia: insights from songbirds. *Journal of Physiology Paris* 107: 219–229.

58. Gadagkar V, Puzerey PA, Chen R, Baird-Daniel E, Farhang AR, Goldberg JH (2016) Dopamine neurons encode performance error in singing birds. *Science* 354: 1278–1282.

59. Whether incentive stimuli are unconditioned or conditioned is not a simple matter. Animals generally have a social and conditioning history prior to their participation in neuroscience experiments. Are sexually mature female conspecifics unconditionally attractive to males or has their prior social experience led to learning that underlies this attraction? I suggested in the text that the taste of food to a rat is unconditioned, but it is well known that flavor preferences can be conditioned, as discussed in Chapter 7. A newborn mammal shows an unconditioned attraction to its mother's teat and perhaps to the taste of her milk. From then on, learning, including incentive learning will begin to operate, honing the stimuli to which the individual responds. There appears to be an unconditioned natural proclivity to respond to certain stimuli over others, as demonstrated by the ethologists (Note 10 in Chapter 2), for example, but learning mechanism quickly modify responses to stimuli making the distinction between unconditioned and conditioned stimuli often fuzzy.

60. Simonyan K, Horwitz B, Jarvis ED (2012) Dopamine regulation of human speech and bird song: a critical review. *Brain and Language* 122: 142–150.

See also:

Warlaumont AS, Finnegan MK (2016) Learning to produce syllabic speech sounds via reward-modulated neural plasticity. *PLOS ONE* 11: e0145096.

61. Skinner BF (1957) *Verbal Behavior*. Appleton-Century-Crofts: New York.

62. Chomsky N (1959) Verbal behavior. By B. F. Skinner. *Language* 35: 26–58.

63. Kleitz-Nelson H, Dominquez JM, Cornil CA, Ball GF (2010) Is sexual motivational state linked to dopamine release in the medial preoptic area? *Behavioral Neuroscience* 124: 300–304.

64. Kleitz-Nelson H, Cornil CA, Balthazart J, Ball GF (2010) Differential effects of central injections of D1 and D2 receptor agonists and antagonists on male sexual behavior in Japanese quail. *European Journal of Neuroscience* 32: 118–129.

65. Woolley SC, Sakata JT, Gupta A, Crews D (2001) Evolutionary changes in dopaminergic modulation of courtship behavior in *Cnemidophorus* whiptail lizards. *Hormones and Behavior* 40: 483–489.

    There are further complexities in this study that I did not discuss in the main text. *C. uniparens* is a parthenogenetic (all-female) species, but individuals display both male- and female-typical sexual behaviors. *Cnemidophorus inornatus* is a sexual species. In spite of their evolutionary divergence, the sexual behavior of both species was similarly affected by manipulations of dopaminergic neurotransmission.

66. Woolley SC, Sakata JT, Crews D (2004) Evolutionary insights into the regulation of courtship behavior in male amphibians and reptiles. *Physiology and Behavior* 83: 347–360.

67. Korzan WJ, Forster GL, Watt MJ, Summers CH (2006) Dopaminergic activity modulation via aggression, status, and a visual social signal. *Behavioral Neuroscience* 120: 93–102.

68. Sakata JT, Crews D (2003) Embryonic temperature shapes behavioural change following social experience in male leopard geckos, *Eublepharis macularius*. *Animal Behaviour* 66: 839–846.

69. Dias BG, Ataya RS, Rushworth D, Zhao J, Crews D (2007) Effect of incubation temperature and androgens on dopaminergic activity in the leopard gecko, *Eublepharis macularius*. *Developmental Neurobiology* 67L: 630636.

70. Creighton A, Satterfield D, Chu J (2013) Effects of dopamine agonists on calling behavior in the green tree frog, *Hyla cinerea*. *Physiology and Behavior* 116: 54–59.

71. Endepoles H, Schul J, Gerhardt HC, Walkowiak W (2004) 6-Hydroxydopamine lesions in anuran amphibians: a new model system for Parkinson's disease? *Journal of Neurobiology* 60: 395–410.

72. Barbeau A, Dallaire L, Buu NT, Poirier J, Rucinska E (1985) Comparative behavioral, biochemical and pigmentary effects of MPTP, MPP+ and paraquate in *Rana pipiens*. *Life Sciences* 37: 1529–1538.

    Barbeau A, Dallaire L, Buu NT, Veilleux F, Boyer H, de Lanney LE, et al. (1985) New amphibian models for the study of 1-methyl-4-phenyl-1,2,3,6-tetrahydropyridine (MPTP). *Life Sciences* 36: 1125–1134.

73. Moncalvo VGR, Burmeister SS, Pfenning KS (2013) Social signals increase monoamine levels in the tegmentum of juvenile Mexican spadefoot toads (*Spea multiplicata*). *Journal of Comparative Physiology A* 199: 681–691.

74. Seghers BH (1974) Schooling behavior in the guppy (*Poecilia reticulate*): an evolutionary response to predation. *Evolution* 28: 486–489.

75. Buske C, Gerlai R (2012) Maturation of shoaling behavior is accompanied by changes in the dopaminergic and serotonergic systems in zebrafish. *Developmental Psychobiology* 54: 28–35.

76. Engeszer RE, Barbiano LA, Ryan MJ, Parichy DM (2007) Timing and plasticity of shoaling behaviour in the zebrafish, *Danio rerio*. *Animal Behaviour* 74: 1269–1275.

77. Al-Imari L, Gerlai R (2008) Sight of conspecifics as reward in associative learning in zebrafish (*Danio rerio*). *Behavioural Brain Research* 189: 216–219.

78. Scerbina T, Chatterjee D, Gerlai R (2012) Dopamine receptor antagonism disrupts social preference in zebrafish: a strain comparison study. *Amino Acids* 43: 2059–2072.

79. Saif, M, Chatterjee D, Buske C, Gerlai R (2013) Sight of conspecific images induces changes in neurochemistry in zebrafish. *Behavioural Brain Research* 243: 294–299.

80. Winberg S, Nilsson GE (1992) Induction of social dominance by L-dopa treatment in Arctic charr. *NeuroReport* 3: 243–246.

81. Teles MC, Dahlbom SJ, Winberg S, Oliveira RF (2013) Social modulation of brain mono-amine levels in zebrafish. *Behavioural Brain Research* 253: 17–24.

    See also:

    Winberg S, Nilsson GE, Olsen KH (1991) Social rank and brain levels of monoamines and monoamine metabolites in Arctic charr, *Salvelinus alpinus* (L.). *Journal of Comparative Physiology A* 168: 241–246.

82. Perry CJ, Barron AB (2013) Neural mechanisms of reward in insects. *Annual Review of Entomology* 58: 543–562.

    Waddell S (2013) Reinforcement signalling in *Drosophila*; dopamine does it all after all. *Current Opinion in Neurobiology* 23: 324–329.

83. Strausfeld NJ, Hirsh F (2013) Deep homology of arthropod central complex and verte-brate basal ganglia. *Science* 340: 157–161.

84. Alekseyenko OV, Lee C, Kravitz EA (2010) Targeted manipulation of serotonergic neuro-transmission affects the escalation of aggression in adult male *Drosophila melanogaster*. *PLOS ONE* 5: e10806.

85. Sasaki K, Nagao T (2013) Juvenile hormone-dopamine systems for the promotion of flight activity in males of the large carpenter bee *Xylocopa appendiculata*. *Naturwissenschaften* 100: 1183–1186.

86. Ma Z, Guo W, Guo X, Wang X, Kang L (2011) Modulation of behavioral phase changes of the migratory locust by the catecholamine metabolic pathway. *Proceedings of the National Academy of Sciences of the United States of America* 108: 3882–3887.

    Yang M, Wei Y, Jiang F, Wang Y, Guo X, He J, Kang L (2014) Micro-RNA-133 inhibits behavioral aggregation by controlling dopamine synthesis in locusts. *PLOS ONE* 10: e1004206.

Chapter 9

1. Kraepelin E (1919) *Dementia Praexox and Paraphrenia*. Translated by Barclay RM, edited by Robertson GM and reprinted in 1971 by Robert E Krieger Publishing Co. Inc.: Huntington, NY; originally published in German in Kraepelin E (1913) *Psychiatrie*.

Ein Lehrbuch für Studierende und Ärzte. Achte, vollständig umgearbeitete Auflage, III. Band, II. Teil. Klinische Psychiatrie. Johann Ambrosius Barth: Leipzig.

2. Bleuler E (1911) *Dementia Praecox or the Group of Schizophrenias.* Translated by Zinkin J and published in 1950 by International Universities Press: New York; originally published as *Dementia Praecox oder Gruppe der Schizophrenien.* Franz Deuticke: Leipzig

3. American Psychiatric Association (2000) *Diagnostic and Statistical Manual of Mental Disorders, Fourth Edition, Text Revision.* American Psychiatric Association: Washington, DC.

4. American Psychiatric Association (2013) *Diagnostic and Statistical Manual of Mental Disorders, Fifth Edition.* American Psychiatric Association: Washington, DC.

5. Bowie CR, Jaga K (2007) Methods for treating cognitive deficits in schizophrenia. *Expert Review in Neurotherapeutics* 7: 281–287.

   Frangou S (2010) Cognitive function in early onset schizophrenia: a selective review. *Frontiers in Human Neuroscience* 3: article 79.

   Keefe RSE, Harvey PD (2012) Cognitive impairment in schizophrenia. In: Geyer MA, Gross G, eds., *Novel Antischizophrenia Treatments, Handbook of Experimental Pharmacology.* Springer: Berlin, pp. 11–37.

   Sip E, Chouinard S, Boulay LJ (2005) On the trail of a cognitive enhancer for the treatment of schizophrenia. *Progress in Neruo-Psychopharmacology & Biological Psychiatry* 29: 219–232.

   Young JW, Powell S, Risbrough V, Marston HM, Geyer MA (2009) Using the MATRICS to guide development of a preclinical cognitive test battery for research in schizophrenia. *Pharmacology and Therapeutics* 122: 150–202.

6. Parkinson J (2002) An essay on the shaking palsy. *Journal of Neuropsychiatry and Clinical Neuroscience* 14: 223–236; originally published in 1817 as a monograph of the same title by Sherwood, Neely, and Jones.

7. Doyle R (2004) The history of adult attention-deficit/hyperactivity disorder. *Psychiatric Clinics of North America* 27: 203–214.

8. Crichton A (2008) An inquiry into the nature and origin of mental derangement. On attention and its diseases. *Journal of Attention Disorders* 12: 200–204; originally published as: Crichton A (1798) *An Inquiry into the Nature and Origin of Mental Derangement: Comprehending a Concise System of the Physiology and Pathology of the Human Mind and a History of the Passions and their Effects.* Cadell T Jr, Davies W: London.

9. Lange KW, Reichi S, Lange KM, Tucha L, Tucha O (2010) The history of attention deficit hyperactivity disorder. *Attention Deficit Hyperactivity Disorder* 2: 241–255.

10. The term "dopamine hypothesis of schizophrenia" is seen frequently in the literature. However, as discussed in the text, schizophrenia is characterized by positive, negative, and cognitive symptoms. Medications used to treat schizophrenia are very effective at reducing positive symptoms, i.e., hallucinations and delusions, but much less effective at ameliorating negative and cognitive symptoms. This suggests that the term "dopamine hypothesis of psychosis" might be more appropriate, and some authors have used this

term. Because of general use, I have employed "dopamine hypothesis of schizophrenia" or, more briefly, "dopamine hypothesis" in the text.

See also:

Brisch R, Saniotis A, Wolf R, Bielau H, Bernstein H-G, Steiner J, et al. (2014) The role of dopamine in schizophrenia from a neurobiological and evolutionary perspective: old fashioned, but still in vogue. *Frontiers in Psychiatry* 5: article 47.

Davis KL, Kahn RS, Ko G, Davidson M (1991) Dopamine in schizophrenia: a review and reconceptualization. *American Journal of Psychiatry* 148: 1474–1486.

Miller R (1981) Major psychosis and dopamine: controversial features and some suggestions. *Psychological Medicine* 14: 779–789.

11. See Note 13 in Chapter 7.

12. Ban TA (2007) Fifty years chlorpromazine: a historical perspective. *Neuropsychiatric Disease and Treatment* 3: 495–500.

13. Iyo M, Tadokoro S, Kanahara N, Hashimoto T, Nitsu T, Watanabe H, Hashimoto K (2013) Optimal extent of dopamine D2 receptor occupancy by antipsychotics for treatment of dopamine supersensitivity psychosis and late-onset psychosis. *Journal of Clinical Psychopharmacology* 33: 398–404.

Toda M, Abi-Dargham A (2007) Dopamine hypothesis of schizophrenia: making sense of it all. *Current Psychiatry Reports* 9: 329–336.

See also Note 19 in Chapter 7.

14. Post RM (1975) Cocaine psychoses: a continuum model. *American Journal of Psychiatry* 132: 225–231.

Post RM, Kopanda RT (1976) Cocaine, kindling, and psychosis. *American Journal of Psychiatry* 133: 627–632.

Snyder SH (1972) Catecholamines in the brain as mediators of amphetamine psychosis. *Archives of General Psychiatry* 27: 169–179.

15. Moskovitz C, Moses H, Klawans HL (1978) Levodopa-induced psychosis: a kindling phenomenon. *American Journal of Psychiatry* 135: 669–675.

16. Lee T, Seeman P (1980) Elevation of brain neuroleptic/dopamine receptors in schizophrenia. *American Journal of Psychiatry* 137: 191–197.

Lee T, Seeman P, Tourtellotte WW, Farley IJ, Hornykiewicz O (1978) Binding of ^{3}H-neuroleptics and ^{3}H-apomorphine in schizophrenic brains. *Nature* 274: 897–900.

17. See Note 15 in Chapter 7.

18. Cross AJ, Crow TJ, Owen F (1981) ^{3}H-flupenthixol binding in post-mortem brains of schizophrenics: evidence for a selective increase in dopamine D2 receptors. *Psychopharmacology* 74: 122–124.

Owen F, Cross AJ, Crow TJ, Longden A, Poulter M, Riley GJ (1978) Increased dopamine-receptor sensitivity in schizophrenia. *Lancet* 312: 223–225.

Owen R, Owen F, Poulter M, Crow TJ (1984) Dopamine D$_2$ receptors in substantia nigra in schizophrenia. *Brain Research* 299: 152–154.

19. Seeman P (1987) Dopamine receptors and the dopamine hypothesis of schizophrenia. *Synapse* 1: 133–152.

20. Abi-Dargham A, Rodenhiser J, Printz D, Zea-Ponce Y, Gil R, Kegeles LS, et al. (2000) Increased baseline occupancy of D_2 receptors by dopamine in schizophrenia. *Proceedings of the National Academy of Sciences of the United States of America* 97: 8104–8109.

21. Abi-Dargham A (2004) Do we still believe the dopamine hypothesis? New data bring new evidence. *International Journal of Neuropharmacology* 7(Suppl. 1): S1–S5.

    Howes OD (2012) From the prodrome to chronic schizophrenia: the neurobiology underlying psychotic symptoms and cognitive impairments. *Current Pharmacological Design* 18: 459–465.

    Kuepper R (2012) The dopamine dysfunction in schizophrenia revisited: new insights into topography and course. *Handbook of Experimental Pharmacology* 212: 1–26.

    Lyon GJ, Abi-Dargham A, Moore H, Lieberman JA, Javitch JA, Sulzer D (2011) Presynaptic regulation of dopamine transmission in schizophrenia. *Schizophrenia Bulletin* 37: 108–117.

    Miyake N, Thompson J, Skinbjerg M, Abi-Dargham A (2010) Presynaptic dopamine in schizophrenia. *CNS Neuroscience & Therapeutics* 17: 104–109.

22. Allen NC, Bagade S, McQueen MB, Ioannidis JPA, Kavvoura FK, Khoury MJ, et al. (2008) Systematic meta-analyses and field synopsis of genetic association studies in schizophrenia: the SzGene database. *Nature Genetics* 40: 827–834.

23. Sanders AR, Duan J, Levinson DF, Shi J, He D, Hou C, et al. (2008) No significant association of 14 candidate genes with schizophrenia in a large European ancestry sample: implications for psychiatric genetics. *American Journal of Psychiatry* 165: 497–506.

24. Greenwood TA, Light GA, Swerdlow NR, Radant AD, Braff DL (2012) Association analysis of 94 candidate genes and schizophrenia-related endophenotypes. *PLOS ONE* 7: e29630.

    Lencz T and multiple coauthors (2014) Molecular genetic evidence for overlap between general cognitive ability and risk for schizophrenia: a report from the Cognitive Genomics consorTium (COGENT). *Molecular Genetics* 19: 168–174.

25. Liang SG, Greenwood TA (2015) The impact of clinical heterogeneity in schizophrenia on genomic analyses. *Schizophrenia Research* 161: 490–495.

    Mowrey BJ, Gratton J (2013) The emerging spectrum of allelic variation in schizophrenia: current evidence and strategies for the identification and functional characterization of common and rare variants. *Molecular Psychiatry* 18: 38–52.

26. Kim Y, Zerwas S, Trace SE, Sullivan PF (2011) Schizophrenia genetics: what next? *Schizophrenia Bulletin* 37: 456–463.

    See Mowrey and Gratton in Note 25.

27. Schizophrenia Psychiatric Genome-Wide Association Study (GWAS) Consortium (2011) Genome-wide association study identifies five new schizophrenia loci. *Nature Genetics* 45: 969–976.

28. See Beninger references, sometimes with co-authors, in Notes 14 and 15 in Chapter 2 and:

    Beninger RJ (1988) The slow therapeutic action of antipsychotic drugs: a possible mechanism involving the role of dopamine in incentive learning. In: Simon P, Soubrié P,

Wildlocher D, eds., *Animal Models of Psychiatric Disorders Volume 1: Selected Models of Anxiety, Depression and Psychosis*. Karger: Basel, pp. 36–51.

29. Heinz A, Schlagenhauf F (2010) Dopaminergic dysfunction in schizophrenia: salience attribution revisited. *Schizophrenia Bulletin* 36: 472–485.

    See also:

    Juckel G, Schlagenhauf F, Koslowski M, Wüstenberg T, Villringer A, Knutson B, et al. (2006) Dysfunction of ventral striatal reward prediction in schizophrenia. *NeuroImage* 29: 409–416.

30. Schlagenhauf F, Sterzer P, Schmack K, Ballmaier M, Rapp M, Warse J, et al. (2009) Reward feedback alterations in unmedicated schizophrenia patients: relevance to delusions. *Biological Psychiatry* 65: 1032–1039.

31. There is another set of studies that produced results consistent with the idea of excessive incentive learning in schizophrenia. Andrew McGhie (1926–1988) and James Chapman, working at the Dundee Royal Mental Hospital in Scotland, UK, in the 1950s and 1960s interviewed a large number of patients with schizophrenia and evaluated their performance on tests requiring focus on a particular target in an array of stimuli. They found that patients were highly distracted by other (non-target) stimuli in the array and concluded that patients suffered from a deficient filter, being impaired in their ability to ignore irrelevant stimuli. Although McGhie and Chapman did not relate this deficit to excessive incentive learning, it is entirely consistent with excessive incentive learning. I discuss the work of Chapman and McGhie further in Chapter 13.

32. There were some studies of incentive learning in humans and the effects of dopamine receptor-blocking drugs. Marianne Fischman (1939–2001) and colleagues from the University of Chicago, for example, tested normal participants in a point-loss avoidance task and found that performance was impaired by the antipsychotic drug chlorpromazine. We found similar results in patients with schizophrenia, linking dopamine receptor blockade by antipsychotic medication to impaired avoidance learning. These studies implicated dopamine in reward-related incentive learning in humans but involved avoidance learning, making them more difficult to interpret because the role of reward in avoidance learning was not widely understood or agreed upon at the time (see Chapters 2 and 3):

    Cutmore TRH, Beninger RJ (1990) Do neuroleptics impair learning in schizophrenic patients? *Schizophrenia Research* 3: 173–186.

    Fischman MW, Schuster CR (1979) The effects of chlorpromazine and pentobarbital on behavior maintained by electric shock or point loss avoidance in humans. *Psychopharmacology* 66: 3–11.

    Fischman MW, Smith RC, Schuster CR (1976) Effects of chlorpromazine on avoidance and escape responding in humans. *Pharmacology, Biochemistry and Behavior* 4: 111–114.

33. Miller R (1976) Schizophrenia psychology, associative learning and the role of forebrain dopamine. *Medical Hypotheses* 2: 203–211.

34. Kim K-i, Zhang LD, Lu MK, Park KK, Hwang T-J, Kim D, Park Y-C (2001) Schizophrenia delusions in Seoul, Shanghai and Taipei: a transcultural study. *Journal of Korean Medical Science* 16: 88–94.

35. Suhail K, Cochrane R (2002) Effect of culture and environment on the phenomenology of delusions and hallucinations. *International Journal of Social Psychiatry* 48: 126–138.

    See also:

    Suhail K (2003) Phenomenology of delusions in Pakistani patients: effect of gender and social class. *Psychopathology* 36: 195–199.

36. Škodlar B, Dernovšek MZ, Kocmur M (2008) Psychopathology of schizophrenia in Ljubljana (Slovenia) from 1881–2000: changes in the content of delusions in schizophrenia patients related to various sociopolitical, technical and scientific changes. *International Journal of Social Psychiatry* 54: 101–111.

37. Miller R (1993) Striatal dopamine in reward and attention: a system for understanding symptomatology of acute schizophrenia and mania. *International Review of Neurobiology* 35: 161–278.

    Miller R (2008) *A Neurodynamic Theory of Schizophrenia and Related Disorders.* Robert Miller: Dunedin.

38. Axelsson R, Ohman R (1987) Patterns of response to neuroleptic treatment: factors influencing the amelioration of individual symptoms in psychotic patients. *Acta Psychiatrica Scandinavica* 76: 707–714.

    Johnstone EC, Crow TJ, Frith CD, Carney MWP, Price JS (1978) Mechanism of the antipsychotic effect in the treatment of acute schizophrenia. *Lancet* 311: 848–851.

    Singh MM, Smith JM (1973) Kinetics and dynamics of response to haloperidol in acute schizophrenia—a longitudinal study of the therapeutic process. *Comprehensive Psychiatry* 14: 393–414.

    Zemlan FP, Hirschowitz J, Sautter R, Garver DL (1986) Relationship of psychotic symptom clusters in schizophrenia to neuroleptic treatment and growth hormone response to apomorphine. *Psychiatry Research* 18: 239–255.

39. See Suhail and Cochrane (2002) in Note 35

40. Gecici O, Kuloglu M, Guler O Ozbulut O, Kurt E, Onen S, Ekinci O, et al. (2010) Phenomenology of delusions and hallucinations in patients with schizophrenia. *Bulletin of Clinical Psychopharmacology* 20: 204–212.

41. The disease classification of hebephrenia was described by the German psychiatrist Ewald Hecker in 1871 and was eventually incorporated by Emil Kraepelin into his classification system of dementia praecox. Several papers by Abdullah Kramm from St James University Hospital in Leeds, UK, provide background to this influential work and reproduce, for the first time, Hecker's complete paper in an English translation. See:

    Kramm A (2004) On the origin of clinical standpoint in psychiatry. *History of Psychiatry* 15: 345–360.

    Kramm A (2009) "Hebephrenia. A contribution to clinical psychiatry" by Dr. Ewald Hecker in Görlitz (1871). *History of Psychiatry* 20: 87–106.

    Kramm A, Phillips P (2012) Hebephrenia: a conceptual history. *History of Psychiatry* 23: 387–403.

42. Akbarian B, Kim JJ, Potkin SG, Hagman JO, Tafazzoli A, Bunney WE Jr, Jones EG (1995) Gene expression for glutamic acid decarboxylase is reduced without loss of neurons in prefrontal cortex of schizophrenia. *Archives of General Psychiatry* 52: 258–266.

Beasley CL, Reynolds GP (1997) Parvalbumin-immunoreactive neurons are reduced in the prefrontal cortex of schizophrenia. *Schizophrenia Research* 24: 349–355.

Benes FM, Khan Y, Vincent SL, Wickramasinghe R (1996) Differences in the subregional and cellular distribution of $GABA_A$ receptor binding in the hippocampal formation of schizophrenic brain. *Synapse* 22: 338–349.

Benes FM, McSparren J, Bird ED, SanGiovanni JP, Vincent SL (1991) Deficits in small interneurons in prefrontal and cingulate cortices of schizophrenic and schizoaffective patients. *Archives of General Psychiatry* 48: 996–1001.

Benes FM, Vincent SL, Alsterberg G, Bird ED, SanGiovanni JP (1992) Increased $GABA_A$ receptor binding in superficial layers of cingulate cortex in schizophrenics. *Journal of Neuroscience* 12: 924–929.

Reynolds GP, Czudek C, Andrews HB (1990) Deficit and hemispheric asymmetry of GABA uptake sites in the hippocampus in schizophrenia. *Biological Psychiatry* 27: 1038–1044.

Volk DW, Austin MC, Pierri JN, Sampson AR, Lewis DA (2000) Decreased GAD_{67} mRNA expression in a subset of prefrontal cortical GABA neurons in subjects with schizophrenia. *Archives of General Psychiatry* 57: 237–245.

43. Duncan GE, Miyamoto S, Leipzig JN, Lieberman JA (2000) Comparison of the effects of clozapine, risperidone, and olanzapine on ketamine-induced alterations in regional brain metabolism. *Journal of Pharmacology and Experimental Therapeutics* 293: 8–14.

Javitt DC, Zukin SR (1991) Recent advances in the phencyclidine model of schizophrenia. *American Journal of Psychiatry* 148: 1301–1308.

Olney JW, Farber NM (1995) Glutamate receptor dysfunction in schizophrenia. *Archives of General Psychiatry* 52: 998–1007.

Jentsch JD, Roth RH (1999) The neuropsychopharmacology of phencyclidine: from NMDA receptor hypofunction to the dopamine hypothesis of schizophrenia. *Neuropsychopharmacology* 20: 201–225.

Moghaddam B, Adams BW (1998) Reversal of phencyclidine effects by a group II metabotropic glutamate receptor agonist in rats. *Science* 281: 1349–1352.

44. Grace AA (2012) Dopamine system dysregulation by the hippocampus: implications for the pathophysiology and treatment of schizophrenia. *Neuropharmacology* 62: 1342–1348.

45. da Silva Alves F, Figee M, van Amelsvoort T, Veltman D, de Haan L (2009) The revised dopamine hypothesis of schizophrenia: evidence from pharmacological MRI studies with atypical antpsychotic medication. *Psychopharmacology Bulletin* 41: 121–132.

Pogarell O, Koch W, Karch S, Dehning S, Müller N, Tatsch K, et al. (2012) Dopaminergic neurotransmission in patient with schizophrenia in relation to positive and negative symptoms. *Pharmacopsychiatry* 45(Suppl. 1): S36–S41.

Walter H, Krammerer H, Frasch K, Spitzer M, Abler B (2009) Altered reward functions in patients on atypical antipsychotic medication in line with the revised dopamine hypothesis of schizophrenia. *Psychopharmacology* 206: 121–132.

Weinstein JJ, Chohan MO, Silfstein M, Kegeles, LS, Moore H, Abi-Dargham A (2017) Pathway-specific dopamine abnormalities in schizophrenia. *Biological Psychiatry* 81: 31–42.

See also Brisch et al. in Note 10.

46. Sawaguchi T, Goldman-Rakic PS (1994) The role of D1-dopamine receptor in working memory: local injections of dopamine antagonists into the prefrontal cortex of rhesus monkeys performing an oculomotor delayed-response task. *Journal of Neurophysiology* 71: 515–528.

47. Barch DM, Ceaser A (2012) Cognition in schizophrenia: core psychological and neural mechanisms. *Trends in Cognitive Sciences* 16: 27–s34.

48. Apud JA, Weinberger DR (2007) Treatment of cognitive deficits associated with schizophrenia: potential role of catechol-O-methyltransferase inhibitors. *CNS Drugs* 21: 535–557.

49. Pycock CJ, Carter CJ, Kerwin RW (1980) Effect of 6-hydroxydopamine lesions of the medial prefrontal cortex on neurotransmitter systems in subcortical sites in the rat. *Journal of Neurochemistry* 34: 91–99.

   Pycock CJ, Kerwin RW, Carter CJ (1980) Effects of lesions of the cortical dopamine terminals on subcortical dopamine receptors in rats. *Nature* 286: 74–77.

50. Rosenbaum RB (2006) *Understanding Parkinson's Disease: A Personal and Professional View*. Greenwood Publishing Group: Portsmouth, NH.

51. Kaminsky TA, Dudgeon BJ, Billingsley FF, Mitchell PH, Weghorst SJ (2007) Virtual cues and functional mobility of people with Parkinson's disease: a single-subject pilot study. *Journal of Rehabilitation Research & Development* 44: 437–448.

   Thaut MH, McIntosh GC, Rice RR, Miller RA, Rathbun J, Brault JM (1996) Rhythmic auditory stimulation in gait training for Parkinson' disease patients. *Movement Disorders* 11: 193–200.

52. Bowers D, Miller K, Bosch W, Gokcay D, Pedraza O, Springer U, Okun M (2006) Faces of emotion in Parkinsons disease: micro-expressivity and bradykinesia during voluntary facial expressions. *Journal of the International Neuropsychological Society* 12: 765–773.

   Marsili L, Agostino R, Bologna M, Belvisi D, Palma A, Fabbrini G, Berardelli A (2014) Bradykinesia of posed smiling and voluntary movement of the lower face in Parkinson's disease. *Parkinsonism and Related Disorders* 20: 370–375.

   Simons G, Pasqualini MCS, Reddy V, Wood J (2004) Emotional and nonemotional facial expressions in people with Parkinson's disease. *Journal of the International Neuropsychological Society* 10: 521–535.

53. Martin JP (1967) *The Basal Ganglia and Posture*. Pitman Medical Publishing Co.: London.

54. Carlsson A, Lindqvist M, Magnusson T (1957) 3,4-Dihydroxyphenylalanine and 5-hydroxytryptophan as reserpine antagonists. *Nature* 180: 1200.

55. See Note 7 in Chapter 7.

56. See Note 8 in Chapter 4.

57. Birkmayer W, Birkmayer JGD (1989) The L-dopa story. In: Calne DB, Crippa D, Comi G, Horowski R, Trabucchi M, eds., *Parkinsonism and Aging; Aging Volume 36*. Raven Press: New York, pp. 1–7.

58. Carlsson A (2001) A paradigm shift in brain research. *Science* 294: 1021–1024.

59. See Note 22 in Chapter 2.

60. Choi WY, Balsam PD, Horvitz JC (2005) Extended habit training reduces dopamine mediation of appetitive response expression. *Journal of Neuroscience* 25: 6729–6733.

See Horvitz et al. (2007) in Note 15 of Chapter 2.

61. I read a number of journal articles that discussed the effectiveness of various "tricks" involving using patterned sensory input to help patients with Parkinson's disease initiate movement, but none of them commented about the effectiveness of these tricks with repeated use. In a 2009 article on tips to help patients with Parkinson's disease deal with freezing episodes, journalist Dennis Thompson, Jr., writing online for *everyday HEALTH* stated with regard to a number of these tricks that "Parkinson's disease patients may find that they have to rotate through these strategies as each may lose its effectiveness over time." The website of the Parkinson's Disease Foundation in the USA has a question-and-answer section where they provide an answer to the question of how to deal with freezing. In the answer they mention the tricks discussed by J.P. Martin (see Note 53) and at the end of their answer they write, "Unfortunately, the effectiveness of such tricks often fades over time."

62. Hornykiewicz O, Pifl C, Kish SJ, Shannak K, Schingnitz G (1989) Biochemical changes in idiopathic Parkinson's disease, aging and MPTP parkinsonism: similarities and differences. In: Calne DB, Crippa D, Comi G, Horowski R, Trabucchi M, eds., *Parkinsonism and Aging; Aging Volume 36*. Raven Press: New York, pp. 57–67.

63. Frank MJ, Seeberger LC, O'Reilly RC (2004) By carrot or by stick: cognitive reinforcement learning in Parkinsonism. *Science* 306: 1940–1943.

Although they did not refer to it as inverse incentive learning, in subsequent preclinical studies using mice, Frank and co-workers showed that learning of a motor skill was impaired by dopamine D2 receptor blockade. This learning led to retarded acquisition of the same skill once the D2 receptor blockade was removed. See:

Beeler JA, Frank MJ, McDaid J, Alexander E, Turkson S, Bernandez MS, et al. (2012) A role for dopamine-mediated learning in the pathophysiology and treatment of Parkinson's disease. *Cell Reports* 2: 1747–1761.

64. See Note 11 in Chapter 4.

65. See Note 9 in Chapter 4.

66. Kaasinen V, Jokinen P, Joutsa J, Eskola O, Rinne JO (2012) Seasonality of striatal dopamine synthesis capacity in Parkinson's disease. *Neuroscience Letters* 530: 80–84.

67. Deniker and Delay published their groundbreaking findings in 1952 in French in a series of six clinical reports. See Note 12 and:

Moncrieff J (2013) Magic bullets for mental disorders: the emergence of the concept of an "antipsychotic" drug. *Journal of the History of the Neurosciences* 22: 30–46.

68. López-Muñoz F, Alamo C (2009) The consolidation of neuroleptic therapy: Janssen, the discovery of haloperidol and its introduction into clinical practice. *Brain Research Bulletin* 79: 130–141.

69. See Note 13 in Chapter 7.

70. Psychiatrist David Healy from Bangor University in the UK provides an excellent account of the impact of chlorpromazine on the asylums in his book:

    Healy D (2002) *The Creation of Psychopharmacology*. Harvard University Press: Cambridge, MA.

    Author and journalist Simon Winchester provides great insight into the life of a person with schizophrenia living in an asylum in the pre-phenothiazine era in his best-selling book:

    Winchester S (1998) *The Professor and the Madman: A Tale of Murder, Insanity and the Making of the Oxford English Dictionary*. HarperCollins: New York.

71. López-Muñoz F, Alamo C, Cuenca E, Shen WW, Clervoy P, Rubio R (2005) History of the discovery and clinical introduction of chlorpromazine. *Annals of Clinical Psychiatry* 17: 113–135.

72. Meyer JM, Simpson GM (1997) From chlorpromazine to olanzapine: a brief history of antipsychotics. *Psychiatric Services* 48: 1137–1139.

73. Crilly J (2007) The history of clozapine and its emergence in the US market: a review and analysis. *History of Psychiatry* 18: 39–60.

    Hippius H (1989) The history of clozapine. *Psychopharmacology* 99: S3–S5.

    Kerwin RW (1995) Clozapine: back to the future for schizophrenia research. *Lancet* 345: 1063–1064.

74. Lieberman JA, Golden R, Stroup S, McEvoy J (2000) Drugs of the psychopharmacological revolution in clinical psychiatry. *Psychiatric Services* 51: 1254–1258.

75. Inoue A, Miki S, Seto M, Kikuchi T, Morita S, Ueda H, et al. (1997) Aripiprazole, a novel antipsychotic drug, inhibits quinpirole-evoked GTPase activity but does not up-regulate dopamine D_2 receptor following repeated treatment in the rat striatum. *European Journal of Pharmacology* 321: 105–111.

    Toru M, Miura S, Kudo Y (1994) Clinical experience of OPC-14597, a dopamine autoreceptor agonist in schizophrenia patients. *Neuropsychopharmacology* 10: 122S.

76. Bodén R, Edman G, Reutfors J, Österson C-G, Ösby U (2013) A comparison of cardiovascular risk factors for ten antipsychotic drugs in clinical practice. *Neuropsychiatric Disease and Treatment* 9: 371–377.

    Rummel-Kluge C, Komossa K, Schwarz S, Hunger H, Schmid F, Lobos CA, et al. (2010) Head-to-head comparisons of metabolic side effects of second generation antipsychotics in the treatment of schizophrenia: a systematic review and meta-analysis. *Schizophrenia Review* 123: 225–233.

    Werner F-M, Coveñas R (2014) Safety of antipsychotic drugs: focus on therapeutic and adverse effects. *Expert Opinion on Drug Safety* 13: 1031–1042.

77. Geddes J, Freemantle N, Harrison P, Beddington P (2000) Atypical antipsychotics in the treatment of schizophrenia: systematic overview and meta-regression analysis. *BMJ* 321: 1371–1376.

    Leucht S, Pitschel-Walz G, Abraham D, Kissling W (1999) Efficacy and extrapyramidal side-effects of the new antipsychotics olanzapine, quetiapine, risperidone, and sertindole compared to conventional antipsychotics and placebo. A meta-analysis of randomized controlled trials. *Schizophrenia Research* 35: 51–68.

Stip E (2002) Happy birthday neuroleptics! 50 years later: *la folie du doute. European Psychiatry* 17: 115–119.

78. Casey JF, Bennett IF, Lindley CJ, Hollister LE, Gordon MH, Springer NN (1960) Drug therapy in schizophrenia. A controlled study of the relative effectiveness of chlorpromazine, promazine, phenobarbital and placebo. *Archives of General Psychiatry* 2: 210–220.

   Elkes J, Elkes C (1954) Effect of chlorpromazine on the behaviour of chronically overactive psychotic patients. *British Medical Journal* 2: 560–565.

   Winkelman NW (1954) Chlorpromazine in the treatment of neuropsychiatric disorders. *Journal of the American Medical Association* 155: 18–21.

79. Chiodo LA, Bunney BS (1983) Typical and atypical neuroleptics: differential effects of chronic administration on the activity of A9 and A10 midbrain dopaminergic neurons. *Journal of Neuroscience* 3: 1607–1619.

80. Kuhar MJ, Joyce AR (2002) Slow onset of CNS drugs: can changes in protein concentration account for the delay? *Trends in Pharmacological Sciences* 22: 450–456.

81. Miller R (1987) The time course of neuroleptic therapy for psychosis: role of learning processes and implications for concepts of psychotic illness. *Psychopharmacology* 92: 405–415.

82. See Note 17 in Chapter 3.

83. Tarrier N, Barrowclough C (1990) Family interventions for schizophrenia. *Behavior Modification* 14: 408–440.

84. Christensen JK (1974) A 5-year follow-up study of male schizophrenics: evaluation of factors influencing success and failure in the community. *Acta Psychiatrica Scandanavica* 50: 60–72.

   Leff J, Berkowitz R (1996) Working with the families of schizophrenic patients. *The Psychotherapy Patient* 9: 185–211.

85. Lucksted A, McFarlane W, Downing D, Dixon L, Adams C (2012) Recent developments in family psychoeducation as an evidence-based practice. *Journal of Marital and Family Therapy* 38: 101–121.

86. Lefley, HP (1992) Expressed emotion: conceptual, clinical and social policy issues. *Hospital and Community Psychiatry* 43: 591–598.

   My former PhD student, Tom Ehmann, who is now a consulting psychologist in Vancouver, British Columbia, provides an excellent summary of psychoeducation and expressed emotion studies in a chapter in his co-edited book:

   Ehmann T, Hanson L (2004) Social and psychological interventions. In: Ehmann T, MacEwan GW, Honer WG, eds., *Best Care in Early Psychosis Intervention*. Taylor & Francis: New York, pp. 61–84.

87. Beninger RJ, Baker TW, Florczynski MM, Banasikowski T (2010) Regional differences in the action of antipsychotic drugs: implications for cognitive effects in schizophrenic patients. *Neurotoxicity Research* 18: 229–243.

88. See Note 9 in Chapter 4.

89. See Note 12 in Chapter 4.

90. Beninger RJ, Wasserman JI, Zanibbi K, Charbonneau D, Mangels J, Beninger BV (2003) Typical and atypical antipsychotic medications differentially affect two nondeclarative

memory tasks in schizophrenic patients: a double dissociation. *Schizophrenia Research* 61: 281–292.

91. Fujimura M, Hashimoto K, Yamagami K (2000) The effect of the antipsychotic drug mosapramine on the expression of Fos protein in the brain: comparison with halo-peridol, clozapine and risperidone. *Life Sciences* 67: 2865–2872.

    Robertson GS, Matsumura H, Fibiger HC (1994) Induction patterns of Fos-like immunoreactivity in the forebrain as predictors of atypical antipsychotic activity. *Journal of Pharmacology and Experimental Therapeutics* 271: 1058–1066.

    Scherer H, Bedard M-A, Stip E, Paquet F, Richer F, Bériault M, et al. (2004) Procedural learning in schizophrenia can reflect the pharmacologic properties of the antipsychotic treatments. *Cognition & Behavioral Neurology* 17: 32–40.

92. Wasserman JI, Barry RJ, Bradford L, Delva NJ, Beninger RJ (2012) Probabilistic classi-fication and gambling in patients with schizophrenia receiving medication: comparison of risperidone, olanzapine, clozapine and typical antipsychotics. *Psychopharmacology* 222: 173–183.

93. Sacks O (1990) *Awakenings*. HarperCollins: New York.

    Note that the patients described by Sacks are thought to have suffered from enceph-alitis *lethargica* or von Economo disease, possibly related to the 1918 flu epidemic. Parkinson's-like symptoms were often seen in these patients and they responded to dopamine-replacement therapy with L-DOPA.

94. Anderson E, Nutt J (2011) The long-duration response to levodopa: phenomenology, potential mechanisms and clinical implications. *Parkinsonism and Related Disorders* 17: 587–592.

95. Heiden P, Heinz A, Romanczuk-Seiferth N (2017) Pathological gambling in Parkinson's disease: what are the risk factors and what is the role of impulsivity? *European Journal of Pharmacology* 45: 67–72.

    Santangelo G, Barone P, Trojano L, Vitale C (2013) Pathological gambling in Parkinson's disease. A comprehensive review. *Parkinsonism and Related Disorders* 19: 645–653.

96. Ray NJ, Miyaski JM, Zurowski M, Ko JH, Cho SS, Pellecchia G, et al. (2012) Extrastriatal dopaminergic abnormalities of DA homeostasis in Parkinson's patients with medication-induced pathological gambling: a [11C] FLB-457 and PET study. *Neurobiology of Disease* 48: 519–525.

    Steeves TDL, Miyaski J, Zurowski M, Lang AE, Pellecchia G, Van Eimeren T, et al. (2009) Increased striatal dopamine release in Parkinsonian patients with pathological gambling: a [^{11}C] raclopride PET study. *Brain* 132: 1376–1385.

97. Kish SJ, Shannak K, Hornykiewicz O (1988) Uneven pattern of dopamine loss in the stri-atum of patients with idiopathic Parkinson's disease. *New England Journal of Medicine* 318: 876–880.

98. Swainson R, Rogers RD, Sahakian BJ, Summers BA, Polkey CE, Robbins TW (2000) Probabilistic learning and reversal deficits in patients with Parkinson's disease or frontal or temporal lobe lesions: possible adverse effects of dopaminergic medication. *Neuropsychologia* 38: 596–612.

99. Weintraub D, Koester J, Potenza MN, Siderowf AD, Stacy M, Voon V, et al. (2010) Impulse control disorder in Parkinson disease: a cross-sectional study with 3090 pa-tients. *Archives of Neurology* 67: 589–595.

100. Voon V, Fernagut P-O, Wickens J, Baunez C, Rodriguez M, Pavon N, et al. (2009) Chronic dopaminergic stimulation in Parkinson's disease: from dyskinesias to impulse control disorders. *Lancet Neurology* 8: 1140–1149.

101. Stefanis N, Bozi M, Christodoulou C, Douzenis A, Gasparinatos G, Stamboulis E, et al. (2010) Isolated delusional syndrome in Parkinson's disease. *Parkinsonism and Related Disorders* 16: 550–552.

102. Seeman P, Madras BK (1998) Anti-hyperactivity medication: methylphenidate and amphetamine. *Molecular Psychiatry* 3: 386–396.

103. Bradley C (1937) The behavior of children receiving benzedrine. *American Journal of Psychiatry* 94: 577–585.

    See also Note 7.

104. Seiden LS, Miller FE, Heffner TG (1989) Neurotransmitters in attention deficit disorder. In: Sagvolden T, Archer T, eds., *Attention Deficit Disorder: Clinical and Basic Research*. Lawrence Erlbaum Associates: Hillsdale, NJ.

105. McCall S, Vilensky JA, Gilman S, Taubenberger JK (2008) The relationship between encephalitis lethargic and influenza: a critical analysis. *Journal of NeuroVirology* 14: 177–185.

    Mortimer PP (2009) Was encephalitis lethargica a post-influenzal or some other phenomenon? Time to re-examine the problem. *Epidemiology & Infection* 137: 449–455.

    Tappe D, Alquezar-Planas DE (2014) Medical and molecular perspectives into a forgotten epidemic: encephalitis lethargica, viruses, and high-throughput sequencing. *Journal of Clinical Virology* 61: 189–195.

106. Vilensky JA, Foley P, Gilman S (2007) Children and encephalitis lethargica: a historical review. *Pediatric Neurology* 37: 79–84.

107. von Economo C (1931) *Encephalitis Lethargica: Its Sequelae and Treatment*. Oxford University Press: London; translated by Newman KO (originally published in 1929 as *Die Encephalitis Lethargica, ihre Nachkrankheiten und ihre Behandlung*. Urban & Schwarzenberg: Berlin).

108. Bond ED, Partridge GE (1926) Post-encephalitic behavior disorders in boys and their management in a hospital. *American Journal of Psychiatry* 83: 25–103.

    See also the following reviews:

    Baumeister AA, Henderson K, Pow JL, Advokat C (2012) The early history of the neuroscience of attention-deficit/hyperactivity disorder. *Journal of the History of the Neurosciences* 21: 263–279.

    Curatolo P, Paloscia C, D'Agati E, Moavero R, Pasini A (2009) The neurobiology of attention deficit/hyperactivity disorder. *European Journal of Paediatric Neurology* 13: 299–304.

109. Max JE, Fox PT, Lancaster P, Kochunov P, Matthews K, Manes FF, et al. (2002) Putamen lesions and the development of attention-deficit/hyperactivity symptomatology. *Journal of the American Academy of Child and Adolescent Psychiatry* 41: 563–571.

110. Shafritz KM, Marchione KE, Gore JC, Shaywitz SE, Shaywitz BA (2004) The effects of methylphenidate on neural systems of attention deficit hyperactivity disorder. *American Journal of Psychiatry* 161: 1990–1997.

Note that performance of an attention task was not correlated with level of activation in the striatum in this study, leaving open interpretation of the observed activation differences.

111. Lou HC, Henriksen L, Bruhn P, Borner H, Nielsen JB (1989) Striatal dysfunction in attention deficit and hyperactivity disorder. *Archives of Neurology* 345: 91–95.

    Vaidya CJ, Austin G, Kirkorian G, Ridlehuber HW, Desmond JE, Glover GH, Gabrieli JDE (1998) Selective effects of methylphenidate in attention deficit hyperactivity disorder: a functional magnetic resonance study. *Proceedings of the National Academy of Sciences of the United States of America* 95: 14494–14499.

    See also the following reviews:

    Baroni A, Castellanos FX (2015) Neroanatomic and cognitive abnormalities in attention-deficit/hyperactivity disorder in the era of "high definition" neuroimaging. *Current Opinions in Neurobiology* 30: 1–8.

    Mehler-Wex C, Reiderer P, Gerlach M (2006) Dopaminergic dysbalance in distinct basal ganglia neurocircuits: implications for the pathophysiology of Parkinson's disease, schizophrenia and attention deficit hyperactivity disorder. *Neurotoxicity Research* 10: 167–179.

112. Volkow ND, Wang G-J, Kollins SH, Wigal TL, Newcorn JH, Telang F, et al. (2009) Evaluating dopamine reward pathway in ADHD. *Journal of the American Medical Association* 302: 1084–1091.

113. Kish SJ, Shannak K, Rajput A, Deck JHN, Hornykiewicz O (1992) Aging produces a specific pattern of striatal dopamine loss: implications for the etiology of idiopathic Parkinson's disease. *Journal of Neurochemistry* 58: 642–648.

114. Fearnley JM, Lees AJ (1991) Ageing and Parkinson's disease: substantia nigra regional selectivity. *Brain* 114: 2283–2301.

    Note: see also many relevant earlier references in this paper

115. Walitza S, Melfsen S, Herhaus G, Scheuerpflug P, Warnke A, Müller T, et al. (2006) Association of Parkinson's disease with symptoms of attention deficit hyperactivity disorder in childhood. *Journal of Neural Transmission* 72(Suppl.): 311–315.

116. Machado L, Devine A, Wyatt N (2009) Distractibility with advancing age and Parkinson's disease. *Neuropsychologia* 47: 1756–1764.

117. Lichter J, Barr CL, Kennedy JL, Van Tol HHM, Kidd KK, Livaka KJ (1993) A hypervariable segment in the human dopamine receptor D_4 (*DRD4*) gene. *Human Molecular Genetics* 2: 767–773.

    Van Tol HHM, Wu CM, Guan H-C, Ohara K, Bunzow JR, Civelli O, et al. (1992) Multiple dopamine D4 receptor variants in the human population. *Nature* 358: 149–152.

118. LaHoste GJ, Swanson JM, Wigal SB, Glabe C, Wigal T, King N, Kennedy JL (1996) Dopamine D4 receptor gene polymorphism is associated with attention deficit hyperactivity disorder. *Molecular Psychiatry* 1: 121–124.

    See review by:

    Gizer IR, Ficks C, Waldman ID (2009) Candidate gene studies of ADHD: a meta-analytic review. *Human Genetics* 126: 51–59.

119. Akutagava-Martins GC, Salatino-Oliveira A, Kieling CC, Rohde L, Hutz MH (2009) Genetics of attention-deficit/hyperactivity disorder: current findings and future directions. *Expert Review of Neurotherapeutics* 13: 435.

See also:

Gallo EF, Posner J (2016) Moving towards causality in attention-deficit hyperactivity disorder: overview of neural and genetic mechanisms. *Lancet Psychiatry* 3: 555–567.

120. Asghari V, Schoots O, van Kats S, Ohara K, Jovanovic V, Guan HC, et al. (1994) Dopamine D4 receptor repeat: analysis of different native and mutant forms of the human and rat genes. *Molecular Pharmacology* 46: 364–373.

Asghari V, Sanyal S, Buchwaldt S, Paterson A, Jovanovic V, Van Tol HH (1995) Modulation of intracellular cyclic AMP levels by different human dopamine D4 receptor variants. *Journal of Neurochemistry* 65: 1157–1165.

121. See Note 133 in Chapter 7.

122. Nederhof E, Creemers HE, Huizink AC, Ormel J, Oldehinkel AJ (2011) L-DRD4 genotype not associated with sensation seeking, gambling performance and startle reactivity in adolescents: the TRAILS study. *Neuropsychologia* 49: 1359–1362.

123. Kruger AN, Siegfried Z, Ebstein RP (2002) A meta-analysis of the association between DRD4 polymorphism and novelty seeking. *Molecular Psychiatry* 7: 712–717.

124. Matthews LJ, Butler PM (2011) Novelty-seeking DRD4 polymorphisms are associated with human migration distance our-of-Africa after controlling for neutral population gene structure. *American Journal of Physical Anthropology* 145: 382–389.

125. Wang, E, Ding Y-C, Flodman P, Kidd JR, Kidd KK, Grady DL, et al. (2004) The genetic architecture of selection at the human dopamine receptor D4 (*DRD4*) gene locus. *American Journal of Human Genetics* 74: 931–944.

126. Oades RD (1982) *Attention and Schizophrenia: Neurobiological Bases*. Pitman Advanced Publishing Program: London.

127. Carli M, Evenden JL, Robbins TW (1985) Depletion of unilateral striatal dopamine impairs initiation of contralateral actions and not sensory attention. *Nature* 313: 679–682.

128. Beninger RJ (1989) Dopamine and learning: Implications for attention deficit disorder and hyperkinetic syndrome. In: T Sagvolden, T Archer, eds., *Attention Deficit Disorder, Clinical and Basic Research*. Lawrence Erlbaum Associates: Hillsdale, NJ, pp. 323–337.

Chapter 10

1. See Note 11 in Chapter 3 and:

Robbins TW, Everitt BJ (1996) Neurobehavioural mechanisms of reward and motivation. *Current Opinions in Neurobiology* 6: 228–236.

2. Dalley JW, Everitt BJ (2009) Dopamine receptors in the learning, memory and drug reward circuitry. *Seminars in Cell & Developmental Biology* 20: 403–410.

3. Ito R, Dalley JW, Howes SR, Robbins TW, Everitt BJ (2000) Dissociation in conditioned dopamine release in the nucleus accumbens core and shell in response to cocaine cues and during cocaine-seeking behavior in rats. *Journal of Neuroscience* 20: 7489–7495.

Schiff SR (1982) Conditioned dopaminergic activity. *Biological Psychiatry* 17: 135–154.

Also see:

Fontana et al. (1993) in Note 34 of Chapter 5

4. Clark MSG (1969) Self-administration of nicotine solutions preferred to placebo by the rat. *British Journal of Pharmacology* 35: P367.

   Fudala PJ, Teoh KW, Iwamoto ET (1985) Pharmacologic characterization of nicotine-induced conditioned place preference. *Pharmacology, Biochemistry and Behavior* 22: 237–241.

5. Black RW, Albiniak T, Davis M, Schumpert J (1973) A preference in rats for cues associated with intoxication. *Bulletin of the Psychonomic Society* 2: 423–424.

   Deneau G, Yanagita T, Seevers MH (1969) Self-administration of psychoactive substances by the monkey. *Psychopharmacologia* 16: 30–48.

6. Lepore M, Vorel SR, Lowinson J, Gardner EL (1995) Conditioned place preference induced by Δ^9-tetrahydrocannabinol: comparison with cocaine, morphine, and food reward. *Life Sciences* 56: 2073–2080.

   Takahashi RN, Singer G (1979) Self-administration of Δ^9-tetrahydrocannabinol by rats. *Pharmacology, Biochemistry and Behavior* 11: 737–740.

7. Pickens R, Harris W (1968) Self-administration of d-amphetamine by rat. *Psychopharmacologia* 12: 158–163.

   Reicher MA, Holman EW (1977) Location preference and flavor aversion reinforced by amphetamine in rats. *Animal Learning & Behavior* 5: 343–346.

8. Pickens R, Thompson T (1968) Cocaine-reinforced behavior in rats: effects of reinforcement magnitude and fixed-ratio size. *Journal of Pharmacology and Experimental Therapeutics* 161: 122–129.

   Spyraki C, Fibiger HC, Phillips AG (1982) Cocaine-induced place preference conditioning: lack of effects of neuroleptics and 6-hydroxydopamine lesions. *Brain Research* 253: 195–203.

9. Rossi NA, Reid LD (1976) Affective states associated with morphine injection. *Physiological Psychology* 4: 269–274.

   Weeks JR (1962) Experimental morphine addiction: method for automatic intravenous injections in unrestrained rats. *Science* 138: 143–144.

10. Bozarth MA, Wise RA (1981) Heroin reward is dependent on a dopaminergic substrate. *Life Sciences* 29: 1881–1886.

    Van Ree JM, De Wied D (1977) Modulation of heroin self-administration by neurohypophyseal principles. *European Journal of Pharmacology* 43: 199–202.

11. Shuster CR, Thompson T (1969) Self administration of and behavioral dependence on drugs. *Annual Reviews of Pharmacology* 9: 483–502.

    Tzschentke TM (1998) Measuring reward with the conditioned place preference paradigm: a comprehensive review of drug effects, recent progress new issues. *Progress in Neurobiology* 56: 613–672.

    Tzschentke TM (2007) Measuring reward with the conditioned place preference (CPP) paradigm: update of the last decade. *Addiction Biology* 12: 227–462.

12. Ferris RM, Tang FLM, Maxwell RA (1972) A comparison of the capacities of isomers of amphetamine, deoxypipradrol and methylphenidate to inhibit the uptake of tritiated catecholamines into rat cerebral cortex slices, synaptosomal preparations of rat cerebral cortex, hypothalamus and striatum and into adrenergic nerves of rabbit aorta. *Journal of Pharmacology and Experimental Therapeutics* 181: 407–416.

 Van Rossum JM, Hurkmans TATM (1964) Mechanism of action of psychomotor stimulant drugs. *International Journal of Neuropharmacology* 3: 227–239.

13. Imperato A, Di Chiara G (1984) Trans-striatal dialysis coupled to reverse phase high performance liquid chromatography with electrochemical detection: a new method for the study of the *in vivo* release of endogenous dopamine and metabolites. *Journal of Neuroscience* 4: 966–977.

 Zetterström T, Sharp T, Marsden CA, Ungerstedt U (1983) *In vivo* measurement of dopamine and its metabolites by intracerebral dialysis: changes after *d*-amphetamine. *Journal of Neurochemistry* 41: 1769–1773.

14. Condi JC, Strope E, Adams RN, Marsden CA (1978) Voltammetry in brain tissue: chronic recording of stimulated dopamine and 5-hydroxytryptamine release. *Life Sciences* 23: 2705–2716.

 Stamford JA, Kruk ZL, Miller J (1988) Stimulated limbic and striatal dopamine release measured by fast cyclic voltammetry: anatomical, electrochemical and pharmacological characterization. *Brain Research* 454: 282–288.

15. Dewey SL, Logan J, Wolf AP, Brodie JD, Angrist B, Fowler JS, Volkow ND (1991) Amphetamine induced decreases in (^{18}F)-N-methylspiroperidol binding in baboon brain using positron emission tomography (PET). *Synapse* 7: 324–327.

 Volkow ND, Ding Y-S, Fowler JS, Wang G-J (1996) Cocaine addiction: hypothesis derived from imaging studies with PET. *Journal of Addictive Diseases* 15: 55–71.

16. Dale HH (1914) The action of certain esters and ethers of choline, and their relation to muscarine. *Journal of Pharmacology* 6: 147–190.

17. Imperato A, Mulas A, Di Chiara G (1986) Nicotine preferentially stimulates dopamine release in the limbic system of freely moving rats. *European Journal of Pharmacology* 132: 337–338.

18. Brazell MP, Mitchell SN, Joseph MH, Gray JA (1990) Acute administration of nicotine increases the *in vivo* extracellular levels of dopamine, 3,4-dihydroxyphenylacetic acid and ascorbic acid preferentially in the nucleus accumbens of the rat: comparison with caudate-putamen. *Neuropharmacology* 29: 1177–1185.

19. Tsukada H, Miyasato K, Harada N, Nishiyama S, Fukumoto D, Kakiuchi T (2005) Nicotine modulates dopamine synthesis rate as determined by L-[β-^{11}C]DOPA: PET studies compared with [^{11}C]raclopride binding in the conscious monkey brain. *Synapse* 57: 120–122.

20. Brody AL, Olmstead RE, London ED, Farahi J, Grossman P, Lee GS, et al. (2004) Smoking-induced ventral striatum dopamine release. *American Journal of Psychiatry* 161: 1211–1218.

21. Gallegos RA, Lee R-S, Criado JR, Henriksen SJ, Steffensen SC (1999) Adaptive responses of γ-aminobutyric acid neurons in the ventral tegmental area to chronic ethanol. *Journal of Pharmacology and Experimental Therapeutics* 291: 1045–1053.

22. Carlsson A, Engel J, Strömbom U, Svensson TH, Waldeck B (1974) Suppression by dopamine-agonists of the ethanol-induced stimulation of locomotor activity and brain dopamine synthesis. *Naunyn-Schmiedeberg's Archives of Pharmacology* 283: 117–128.

Di Chiara G, Imperato A (1985) Ethanol preferentially stimulates dopamine release in the nucleus accumbens of freely moving rats. *European Journal of Pharmacology* 115: 131–132.

23. Gessa GL, Muntoni F, Collu M, Vargiu L Mereu G (1985) Low doses of ethanol activate dopaminergic neurons in the ventral tegmental area. *Brain Research* 348: 201–203.

Mereu G, Fadda R, Gessa GL (1984) Ethanol stimulates the firing rate of nigral dopaminergic neurons in unanesthetized rats. *Brain Research* 292: 63–69.

24. Boileau I, Assaad J-M, Pihl RO, Benkelfat C, Leyton M, Diskic RE, et al. (2003) Alcohol promotes dopamine release in the human nucleus accumbens. *Synapse* 49: 226–231.

25. Gaoni Y, Mechoulam R (1964) Isolation, structure, and partial synthesis of an active constituent of hashish. *Journal of the American Chemical Society* 86: 1646–1647.

26. Devane WA, Dysarz FA III, Johnson R, Melvin LS, Howlett AC (1988) Determination and characterization of a cannabinoid receptor in rat brain. *Molecular Pharmacology* 34: 606–613.

27. Devane WA, Hanuš L, Breuer A, Pertwee RG, Stevenson LA, Griffin G, et al. (1992) Isolation and structure of a brain constituent that binds to the cannabinoid receptor. *Science* 258: 1946–1949.

28. Mechoulam R, Ben-Shabat S, Hanuš L, Ligumsky M, Kaminski NE, Schatz AR, et al. (1995) Identification of an endogenous 2-mono-glyceride, present in canine gut, that binds to cannabinoid receptors. *Biochemical Pharmacology* 50: 83–90.

See also:

Mechoulam R, Fride E, Di Marzo V (1998) Endocannabinoids. *European Journal of Pharmacology* 359: 1–18.

29. Poddar MK, Dewey WL (1980) Effects of cannabinoids on catecholamine uptake and release in hypothalamic and striatal synaptosomes. *Journal of Pharmacology and Experimental Therapeutics* 214: 63–67.

30. Ton NMNC, Gernardt GA, Friedemann M, Etgen AM, Rose GM, Sharpless NS, Gardner EL (1988) The effects of Δ^9-tetrahydrocannabinol on potassium-evoked release of dopamine in the rat caudate nucleus: an in vivo electrochemical and in vivo microdialysis study. *Brain Research* 451: 59–68.

31. Voruganti LNP, Slomka P, Zabel P, Mattar A, Awad AG (2001) Cannabis induced dopamine release: an in-vivo SPECT study. *Psychiatry Research: Neuroimaging Section* 107: 173–177.

32. Bossong MG, van Berckel BNM, Boellaard R, Zuuman L, Schuit RC, Windhorst AD, et al. (2009) Δ^9-Tetrahydrocannabinol induces dopamine release in the human striatum. *Neuropsychopharmacology* 34: 759–766.

33. Pert CB, Snyder SH (1973) Opiate receptor: demonstration in nervous tissue. *Science* 179: 1011–1014.

Almost simultaneously, two other groups made similar discoveries:

Simon EJ, Hiller JM, Edelman I (1973) Stereospecific binding of the potent narcotic analgesic [^{3}H] endorphine to rat-brain homogenate. *Proceedings of the National Academy of Sciences of the United States of America* 70: 1947–1949.

Terenius L (1973) Characteristics of the "receptors" for narcotic analgesics in synaptic plasma membrane fraction from rat brain. *Acta Pharmacologica et Toxicologica* 33: 377–384.

34. Hughs J, Smith TW, Kosterlitz HW, Fothergill LA, Morgan BA, Morris HR (1975) Identification of two related pentapeptides from the brain with potent opiate agonist activity. *Nature* 258: 577–579.

35. Bradbury AF, Smyth DG, Snell CR, Birdsall NJM, Hulme EC (1976) C fragment of lipotropin has a high affinity for brain opiate receptors. *Nature* 260: 793–795.

36. Di Chiara G, Imperato A (1986) Preferential stimulation of dopamine release in the nucleus accumbens by opiates, alcohol, and barbiturates: studies with transcerebral dialysis in freely moving rats. *Annals of the New York Academy of Sciences* 473: 367–381.

37. Acquas E, Carboni E, Leone P, Di Chiara G (1989) SCH23390 blocks drug-conditioned place-preference and place-aversion: anhedonia (lack of reward) or apathy (lack of motivation) after dopamine receptor blockade? *Psychopharmacology* 99: 151–155.

38. Sellings LH, Baharnouri G, McQuade LE, Clarke PBS (2008) Rewarding and aversive effects of nicotine are segregated within the nucleus accumbens. *European Journal of Neuroscience* 28: 342–352.

    Spina L, Fenu S, Longoni R, Rivas E, Di Chiara G (2006) Nicotine-conditioned single-trial place preference: selective role of nucleus accumbens shell dopamine D1 receptors in acquisition. *Psychopharmacology* 184: 447–455.

39. Corrigall WA, Franklin KBJ, Coen KM, Clarke PBS (1992) The mesolimbic dopaminergic system is implicated in the reinforcing effects of nicotine. *Psychopharmacology* 107: 285–289.

40. Besson M, David B, Baudonnat M, Cazala P, Guilloux J-P, Reperant C, et al. (2012) Alpha7-nicotinic receptors modulate nicotine-induces reinforcement and extracellular dopamine outflow in the mesolimbic system in mice. *Psychopharmacology* 220: 1–14.

    Gotti C, Guiducci S, Tedesco V, Corbioli S, Zanetti L, Moretti M, et al. (2010) Nicotinic acetylcholine receptors in the mesolimbic pathway: primary role of ventral tegmental area α6β2* receptors in mediating systemic nicotine effects on dopamine release, locomotion, and reinforcement. *Journal of Neuroscience* 30: 5311–5325

41. Wang LP, Li F, Shen X, Tsien JZ (2010) Conditional knockout of NMDA receptors in dopamine neurons prevents nicotine-conditioned place preference. *PLOS ONE* 5: e8616.

42. Berrendero F, Plaza-Zabala A, Galeote L, Flores Á, Bura SA, Kieffer BL, Maldonado R (2012) Influence of δ-opioid receptors in the behavioral effects of nicotine. *Neuropsychopharmacology* 37: 2332–2344.

43. Matsuzawa S, Suzuki T, Misawa M, Nagase H (1999) Involvement of dopamine D1 and D2 receptors in the ethanol-associated place preference in rats exposed to conditioned fear stress. *Brain Research* 835: 298–305.

    An unusual feature of this study was that the rats were exposed to a conditioned aversive stimulus (a chamber where they had previously received electric foot shocks) prior to the pairing sessions of one side of the place-conditioning chamber with ethanol.

44. Bahi A, Dreyer J-L (2012) Involvement of nucleus accumbens dopamine D1 receptors in ethanol drinking, ethanol-induced conditioned place preference, and ethanol-induced psychomotor sensitization in mice. *Psychopharmacology* 222: 141–153.

45. Pfeffer AO, Samson HH (1986) Effect of pimozide on home cage ethanol drinking in the rat: dependence on drinking session length. *Drug and Alcohol Dependence* 17: 47–55.

46. Pfeffer AO, Samson HH (1988) Haloperidol and apomorphine effects on ethanol reinforcement in free feeding rats. *Pharmacology, Biochemistry and Behavior* 29: 343–350.

47. Koob GF (1992) Drugs of abuse: anatomy, pharmacology and function of reward pathways. *Trends in Pharmacological Sciences* 13: 177–184.

    Koob GF, Roberts AJ, Schulteis G, Parsons LH, Heyser CJ, Hyytiä P, et al. (1998) Neurocircuitry targets in ethanol reward and dependence. *Alcoholism: Clinical and Experimental Research* 22: 3–9.

    Weiss F, Hurd YL, Ungerstedt U, Markou A, Plotsky PM, Koob GF (1992) Neurochemical correlates of cocaine and ethanol self-administration. *Annals of the New York Academy of Sciences* 954: 220–241.

48. Fadda P, Scherma M, Spano MS, Salis P, Melis V, Fattore L, Fratta W (2006) Cannabinoid self-administration increases dopamine release in the nucleus accumbens. *NeuroReport* 17: 1629–1632.

49. Valjent E, Pagès C, Rogard M, Besson M-J, Maldonado R, Caboche J (2001) Δ⁹-tetrahydrocannabinol-induced MAPK/ERK and Elk-1 activation *in vivo* depends on dopaminergic transmission. *European Journal of Neuroscience* 14: 342–352.

50. Gerdjikov TV, Ross G, Beninger RJ. (2004) Place preference induced by nucleus accumbens amphetamine is impaired by antagonists of ERK or p38 MAP kinases in rats. *Behavioral Neuroscience* 118: 740–750.

51. Scherma M, Justinova Z, Zanettini C, Panlilio LV, Mascia P, Fadda P, et al. (2012) The anandamide transport inhibitor AM404 reduces the rewarding effects of nicotine and nicotine-induced dopamine elevations in the nucleus accumbens shell in rats. *British Journal of Pharmacology* 165: 2539–2548.

52. See Pickens and Harris (1968) in Note 7 and Pickens and Thompson (1968) in Note 8.

53. Wilson MC, Hitomi M, Schuster CR (1971) Psychomotor stimulant self administration as a function of dosage per injection in the rhesus monkey. *Psychopharmacologia* 22: 271–281.

54. Yokel RA, Wise RA (1975) Increased lever pressing for amphetamine after pimozide in rats: implications for a dopamine theory of reward. *Science* 187: 547–549.

55. De Wit H, Wise RA (1977) Blockade of cocaine reinforcement in rats with the dopamine receptor blocker pimozide, but not with the noradrenergic blockers phentolamine or phenoxybenzamine. *Canadian Journal of Psychology* 31: 195–203.

56. Bozarth MA, Wise RA (1981) Heroin reward is dependent on a dopaminergic substrate. *Life Sciences* 29: 1881–1886.

57. Hanson HM, Cimini-Venema CA (1972). Effects of haloperidol on self-administration of morphine in rats. *Federation Proceedings*, **31**: 503.

58. Bozarth MA, Wise RA (1981) Brain substrates for reinforcement and drug self-administration. *Progress in Neuro-Psychopharmacology* 5: 467–474.

    University of Toronto neuroscientist Derek van der Kooy and co-workers have also reported dopamine-independent opiate reward-related learning. See:

Ting-A-Kee R, van der Kooy D (2012) The neurobiology of opiate motivation. *Cold Spring Harbor Perspectives in Medicine* 2: a012096.

59. See the discussion of the work of Massachusetts Institute of Technology in Cambridge neuroscientist Ann Graybiel and co-workers in Chapter 5, cited in Note 85 of that chapter, for a brief description of how incentive learning can lead to a chain of conditioning whereby incentive stimuli most proximal to the primary reward act backwards in time to give less proximal stimuli an increased ability to elicit approach and other responses.

60. Morgan MJ (1974) Resistance to satiation. *Animal Behaviour* 22: 449–466.

61. Kimble GA (1951) Behavior strength as a function of the intensity of the hunger drive. *Journal of Experimental Psychology* 41: 341–348.

    See also:

    Beninger RJ (1989) Methods for determining the effects of drugs on learning. In: Boulton AA, Baker GB, Greenshaw AJ, eds., *Neuromethods: Psychopharmacology*. Humana Press: Clifton, NJ, pp. 623–685.

62. See Skinner in Note 1 of Chapter 2.

63. See Bassareo et al. (2007) in Note 34 of Chapter 5. For a recent review of studies showing that drug-associated cues can elicit dopamine release see:

    Leyton M, Vezina P (2013) Striatal ups and downs: their roles in vulnerability to addictions in humans. *Neuroscience and Biobehavioral Reviews* 37: 1999–2014.

64. Dar R, Rosen-Korakin N, Shapira O, Gottlieb Y, Frenk H (2010) The craving to smoke in flight attendants: relations with smoking deprivation, anticipation of smoking, and actual smoking. *Journal of Abnormal Psychology* 119: 248–253.

65. Nutt DJ, Lingford-Hughes A, Erritzoe D, Stokes RA (2015) The dopamine theory of addictions: 40 years of highs and lows. *Nature Neuroscience* 16: 305–312.

66. Khantzian EJ, McKenna GJ (1979) Acute toxic and withdrawal reactions associated with drug use and abuse. *Annals of Internal Medicine* 90: 361–372.

67. The strength of the need state associated with chronic marijuana intake may vary depending on the THC content of the consumed drug, the ratio of THC to cannabidiol, and the frequency of use. In many countries, including the USA and the UK, for example, the THC content of street marijuana has increased in recent years and the cannabidiol content has decreased; reports of greater drug dependency and more severe withdrawal symptoms have increased in parallel. See:

    Di Forti M, Morgan C, Dazzan P, Pariante C, Mondelli V, Marques TR, et al. (2009) High-potency cannabis and the risk of psychosis. *British Journal of Psychiatry* 195: 488–491.

    Hall W, Degenhardt L (2009) Adverse effects of non-medical cannabis use. *The Lancet* 374: 1383–1391.

68. Gawin FH, Ellinwood EH, Jr. (1988) Cocaine and other stimulants. *New England Journal of Medicine* 318: 1173–1182.

69. Volkow ND, Wang G-J, Telang F, Fowler JS, Logan J, Childress A-R, et al. (2006) Cocaine cues and dopamine in dorsal striatum: mechanisms of craving in cocaine addiction. *Journal of Neuroscience* 26: 6583–6588.

70. Zijlstra F, Booij J, van den Brink W, Franken IHA (2008) Striatal dopamine D2 receptor binding and dopamine release during cue-elicited craving in recently abstinent opiate-dependent males. *European Neuropsychopharmacology* 18: 262–270.

71. Kokkinidis L, McCarter BD (1990) Postcocaine depression and sensitization of brain-stimulation reward: analysis of reinforcement and performance effects. *Pharmacology, Biochemistry and Behavior* 36: 463–471.

    Leith NJ, Barrett RJ (1976) Amphetamine and the reward system: evidence for tolerance and post-drug depression. *Psychopharmacologia* 46: 19–25.

72. Epping-Jordan MP, Watkins SS, Koob GS, Markou A (1998) Dramatic decreases in brain reward function during nicotine withdrawal. *Nature* 393:76–79.

73. Schulteis G, Markou A, Cole M, Koob GF (1995) Decreased brain reward produced by ethanol withdrawal. *Proceedings of the National Academy of Sciences of the United States of America* 92: 5880–5884.

74. Schulteis G, Markou A, Gold LH, Stinus L, Koob GF (1994) Relative sensitivity to na-loxone of multiple indices of opiate withdrawal: a quantitative dose-response analysis. *Journal of the Experimental Analysis of Behavior* 271: 1391–1398.

75. Robertson MW, Leslie CA, Bennett JP Jr (1991) Apparent synaptic dopamine deficiency induced by withdrawal from chronic cocaine treatment. *Brain Research* 538: 337–339.

76. Rossetti Z, Hmaidan Y, Gessa GL (1992) Marked inhibition of mesolimbic dopamine re-lease: a common feature of ethanol, morphine, cocaine and amphetamine abstinence in rats. *European Journal of Pharmacology* 221: 227–234.

77. Ackerman JM, White FJ (1992) Decreased activity of rat A10 dopamine neurons following withdrawal from repeated cocaine. *European Journal of Pharmacology* 218: 171–173.

78. Liu Z-H, Jin W-Q (2004) Decrease in ventral tegmental area dopamine neuronal activity in nicotine withdrawal in rats. *NeuroReport* 15: 1479–1481.

79. Shen R-Y (2003) Ethanol withdrawal reduces the number of spontaneously active ventral tegmental area dopamine neurons in conscious animals. *Journal of Pharmacology and Experimental Therapeutics* 307: 566–572.

80. Diana M, Melis M, Muntoni AL, Gessa GL (1998) Mesolimbic dopaminergic decline after cannabinoid withdrawal. *Proceedings of the National Academy of Sciences of the United States of America* 95: 10269–10273.

81. Diana M, Muntoni AL, Pistis M, Melis M, Gessa GL (1999) Lasting reduction in mesolimbic dopamine neuronal activity after morphine withdrawal. *European Journal of Neuroscience* 11: 1037–1041.

82. Volkow ND, Fowler JS, Wang GJ (2003) The addicted human brain: insights from im-aging studies. *Journal of Clinical Investigations* 111: 1444–1451.

83. Koob GF, Le Moal M (2006) *Neurobiology of Addiction*. Elsevier: Amsterdam.

84. Koob GF, Le Moal M (2001) Drug addiction, dysregulation of reward, and allostasis. *Neuropsychopharmacology* 24: 97–129.

85. Koob GF (2013) Addiction is a reward deficit and stress surfeit disorder. *Frontiers in Psychiatry* 4: 1–18.

86. Welsh I (1993) *Trainspotting*. Vintage Books: London.

87. The comment of Koob and Le Moal (2001; see Note 84) that "Addicted patients ... are remarkably unencumbered by the memory of negative consequences of drug-taking" (p. 98), reminded me of Renton's apparent abandonment when he said yes to Seeker's smack.

88. Preller KH, Wagner M, Sulbach C, Hoenig K, Neubauer J, Franke PE, et al. (2013) Sustained incentive value of heroin-related cues in short- and long-term abstinent heroin users. *European Neuropsychopharmacology* 23: 1270–1279.

    An interesting aspect of this paper was that they showed the sustained incentive value of heroin-related stimuli using an implicit memory task, i.e., the participants were not conscious of this effect. In fact, when the former heroin-user participants were asked to explicitly rate the valence (pleasantness) of the heroin-related stimuli, their ratings were at control levels. These results support the distinction made in Chapter 4 between declarative (explicit) and non-declarative (implicit) memories and are consistent with incentive learning being non-declarative. They show that incentive learning can affect behavior without the individual being aware of it.

89. Robins LN (1993) Vietnam veterans' rapid recovery from heroin addiction: a fluke or normal expectation? *Addiction* 88: 1041–1054.

    Robins LN, Davis DH, Goodwin DW (1974) Drug use by U.S. army enlisted men in Vietnam: a follow-up on their return home. *American Journal of Epidemiology* 99: 235–249.

    Robins LN, Helzer JE, Davis DH (1975) Narcotic use in southeast Asia and afterward. *Archives of General Psychiatry* 32: 955–961.

    Robins LN, Helzer JE, Hasselbrook M, Wish E (2010) Vietnam veterans three years after Vietnam: how our study changed our view of heroin. *American Journal on Addictions* 19: 203–211 (originally published in *Problems of Drug Dependence, 1977, Proceedings of the Thirty-Ninth Annual Meetings of the Committee on Problems of Drug Dependence*).

90. Rosenbaum BJ (1971) Heroin: influence of method of use. *New England Journal of Medicine* 285: 299–300.

91. Siegel S, Hinson RE, Krank MD, McCully J (1982) Heroin "overdose" death: contribution of drug-associated environmental cues. *Science* 216: 436–437.

92. See Figure 4 in Robins (1993) in Note 89.

93. Wikler A (1973) Dynamics of drug dependence: implications of a conditioning theory for research and treatment. *Archives of General Psychiatry* 28: 611–616.

94. Childress AR, McLellan AT, O'Brien CP (1985) Behavioral therapies for substance abuse. *International Journal of the Addictions* 20: 947–969.

95. Myers KM, Carlezon WA Jr (2010) Extinction of drug- and withdrawal-paired cues in animal models: relevance to the treatment of addiction. *Neuroscience and Biobehavioral Reviews* 35: 285–302.

96. Saunders BT, Robinson TE (2013) Individual differences in resisting temptation: implications for addiction. *Neuroscience and Biobehavioral Reviews* 37: 1955–1975.

97. Everitt BJ (2014) Neural and psychological mechanisms underlying compulsive drug seeking habits and drug memories—indications for novel treatment of addiction. *European Journal of Neuroscience* 40: 2163–2182.

Chapter 11

1. Jhou TC, Geisler S, Marinelli M, DeGarmo BA, Zahm DS (2009) The mesopontine rostromedial tegmental nucleus: a structure targeted by the lateral habenula that projects to the ventral tegmental area of Tsai and substantia nigra compacta. *Journal of Comparative Neuroanatomy* 513: 566–596.

2. Bargmann C, Marder E (2013) From the connectome to brain function. *Nature Methods* 10: 483–490.

3. Cohen N, Sanders T (2014) Nematode locomotion: dissecting the neuronal-environmental loop. *Current Opinion in Neurobiology* 25: 99–106.

4. Hubel DH, Wiesel TN (1960) Receptive fields of the optic nerve fibres in the spider monkey. *Journal of Physiology* 154: 572–580.

5. Hubel DH, Wiesel TN (1962) Receptive fields, binocular interaction and functional architecture in the cat's visual cortex. *Journal of Physiology* 160: 106–154.

6. Hubel DH, Wiesel TN (1965) Receptive fields and functional architecture in two nonstriate visual areas (18 and 19) of the cat. *Journal of Neurophysiology* 28: 229–289.

7. Konorski J (1967) *Integrative Activity of the Brain: An Interdisciplinary Approach.* University of Chicago Press: Chicago, IL.

8. Gross CG, Rocha-Miranda CE, Bender DB (1972) Visual properties of neurons in inferotemporal cortex of the macaque. *Journal of Neurophysiology* 35: 96–111.

   See also this review:

   Desimone R (1991) Face-selective cells in the temporal cortex of monkeys. *Journal of Cognitive Neuroscience* 3: 1–8.

9. Tsao DY, Freiwald WA, Tootell RBH, Livingstone MS (2006) A cortical region consisting entirely of face-selective cells. *Science* 311: 670–674.

10. Freiwald WA, Tsao DY, Livingstone MS (2009) A face feature space in the macaque temporal lobe. *Nature Neuroscience* 12: 1187–1198.

11. Oliver Sacks (1933–2015) provides an engaging account of a patient suffering from prosopagnosia in his story of Dr. P, the eponymous chapter in his excellent 1985 book,

    The Man who Mistook his Wife for a Hat and Other Clinical Tales. Harper & Row: New York, pp. 1–22.

12. Hebb DP (1949) *Organization of Behavior: a Neuropsychological Theory.* Wiley Books: New York.

    See also:

    Carrillo-Reid L, Yang W, Bando Y, Peterka DS, Yuste R (2016) Imprinting and recalling cortical ensembles. *Science* 353: 691–694.

13. See Bindra (1976) in Note 13, Chapter 2.

14. Galambos R, Davis H (1943) The response of single auditory nerve fibers to acoustic stimulation. *Journal of Neurophysiology* 6: 39–57.

    Kiang NY-S (1965) *Discharge Patterns of Single Fibers in the Cat's Auditory Nerve.* MIT Press: Cambridge, MA.

15. Clopton BM, Winfield JA, Flammino RJ (1974) Tonotopic organization: review and analysis. *Brain Research* 76: 1–20.

16. Perrodin C, Kayser C, Logothetis NK, Petkov CI (2011) Voice cells in the primate temporal lobe. *Current Biology* 21: 1408–1415.

17. Wu SM (2010) Synaptic organization of the vertebrate retina: general principles and species-specific variations. *Investigative Ophthalmology & Visual Science* 51: 1264–1274.

18. Corwin JT, Warchol ME (1991) Auditory hair cells: structure, function, development and regeneration. *Annual Review of Neuroscience* 14: 301–333.

19. Fex J, Altschuler RA (1986) Neurotransmitter-related immunocytochemistry of the organ of corti. *Hearing Research* 22: 249–263.

    Klinke R (1986) Neurotransmission in the inner ear. *Hearing Research* 22: 235–243.

20. Buck L, Axel R (1991) A novel multigene family may encode odorant receptors: a molecular basis for odor recognition. *Cell* 65: 175–187.

21. Mombaerts P, Wang F, Dulac C, Chao SK, Nemes A, Mendelsohn M, et al. (1996) Visualizing an olfactory sensory map. *Cell* 87: 675–686.

22. The following paper provides an excellent review of olfactory reception and circuitry. The authors emphasize the remarkable similarity in the organizations of olfactory systems across species ranging from insects to mammals:

    Su, C-Y, Menuz K, Carlson JR (2009) Olfactory perception: receptors, cells, and circuits. *Cell* 139: 45–59.

23. Poo C, Isaacson JS (2009) Odor representations in olfactory cortex: "sparse" coding, global inhibition, and oscillations. *Neuron* 62: 850–861.

24. Apicella A, Yuan Q, Scanziani M, Isaacson JS (2010) Pyramidal cells in piriform cortex receive convergent input from distinct olfactory bulb glomeruli. *Journal of Neuroscience* 30: 14255–14260.

    Wilson DA (2001) Receptive fields in the rat piriform cortex. *Chemical Senses* 26: 577–584.

25. Poo C, Isaacson JS (2011) A major role for intracortical circuits in the strength and tuning of odor-evoked excitation in olfactory cortex. *Neuron* 72: 41–48.

26. Giessel AJ, Datta SR (2014) Olfactory maps, circuits and computations. *Current Opinions in Neurobiology* 24: 120–132.

    Uchida N, Poo C, Haddad R (2014) Coding and transformations in the olfactory system. *Annual Review of Neuroscience* 37: 363–385.

27. Pfaffman C (1959) The afferent code for sensory quality. *American Psychologist* 14: 226–232.

28. Smith DV, St John S (1999) Neural coding of gustatory information. *Current Opinion in Neurobiology* 9: 427–435.

29. Simon SA, de Araujo IE, Gutierrez R, Nicolelis MAL (2006) The neural mechanisms of gustation: a distributed processing code. *Natures Reviews Neuroscience* 7: 890–901.

30. Scott TR, Yaxley S, Stienkiewica ZJ, Rolls ET (1986) Taste responses in the nucleus tractus solitarius of the behaving monkey. *Journal of Neurophysiology* 55: 182–200.

31. Hanamori T, Kunitake T, Kato K, Kannan H (1998) Responses of neurons in the insular cortex to gustatory, visceral and nociceptive stimuli in rats. *Journal of Neurophysiology* 79: 2535–2545.

32. Yamamoto T (2006) Neural substrates for the processing of cognitive and affective aspects of taste in the brain. *Archives of Histology and Cytology* 69: 243–255.

    See also:

    Accolla R, Bathellier B, Petersen CC, Carleton A (2007) Differential spatial representation of taste modalities in the rat gustatory cortex. *Journal of Neuroscience* 27: 1396–1404.

33. Lemon CH, Katz DB (2007) The neural processing of taste. *BMC Neuroscience* 8 (Suppl. 2): S5.

34. Jones LM, Fontanini A, Katz DB (2006) Gustatory processing: a dynamic systems approach. *Current Opinions in Neurobiology* 16: 420–428.

35. Sherrington CS (1906) *The Integrative Action of the Nervous System*. Charles Scribner's Sons: New York.

36. Johnson KO (2001) The roles and functions of cutaneous mechanoreceptors. *Current Opinion in Neurobiology* 11: 455–461.

37. Ekedahl R, Frank O, Hallin RG (1997) Peripheral afferents with common function cluster in the median nerve and somatotopically innervate the human palm. *Brain Research Bulletin* 42: 367–376.

38. Dykes RW, Rasmusson DD, Sretavan D, Rehman NB (1982) Submodality segregation and receptive-field sequences in cuneate, gracile, and external cuneate nuclei of the cat. *Journal of Neurophysiology* 47: 389–416.

39. Saal HP, Bensmaia SJ (2014) Touch is a team effort: interplay of submodalities in cutaneous sensitivity. *Trends in Neuroscience* 37: 689–697.

40. Mountcastle VB (1978) An organizing principle for cerebral function: the unit model and the distributed system. In: Edelman GM, Mountcastle VB, eds., *The Mindful Brain*. MIT Press: Cambridge, MA.

41. Pubols LM, Leroy RF (1977) Orientation detectors in the primary somatosensory neocortex of the raccoon. *Brain Research* 129: 61–74.

42. Pei Y-C, Denchev PV, Hsiao SS, Craig JC, Bensmaia SJ (2009) Convergence of submodality-specific input onto neurons in primary somatosensory cortex. *Journal of Neurophysiology* 102: 1843–1853.

43. Pandya DN, Seltzer B (1982) Association areas of the cerebral cortex. *Trends in Neuroscience* 5: 386–390.

44. Wallace MT, Meredith MA, Stein BF (1992) Integration of multiple sensory modalities in cat cortex. *Experimental Brain Research* 91: 484–488.

45. Schroeder CE, Lindsley RW, Specht C, Marcovici A, Smiley JF, Javitt DC (2001) Somatosensory input to auditory association cortex in the macaque monkey. *Journal of Neurophysiology* 85: 1322–1327.

46. Brett-Green B, Fifková E, Larue DT, Winer JW, Barth DS (2003) A multisensory zone in rat parietotemporal cortex: intra- and extracellular physiology and thalamocortial connections. *Journal of Comparative Neurology* 460: 223–237.

47. Samuelsen CL, Gardner MPH, Fontanini A (2012) Effects of cue-triggered expectation on cortical processing of taste. *Neuron* 74: 410–422.

48. Romanski LM, Hwang J (2012) Timing and audiovisual inputs to the prefrontal cortex and multisensory integration. *Neuroscience* 214: 36–48.

49. See Note 22 of Chapter 4.

50. O'Keefe J, Burgess N (1996) Geometric determinants of the place fields of hippocampal neurons. *Nature* 381: 425–428.

51. O'Keefe J, Recce ML (1993) Phase relationship between hippocampal place units and the EEG theta rhythm. *Hippocampus* 3: 317–330.

52. Hafting T, Flynn M, Molden S, Moser M-B, Moser EI (2005) Microstructure of a spatial map in the entorhinal cortex. *Nature* 436: 801–896.

53. Buzsáki G (2015) Our skewed sense of space. *Science* 347: 612–613.

54. Seghier M (2013) The angular gyrus: multiple functions and multiple subdivisions. *The Neuroscientist* 19: 43–61.

    Sereno MI, Huang R-S (2014) Multisensory maps in parietal cortex. *Current Opinions in Neurobiology* 24: 39–46.

55. Calvert GA, Campbell R, Brammer MJ (2000) Evidence from functional magnetic resonance imaging of crossmodal binding in the human heteromodal cortex. *Current Biology* 10: 649–657.

56. Parent A (1995) *Carpenter's Human Neuroanatomy* (9th ed.). Williams & Wilkins: Baltimore, MD.

57. See Note 47 in Chapter 8. See also:

    Redgrave P, Gurney K (2006) The short-latency dopamine signal: a role in discovering novel actions? *Nature Reviews Neuroscience* 7: 967–975.

58. See Note 24 of Chapter 4.

59. Butler AB, Hodos W (1996) *Comparative Vertebrate Neuroanatomy: Evolution and Adaptation.* John Wiley & Sons: New York.

60. Chow KL, Leiman AL (1970) Aspects of the structural and functional organization of the neocortex. *Neurosciences Research Progress Bulletin* 8: 157–220.

    See also:

    Butler AB, Reiner A, Karten HJ (2011) Evolution of the amniote pallium and the origins of mammalian neocortex. *Annals of the New York Academy of Sciences* 1225: 14–27.

61. Aboitiz F, Morales D, Montiel J (2003) The evolutionary origin of the mammalian isocortex: toward an integrated developmental and functional approach. *Behavioral and Brain Sciences* 26: 535–586.

    Smeets WJAJ, Marín O, González A (2000) Evolution of the basal ganglia: new perspectives through a comparative approach. *Journal of Anatomy* 196: 501–517.

62. Even in primates, there are important projections from the basal ganglia to the tectum that play a major role in controlling the speed and direction of gaze by influencing saccades. See:

    Kim HF, Hikosaka O (2015) Parallel basal ganglia circuits for voluntary and automatic behaviour to reach rewards. *Brain* 138: 776–800.

63. Schoen JHR (1964) Comparative aspects of the descending fibre systems in the spinal cord. *Progress in Brain Research* 11: 203–222.

64. Lawrence DG, Kuypers HGJM (1968) The functional organization of the motor system in the monkey. I. The effects of bilateral pyramidal lesions. *Brain* 91: 1–14.

    See also:

    van Gijn J (2006) From the archives. *Brain* 129: 557–560.

65. Nauta WJH, Mehler WR (1966) Projections of the lentiform nucleus in the monkey. *Brain Research* 1: 3–42.

66. Benarroch EE (2013) Pedunculopontine nucleus: functional organization and clinical implications. *Neurology* 80: 1148–1155.

    Garcia-Rill E, Hyde J, Kezunovic N, Urbano FJ, Petersen E (2015) The physiology of the pedunculopontine nucleus: implications for deep brain stimulation. *Journal of Neural Transmission* 122: 225–235.

    Winn P (2006) How best to consider the structure and function of the pedunculopontine tegmental nucleus: evidence from animal studies. *Journal of the Neurological Sciences* 248: 234–250.

67. ten Donkelaar HJ (1988) Evolution of the red nucleus and rubrospinal tract. *Behavioural Brain Research* 28: 9–20.

68. Hicks TP, Onodera S (2012) The mammalian red nucleus and its role in motor systems, including the emergence of bipedalism and language. *Progress in Neurobiology* 96: 165–175.

69. Barton RA, Dean P (1993) Comparative evidence indicating neural specialization for predatory behaviour in mammals. *Proceedings of the Royal Society of London (Biology)* 254: 63–68.

70. Rose PK, Abrahams VC (1978) Tectospinal and tectoreticular cells: their distribution and afferent connections. *Canadian Journal of Physiology and Pharmacology* 56: 650–658.

71. Stephenson-Jones M, Samuelsson E, Ericsson J, Robertson B, Grillner S (2011) Evolutionary conservation of the basal ganglia as a common vertebrate mechanism for action selection. *Current Biology* 21: 1081–1090.

72. Strausfeld NJ (2012) *Arthropod Brains: Evolution, Functional Elegance, and Historical Significance.* Belknap Press of Harvard University Press: Cambridge, MA.

    See also Note 83, Chapter 8.

73. Qin J, Wheeler AR (2007) Maze exploration and learning in *C. elegans. Lab on a Chip* 7: 186–192.

74. Kusayama T, Watanabe S (2000) Reinforcing effects of amphetamine in planarians. *NeruoReport* 11: 2511–2513.

75. Brembs B, Lorenzetti FD, Reyes FD, Baxter DA, Bryne JH (2002) Operant reward learning in *Aplysia*: neuronal correlates and mechanism. *Science* 296: 1706–1709.

76. Kabotyanski EA, Baster DA, Cushman SJ, Byrne JH (2000) Modulation of fictive feeding by dopamine and serotonin in *Aplysia. Journal of Neurophysiology* 83: 374–392.

77. Barron AB, Søvik E, Cronish JL (2010) The roles of dopamine and related compounds in reward-seeking behaviors across animal phyla. *Frontiers in Behavioral Neuroscience* 4: article 163.

78. Falck B, Hillarp NÅ, Thieme G, Torp A (1962) Fluorescence of catechol amines and related compounds condensed with formaldehyde. *Journal of Histochemistry and Cytochemistry* 10: 348–354.

79. See Note 19 in Chapter 2.

80. This description of the brain's dopamine systems is a convenient heuristic for what is now known to be a far more complex anatomical picture. See:

    Björklund A, Dunnett SB (2007) Dopamine neuron systems in the brain: an update. *Trends in Neuroscience* 30: 194–202.

    Lookingland KJ, Moore KE (2005) Functional neuroanatomy of hypothalamic dopaminergic neuroendocrine systems. In: Dunnett SB, Bentivoglio M, Björklund A, Hökfelt T, eds., *Handbook of Chemical Neuroanatomy Volume 21 Dopamine.* Elsevier: Amsterdam, pp. 435–523.

81. See Schultz (1998) in Note 60, Chapter 5.

82. Kemp JM, Powell TPS (1971) The synaptic organization of the caudate nucleus. *Philosophical Transactions of the Royal Society of London (Biology)* 262: 403–412.

    The other approximately 5% of neurons in the striatum include not only large aspiny cholinergic interneurons, but also five subtypes of interneurons that use GABA as their neurotransmitter. These GABAergic interneurons include parvalbumin-expressing fast-spiking interneurons; neurons that co-express neuropeptide Y, somatostatin, and nitric oxide synthase along with GABA and are termed low-threshold spiking interneurons; GABA and neuropeptide Y-only-expressing neurogliaform interneurons; tyrosine hydroxylase-expressing interneurons; and calretinin-expressing interneurons. The function of these interneurons is not well understood. See Chapter 12 and:

    Tritsch NX, Sabatini BL (2012) Dopamine modulation of synaptic transmission in cortex and striatum. *Neuron* 76: 33–50.

83. Pasik P, Pasik T, DiFiglia M (1976) Quantitative aspects of neuronal organization in the neostriatum of macaque monkey. In: Yahr MD, ed., *The Basal Ganglia: Association for Research in Nervous and Mental Disease Volume 55.* Raven Press: New York, pp. 57–90.

84. Kincaid AE, Zheng T, Wilson CJ (1998) Connectivity and convergence of single corticospinal axons. *Journal of Neuroscience* 18: 4722–4731.

85. Freund TF, Powell JF, Smith AD (1984) Tyrosine hydroxylase-immunoreactive boutons in synaptic contact with identified striatonigral neurons, with particular reference to dendritic spines. *Neuroscience* 13: 1189–1215.

86. Wickens J (1993) *A Theory of the Striatum.* Pergamon Press: Oxford.

    Wickens J, Kötter R (1995) Cellular models of reinforcement. In: Houk JC, Davis JL, Beiser DG, eds., *Models of Information Processing in the Basal Ganglia.* MIT Press: Cambridge, MA: pp. 187–214.

87. Zheng T, Wilson CJ (2002) Corticostriatal combinatorics: the implications of corticostriatal axonal arborizations. *Journal of Neurophysiology* 87: 1007–1017.

88. Kemp JM, Powell TPS (1971) The site of termination of afferent fibres in the caudate nucleus. *Philosophical Transactions of the Royal Society of London (Biology)* 262: 413–427.

89. Bentivoglio M, Morelli M (2005) The organization and circuits of mesencephalic dopaminergic neurons and the distribution of dopamine receptors in the brain. In: Dunnett

SB, Bentivoglio M, Björklund A, Hökfelt T, eds., *Handbook of Chemical Neuroanatomy Volume 21 Dopamine*. Elsevier: Amsterdam, pp. 1–107.

90. Andén NE, Fuxe K, Hamberger B, Hökfelt TA (1966) A quantitative study of the nigro-neostriatal dopamine neurons. *Acta Physiologica Scandinavica* 67: 306–312.

91. Moss J, Bolam JP (2010) The relationship between dopaminergic axons and glutamatergic synapses: structural considerations. In: Iversen LL, Iversen SD, Dunnett SB, Björklund A, eds., *Dopamine Handbook*. Oxford University Press: Oxford, pp. 49–59.

These authors also discuss *thalamo*striatal projections. These originate from the intralaminar thalamus and project to the caudate-putamen. Thalamostriatal glutamatergic neurons originating from the centromedian, central medial, and paracentral nucleus (centromedian and parafascicular nucleus in rodents) make about as many axospinous contacts with striatal medium spiny neurons as corticostriatal afferents and the plasticity of these synapses, like that of corticospinal synapses, may depend on dopamine. Unlike the relatively sparse connection of any one corticostriatal afferent with a single medium spiny neuron, individual thalamostriatal afferents may make multiple contacts with a single medium spiny neuron; this suggests that the nature of the influence of thalamostriatal afferents on medium spiny neurons may be different from that of corticostriatal afferents. The thalamostriatal projections have received much less attention from researchers than the corticostriatal projections. See also Redgrave and Gurney in Note 57 and:

Bennett BD, Wilson CJ (2000) Synaptology and physiology of neostriatal neurones. In: Miller R, Wickens JR, eds., *Brain Dynamics and the Striatal Complex*. Harwood Academic Publishers: Amsterdam, pp. 111–140.

92. Albin RL, Young AB, Penney JB (1989) The functional anatomy of basal ganglia disorders. *Trends in Neuroscience* 12: 366–375.

Gerfen CR (2000) Molecular effects of dopamine in striatal-projection pathways. *Trends in Neuroscience* 23: S64–S70.

Smith Y, Bevan MD, Shink E, Bolam JP (1998) Microcircuitry of the direct and indirect pathways of the basal ganglia. *Neuroscience* 86: 353–387.

93. Lei W, Jiao Y, Del Mar N, Reiner A (2004) Evidence for differential cortical input to direct pathway versus indirect pathway striatal projection neurons in rats. *Journal of Neuroscience* 24: 8289–8299.

94. Reiner A, Medina L, Veenman CL (1998) Structural and functional evolution of the basal ganglia in vertebrates. *Brain Research Reviews* 28: 235–285.

95. Humphries MD, Prescott TJ (2010) The ventral basal ganglia, a selection mechanism at the crossroads of space, strategy, and reward. *Progress in Neurobiology* 90: 385–417.

96. MacAskill A, Little JP, Cassel JM, Carter AG (2012) Subcellular connectivity underlies pathway-specific signaling in the nucleus accumbens. *Nature Neuroscience* 15: 1624–1626.

97. Haber SN, Fudge JL, McFarland NR (2000) Striatonigrostriatal pathways in primates form an ascending spiral from the shell to the dorsolateral striatum. *Journal of Neuroscience* 20: 2369–2382.

See also:

Haber SN (2014) The place of dopamine in the cortico-basal ganglia circuit. *Neuroscience* 282: 248–257.

Robbins TW, Cador M, Taylor JR, Everitt BJ (1989) Limbic-striatal interactions in reward-related processes. *Neuroscience and Biobehavioral Reviews* 13: 155–162.

98. Burton AC, Nakamura K, Roesch MR (2015) From ventral-medial to dorsal-lateral striatum: neural correlates of reward-guided decision-making. *Neurobiology of Learning and Memory* 117: 51–59.

    See also:

    Rueda-Orozoco P, Robbe D (2015) The striatum multiplexes contextual and kinematic information to constrain motor habits execution. *Nature Neuroscience* 18: 453–460.

99. Williams GV, Rolls ET, Leonard CM, Stern C (1993) Neuronal responses in the ventral striatum of the behaving macaque. *Behavioural Brain Research* 55: 243–252.

100. Koya E, Golden SA, Harvey BK, Guez-Barber DH, Berkow A, Simmons DE, et al. (2009) Targeted disruption of cocaine-activated nucleus accumbens neurons prevents context-specific sensitization. *Nature Neuroscience* 12: 1069–1073.

    In this interesting paper the authors showed that rats given an injection of cocaine in an environment previously paired with cocaine showed a sensitized locomotor activity response versus control rats also tested in that environment but with a similar history of cocaine injections paired with another environment. Although they failed to observe a significant conditioned activity effect in a saline test, the result from the cocaine test is consistent with incentive learning about the cues in the cocaine-paired environment (Chapter 3). They showed that a small subset of sparsely distributed nucleus accumbens neurons was activated by exposure to cocaine in the environment previously paired with cocaine. They used transgenetic rats that allowed them to specifically inactivate those neurons and found that this manipulation eliminated the sensitized response to cocaine in the cocaine-paired environment. They concluded that environmental stimuli were encoded by a small subset of nucleus accumbens neurons and that those neurons were necessary for the observation of a sensitized response to cocaine. The sensitized response to cocaine observed only in the environment previously paired with cocaine is an example of incentive learning, those stimuli having an increased ability to elicit approach and other responses.

101. Miller R (1981) *Meaning and Purpose in the Intact Brain*. Oxford University Press: Oxford.

102. Perin CT (1943) A quantitative investigation of the delay-of-reinforcement gradient. *Journal of Experimental Psychology* 32: 37–51.

103. Ellison GD (1964) Differential salivary conditioning to traces. *Journal of Comparative and Physiological Psychology* 57: 373–380.

Chapter 12

1. Recall from Chapter 4 that incentive learning is only one type of learning. The fox may learn the cognitive map of the region in which it is foraging, for example, and dopamine may not be necessary for this type of learning. The likelihood of certain responses, e.g. clearing reeds with the muzzle or biting the eggs in a particular way, may be enhanced by incentive learning, but the cortical neuronal cell assemblies activated by those responses may also be partially activated by dopamine-independent associative learning mechanisms that link contiguously activated cell assemblies.

2. Yao W-D, Spealman RD, Zhang J (2008) Dopaminergic signaling in dendritic spines. *Biochemical Pharmacology* 75: 2055–2069.

3. Girault J-A, Valjent E, Caboche J, Hervé D (2007) ERK2: a logical AND gate critical for drug-induced plasticity? *Current Opinion in Pharmacology* 7: 77–85.

4. Shiflett MW, Balleine BW (2011) Molecular substrates of action control by cortico-striatal circuits. *Progress in Neurobiology* 95: 1–13.

5. Eccles JC (1981) Calcium in long-term potentiation as a model of memory. *Neuroscience* 10: 1071–1081

   Sir John Eccles (1903–1997) received the 1963 Nobel Prize in Physiology or Medicine for his pioneering work on the synapse and his subsequent discovery of chemical neurotransmission. Note that metabotropic glutamate receptors are also found at corticostriatal axospinous synapses stimulated by glutamate; they can activate phospholipase C that, in turn, increases the formation of inositol triphosphate leading to the release of intracellular calcium, providing a parallel route for increasing intracellular calcium concentration following activity at glutamatergic synapses.

6. Wickens J (1990) Striatal dopamine in motor activation and reward-mediated learning, steps towards a unifying model. *Journal of Neural Transmission* 80: 9–31.

7. Wickens J (1988) Electrically coupled but chemically isolated synapses: dendritic spines and calcium in a rule for synaptic modification. *Progress in Neurobiology* 31: 507–528.

   See also:

   Koch C, Zador A (1993) The function of dendritic spines: devices subserving biochemical rather than electrical compartmentalization. *Journal of Neuroscience* 13: 413–422.

8. Kennedy MB (2000) Signal-processing machines at the postsynaptic density. *Science* 290: 750–754.

   Soderling TR, Derkach VA (2000) Postsynaptic protein phosphorylation and LTP. *Trends in Neuroscience* 23: 75–80.

9. Kim J, Jung SC, Clemens AM, Petralia RS, Hoffman DA (2007) Regulation of dendritic excitability by activity-dependent trafficking of the A-type K+ channel subunit Kv4.2 in hippocampal neurons. *Neuron* 54: 933–947.

   Lei Z, Deng P, Xu ZC (2008) Regulation of Kv4.2 channels by glutamate in cultured hippocampal neurons. *Journal of Neurochemistry* 106: 182–192.

10. Lucchesi W, Mizuno K, Giese KP (2011) Novel insights into CaMKII function and regulation during memory formation. *Brain Research Bulletin* 85: 2–8.

11. Barria A, Derkach V, Soderling T (1997) Identification of the Ca^{2+}/calmodulin-dependent protein kinase II regulatory phosphorylation site in the α-amino-3-hydroxy-5-methyl-4-isoxazole-propionate-type glutamate receptor. *Journal of Biological Chemistry* 272: 32727–32730.

    Lee H-K, Barbarosie M, Kameyama K, Baer MF, Huganir RL (2000) Regulation of distinct AMPA receptor phosphorylation sites during bidirectional plasticity. *Nature* 405: 955–959.

    Lisman J, Schulman H, Cline H (2002) The molecular basis of CaMKII function in synaptic and behavioural memory. *Nature Reviews Neuroscience* 3: 175–190.

12. Lüscher C, Nicoll RA, Malenka RC, Muller D (2000) Synaptic plasticity and dynamic modulation of the postsynaptic membrane. *Nature Neuroscience* 3: 545–550.

The neurotrophin, brain-derived neurotrophic factor (BDNF) has been implicated in AMPA receptor trafficking and synaptic plasticity. Further studies are needed to understand the possible role of BDNF in striatal synaptic plasticity. See:

Li X, Wolf ME (2015) Multiple faces of BDNF in cocaine addiction. *Behavioural Brain Research* 279: 240–254.

13. Birnbaum SG, Varga AW, Yuan LL, Anderson AE, Sweatt JD, Schrader LA (2004) Structure and function of Kv4-family transient potassium channels. *Physiological Review* 84: 803–833.

14. Lu L, Koya E, Zhai H, Hope BT, Shaham Y (2006) Role of ERK in cocaine addiction. *Trends in Neuroscience* 29: 695–703.

15. Greengard P, Allen PB, Nairn AC (1999) Beyond the dopamine receptor: the DARPP-32/ protein phosphatase-1 cascade. *Neuron* 23: 435–447.

See also:

Walaas SI, Hemmings HC Jr., Greengard P, Nairn AC (2011) Beyond the dopamine receptor: regulation and roles of serine/threonine protein phosphatases. *Frontiers of Neuroanatomy* 5: article 50.

16. Dash PK, Moore AN, Kobori N, Runyan JD (2007) Molecular activity underlying working memory. *Learning & Memory* 14: 554–563.

17. Baumgärtel K, Mansuy IM (2012) Neural functions of calcineurin in synaptic plasticity and memory. *Learning and Memory* 19: 375–384.

18. Nishi A, Bibb JA, Matsuyama S, Hamada M, Higashi H, Nairn AC, Greengard P (2002) Regulation of DARPP-32 phosphorylation at PKA- and Cdk5-sites by NMDA and AMPA receptors: distinct roles of calcineurin and protein phosphatase-2A. *Journal of Neurochemistry* 81: 832–841.

Nishi A, Bibb JA, Snyder GL, Higashi H, Nairn AC, Greengard P (2000) Amplification of dopaminergic signaling by a positive feedback loop. *Proceedings of the National Academy of Sciences of the United States of America* 97: 12840–12845.

See also Walaas et al. in Note 15

19. Paul S, Nairn AC, Wang P, Lombroso PJ (2003) NMDA-mediated activation of the tyrosine phosphatase STEP regulates the duration of ERK signaling. *Nature Neuroscience* 6: 34–42.

20. Lin AH, Onyike CU, Abrams TW (1998) Sequence-dependent interaction between transient calcium and transmitter stimuli in activation of mammalian adenylyl cyclase. *Brain Research* 800: 300–307.

Yovell Y, Kandel ER, Dudai Y, Abrams TW (1992) A quantitative study of the Ca^{2+}/ calmodulin sensitivity of adenylyl cyclase in *Aplysia*, *Drosophila*, and rat. *Journal of Neurochemistry* 59: 1736–1744.

Zhang J, Xu T-W, Hallett PJ, Watanabe M, Grant SGN, Isacson O, Yao W-D (2009) PSD-95 uncouples dopamine-glutamate interactions in the D_1/PSD-95/NMDA receptor complex. *Journal of Neuroscience* 29: 2948–2960.

Note that Zhang et al. (2009) discuss mechanisms for NMDA-D1 receptor cooperation. They note that NMDA receptor stimulation mediates D1 receptor signaling enhancement.

21. In hippocampus:

Pei L, Lee FJS, Moszczynska A, Vukusic B, Liu F (2004) Regulation of dopamine D1 receptor function by physical interaction with the NMDA receptor. *Journal of Neuroscience* 24: 1149–1158.

In striatum:

Scott L, Kruse MS, Forssberg H, Brismar H, Greengard P, Aperia A (2002) Selective up-regulation of dopamine D1 receptors in dendritic spines by NMDA receptor activation. *Proceedings of the National Academy of Sciences of the United States of America* 99: 1661–1664.

22. Abrams TW, Kandel ER (1988) Is contiguity in classical conditioning a system or a cellular property? Learning in *Aplysia* suggests a possible molecular site. *Trends in Neuroscience* 11: 128–135.

Abrams TW, Karl KA, Kandel ER (1991) Biochemical studies of stimulus convergence during classical conditioning in *Aplysia*: dual regulation of adenylate cyclase by Ca^{2+}/calmodulin and transmitter. *Journal of Neuroscience* 11: 2655–2665.

Eliot LS, Hawkins RD, Kandel ER, Schacher S (1994) Pairing-specific, activity-dependent presynaptic facilitation at *Aplysia* sensory-motor neuron synapses in isolated cell culture. *Journal of Neuroscience* 14: 368–383.

23. Hawkins RD, Abrams TW, Carew TJ, Kandel ER (1983) A cellular mechanism of classical conditioning in *Aplysia*: activity-dependent amplification of presynaptic facilitation. *Science* 219: 400–405.

24. Brunelli M, Castellucci V, Kandel ER (1976) Synaptic facilitation and behavioral sensitization in *Aplysia*: possible role of serotonin and cAMP. *Science* 194: 1178–1181.

25. Kawagoe KT, Garris PA, Wiedemann DJ, Wightman RM (1992) Regulation of transient dopamine concentration gradients in the microenvironment surrounding nerve terminals in the rat striatum. *Neuroscience* 51: 55–64.

26. Wolfram Schultz (1998), on pages 8–11 of the paper cited in Note 60 of Chapter 5, provides an excellent discussion of phasic dopamine's influence on target structures. He cites the work of many researchers and discusses details of the timing of changes in dopamine concentration associated with reward-related phasic bursts of activity in dopamine neurons and the mechanisms for rapidly decreasing dopamine concentrations. See also:

Pawlak V, Wickens JR, Kirkwood A, Kerr NJD (2010) Timing is not everything: neuromodulation opens the STDP gate. *Frontiers in Synaptic Neuroscience* 2: article 146.

27. Price CJ, Kim P, Raymond LA (1999) D1 dopamine receptor-induced cyclic AMP-dependent protein kinase phosphorylation and potentiation of striatal glutamate receptors. *Journal of Neurochemistry* 73: 2441–2446.

28. Kessels HW, Malinow R (2009) Synaptic AMPA receptor plasticity and behavior. *Neuron* 61: 340–350.

29. See the following review for many references and details of ERK signaling:

Wiegert JS, Bading H (2011) Activity-dependent calcium signaling in ERK-MAP kinases in neurons: a link to structural plasticity of the nucleus and gene transcription regulation. *Cell Calcium* 49: 296–305.

See also:

Day JJ (2008) Extracellular signal-regulated kinase activation during natural reward learning: a physiological role for phasic nucleus accumbens dopamine? *Journal of Neuroscience* 28: 4295–4297.

Jenab S, Festa ED, Nazarian A, Wu HBK, Sun WL, Hazim R, Russo SJ, Quinones-Jenab V (2005) Cocaine induction of ERK proteins in dorsal striatum of Fischer rats. *Molecular Brain Research* 142: 134–138.

Matamales M, Girault J-A (2011) Signaling from the cytoplasm to the nucleus of striatal medium-sized spiny neurons. *Frontiers in Neuroanatomy* 5: 37.

Valjent E, Pascoli V, Svenningsson P, Paul S, Enslen H, Corvol JC, et al. (2005) Regulation of protein phosphatase cascade allows convergent dopamine and glutamatergic signals to activate ERK in the striatum. *Proceedings of the National Academy of Sciences of the United States of America* 102: 491–496.

30. Huang F, Chotiner JK, Steward O (2007) Actin polymerization and ERK phosphorylation are required for Arc/Arg3.1 mRNA targeting to activated synaptic sites on dendrites. *Journal of Neuroscience* 27: 9054–9067.

31. Frank DA, Greenberg ME (1994) CREB: a mediator of long-term memory from mollusks to mammals. *Cell* 79: 5–8.

32. Ciccarelli A, Giustetto M (2014) Role of ERK signaling in activity-dependent modifications of histone proteins. *Neuropharmacology* 80: 34–44.

Stipanovich A, Valjent E, Matamales M, Nishi A, Ahn J-H, Maroteaux M, et al. (2008) A phosphatase cascade by which rewarding stimuli control nucleosomal response. *Nature* 453: 879–884.

33. Beninger RJ, Gerdjikov TV (2004) The role of signaling molecules in reward-related incentive learning. *Neurotoxicity Research* 6: 91–104.

See also:

Beninger and Nakonechny (1996) in Note 35 of Chapter 7

34. Bodetto SP, Romieu P, Sartori M, Tesone-Colho C, Majchrzak M, Barbelivien A, et al. (2014) Differential regulation of MeCP2 and PP1 in passive or voluntary administration of cocaine or food. *International Journal of Neuropsychopharmacology* 17: 2031–2044.

35. Tropea TF, Kosofsky BE, Rajadhyaksha AM (2008) Enhanced CREB and DARPP-32 phosphorylation in the nucleus accumbens and CREB, ERK, and GluR1 phosphorylation in the dorsal hippocampus is associated with cocaine-conditioned place preference behavior. *Journal of Neurochemistry* 106: 1780–1790.

See also:

Segovia KN, Correa M, Lennington JB, Conover JC, Salamone JD (2012) Changes in nucleus accumbens and neostriatal c-Fos and DARPP-32 immunoreactivity during different stages of food-reinforced instrumental learning. *European Journal of Neuroscience* 35: 1354–1367.

36. Kirschmann EKZ, Mauna JC, Willis CM, Foster RL, Chipman AM, Thiels E (2014) Appetitive cue-evoked ERK signaling in the nucleus accumbens requires NMDA and D1 dopamine receptor activation and regulates CREB phosphorylation. *Learning & Memory* 21: 606–615.

See also:

Fricks-Gleason A, Marashll JF (2011) Role of dopamine D1 receptors in the activation of nucleus accumbens extracellular signal-regulated kinase (ERK) by cocaine-paired contextual cues. *Neuropsychopharmacology* 36: 434–444.

Sun W-L, Zhou L, Hazim R, Quinones-Jenab V, Jenab S (2007) Effects of acute cocaine on ERK and DARPP-32 phosphorylation pathways in the caudate-putamen of Fischer rats. *Brain Research* 1178: 12–19.

37. Rajan KE, Thangaleela S, Balasundaram C (2015) Spatial learning associated with stimulus response in goldfish *Carassius auratus*: relationship to activation of CREB signaling. *Fish Physiology and Biochemistry* 41: 685–694.

38. Kim YC, Lee HG, Han KA (2007) D1 dopamine receptor dDA1 is required in the mushroom body neurons for aversive and appetitive learning in *Drosophila*. *Journal of Neuroscience* 27: 7640–7647.

See also:

Waddell S (2013) Reinforcement signalling in *Drosophila*; dopamine does it all after all. *Current Opinion in Neurobiology* 23: 324–329.

Dubnau J, Tully T (1998) Gene discovery in *Drosophila*: new insights for learning and memory. *Annual Review of Neuroscience* 21: 407–444.

39. Waddell S, Quinn WG (2001) Flies, genes, and learning. *Annual Review of Neuroscience* 24: 1283–1309.

40. Guan Z, Buhl LK, Quinn WG, Littleton JT (2011) Altered gene regulation and synaptic morphology in *Drosophila* learning and memory mutants. *Learning & Memory* 18: 191–206.

41. Davis RL (2005) Olfactory memory formation in *Drosophila*: from molecular to systems neuroscience. *Annual Review of Neuroscience* 28: 275–302.

42. Bédécarrrats A, Cornet C, Simmers J, Nargeot R (2013) Implication of dopaminergic modulation in operant reward learning and the induction of compulsive-like feeding behavior in *Aplysia*. *Learning & Motivation* 20: 318–327.

See also Note 75 in Chapter 11

43. Nargeot R, Simmers J (2011) Neural mechanisms of operant conditioning and learning-induced behavioral plasticity in *Aplysia*. *Cellular and Molecular Life Sciences* 68: 803–816.

44. Bliss TVP, Lømo T (1973) Long-lasting potentiation of synaptic transmission in the dentate area of the anaesthetized rabbit following stimulation of the perforant path. *Journal of Physiology (London)* 232: 331–356.

Lømo T (2003) The discovery of long-term potentiation. *Philosophical Transactions of the Royal Society of London B* 358: 617–620.

45. Mayford M, Siegelbaum SA, Kandel ER (2012) Synapses and memory storage. *Cold Spring Harbor Perspectives in Biology* 4: a005751.

Nguyen PV, Kandel ER (1997) Brief θ-burst stimulation induces a transcription-dependent late phase of LTP requiring cAMP in area CA1 of the mouse hippocampus. *Learning & Memory* 4: 230–243.

46. Coultrap SJ, Bayer KU (2012) CaMKII regulation in information processing and storage. *Trends in Neuroscience* 35: 607–618.

Lemieux M, Labrecque S, Tardif C, Labrie-Dion É, LeBel É, De Koninck P (2012) Translocation of CaMKII to dendritic microtubules supports the plasticity of local synapses. *Journal of Cell Biology* 198: 1055–1073.

47. Sweatt JD (2001) The neuronal MAP kinase cascade: a biochemical signal integration system subserving synaptic plasticity and memory. *Journal of Neurochemistry* 76: 1–10.

48. Hinz FI, Aizerberg M, Tushev G, Schuman EM (2013) Protein synthesis-dependent associative long-term memory in larval zebrafish. *Journal of Neuroscience* 33: 15382–15387.

49. Reymann KG, Frey JU (2007) The late maintenance of hippocampal LTP: requirements, phases, "synaptic tagging," "late-associativity" and implications. *Neuropharmacology* 52: 24–40.

50. Hyman SE, Malenka RC, Nestler EJ (2006) Neural mechanisms of addiction: the role of reward-related learning and memory. *Annual Review of Neuroscience* 29: 565–598.

    Pitchers KK, Vialou V, Nestler EJ, Laviolette SR, Lehman MN, Coolen LM (2013) Natural and drug rewards act on common neural plasticity mechanisms with ΔFosB as a key mediator. *Journal of Neuroscience* 33: 3434–3442.

51. Girault J-A (2012) Signaling in striatal neurons: the phosphoproteins of reward, addiction, and dyskinesia. *Progress in Molecular Biology and Translational Science* 106: 33–62.

    Rogge GA, Singh H, Dang R, Wood MA (2013) HDAC3 is a negative regulator of cocaine-context-associated memory formation. *Journal of Neuroscience* 33: 6623–6632.

52. Kalivas PW (2004) Glutamate systems in cocaine addiction. *Current Opinion in Pharmacology* 4: 23–29.

    Kalivas PW, Volkow N, Seamans J (2005) Unmanageable motivation in addiction: a pathology in prefrontal-accumbens glutamate transmission. *Neuron* 45: 647–650.

53. Norrholm SC, Bibb JA, Nestler EJ, Ouimet CC, Taylor JR, Greengard P (2003) Cocaine-induced proliferation of dendritic spines in nucleus accumbens is dependent on the activity of cyclin-dependent kinase-5. *Neuroscience* 116: 19–22.

54. Berke JD, Paletzki RF, Aronson GJ, Hyman SE, Gerfen CR (1998) A complex program of striatal gene expression induced by dopaminergic stimulation. *Journal of Neuroscience* 18: 5301–5310.

    McClung CA, Nestler EJ (2003) Regulation of gene expression and cocaine reward by CREB and ΔFosB. *Nature Neuroscience* 11: 1208–1215.

55. Robinson TE, Kolb B (2004) Structureal plasticity associated with exposure to drugs of abuse. *Neuropharmacology* 47: 33–46.

    See also:

    Li J, Liu N, Lu K, Zhang L, Gu J, Guo F, et al. (2012) Cocaine-induced dendritic remodeling occurs in both D1 and D2 dopamine receptor-expressing neurons in the nucleus accumbens. *Neuroscience Letters* 517: 118–122.

56. Yagishita S, Hayashi-Takagi A, Ellis-Davies GCR, Urakubo H, Ishii S, Kasai H (2014) A critical time window for dopamine actions on the structural plasticity of dendritic spines. *Science* 345: 1616–1620.

    See also:

Fisher SD, Robertson PB, Black MJ, Redgrave P, Sagar MA, Abraham WC, Reynolds JNL (2017) Reinforcement determines the timing dependence of corticostriatal synaptic plasticity in vivo. *Nature Communications* 8: 334.

57. See Note 130 of Chapter 7.

58. Sokoloff P, Leriche L, Diaz J, Louvel J, Pumain R (2013) Direct and indirect interactions of the dopamine D3 receptor with glutamate pathways: implications for the treatment of schizophrenia. *Naunyn-Schmiedeberg's Archives of Pharmacology* 386: 107–124.

59. Beninger RJ, Gerdjikov TV (2005) Dopamine-glutamate interactions in reward-related incentive learning. In: Schmidt WJ, Reith MEA, eds., *Dopamine and Glutamate in Psychiatric Disorders*. Humana Press: Totowa, NJ, pp. 319–354.

60. Zhang F, Tsai H-C, Airan RD, Stuber GD, Adamantidis AR, de Lecea L, et al. (2015) Optogenetics in freely moving mammals: dopamine and reward. *Cold Spring Harbor Protocols*: doi: 10.1101/pdb.top086330.

    See also:

    Steinberg EE, Janak PH (2013) Establishing causality for dopamine in neural function and behavior with optogenetics. *Brain Research* 1511: 46–64.

61. Kravitz AV, Freeze BS, Parker PRL, Kay K, Thwin MT, Deisseroth K, Kreitzer AC (2010) Regulation of parkinsonian motor behaviours by optogenetic control of basal ganglia circuitry. *Nature* 466: 622–626.

    The results in this paper are based on global manipulations of the direct or indirect pathway. In a normally behaving animal, both pathways appear to be involved in action selection, with the direct pathway promoting the effective motor program and the indirect pathway inhibiting competing motor programs. This view is not inconsistent with that of Kravitz et al. but is a refinement on their findings. See:

    Cui G, Jun SB, Jin X, Pham MD, Vogel SS, Lovinger DM, Costa RM (2013) Concurrent activation of striatal direct and indirect pathways during action initiation. *Nature* 494: 238–242.

62. Calabresi P, Picconi B, Tozzi A, Di Filippo M (2007) Dopamine-mediated regulation of corticostriatal synaptic plasticity. *Trends in Neuroscience* 30: 211–219.

63. Cerovic M, d-Isa R, Tonini R, Brambilla R (2013) Molecular and cellular mechanisms of dopamine-mediated behavioral plasticity in the striatum. *Neurobiology of Learning and Memory* 105: 63–80.

    See also:

    Bateup HS, Svenningsson P, Kuroiwa M, Gong S, Nishi A, Heintz N, Greengard P (2008) Cell type-specific regulation of DARPP-32 phosphorylation by psychostimulant and antipsychotic drugs. *Nature Neuroscience* 11: 932–939.

    Lovinger DM (2010) Neurotransmitter roles in synaptic modulation, plasticity and learning in the dorsal striatum. *Neuropharmacology* 58: 951–961.

    Reynolds JNJ, Wickens JR (2000) Substantia nigra dopamine regulates synaptic plasticity and membrane potential fluctuations in the rat neostriatum, *in vivo*. *Neuroscience* 99: 199–203.

    Schultz W (2013) Updating dopamine reward signals. *Current Opinion in Neurobiology* 23: 229–2238.

Wickens JR (2009) Synaptic plasticity in the basal ganglia. *Behavioural Brain Research* 199: 119–128.

64. Dupuis JP, Bioulac BH, Baufreton J (2014) Long-term depression at distinct glutamatergic synapses in the basal ganglia. *Reviews in the Neurosciences* 25: 741–754.

Uchigashima M, Narushima M, Fukaya M, Katona I, Kano M, Watanabe M (2007) Subcellular arrangement of molecules for 2-archidonyl-glycerol-mediated retrograde signaling and its physiological contribution to synaptic modulation in the striatum. *Journal of Neuroscience* 27: 3663–3676.

65. Lobo MK, Covington HE, Chaudhury D, Friedman AK, Sun H, Damez-Werno D, et al. (2010) Cell type-specific loss of BDNF signaling mimics optogenetic control of cocaine reward. *Science* 330: 385–390.

Steinberg EE, Boivin JR, Saunders BT, Witten IB, Deisseroth K, Janak PH (2014) Positive reinforcement mediated by midbrain dopamine neurons requires D1 and D2 receptor activation in the nucleus accumbens. *PLOS ONE* 9: e94771.

66. Calipari ES, Bagot RC, Purushothaman I, Davidson TJ, Yorgason JT, Peña CJ, et al. (2016) In vivo imaging identifies temporal signature of D1 and D2 medium spiny neurons in cocaine reward. *Proceedings of the National Academy of Sciences of the United States of America* 113: 2726–2731.

One study in this excellent paper uses designer receptors exclusively activated by designer drugs to inactivate D1 receptor-expressing medium spiny neurons during the expression of conditioned place preference based on cocaine in mice. They observed that conditioned place preference was blocked. This led the authors to conclude "that D1 signaling is the critical mediator of drug-context learning" (pp. 2728–2729). However, this conclusion is not justified by the findings. The findings clearly show that activity in D1 receptor-expressing neurons is necessary for the expression of incentive learning but do not show that D1 receptor stimulation is required. As discussed at great length in this chapter, incentive learning appears to involve strengthening of corticostriatal glutamatergic synapses onto D1 receptor-expressing neurons. Once incentive learning has taken place, its expression is possible, even when dopamine receptors are blocked. In spite of their earlier statement, the authors go on in their Discussion to say that dopamine-mediated learning involves strengthening of glutamatergic synapses onto medium spiny neurons and that this could underlie some of the changes in responding to conditioned incentive stimuli. The data support this claim.

67. Beaulieu J-M, Gainetdinov RR (2011) The physiology, signaling, and pharmacology of dopamine receptors. *Pharmacological Reviews* 63: 182–217.

68. Miller JS, Barr JL, Harper LJ, Poole RL, Gould TJ, Unterwald EM (2014) The GSK3 signaling pathway is activated by cocaine and is critical for cocaine conditioned reward in mice. *PLOS ONE* 9: e88026.

69. Wickens R, Quartarone SE, Beninger RJ. (2017) Inhibition of GSK3 by SB 216763 affects acquisition at lower doses than expression of amphetamine-conditioned place preference in rats. *Behavioural Pharmacology* 28: 262–271.

70. Nelson CD, Kim MJ, Hsin H, Chen Y, Sheng M (2013) Phosphorylation of threonine-19 of PSD-95 by GSK-3β is required for PSD-95 mobilization and long-term depression. *Journal of Neuroscience* 33: 12122–12135.

71. Beaulieu J-M, Gainetdinov RP, Caron MG (2007) The Akt-GSK-3 signaling cascade in the actions of dopamine. *Trends in Pharmacological Sciences* 28: 166–172.

    Beaulieu J-M, Sotnikova TD, Yao W-D, Kockeritz L, Woodgett JR, Gainetdinov PR, Caron, MG (2004) Lithium antagonizes dopamine-dependent behaviors mediated by an AKT/glycogen synthase kinase 3 signaling cascade. *Proceedings of the National Academy of Sciences of the United States of America* 101: 5099–5104.

72. Inestrosa NC, Varela-Nallar L (2014) Wnt signaling in the nervous system and in Alzheimer's disease. *Journal of Molecular Cell Biology* 6: 64–74.

73. Logan CY, Nusse R (2004) The Wnt signaling pathway in development and disease. *Annual Review of Cell and Developmental Biology* 20: 781–810.

74. Chen J, Park CS, Tang S-J (2006) Activity-dependent synaptic Wnt release regulates hippocampal long term potentiation. *Journal of Biological Chemistry* 281: 11910–11916.

75. Islam F, Xu K, Beninger RJ (2017) Inhibition of Wnt signalling dose-dependently impairs the acquisition and expression of amphetamine-induced conditioned place preference. *Behavioural Brain Research* 326: 217–225.

76. Svenningsson P, Le Moine C, Fisone G, Fredholm BB (1999) Distribution, biochemistry and function of striatal A_{2A} receptors. *Progress in Neurobiology* 59: 355–396.

77. See Schultz (1998) in Note 60 of Chapter 5.

78. See Note 46 of Chapter 6.

79. Nair AG, Gutierrez-Arenas O, Eriksson O, Vincent P, Kotaleski JH (2015) Sensing positive versus negative reward signals through adenylyl cyclase-coupled GPCRs in direct and indirect pathway striatal medium spiny neurons. *Journal of Neuroscience* 35: 14017–14030.

80. Flajolet M, Wang Z, Futter M, Shen W, Nuangchamnong N, Bender J, et al. (2008) FGF acts as a co-transmitter through adenosine A_{2A} receptor to regulate synaptic plasticity. *Nature Neuroscience* 11: 1402–1409.

    Shen W, Flajolet M, Greengard P, Surmeier DJ (2008) Dichotomous dopaminergic control of striatal synaptic plasticity. *Science* 321: 848–851.

81. See Banasikowski and Beninger (2012) in the *International Journal of Neuropsychopharmacology* in Note 34 of Chapter 6

82. Adermark L, Lovinger DM (2007) Combined activation of L-type Ca^{2+} channels and synaptic transmission is sufficient to induce striatal long-term depression. *Journal of Neuroscience* 27: 6781–6787.

    Bagetta V, Picconi B, Marinucci S, Sgobio C, Pendolino V, Ghiglieri V, et al. (2011) Dopamine-dependent long-term depression is expressed in striatal spiny neurons of both direct and indirect pathways: Implications for Parkinson's Disease. *Journal of Neuroscience* 31: 12513–12522.

83. Wang Z, Kai L, Day M, Ronesi J, Yin HH, Ding J, et al. (2006) Dopaminergic control of corticostriatal long-term synaptic depression in medium spiny neurons is mediated by cholinergic interneurons. *Neuron* 50: 443–452.

84. See Note 82 of Chapter 11.

85. Gerfen CR, Surmeier DJ (2011) Modulation of striatal projection systems by dopamine. *Annual Review of Neuroscience* 34: 441–466.

Surmeier DJ, Ding J, Day M, Wang Z, Shen W (2007) D1 and D2 dopamine-receptor modulation of striatal glutamatergic signaling in striatal medium spiny neurons. *Trends in Neuroscience* 30: 228–235.

86. The axons of direct and indirect pathway medium spiny projection neurons of the striatum branch extensively and make contact with neighboring medium spiny projection neurons. This connectivity provides another means for crosstalk between the two projection pathways but it is difficult to study because the contacts are with distal dendrites making their influence at somatic recording electrodes weak. See Note 82 of Chapter 11.

87. Josselyn S Beninger RJ (1993) Neuropeptide Y: intra-accumbens injections produce a place preference that is blocked by *cis*-flupenthixol. *Pharmacology, Biochemistry and Behavior* 46:543–552.

88. Martin R, Bajo-Grañeras R, Moratalla R, Perea G, Araque A (2015) Circuit-specific signaling in astrocyte-neuron networks in basal ganglia pathways. *Science* 349: 730–734.

    See also:

    Gittis AH, Brasier DJ (2015) Astrocytes tell neurons when to listen up. *Science* 349: 690–691.

89. See Mackintosh (1974) in Note 1 of Chapter 2.

90. See Note 5 of Chapter 6.

91. See Horvitz et al. (2007) in Note 15 of Chapter 2.

92. Bozogrmehr T, Ardiel EL, McEwan AH, Rankin CH (2013) Mechanisms of plasticity in *Caenorhabditis elegans* mechanosensory circuit. *Frontiers of Physiology* 4: 88.

    Holmes G, Herdegen S, Schuon J, Cyriac A, Lass J, Conte C, et al. (2015) Transcriptional analysis of a whole-body form of long-term habituation in *Aplysia californica*. *Learning & Memory* 22: 11–23.

    Kandel ER (2005) The molecular biology of memory storage: a dialogue between genes and synapses. *Bioscience Reports* 24: 477–522.

    Roberts AC, Bill BR, Glanzman DL (2013) Learning and memory in zebrafish larvae. *Frontiers in Neural Circuits* 7: 126.

    Roberts AC, Pearce KC, Choe RC, Alzagatiti JB, Yeung AK, Bill BR, Glanzman DL (2016) Long-term habituation of the C-start escape response in zebrafish larvae. *Neurobiology of Learning and Memory* 134: 360–368.

93. See Notes 37 and 39 of Chapter 6.

94. Wise RA, Schwartz HV (1981) Pimozide attenuates acquisition of lever-pressing for food in rats. *Pharmacology, Biochemistry and Behavior* 15: 655–656.

95. See Note 22 of Chapter 3.

96. See Note 24 of Chapter 2.

97. See Note 21 of Chapter 3.

98. Ranaldi R (2014) Dopamine and reward seeking: the role of ventral tegmental area. *Reviews in the Neurosciences* 25: 1–10.

99. Tian J, Huang R, Cohen JY, Osakada F, Kobak D, Machens CK, et al. (2016) Distributed and mixed information in monosynaptic inputs to dopamine neurons. *Neuron* 91: 1374–1389.

100. Pan B, Zhong P, Sun D, Liu Q-s (2011) Extracellular signal-regulated kinase signaling in the ventral tegmental area mediates cocaine-induced synaptic plasticity and rewarding effects. *Journal of Neuroscience* 31: 11244–11255.

101. Nisanov R, Galaj E, Ranaldi R (2016) Treatment with a muscarinic acetylcholine receptor antagonist impairs the acquisition of conditioned reward learning in rats. *Neuroscience Letters* 614: 95–98.

102. Barco A, Bailey CH, Kandel ER (2006) Common molecular mechanisms in explicit and implicit memory. *Journal of Neurochemistry* 97: 1520–1533.

    McNamara CG, Tejero-Cantero Á, Trouche S, Campo-Urriza N, Dupret D (2014) Dopaminergic neurons promote hippocampal reactivation and spatial memory persistence. *Nature Neuroscience* 17: 1658–1660.

    Rossato JI, Bevilaqua LRM, Izquierdo I, Medina JH, Cammarota M (2009) Dopamine controls persistence of long-term memory storage. *Science* 325: 1017–1020.

    Tran AH, Uwano T, Kimura T, Hori E, Katsuki M, Nishijo H, Ono T (2008) Dopamine D1 receptor modulates hippocampal representation plasticity to spatial novelty. *Journal of Neuroscience* 28: 13390–13400.

    Also see Note 94 of Chapter 7.

103. Kruse MS, Prémont J, Krebs M-O, Jay TM (2009) Interaction of dopamine D1 with NMDA NR1 receptors in rat prefrontal cortex. *European Neuropsychopharmacology* 19: 296–304.

Chapter 13

1. Neisser U (1967) *Cognitive Psychology*. Appleton-Century-Crofts: New York.

2. See the historical references in:

    Feindel W, Leblanc R, de Almeida AN (2009) Epilepsy surgery: historical highlights 1909–2009. *Epilepsia* 50 Supplement 3: 131–151.

3. Gazzaniga MS, Bogen JE, Sperry RW (1962) Some functional effects of sectioning the cerebral commissures in man. *Proceedings of the National Academy of Sciences of the United States of America* 48: 1765–1769.

4. Sperry RW (1961) Cerebral organization and behavior. *Science* 133: 1749–1757.

5. Gazzaniga MS, Bogen JE, Sperry RW (1965) Observations on visual perception after disconnexion of the cerebral hemispheres in man. *Brain* 88: 221–236.

6. Sperry RW (1968) Hemisphere disconnection and the unity of conscious awareness. *American Psychologist* 23: 723–733.

7. Goodale MA, Millner AD, Jakobson LS, Carey DP (1991) A neurological dissociation between perceiving objects and grasping them. *Nature* 349: 154–156.

    Milner AD, Goodale MA (1996) *The Visual Brain in Action*. Oxford University Press: Oxford.

    Milner AD, Perrett DI, Johnston RS, Benson PJ, Jordan TR, Heeley DW, et al. (1991) Perception and action in "visual form agnosia." *Brain* 114: 405–428.

8. Perenin M-T, Vighetto A (1988) Optic ataxia: a specific disruption in visuomotor mechanisms: 1. Different aspects of the deficit in reaching for objects. *Brain* 111: 643–674.

9. Goodale MA, Milner AD (1992) Separate visual pathways for perception and action. *Trends in Neurosciences* 15: 20–25.

10. Horsley V (1886) Brain surgery. *British Medical Journal* 2: 670–675.

11. Jasper HH, Carmichael L (1935) Electrical potentials from the intact human brain. *Science* 81: 51–53.

12. Penfield W (1975) *The Mystery of the Mind*. Princeton University Press: Princeton, NJ.

13. Selimbeyoglu A, Parvizi J (2010) Electrical stimulation of the human brain: perceptual and behavioral phenomena reported in the old and new literature. *Frontiers in Human Neuroscience* 4: article 46.

14. Valenstein ES (1973) *Brain Control: A Critical Examination of Brain Stimulation and Psychosurgery*. John Wiley & Sons: New York.

15. Olsen RW, Hanchar HJ, Meera P, Wallner M (2007) GABA$_A$ receptor subtypes: the "one glass of wine" receptors. *Alcohol* 41: 201–209.

16. Schulte T, Oberlin BG, Kareken DA, Marinkovic K, Müller-Oehring EM, Meyerhoff DJ, Tapert S (2012) How acute and chronic alcohol consumption affect brain networks: insights from multimodal neuroimaging. *Alcoholism: Clinical and Experimental Research* 36: 2017–2027.

17. Martin CS, Earleywine M, Musty RE, Perrine MW, Swift RM (1993) Development and validation of the biphasic alcohol effects scale. *Alcoholism: Clinical and Experimental Research* 17: 140–146.

18. Hoffman A (1994) Notes and documents concerning the discovery of LSD. *Agents and Actions* 43: 79–81.

19. Hoffman A (1979) How LSD originated. *Journal of Psychedelic Drugs* 11: 53–60.

20. Tylš F, Páleníček T, Horáček J (2014) Psilocybin—summary of knowledge and new perspectives. *European Neuropsychopharmacology* 24: 342–356.

21. Aldus Huxley writes about his "self-experiments" with mescaline in: Huxley A (1954) *The Doors of Perception*. Harper & Row: New York.

22. Brawley P, Duffield JC (1972) The pharmacology of hallucinogens. *Pharmacological Reviews* 24: 31–66.

23. Much has been written about the history of psychedelic drugs. The following paper provides a brief history of LSD and many relevant references:

    Smith DE, Raswyck GE, Davidson LD (2014) From Hofmann to the Haight Ashbury, and into the future: the past and potential of lysergic acid diethylaminde. *Journal of Psychoactive Drugs* 46: 3–10.

24. Volkow ND, Wang G-J, Fischman MW, Foltin RW, Fowler JS, Abumrad NN, t al. (1997) Relationship between subjective effects of cocaine and dopamine transporter occupancy. *Nature* 386: 827–830.

    See related findings in:

    Volkow ND, Wang G-J, Fowler JS, Logan J, Gaeley SJ, Wong C, et al. (1999) Reinforcing effects of psychostimulants in humans are associated with increases in brain dopamine and occupancy of D$_2$ receptors. *Journal of Pharmacology and Experimental Therapeutics* 291: 409–415.

25. See Note 110 in Chapter 5.

26. Volkow ND, Wang G-J, Telang F, Fowler JS, Logan J, Childress A-R, et al. (2006) Cocaine cues and dopamine in dorsal striatum: mechanism of craving in cocaine addiction. *Journal of Neuroscience* 26: 6583–6588.

See also:

Wong DF, Kuwabara H, Schretlen DJ, Bonson KR, Zhou Y, Nandi A et al. (2006) Increased occupancy of dopamine receptors in human striatum during cue-elicited cocaine craving. *Neuropsychopharmacology* 31: 2716–2727.

27. Volkow ND, Wang G-J, Fowler JS, Logan J, Jayne M, Franceschi D, et al. (2002) "Nonhedonic" food motivation in humans involves dopamine in the dorsal striatum and methylphenidate amplifies the effect. *Synapse* 44: 175–180.

28. For a review see:

Leyton M (2008) The neurobiology of desire: dopamine and the regulation of mood in motivational states in humans. In: Kringelback ML, Berridge KC, eds., *Pleasure of the Brain*. Oxford University Press: Oxford, pp. 1–35.

29. Volkow ND, Wang G-J, Telang R, Fowler JS, Logan J, Childress A-R, et al. (2008) Dopamine increases in striatum do not elicit craving in cocaine abusers unless they are coupled with cocaine cues. *NeuroImage* 39: 1266–1273.

See also the review by Leyton and Vezina in Note 63 of Chapter 10.

30. Evans SM, Walsh SL, Levin FR, Foltin RW, Fishman MW, Bigelow GE (2001) Effect of flupenthixol on subjective and cardiovascular responses to intravenous cocaine in humans. *Drug and Alcohol Dependence* 64: 271–283.

Nann-Vernotica E, Donny EC, Bigelow GE, Walsh SL (2001) Repeated administration of the $D_{1/5}$ antagonist ecopipam fails to attenuate the subjective effects of cocaine. *Psychopharmacology* 155: 338–347.

31. Volkow ND, Fowler JS, Wang G-J (1999) Imaging studies on the role of dopamine in cocaine reinforcement in addiction in humans. *Journal of Psychopharmacology* 13: 337–345.

32. McGhie A (1977) Attention and perception in schizophrenia. In: Maher BA, ed., *Contributions to the Psychopathology of Schizophrenia*. Academic Press: New York, pp. 57–96.

33. McGhie A, Chapman J (1961) Disorders of attention and perception in early schizophrenia. *British Journal of Medical Psychology* 34: 103–116.

For some additional case reports of the mental experiences of people in the early stages of psychosis see Cases 1–6 in:

Bowers MB, Freedman DX (1966) "Psychedelic" experiences in acute psychoses. *Archives of General Psychiatry* 15: 240–248.

See also:

Chapman J (1966) The early symptoms of schizophrenia. *British Journal of Psychiatry* 112: 225–251.

34. MacDonald N (1960) Living with schizophrenia. *Canadian Medical Association Journal* 82: 218–221.

35. See Note 1 in Chapter 9.

36. See Post (1975) in Note 14, Chapter 9.

37. Grinspoon L, Bakalar JB (1976) *Cocaine: A Drug and its Social Evolution*. Basic Books: New York.

38. See Note 93 in Chapter 9.

39. Leibrich J (1999) *A Gift of Stories: Discovering How to Deal with Mental Illness*. University of Otago Press: Dunedin, New Zealand.

40. See Note 11 in Chapter 11.

41. Colpaert FC, Niemegeers CJE, Janssen PAJ (1976) Cocaine cue in rats as it relates to subjective drug effects: a preliminary report. *European Journal of Pharmacology* 40: 195–199.

42. Barry H III, Steenberg ML, Manian AA, Buckley JP (1974) Effects of chlorpromazine and three metabolites on behavioral responses in rats. *Psychopharmacology* 34: 351–360.

43. Colpaert FC (1999) Drug discrimination in neurobiology. *Pharmacology, Biochemistry and Behavior* 64: 337–345.

44. LeDoux JE (2014) Coming to terms with fear. *Proceedings of the National Academy of Sciences of the United States of America* 111: 2871–2878.

45. Everitt BJ, Robbins TW (2005) Neural systems of reinforcement for drug addiction: from actions to habits to compulsion. *Nature Neuroscience* 8: 1481–1489.

    In Box 1 on p. 1483, this paper provides thoughtful comments on the thorny problem of conflating the description of empirically derived mechanisms for brain functions such as the effects of rewarding stimuli on behavior and the possible association of those mechanisms with mental experience.

46. See Note 24 in Chapter 2.

47. Berridge KC, Robinson TE (2003) Parsing reward. *Trends in Neurosciences* 26: 507–513.

    See also Berridge and Robinson (1998) in Note 15 of Chapter 2.

48. See Note 77 in Chapter 11.

49. See Perry and Barron (2013) in Note 82 in Chapter 8.

50. Perry CJ, Baciadonna L, Chittka L (2016) Unexpected rewards induce dopamine-dependent positive emotion-like changes in bumblebees. *Science* 353: 1529–1531.

    These authors trained bumblebees (*Bombus terrestris*) in a successive color-discrimination task using sucrose reward. They probed with unrewarded ambiguous stimuli and observed standard generalization gradients. If the bees were pre-fed with a small quantity of sucrose before probe trials, generalization gradients shifted toward the positive stimulus (i.e., response latencies to ambiguous stimuli were shorter); this phenomenon has been termed "positive judgment bias." In a second experiment they showed that restraint-produced augmentation of response latency in a foraging task was reduced if the bees were fed sucrose prior to restraint. Treatment with a dopamine receptor antagonist prior to sucrose pre-feeding in either task blocked the effect of sucrose pre-feeding. The authors speculated that sucrose feeding produced a positive emotion-like state in the bumblebees. However, emotional states can only be inferred in these experiments by the observation of behavior. Results provide no information about possible mental experience in bumblebees.

    See also the commentary:

    Mendl MT, Paul ES (2016) Bee happy: bumblebees show decision-making that reflects emotion-like states. *Science* 353: 1499–1500.

Index

Notes
Figures are indicated by an italic f following the page number.
vs. indicates a comparison or differential diagnosis

Abbreviations used
ADHD - attention-deficit hyperactivity disorder
CaMKII - calcium/calmodulin-dependent kinase II
DOPAC - 3,4-dihydroxyphenylacetic acid
GABA - γ-aminobutyric acid
PET - positron emission tomography
THC - Δ^9-tetrahydrocannabinol

A-412997, 173
AB-127, 172
Abi-Darghamm, Anissa, 208
ABT-724, 173, 174
Adams, Ralph, 105–6
adenosine A2A receptor, 19
    D1-/D2-like receptor heterodimers, 175
    dopamine receptors dimer formation, 11
    theophylline, 321
adenylyl cyclase
    CaMKII action, 302
    inhibition by D2-like receptors, 153
    see also cAMP (cyclic 3,5'-adenosine
        monophosphate)
ADHD *see* attention-deficit hyperactivity
        disorder (ADHD)
Adrian, Edgar, 99
agonistic social behavior
    Arctic char *(Salvelinus alpinus)*, 199–200
    rats, 189–90
agoraphobia, two-factor theory treatment,
        37–38
agranulocytosis, 228
Ahlenius, Sven, 82–83, 95
air-puff stimuli, 131–2, 385–6
Ajhajanian, George, 100
alcohol
    mental experience, 334
    reward properties, 54
Al-Imari, Lina, 199
Alpert, Richard, 335
Alzheimer's disease, 85
α-amino-3-hydroxy-5-methyl-4-
        isoxazolepropionic acid (AMPA)
        receptors *see* AMPA receptors
amnesia, 73
    anterograde, 68–69
amnesiac mutant, 310

AMPA receptors, 296–7
    dephosphorylation by calcineurin, 300
    glutamatergic inputs, 304
    long-term incentive learning, 315–16
    phosphorylation, 316
    reward learning mechanisms, 327
    short-term incentive learning, 311, 312
amphetamine
    ADHD treatment, 236–7
    brain stimulation reward experiments, 31
    condition place preference studies, 50–54
    dopamine transporter, reversal of, 52, 53*f*
    drug of abuse as, 15
    incentive learning effects, 161, 162, 255–6
    mechanism of action, 246
    mental experience, 339–40
    non-declarative memory effects, 155
    onset of action, 251
    PET, 115
    place preference, 4
    self-administered drug studies, 246, 250–1
    withdrawal, 256
amygdala
    DOPAC:dopamine ratio, 93
    hippocampus interaction, 86–87
    lateral *see* lateral amygdala
analgesic reward study, 120
anesthetized rats, novel stimuli tests, 124
Angelucci, Luciano, 128–9
angular gyrus, 278–9
anhedonia, 34–35, 42
animal studies
    kinesia paradoxa, 221–2
    laws of learning, 25
    mental experience, 345–50
    training of, 25–26
Annelida, 285
Anolis carolensis (Carolina anoles), 197

anterior ectosylvian gyrus, 277–8
anterograde amnesia, 68–69
antipsychotic drugs, 227
  adverse effects, 227, 228–9
  atypical *see* atypical antipsychotic drugs
  dopamine hypothesis of schizophrenia, 205, 206*f*
  first-generation, 228
  mechanism of action, 151–2, 229–30
  onset of action, 229–30
  reward signalling, 210
  schizophrenia treatment, 14
  second-generation, 228
  third-generation, 228
  typical *see* typical antipsychotic drugs
  see also dopamine receptor antagonist drugs
anxiety disorder treatment, 37–38
Aphelocoma coerulescens (scrub jays), 75
Aplysia
  adenylyl cyclase activation, 302–3
  food reward-related learning, 310
  operant biting response learning, 284
apomorphine, 161, 162
applied behavioral analysis, anxiety/phobia treatment, 38
2-arachidonyl glycerol, 247
Arctic char *(Salvelinus alpinus)*, 199–200
aripiprazole, 228
Aron, Arthur, 179–80
ascending spiral connections, 290
atropine studies, 152
attention-deficit hyperactivity disorder (ADHD), 14–15, 236–42
  aetiology, 237–8
  amphetamine treatment, 236–7
  genetics, 240–1
  history of, 204
  neuroimaging studies, 238–9
  Parkinson's disease, development of, 239–40
  symptoms, 236
    Parkinson's disease *vs.*, 241–2
atypical antipsychotic drugs, 229
  brain regions affected, 232–3
audition, neuroanatomy, 270–2
auditory cortex, 278
aversive conditioning, 358
  see also aversive stimuli; threat conditioning
aversive foot pinch studies, 131
aversive stimuli, 8, 123, 386
  dopamine cell subset firing, 385–6
  dopamine, effects on, 147
avoidance conditioning/learning, 35–41
  behaviorism, problems with, 42–43
  behavior persistence, 37
  classical conditioning as, 36
  definition, 35

  dopamine role, 40–41
  dual-chamber shuttle box experiments, 35–36
  mechanisms of, 359
  response flexibility, 38–39
  two-factor theory, 36–38
avoidance responses, chlorpromazine blocking, 41
avoidance task, one-way version, 358
Awakenings (Sacks), 340–4
Axel, Richard, 273

Babb, Stephanie, 76
Bading, Hilmar, 306
Barron, Andrew, 284–5
bar test, 132
  descent latency sensitization, 132–7, 135*f*, 136*f*, 139, 140*f*
basal ganglia
  incentive learning, 16
  neuroanatomy, 285–93
  Parkinson's disease, 219–20
  tectum projections in primates, 437
Beaulieu, Jean-Martin, 319
behavior
  avoidance learning, 37
  modification consequences, 1–2
  selectionism, 49–50
behavioral contrast, 24–25, 353
behaviorism
  avoidance learning, problems with, 42–43
  development of, 27
  problems with, 26–27
The Behavior of Organisms (Skinner), 26
benzodiazepines, 387
Bernstein, Julius, 99
Berridge, Kent, 348
Berson, Solomon Aaron, 92
bilateral hippocampal damage, 6
bilateral medial temporal lobectomy, 333–4
Bindra, Dalbir, 2
binge eating, 235
bird flocking studies, 195
birdsong, 12–13
  directed *vs.* undirected, 192–6
Birkmayer, Walther, 220
Bito, Laszlo, 96
Blackburn, James, 93–94
black-capped chickadee *(Poecile atricapillus)*, song learning, 87–88
Bleuler, Eugen, 203
The Blind Watchmaker (Dawkins), 50
Bliss, Timothy, 311–12
Bloch, Felix, 113
Blodgett, Hugh Carlton, 83–84
blood oxygenation level-dependent fMRI *see* BOLD
Bobillier, Pierre, 92
Bodnar, Richard, 159

Bolam, Paul, 287–8
BOLD, 8, 91
  ADHD, 238–9
  analgesic reward study, 120
  angular gyrus, 278–9
  cocaine studies, 120–1
  intense romantic love, 180
  monetary reward studies, 119–20
  novel stimuli, 125
  nucleus accumbens, 291
  prisoner's dilemma game, 178
  route recognition tasks, 86
  schizophrenia, 210
  sexual stimuli studies, 118
  weather prediction task, 84–85
Bolles, Robert, 2, 39
Bombus terrestris (bumblebees),
      color-discrimination tasks, 455
Bond, Earl, 238
Bourbonais, Kathy, 94
Bozarth, Michael, 251
Bradley, Charles, 204, 236–7
brain
  damage, 6, 330–4
  electrical stimulation studies, 3, 29
    D3 receptors antagonists, 170
    dopamine-blocking drugs, 30–31
    reward-related learning, 29
    schedule training, 31–32
  feeding dopamine levels, 97
  mapping studies, 29–30
  mental experiences, 19
  mind linkage, 330–5
Brain Control: A Critical Examination of
    Brain Stimulation and Psychotherapy
    (Valenstein), 333
Breese, George, 40–41
Breland, Marian, 25–26
broad tuning, gustation, 274–5
Broca, Paul, 154
bromocriptine
  incentive learning effects, 161, 162–3
  locomotor activity effects, 156
Brown, Lucy, 179–80
Brudzynski, Stefan, 188–9
Buck, Linda, 273
Bugelski, B Richard, 110
bumblebees *(Bombus terrestris)*,
    color-discrimination tasks, 455
Bunney, Benjamin, 100
Buske, Christine, 199

Cabib, Simona, 127
Caenorhabditis elegans, maze
    learning, 284
Calabresi, Paolo, 317
calcineurin, 299, 300
  protein kinase A *vs.*, 305

calcium/calmodulin-dependent kinase II
    (CaMKII), 297, 302
  D1-like receptors, 305
  short-term incentive learning, 311
Calne, Donald, 153
cAMP (cyclic 3′,5′-adenosine
    monophosphate)
  antipsychotic drugs, 151
  chlorpromazine effects, 151
  D1-/D2-like receptors, 9, 18–19
  haloperidol effects, 151
Capecchi, Mario, 164
Carassius auratus (goldfish), 309
β-carbolines, 387
Carelli, Regina, 107–8
Carlsson, Arvid, 41, 95, 220, 234
Carolina anoles *(Anolis carolensis),* 197
carpenter bee *(Xylocopa appendicularis),* 201
Casolini, Paola, 128–9
catechol-*O*-methyltransferase (COMT), 182, 184
β-catenin inhibition, 319
caudate nucleus
  cortical glutamatergic neurons, 287
  expert persuasion, 180–1
  human social cooperation, 179, 182
  Huntington's disease, 86
  incentive learning, 16
  maternal love, 180
  motor system, 280
  paired associate learning, 84
  Parkinson's disease, 220
  route recognition tasks, 86
  schizophrenia, 207, 217
CB1 receptor, 247
celebrities, 182
cerebral cortex
  incentive learning, 16, 17
  motor system, 280
c-Fos, 314–15
channelrhodopsin, 316
Charbonneau, Danielle, 73–74, 224–5
Charcot, Jean-Martin, 341
Cheer, Joseph, 130
Childress, Anna Rose, 263–4
Chiodo, Louis, 124
chlorpromazine
  avoidance responses blocking, 41
  discovery, 226
  effects of, 226–7
  mechanism of action, 151
  mental experiences, 346
Chomsky, Noam, 196
Church, William, 96–97
Ciovelli, Robert, 154
circadian rhythm, postmortem dopamine
    assessment, 92
classical conditioning, 36
Clayton, Nicola, 75

clozapine, 228
  adverse effects, 228–9
  brain regions affected, 233
Cnemidophorus inornatus (little striped
      whiptail lizard), 196–7, 410
Cnemidophorus uniparens see desert grassland
      whiptail lizard *(Cnemidophorus
      uniparens)*
Cnidaria, 285
cocaine, 15
  BOLD studies, 120–1
  conditioned activity studies, 54–58,
      57*f*, 173
  environmental effects, 441
  incentive learning effects, 255–6
  mechanism of action, 246
  mental experience, 336–7, 339–40
  onset of action, 251
  psychoactive drug as, 19
  self-administered drug studies, 170, 171,
      246, 250–1
  in vivo electrochemistry, 109
  withdrawal, 256
cochlear nucleus, 271
cognitive map development, lever pressing for
      food studies, 45–46
Cohen, Jonathan, 177–9
Colpaert, Francis, 346
Colurnix japonica (galliform Japanese
      quail), 196
compulsive shopping, 235
computed tomography (CT), 111–12
COMT, 182
COMT (catechol-*O*-methyltransferase),
      182, 184
conditioned activity
  cocaine-based, 54–58, 57*f*, 173
  D3 receptor antagonist studies, 172
  definition, 55
  dopamine-receptor knockout mice, 172
conditioned aversive stimuli, 429
  pharmacology and, 358–9
conditioned avoidance learning
  D1-like receptor knockout mice, 166
  incentive learning and, 5
conditioned avoidance responding, 58–66
  apparatus, 59
  conditioned suppression, 63–66, 65*f*
  dopamine receptor blocking drug
      effects, 60
  escape latency, 60–61, 62*f*, 63
  learning curve, 61*f*
  protocol, 59–60
  psychotic drug treatment screening, 58–59
  safety location, 60, 64, 66
  tone–shock association, 64–66
conditioned cue preference task, 77–78, 80

conditioned incentive stimuli, 409
  ADHD *vs.* Parkinson's disease, 241–2
  association with rewards, 253–4
  development of, 4
  dopamine release, 326
  drugs of abuse, 258, 260
  incentive learning, 373
  reduction of, 254
  in vivo electrochemistry, 110–11
conditioned place preference
  D1-/D2-like receptor antagonists, 249
  D3 receptor-knockout mice, 171–2
  dopamine receptor agonists, 163–4
  ethanol, 254–5
  incentive learning, 53*f*
  learning, 4–5
  THC blocking by SL327, 250
conditioned reward, pimozide, 80
conditioned reward responses
  D1-like receptors in incentive learning, 160–1
  definition, 36
conditioned-sensitization-to-morphine
      study, 173
conditioned sexual stimuli in rats, 372
conditioned stimuli, 7
  definition, 36
  dopamine release in nucleus accumbens, 376
conditioned suppression, 63–66, 65*f*
conditioning
  chain of incentive learning, 431
  heroin withdrawal, 261–2
  incentive stimuli, 409
context effect, rewarding stimuli, 24–25
cooperative social interactions, 13
Cooper, Barrett, 40–41
Corkin, Suzanne, 69–70
Cormack, Allan, 111, 113
Cornish, Jennifer, 284–5
corpus callosum, 330–1
cortical cup technique, 95–96
cortical glutamatergic neurons, caudate
      nucleus, 287
corticospinal (pyramidal) tract, 17
  motor system, 280–1
corticotrophin-releasing factor (CRF) system, 257–8
Coryall, Charles, 114
Courvoisier, Simone, 41
creativity, 50
CREB
  gene activation, 306, 307–8*f*
  long-term incentive learning, 312–13
  nucleus accumbens, 309
Crews, David, 197–8
Crichton, Alexander, 204
Crow, Tim, 207–8
Crystal, Johnathon, 76
cued-lever press studies, 158–9

cue tasks
  dopamine neuron firing, 7
  eight-arm radial maze tests, 77
cultural dependence
  delusion content in schizophrenia, 212–14
  hallucinations in schizophrenia, 214–15
cyclic 3′,5′-adenosine monophosphate
      see cAMP (cyclic 3′,5′-adenosine
      monophosphate)

D1-like receptors, 9–10
  adenylyl cyclase activation, 18–19, 148, 149,
      305
  affinity, 304–5
  agonist drugs, 10–11
    rat social cooperation, 187
  antagonist drugs, 10–11, 449
    conditioned place preference, 249
  CaMKII activation, 305
  cAMP signaling, 18–19, 148, 149, 305
  cloning of, 154
  differential incentive learning function,
      158–64
  differential locomotor function, 155–7
  discovery, 149–53, 153–5
  histochemical studies, 150–1
  indirect pathway in incentive learning, 317
  knockout mice, 11, 164, 166
  medium spiny neurons, 18, 288
  phasic stimulation, 305
  protein kinase A, 18–19
  receptor heterodimers, 175, 302
  reward-related learning, 10
D2-like receptors, 9–10
  adenylyl cyclase inhibition, 153
  affinity, 304–5
  agonist drugs, 10–11
  antagonist drugs, 10–11
    conditioned place preference, 249
  cloning of, 154
  differential incentive learning function,
      158–64
  differential locomotor function, 155–7
  direct pathway, effects on, 321–2
  discovery, 149–53, 153–5
  haloperidol-induced stimulation decreases,
      320–1
  human social cooperation, 184
  indirect pathway in incentive learning,
      317–19
  inverse incentive learning, 320, 321
  knockout mice, 11, 164, 166
  medium spiny neurons, 18
  plasticity of, 319
  receptor heterodimers, 175–6
  reward-related learning, 10
  schizophrenia, 208

D3 receptors, 11
  agonist drug studies, 170, 171
  antagonist drug studies, 170–1, 172–3
  cocaine-based conditioned activity, 173
  D1-like receptor heterodimers, 175
  incentive learning, 315
  knockout mice, 164, 166–7, 171–2
  psychopharmacology, 167–74
D4 receptors
  agonist drug studies, 173–4
  antagonist drug studies, 173–4
  cloning of, 154
  genetics, 240–1
    gene polymorphism, 174
  incentive learning, 173
  knockout mice, 164, 166
  psychopharmacology, 167–74
D5 receptors
  cloning of, 154
  knockout mice, 164, 166
Dagher, Alain, 335–6
Dahlström, Annica, 3, 29–30, 285
Danio rerio see zebrafish *(Danio rerio)*
DARPP-32 *see* dopamine and cAMP-regulated
      phosphoprotein-32 (DARPP-32)
Darwin, Charles, 1
Dawkins, Richard, 50
declarative memory, 5–6
  Alzheimer's disease, 85
  brain areas, 68, 85
  brain damage effects, 6
  cultural norms, 214
  definition, 70, 205
  inverse incentive learning, 144–5
  non-declarative memory *vs.*, 89–90
  Parkinson disease, 6
  seed caching in birds, 88
  see also episodic memory; paired associate
      learning; semantic memory
Delay, Jean, 226
Delgado, José Manuel Rodriguez, 96
delusion content, schizophrenia, 212–14
Delva, Nicholas, 233
Dementia Praecox and Paraphrenia
      (Kraepelin), 339
dendritic spines, medium spiny neurons,
      286–7
Deniker, Pierre, 226
descent latency
  bar test, 132–7, 135*f*, 136*f*, 139, 140*f*
  conditioned increases, 137–9
  sensitization and conditioning, 141–8
desert grassland whiptail lizard
      (Cnemidophorus uniparens)
  sexual behavior, 410
  social cooperation studies, 196
De Wit, Harriet, 32–35, 251

Diagnostic and Statistical Manual of Mental Disorders IV (DSM-IV), schizophrenia, 215–16
diazepam (Valium), 387
Di Ciano, Patricia, 168
Di Chiara, Gaetano, 97, 249
Dickinson, Anthony, 75
3,4-dihydroxyphenylacetic acid (DOPAC)
  aversive stimuli studies, 129–30
  dopamine ratio, 366
    fed *vs.* starved rats, 93–94
    sexual stimuli, 95
  foot-restricted rat studies, 366
  postmortem dopamine assessment, 92–94
  in vivo electrochemistry, 106–7
3,4-dihydroxyphenylalanine *see* DOPA (3,4-dihydroxyphenylalanine)
direct pathway
  dorsal striatum, 288–9
  inverse incentive learning, 321, 322
  nucleus accumbens, 289
discrimination tasks, pigeon pecking keys, 40
Dolan, Raymond, 86–87
dominance relationships, reptiles, 197
door-opening stimuli, electrophysiology in monkeys, 101–2
DOPA (3,4-dihydroxyphenylalanine), 14
  Parkinson's disease treatment, 207
  see also L-DOPA
DOPAC *see* 3,4-dihydroxyphenylacetic acid (DOPAC)
[³H]dopamine, 153
dopamine and cAMP-regulated phosphoprotein-32 (DARPP-32), 298, 299*f*, 300, 309
  protein kinase A action, 305
dopamine receptor(s), 9–10
  amphetamine-produced condition place preference, 52, 54
  conditioned-sensitization-to-morphine study, 173
  dimer formation, 11
  identification of, 152
  knockout mice, incentive learning, 164–7
  radio-receptor binding technology, 152
  subtype functions, 11–12
  subtypes, 149–76
  see also D1-like receptors; D2-like receptors; D2 receptors; D3 receptors; D4 receptors; D5 receptors
dopamine receptor agonist drugs, 234–6
  adverse effects, 235–6
  conditioned place preference, 163–4
  incentive learning effects, 161, 162–4
  locomotor activity effects, 156
  see also L-DOPA; pramipexole; ropinirole

dopamine receptor antagonist drugs, 226–34
  brain stimulation rewards, 30–31
  food reward response decline, 347–8
  incentive learning effects, 415
  kinesia paradoxa animal studies, 221–2
  latent learning in maze running tasks, 83–84
  locomotor activity effects, 156
  mental experience, 340, 344–5
  reward-related learning blocking, 249
  see also antipsychotic drugs; chlorpromazine; haloperidol
dorsal striatum
  direct pathway, 288–9
  eight-arm radial maze tests, 78, 79*f*
  indirect pathway, 288
  information processing, 80
  lesions of, 363
    stimulus–response learning tasks, 82
  medium spiny neuron inputs, 288–9
  paired associate learning, 84
DRD1, 208
DRD2, 184, 208
DRD4, 240–1
Drosophila melanogaster
  D1 receptor knockouts, 309–10
  dopamine disruption studies, 200–1
  social stimuli learning, 284
drug discrimination studies, 346
drugs of abuse, 15–16, 245–65
  conditioned incentive stimuli, 251–6, 258, 260
  conditioned place preference, 50–51
  dopamine reduction in nucleus accumbens, 257
  dopaminergic neurotransmission, 246–8
  incentive learning, 248–51
  need state mechanisms, 256–8
  reward-related learning, 245–6
  reward threshold elevations, 257
  treatment, 258–64
    environmental cues, 262–3
    extinction techniques, 263–4
  Vietnam war (1955-1975), 260–1, 262
dual-chamber shuttle box studies, 35–36
du Bois-Reymond, Emil, 99
Dugesia japonica, conditioned preferences, 284
dumb mutant, 309
dunce mutant, 309–10
dynorphin, 288
dynorphin-κ opioid system, 257–8

Eccles, John, 99, 442
EGR1, 314–15
Ehringer, Herbert, 150, 220
eight-arm radial maze tests
  conditioned cue preference task, 77–78, 80

episodic memory, 76–77
incentive learning, 78, 80
spatial learning, 77–78
electrical stimulation studies *see* brain
electric foot shock, 8
electrophysiology, 7, 99–105
aversive stimuli studies, 126, 147–8
development of, 99–100
humans, substantia nigra, 103
Macaca fascicularis monkeys, 100–2
novel stimuli, 8, 125
reward withholding, 146–7
somatosensation, 276
trained, water-restricted rats, 104
see also in vivo electrochemistry; in vivo
voltammetry studies
encephalitis lethargica, 237–8
endogenous cannabinoid system, 18–19
discovery of, 248
environmental stimuli
cocaine effects, 441
descent latency sensitization, 138–9
drug addiction, 15–16
incentive learning, 15, 17
nicotine, 252
epileptic focus, 332–3
episodic memory, 75
eight-arm radial maze tests, 76–77
ERK1/2 *see* extracellular signal-regulated
protein kinase 1/2 (ERK1/2)
Ernst, Richard, 113
escape latency, conditioned avoidance
responding, 60–61, 62*f*, 63
estrildid finches, social cooperation studies,
193–4
ethanol, 15, 247, 250
conditioned place preference, 249,
254–5
onset of action, 251
self-administered drug studies, 246
Eublepharis macularius (leopard gecko),
197–8
European starling *(Sturnus vulgaris),* 193, 194
Everitt, Barry, 263–4
expert persuasion, 180–1, 182
extinction, 56
definition, 32–35
drugs of abuse treatment, 263–4
extracellular signal-regulated protein kinase
1/2 (ERK1/2), 297–8
activation, 305–6
blockade of, 309
long-term incentive learning, 312–13
targets of, 306
extrapyramidal motor system, 280
extrapyramidal side effects, antipsychotic
drugs, 227

face identification, 270
facial attraction studies, 118–19
Falk–Hillarp formaldehyde histofluorescence
technique, 285
family psychoeducation/therapy,
schizophrenia, 231
fast-scan cyclic voltammetry, aversive stimuli
studies, 130
fear conditioning, neurobiology, 347
feeding studies
electrophysiology in *Macaca fascicularis*
monkeys, 101
food-related color discrimination incentive
learning task, 309
food-restricted rats, DOPAC, rise in, 366
incentive learning, 252–3
intracerebral microdialysis, 97
lever-press response *see* lever-press response
for food studies
PET, 114–15
response decline, dopamine receptor
antagonist drugs, 347–8
visual stimulus study and, fMRI, 118
in vivo electrochemistry, 108
fiber photometry, 7
D2-like receptors incentive learning,
317–18
mice social cooperation, 188
Fibiger, Hans Chris, 93–95, 98
finches, models as, 12–13
Fiorillo, Christopher, 126
Fisher, Helen, 179–80, 186
flashing lights, brain stimulation experiments,
31–32
Fleming, Alison, 187
Floresco, Stan, 174
flumazenil, 387
fluphenazine, 226
fMRI *see* functional magnetic resonance
imaging (fMRI)
Fogel, Stuart, 39–40
food-storing birds, seed caching, 87–89
foot pinch studies, 131
fornix lesions, stimulus–response learning
tasks, 82
FOSB, 314–15
Fowler, Stephen, 158
Franklin, Keith, 31–32
Frank, Michael, 224
Freedman, Nelson, 32
frequency range, audition, 270–1
Freud, Sigmund, 234
frontal cortex
DOPAC:dopamine ratio, fed *vs.* starved
rats, 93
schizophrenia, 217
fruitfly *see Drosophila melanogaster*

functional magnetic resonance imaging
(fMRI), 7, 8, 91, 117–21
ADHD, 238–9
dopamine receptor subtype functions,
11–12
facial attraction studies, 118–19
food and visual stimulus study, 118
hippocampus–amygdala interaction, 86–87
human social cooperation, 177–9
intense romantic love, 179–80
novel stimuli, 125
PET vs., 117
primary reward studies, 117–18
weather prediction task, 84–85
see also BOLD
fusiform gyrus, 269–70
Fuxe, Kjell, 3, 29-30, 285

GABA (γ-aminobutyric acid) receptors
drug effects, 387
medium spiny neurons, 288
neurotransmitter as, 439
schizophrenia, 217
galliform Japanese quail (Colurnix japonica),
196
gambling, 235
γ-aminobutyric acid receptors see GABA
(γ-aminobutyric acid) receptors
Gaoni, Y, 247–8
Gerber, Gary, 32–35
Gerdjikov, Todor, 308, 315–16
Gerfen, Charles, 322
Gerlach, Manfred, 239–40
Gerlai, Robert, 199
German, Dwight, 100
ghrelin (GHSR1a) receptor, 175–6
A Gift of Stories: Discovering How to Deal with
Mental Illness (Leibrich), 344–5
globus pallidus, 322–3
glutamate, schizophrenia, 217
glutamatergic inputs, 18
dopaminergic neurons, 19
glutamatergic synapses
corticostriatal dopamine modification, 17
ventral tegmental area, 326–7
glycogen synthase kinase-3 (GSK-3),
318–19
gnostic neurons, 269
goldfish (Carassius auratus), 309
Gonon, François, 106
Goodale, Melvyn, 331
Gore, Bryan, 166
Govoni, Stefano, 153
G protein-coupled receptors (GPCR), 154
G proteins, 391
Grace, Anthony, 217
Grant, Lester, 40–41

Gratton, Alain, 107
Graybiel, Ann, 108–9, 110, 328
gray tree frogs (Hyla versicolor), 198
Greengard, Paul, 150, 220, 298, 302–3
green tree frog (Hyla cinera), 198
Gross, Charles, 269–70
growth hormone secretagogue receptor 1a, 11
GSK-3 (glycogen synthase kinase-3), 318–19
gustation, neuroanatomy, 273–5

Haber, Suzanne, 290
habit learning, 70–71
habituation, 46, 139–41
definition, 8, 139
mechanisms of, 324
hallucinations, 339–40
schizophrenia, 214–15
haloperidol
aversive stimuli studies, 9
D2-like receptor stimulation decreases, 320–1
descent latency sensitization, 141
bar test, 133–4, 135f
discovery, 226
latent learning in maze running tasks, 83–84
locomotor activity effects, 156
mechanism of action, 131, 151–2
place preference blocking, 4–5
social cooperation in hamsters, 191
tritium-labelled studies, 153
halorhodopsin, 316
Hartman, John, 92–93
Hebb, Donald, 270
hebephrenia, 416
Heffner, Thomas, 92–93
Henry Molaison see HM (Henry Molaison)
heroin
conditioned place preference, 251
conditioning in withdrawal, 261–2
implicit memory tasks, 433
reward-related learning, 15
self-administration studies, 246
Heyrovsky, Jaroslav, 105
hierarchical processing mode, visual system,
269–70
Hikosaka, Okihide, 131–2, 290–1
hippocampus
amygdala interaction, 86–87
damage, 6
spatial learning task, 82
declarative memory, 68, 85
eight-arm radial maze tests, 78, 79f
incentive learning, 80
paired associate learning, 84
place cells, 278
route recognition tasks, 86
seed caching in birds, 88
Hirsh, Frank, 200

histochemical studies, D1-like receptors, 150–1
HM (Henry Molaison), 5, 68–70, 89
  anterograde amnesia, 68–69
  mirror-drawing task, 70
  post-bilateral medial temporal lobectomy, 333–4
  pursuit rotor task, 69–70
Hodgkin, Alan, 99
Hoffman, Edward, 113
homovanillic acid (HVA)
  dopamine ratio, 366
  postmortem dopamine assessment, 93–95
  in vivo electrochemistry, 106–7
Honzik, Charles H, 83–84
Hornykiewicz, Oleh, 150, 220
Horsley, Victor, 332–3
Horvitz, Jon, 125, 158–9, 221–2, 323
Hubel, David, 267–9
Hounsfield, Godfrey, 111
Howard, James, 40–41
Hull, Clark, 2, 109
Huntington's disease, 86
Huxley, Andrew, 99
HVA *see* homovanillic acid (HVA)
Hydra japonica, 285
6-hydroxydopamine
  adults *vs.* neonates, 164–5
  descent latency sensitization in bar test, 132–3
  locomotor activity effects, 156
  non-declarative memory effects, 155
  Parkinson-like symptoms, 165
Hyla cinerea (green tree frog), 198
Hyland, Bryan, 104
Hyla versicolor (gray tree frog), 198
hyperdopaminergic, schizophrenia, 231–2
hyperkinesia, 237
hypersexuality, 235
hypothalamus, 93, 94

Ichihara, Kenji, 83–84
imaging *see* neuroimaging
Imperato, Assunta, 128–9
implicit memory tasks, heroin-related stimuli, 433
incentive learning, 28–35, 42, 44–67
  ADHD *vs.* Parkinson's disease, 241
  amphetamine effects, 255–6
    condition place preference, 50–54
  beginning of, 2–3
  behavioral approaches, 3–4
  cocaine effects, 255–6
    conditioned activity, 54–58, 57*f*, 173
  conditioned avoidance responding *see* conditioned avoidance responding
  conditioned incentive stimuli, 373
  conditioned place preference, 53*f*
  conditioning chain, 431
  definition, 2–3, 20, 28, 44, 205, 355, 441
  development of, 3–4
  dopamine
    effects of, 304–7
    importance of, 103
    local enhancement, 302–4
  dopamine receptors, 158–64
    antagonist drugs, 415
    D1 receptor knockout mice, 166
    D2 receptor knockout mice, 166
    D3 receptor knockout mice, 166–7
    D3 receptors, 11, 315
    D4 receptors, 173
  eight-arm radial maze tests, 78, 80
  environmental stimuli, 15, 17
  excessive in schizophrenia, 215, 415
  food-related stimuli, 252–3
  hippocampus, 80
  human social cooperation, 182, 183*f*
  indirect pathway, 316–20
  Iowa gambling task, 74–75
  kinesia paradoxa, 222, 223
  lever pressing for food *see* lever-press response for food studies
  long-term *see* long-term incentive learning
  mechanisms of, 21–22, 295–329
  neuroanatomy, 16–17
  oxytocin/vasopressin, 186
  Parkinson's disease, 14, 73–74, 220–1, 223–4
  reptiles, 197–8
  reward stimuli, 327–8
  schizophrenia, 210–11
  short-term *see* short-term incentive learning
  signaling molecules, 308–10
  song learning in birds, 88
  tasks, development of, 71–72
  timing of, 292–3
  ventral striatal regions, 290
  weather prediction task, 85
  see also inverse incentive learning; reward-related learning
incentive learning, Parkinson disease, 6
incentive-motivational theories, 354–5
indirect pathway
  dorsal striatum, 288
  inverse incentive learning, 321, 322
  nucleus accumbens, 289
inferior colliculus, audition, 271
information processing, brain areas, 80
Ingvar, David, 112
Insel, Thomas, 190
intense romantic love, 179–80, 182
intense stimuli, 123
  inverse incentive learning, 126

intracerebral microdialysis, 7, 95–99
  aversive stimuli studies, 126, 127–9
  brain stimulation reward, 97–98
  feeding dopamine levels, 96–97
  nicotine studies, 246
  self-administered drugs, 98
  sexual behavior, 98
  THC, 247–8
  zebra finches (*Taeniopygia guttata*) singing
    studies, 193
inverse agonists, 387
inverse incentive learning, 123–48
  aversive stimuli, 126–32
  bar test *see* bar test
  D2-like receptors, 321
  D3 receptor antagonist studies, 172–3
  definition, 123, 419
  dopamine receptor agonist drugs, 235
  dopamine role, 144
  intense stimuli, 126
  latent inhibition, 145
  mechanism of action, 144
  novel stimuli, 124–5
  Parkinson's disease, 223–4
  pathways, 320–8
  pre-exposure conditioning and test phase,
    145–6
  see also incentive learning
inverse incentive training, 9
in vivo electrochemistry, 7, 105–11
  aversive stimuli studies, 126
  conditioned incentives, 110–11
  DOPAC measurements, 106–7
  food rewards, 108
  HVA measurements, 106–7
  increased dopamine levels, 106–7
  maze-trained rats, 108–9
  medial prefrontal cortex, 107
  milk reward, 107
  nucleus accumbens, 107, 108
  prediction errors, 109–10
  reward-related learning, 107–8
  sexual behavior, 109
  striatum, 108
  in vivo voltammetry studies, 109
in vivo microdialysis, nucleus accumbens, 12
in vivo voltammetry studies, 109
  aversive stimuli studies, 129–30
  nicotine, 246
  novel stimuli, 124–5
  THC, 247–8
iodobenzamide, 248
Iowa gambling task, 74–75
  schizophrenia patients, 232–3

Jacobs, Barry, 126
Jakubovic, Alexander, 93–94
Janssen, Paul, 226

Jasper, Herbert, 332–3
Jenkins, Bruce, 120–1
Jhamandas, Khem, 95–96
Joiliot-Curie, Frédéric, 112
Joiliot-Curie, Irène, 112
Josselyn, Sheena, 323
Joyce, Andrew, 229
Joyce, Jeffrey, 165
Justice, Joseph, 96–97

kainic acid, 363
Kandel, Eric, 220, 302–3, 311–12, 328
Kebabian, John, 150, 153
Keller, Richard, 106
Kendall, Stephen, 24–25
Kety, Seymour S, 112
kidney fluid retention, vasopressin, 185
kinesia paradoxa, 14, 21, 218–19, 221–2, 223
Kitazawa, Shigeru, 108
Klimkowicz-Mrowic, Aleksandra, 85
Koepp, Matthias, J, 115
Kolb, Bryan, 314
Konorski, Jerzy, 269
Koob, George, 250, 257–8
Kosofsky, Barry, 309
Kraepelin, Emil, 203, 339
Krebs, Edwin, 150
Kuhar, Michael, 229
Kuhl, David E, 111
Kuypers, Hans, 281
Kv4.2 potassium channels, 297, 300
  ERK1/2 target, 306
  short-term incentive learning, 311, 312

L-745,870, 173, 174
language
  acquisition studies, 196
  problems with, 349–50
language-based communication, 20
Lassen, Niels, 112
latent inhibition, inverse incentive learning, 145
latent learning, 82–84
  maze running tasks *see* mazes
lateral amygdala
  eight-arm radial maze tests, 78, 79f
  information processing, 80
  see also amygdala
lateral tongue protrusion, 348
Lauterbur, Paul, 113
law of effect, 23–28
  behaviorism, 27–28
Lawrence, Donald, 281
Lawrence, Ernest O, 112
laws of learning, 354
  animal behavior, 25
  challenges to, 2
  downfall of, 39
  evidence against, 25

L-DOPA
  discovery of, 234
  long-duration response, 234–5
  mechanism of action, 234–5
  mental experience, 340–4
  reserpine *vs.*, 220
  short-duration response, 234–5
learned avoidance responses, 39
learning
  disruption, animal studies, 216–17
  habit learning, 70–71
  motor learning, 235
  paired associate learning, 84–85
  song learning, 87–89
  types of, 441
    see also avoidance conditioning/learning;
      conditioned avoidance learning;
      incentive learning; inverse incentive
      learning; latent learning; long-term
      incentive learning; reward-related
      learning; spatial learning;
      stimulus–response learning
learning curve, conditioned avoidance
    responding, 61*f*
Leary, Timothy, 335
Leblois, Arthur, 194
LeDoux, Joseph, 347, 348–9
Lefkowitz, Robert, 153–4
Le Foll, Bernard, 173, 315
Legault, Mark, 125
Leibrich, Julie, 344–5
Le Moal, Michel, 257–8
leonardo mutant, 310
leopard gecko *(Eublepharis macularius)*,
    197–8
lever-press response for food studies, 45–50
  behavior reinforcement by selectionism,
    49–50
  cognitive map development, 45–46
  creativity, 50
  food introduction, 46
  Macaca fascicularis monkeys
    electrophysiology, 102
  magazine training, 46–47
  pimozide treatment, 32–35
  response shaping, 47, 48*f*, 49
lever-press studies
  avoidance task, 130
  dopamine receptor antagonists
    effects, 158
  shock avoidance–escape studies, 129
light signals, impending electrical shocks, 358
Lindqvist, Margitt, 41
Liou, Jiing-Ren, 158
Lister, Joshua, 133–4
little striped whiptail lizard *(Cnemidophorus
    inornatus)*, 196–7, 410
Livingstone, Margaret, 270

locomotion
  chronic dopamine depletion, 156–7
  dopamine receptor effects, 155–7
Locusta migratoria (migratory locust), 201
long-term incentive learning, 310–16
  AMPA receptors, 315–16
  CREB, 312–13
  ERK1/2, 312–13
  glutamate inputs, 314–15
  protein kinase A (PKA), 312–13
  protein synthesis, 312–14
long-term potentiation, short-term incentive
    learning, 311–12
Lorenz, Konrad, 26–27
love *see* intense romantic love
LSD (lysergic acid diethylamide), 19, 334–5
lurasidone, 228
LY 171555 *see* quinpirole (LY 171555)
lysergic acid diethylamide (LSD), 19, 334–5

macaque *(Macaca fascicularis)*
  electrophysiology, 100–2
    see also electrophysiology
  intense stimuli, 126
  novel stimuli, 124
  Parkinson's disease symptoms from chronic
    dopamine depletion, 157
MacDonald, Norma, 339
Madras, Bertha, 152
magazine training, lever pressing studies, 46–47
Magill, Peter, 131
magnetic resonance imaging (MRI)
  ADHD, 238
  history of, 113–14
    see also functional magnetic resonance
      imaging (fMRI)
Mansfield, Peter, 113
*The Man Who Mistook His Wife for a Hat and
    Other Clinical Tales* (Sacks), 345
marijuana, 15
  associated need state, 431
  onset of action, 251
  use cessation, 255
  see also Δ⁹-tetrahydrocannabinol (THC)
Markou, Athena, 15
Martin, James, 219–20, 222
masked *facies,* Parkinson's disease, 219
Mas, Manuel, 95
maternal behavior, 180
  oxytocin, 185
  rats, 187
Matsumoto, Masayuki, 131–2
Matteuchi, Carlo, 99
mazes
  latent learning, 83–84
  rats, 27–28
    see also eight-arm radial maze tests
McCoy, S N, 31–32

McDonald, Robert, 76–77
McGhie, Andrew, 338–9
McLelland, A Thomas, 263–4
meadow voles *(Microtus pennsylvanicus)*, 185–6
Meaney, Michael, 187
mechanoreception, 275–6
Mechoulam, Raphael, 247–8
medial diencephalic nuclei, 68
medial geniculate area, 271
medial prefrontal cortex
    feeding dopamine levels, 97
    in vivo electrochemistry, 107
medial temporal lobes
    bilateral lobectomy, 333–4
    declarative memory, 6, 68, 85
    HM, removal in, 5
    paired associate learning, 84
medium spiny neurons, 17–18, 286, 295
    dendritic spines, 286–7, 303–4
    direct/indirect pathway, 451
    dopamine receptors, 18, 288
    inputs in dorsal striatum, 288–9
Meissner corpuscles, 276
MEK 1/2 (mitogen-activated protein kinase
    1/2), 305–6
mental experience, 330–51
    amphetamine, 339–40
    animals, 345–50
    brain activity, 19
    brain–mind linkage, 330–5
    cocaine, 339–40
    dopamine and, 335–45
    dopamine receptor antagonist drugs, 340,
        344–5
    language-based communication, 20
    language/terminology problems, 349–50
    L-DOPA, 340–4
    psychoactive drugs, 334–5, 334–6
    schizophrenia, 337–9
Merkel cells, 276
mesoaccumbens system, 286
mesocortical dopaminergic system, 286
Mesocricetus auratus see Syrian hamsters
    (Mesocricetus auratus)
mesolimbic dopaminergic system, 286
    branching of, 287–8
mesolimbocortical system, 286
mesopontine rostromedial temporal
    nucleus, 266
metabotropic glutamate receptors, 442
methamphetamine, 170
1-methyl-4-phenyl-1,2,3,
    6-tetrahydropyridine (MPTP), 156
Mexican spadefoot toad *(Spea multiplicata)*, 198
microdialysis experiments
    aversive stimuli effects, 147
    intracerebral *see* intracerebral microdialysis
    novel stimuli, 125
Microtus monanus (montane voles), 186

Microtus ochrogaster see prairie voles *(Microtus
    ochrogaster)*
Microtus pennsylvanicus (meadow voles), 185–6
Miczek, Klaus, 189–90
migratory locust *(Locusta migratoria)*, 201
Miller, Joseph, 100
Miller, Robert, 158, 214, 215, 229, 292
Milner, Brenda, 5, 89
Milner, David, 331
Milner, Peter, 3, 29, 146
MIR 137, 209
Mirenowicz, Jacques, 130–1
mirror-drawing task, 70
misbehavior, 353
mitogen-activated protein kinase (MEK) 1/2,
    297–8, 305–6
mitogen- and stress-activated kinase-1
    (MSK1), 306
mobility time, descent latency scores, 139,
    140*f*, 141
Molaison, Henry, 333–4
monetary reward studies
    BOLD, 119–20
    PET, 115, 116–17
monkeys *see* macaque *(Macaca fascicularis)*
monoaminergic neurotransmitter systems, 29
montane voles *(Microtus monanus)*, 186
morphine, 15
    onset of action, 251
    self-administered drug studies, 246
Moser, Edvard, 278
Moser, May-Britt, 278
Moss, Jonathan, 287–8
Mosso, Angelo, 112
motor learning, L-DOPA mechanism of
    action, 235
motor system, neuroanatomy, 279–85
Mountcastle, Vernon, 276
Mouret, Jean-Roch, 92
Mowrer, Orval Hobart, 36
MPTP (1-methyl-4-phenyl-1,2,3,
    6-tetrahydropyridine), 156
MRI *see* magnetic resonance imaging (MRI)
MSK1 (mitogen- and stress-activated
    kinase-1), 306
Müller, Johannes, 99
multimodal cortical cells, 277–9
multiple memory systems, 5–6, 68–90
    animals, 75–82
        competition/cooperation between, 82–84
    brain regions, 71*f*
    evolution of, 81–82, 87–89
    humans, 68–75
        competition/cooperation between, 84–87
multi-round trust games, 179
muscarinic cholinergic receptors, 321–2
music, Parkinson's disease, 343
Myers, Robert D, 96
The Mystery of the Mind (Penfield), 333

nafadotride, 172–3
Nakazato, Taizo, 108
naloxone, 248
navigational memory, 86
need state
drugs of abuse, 258
marijuana, 431
negative prediction error, inverse incentive learning, 319
negative reinforcement, 36–37
Neill, Daryl, 96–97
Neisewander, Janet, 169–70, 187–8
Nestler, Eric, 317–18
neuroanatomy, 266–94
audition, 270–2
basal ganglia, 285–93
development across phyla, 282–5
dopamine systems, 285–93
gustation, 273–5
incentive learning, 16–17
multimodal cortical cells, 277–9
olfaction, 272–3
somatosensation, 275–7
vision, 267–70
neuroimaging, 111–21
ADHD, 238–9
dopamine and mental experience, 335
hippocampus interaction amygdala, 86–87
history of, 111–14
paired associate learning, 84–85
schizophrenia, 208, 210
techniques, 7, 8
see also functional magnetic resonance imaging (fMRI); magnetic resonance imaging (MRI)
neuropsychiatric disorders, 34–35
neurotransmitters, 6–7
schizophrenia, 217
NGB 2904, 172–3
Nicolelis, Miguel, 108
nicotine, 15, 246–7
conditioned incentive stimuli, 253
conditioned incentive stimuli reduction, 254
environment of use, 252
onset of action, 251, 252
reward properties, 54
reward-related learning, 249
self-administered drug studies, 170, 246
nigrostriatal dopaminergic system, 285–6
branching of neurons, 287–8
NMDA receptors, 296–7
D1-like receptor heterodimers, 11, 175, 302
glutamatergic inputs, 304
knockout mice, 249
mechanism of action, 297
phosphorylation of, 303–4
reward learning mechanisms, 327
NMR (nuclear magnetic resonance), 113

nociception, 275–6
non-declarative memory, 5–6, 68
Alzheimer's disease, 85
declarative memory vs., 89–90
definition, 70
Iowa gambling task, 74–75
Parkinson's disease, 89
probabilistic classification tasks in Parkinson's disease, 225
subtypes, 6
see also habit learning; incentive learning
non-pyramidal motor systems, 281–2
nose poke training studies, 308–9
novel stimuli, 8, 123, 323
dopamine release, 145
inverse incentive learning, 124–5
nuclear magnetic resonance (NMR), 113
nucleus accumbens
aversive stimuli studies, 127–9, 130
BOLD, 291
CREB, 309
direct pathway, 289
DOPAC:dopamine ratio, 93–94, 94–95
dopamine levels, 95, 98, 257
conditioned stimuli, 376
feeding, 97
human social cooperation, 182
HVA:dopamine ratio, 94–95
incentive learning, 16
indirect pathway, 289
medium spiny neurons, 295, 303–4
microdialysis experiments, 147
motor system, 280
novel stimuli, 124–5
prisoner's dilemma game, 178
protein kinase A, 308
schizophrenia, 217
in vivo electrochemistry, 107, 108, 109
in vivo microdialysis, 12

O'Brien, Charles, 263–4
O'Doherty, John, 118
odor coding, piriform cortex, 273
Ogawa, Seiji, 114
O'Keefe, John, 278
olanzepine, 228
adverse effects, 228–9
brain regions affected, 233
Olds, James, 29
olfaction, 272–3
reception/circuitry, 435
olfactory cortex, 273
olfactory receptors, 273
olfactory tubercule, 273
incentive learning, 16
medium spiny neurons, 295, 303–4
motor system, 280
operant conditioning, 36–37

opiates
  binding sites, 248
  environmental cues, 262–3
optic nerve, 267–9
optogenetics, 316
orofacial expressions, 348
Overmier, Bruce, 147
oxytocin
  animal social cooperation, 184–6
  incentive learning, 186
  maternal behavior, 185
  pair bonding, 185
  uterine contractions, 185

Pacinian corpuscles, 276
pair bonding, oxytocin, 185
paired associate learning, 84–85
Panksepp, Jaak, 189
parabrachial nucleus, 274
parasagittal occipitoparietal region, 331
Pari, Giovana, 73
Parkinson, James, 204
Parkinson's disease, 218–25
  ADHD as precursor, 239–40
  basal ganglia, 219–20
  declarative vs. incentive memory, 6
  diagnostic tests, 218
  dopaminergic neurons, 20, 21
    loss, 220, 222–3
    numbers, 13–14
  facial expressions, 219
  history of, 204
  incentive learning, 14, 73–74, 220–1, 223–4
  inverse incentive learning, 223–4
  kinesia paradoxa, 218–19, 221–2, 223
  masked facies, 219
  music, effects of, 343
  non-declarative memory tasks, 89
  non-declarative probabilistic classification task, 225
  patterned sensory inputs, 419
  point-loss avoidance task, 224–5
  probabilistic classification learning tasks, 73
  probabilistic selection tasks, 224
  symptoms, 218
    ADHD vs., 241–2
    chronic dopamine depletion, 156–7
  treatment, 14
    3,4-dihydroxyphenylalanine, 207
    dopamine receptor agonist drugs see
      dopamine receptor agonist drugs
      see also DOPA
      (3,4-dihydroxyphenylalanine)
    voice quality changes, 195–6
Partridge, George, 238
parvalbumin-expressing fast-spiking
      interneurons, 322–3
pathological gambling, 235

Paton, William, 152
patterned sensory inputs, Parkinson
      disease, 419
Patton, Harry, 99
Pauling, Linus, 114
Pavlov, Ivan, 36, 303
paw licking, 348
PCR (polymerase chain reaction), 391
PD168,077, 174
Penfield, Wilder, 19, 332-3
Perretta, James, 73
Pert, Candace, 152, 248
PET see positron emission tomography (PET)
Pfaus, James, 98
Phelps, Michael, 113
phenothiazines, 151–2
Phillips, Anthony, 80, 93–94, 94–95, 98, 160–1
phobia treatment, 37–38
phosphatases, 298, 300
phospholipase C pathway, 175
phosphorylation, AMPA receptors, 316
picture selection tests, 331
pigeons
  pecking for food, 26
    associated stimuli, 28–29
    response elicitation, 27
  pecking key discrimination task, 40
pigs, coins in piggy bank training, 26
pimozide
  brain stimulation reward experiments,
      30–31
  conditioned reward and, 80
  heroin conditioned place preference
      blocking, 251
  mechanism of action, 151–2, 364
  self-administered cocaine effects, 251
piriform cortex, odor coding, 273
PKA see protein kinase A (PKA)
PKC (protein kinase C), 297–8
place cells, hippocampus, 278
place conditioning apparatus, stimuli
      configuration, 360
place preference
  amphetamine, 4
  blocking, haloperidol, 4–5
Poecile atricapillus (black-capped chickadee),
      song learning, 87–88
point-loss avoidance task, 74
  Parkinson's disease, 224–5
Poldrack, Russell, 84
polymerase chain reaction (PCR), 391
positive social stimuli, BOLD of nucleus
      accumbens, 291
positron emission tomography (PET), 7, 8, 91,
      114–17
  ADHD, 239
  amphetamine studies, 115
  dopamine and mental experience, 335–6

ethanol, 247
fed *vs.* unfed, 114–15
fMRI *vs.*, 117
invention of, 112
monetary reward tasks, 115, 116–17
nicotine studies, 246–7
schizophrenia, 208
social cooperation in cynomolgus moneys
(*Macaca fascicularis*), 186
post-encephalitic behavior disorders, 238
postmortem dopamine assessment, 7, 91,
92–95
aversive stimuli studies, 126, 127
circadian rhythm, 92
HVA, 93–95
Parkinson's disease, 220
schizophrenia, 205, 207–8
sexual stimuli, 95
social cooperation in reptiles, 197
specific brain areas, 92
stimuli predictive of food, 94–95
treadmill running, 95
zebrafish (*Danio rerio*), 199
Post, Robert, 340
PP 1, 309
PP2A (protein phosphatase 2A), 298
prairie voles (*Microtus ochrogaster*)
monogamy-associated behavior, 185
pair bonding studies, 12, 185, 190
pramipexole
adverse effects, 235
cocaine self-administration studies, 171
prediction errors, 104–5
in vivo electrochemistry, 109–10
prefrontal cortex
aversive stimuli studies, 127–9
schizophrenia, 217
primary gustatory cortex, 274
primary somatosensory cortex, 277
primary visual cortex, 268
prisoner's dilemma game, 177–9
probabilistic classification learning tasks, 72–73
schizophrenia patients, 232–3
probabilistic selection tasks, 224
problem-solving behavior, 2
progressive ratio schedule, self-administration
protocols, 169
proprioception, 280
protein kinase A (PKA), 298
calcineurin *vs.*, 305
D1-like receptors, 18–19, 150
DARPP-32 phosphorylation, 305
long-term incentive learning, 312–13
nucleus accumbens, 308
protein kinase C (PKC), 297–8
protein phosphatase 2A (PP2A), 298
protein synthesis, long-term incentive
learning, 312–14

psychoactive drugs, 19
mental experience, 334–5, 334–6
psychogenic drugs, 205–7, 206*f*
psychosis
dopamine hypothesis, 206*f*, 412–13
drug treatment screening *see* conditioned
avoidance responding
Puglisi-Allegra, Stefano, 127–9
Purcell, Edward, 113
purchase incidence, 181
pursuit rotor task, HM (Henry Molaison),
69–70
push–pull cannulae technique, 96
putamen nuclei
dopamine hypothesis of schizophrenia, 207
incentive learning, 16
maternal love, 180
motor system, 280
schizophrenia, 217
Pycock, Christopher, 96
pyramidial motor system, 280

Quartarone, Susan, 318
quetiapine, 228
quinpirole (LY 171555)
cocaine self-administration studies, 171
incentive learning effects, 161, 162–3
locomotor activity effects, 156
Quinsey, Vernon, 189

raccoons, coin in box training, 26
raclopride
incentive learning function effects, 158, 159
radiolabeled studies, 114–16
radial maze tests *see* eight-arm radial maze
tests
radioisotopes, neuroimaging, 112–14
radish mutant, 310
Rall, Ted, 150
Ranaldi, Robert, 98, 326
Rang, Humphrey, 152
rat (*Rattus norvegicus*)
fed *vs.* starved
DOPAC:dopamine ratio, 93–94
HVA:dopamine ratio, 93–94
maternal behavior, 187
maze running, 27–28
reward-related learning and mental
experiences, 348
Rebec, George, 124–5
receptive-field axis, 268–9
receptors
CB1 receptor, 247
ghrelin (GHSR1a) receptor, 175–6
G protein-coupled receptors (GPCR), 154
growth hormone secretagogue receptor 1a, 11
heteromers, 174–6
metabotropic glutamate receptors, 442

receptors (*cont.*)
  muscarinic cholinergic receptors, 321–2
  olfactory receptors, 273
  serotonin receptors, 302–3
  somatosensation, 275
  taste receptors, 273
  see also adenosine A2A receptor; AMPA
      receptors; dopamine receptor(s);
      GABA (γ-aminobutyric acid)
      receptors; NMDA receptors
reinforcers, 23–24
  shift away from, 28
reserpine, 220
resident-intruder tests, 191–2
responses
  avoidance learning, 38–39
  lever pressing for food experiments, 47,
      48*f*, 49
  pigeons pecking for food, 27
restraint freeing, rats social cooperation, 188
rewarding stimuli
  associated stimuli, 28–29
  brain electrical stimulation, 3
  context effect, 24–25
  definition, 1
  descent latency sensitization and
      conditioning, 143
  dopamine neuron firing, 7
  incentive learning, 327–8
  terminology change to, 28
  types of, 21
  ventral tegmental area activation, 326
reward-related learning, 3, 23–43
  D1-like-/D2-like receptors, 10
  direct electrical stimulation of brain, 29
  dopamine effects, 146
  dopamine hypothesis development, 357
  dopamine receptor agonist drugs, 235
  dopaminergic neurotransmission
      activation, 249
  drugs of abuse, 245–6
  ventral tegmental area, 327
  in vivo electrochemistry, 107–8
  see also incentive learning
reward signalling, anti-psychotic drugs, 210
Reynolds, George Stanley, 40
rhythmic midline tongue protrusion, 348
ribosomal S6 kinase2 (RSK2), 306
Richardson, Mark, 86–87
Richardson, Nicole, 107
Rilling, James, 177–9
Riopell, Richard, 73–74
Risberg, Jarl, 112
risperidone, 228, 233
Ritters, Lauren, 193, 194
Robbins, Trevor, 161, 242
Robins, Lee N, 260–1
Robinson, Terry, 263–4, 314

Rocca, Jeffery, 133–4, 321
Rodbell, Martin, 391
Roentgen, Wilhelm Conrad, 111
Roitman, Mitchell, 108
romantic love *see* intense romantic love
ropinirole, 171, 235
route recognition tasks, brain areas, 86
R-SKF 83566, 156
rubrospinal tracts, motor systems, 282, 283
rutabaga mutant, 310

S33138, 167, 170
saccharine, 366
Sacks, Oliver, 340–4, 345
safety location, conditioned avoidance
      responding, 60, 64, 66
Sakata, Jon, 197–8
Salamone, John, 129
Salvelinus alpinus (Arctic char), 199–200
Sanghera, Manjit, 100
Saunders, Benjamin, 263–4
Sclafani, Anthony, 159
SCH 23390
  incentive learning effects, 158, 159
  inverse incentive learning, 321
  locomotor activity effects, 156
Schacter, Daniel, 81–82, 87–89
schedule training, brain stimulation
      experiments, 31–32
Schiff, Stanley, 94
Schimmel, Lexy, 134
schizophrenia, 13, 205–18
  dopamine hypothesis, 205–8, 206*f*, 412–13
  dopaminergic neurotransmission levels, 20, 21
  DSM-IV, 215–16
  excessive incentive learning, 415
  family psychoeducation/therapy, 231
  genetic studies, 208–9
  history of, 203–4
  hyperdopaminergic, 231–2
  incentive learning, 210–11, 215
  mental experience, 337–9
  neuroimaging, 208, 210
  neurotransmitters, 217
  relapse rate, 231
  revised dopamine hypothesis, 217–18
  symptoms, 203–4
    delusions, 212–14
    dopamine receptor agonist drugs, 236
    hallucinations, 214–15
  treatment
    antipsychotic drugs, 14, 227
    chlorpromazine, 41
Schmidt, Werner, 8–9, 132–3
Schultz, Wolfram, 100–2, 104–5, 119
  aversive stimuli studies, 130–1
  inverse incentive learning, 319
  in vivo electrochemistry, 106–7

Scoville, Henry, 68
scrub jays *(Aphelocoma coerulescens)*, 75
seed caching, 87–89
Seeman, Philip, 152
    schizophrenia studies, 205, 207–8
Seiden, Lewis, 92–93, 237
selectionism, behavior reinforcement, 49–50
self-administered drug studies
    amphetamine, 250–1
    cocaine, 170, 171, 246, 250–1
    dopamine receptor knockout studies,
        167–70
    drugs of abuse, 246
    intracerebral microdialysis, 98
    WIN 55, 212-2, 250
Seligman, Martin, 147
semantic knowledge, cultural norms, 214
semantic memory, 75
sensitization, 58
sensory perceptual information processing,
    291–2
sensory/perceptual system, incentive
    learning, 16
serotonin receptors, 302–3
Settler, Paulette, 30–31
sexual behavior
    C uniparens, 410
    intracerebral microdialysis, 98
    in vivo electrochemistry, 109
sexual stimuli studies
    BOLD, 118
    DOPAC:dopamine ratio, 95
    postmortem dopamine assessment, 95
Sherrington, Charles, 276
Sherry, David, 81–82, 87–89
short-term incentive learning, 310–16
    AMPA receptors, 311, 312
    CaMKII, 311
    Kv4.2, 311, 312
    long-term potentiation, 311–12
shuttle box experiments, dual-chamber, 35–36
Siegel, Shepard, 261–2
signal integration, gustation, 274
Simansky, Kevin, 94
single nucleotide polymorphisms (SNPs),
    schizophrenia, 209
SKF 38393
    incentive learning function effects, 161,
        162, 163
    locomotor activity effects, 156
Skinhøj, Erik, 112
Skinner box, 3–4, 45
    see also lever-press response for food studies
Skinner, Burrhus F, 2, 25–26, 45, 49, 196
SL327, 250
Smith, Carlyle, 39–40
Smith, Gerald, 94
Smithies, Oliver, 164

Snyder, Solomon, 150, 152, 248
social cooperation, 177–202
    animals, non-human, 184–201
        amphibians, 198
        birds, 192–6
        fish, 198–200
        insects, 200–1
        monkeys, 186
        prairie voles, 190
        rats, 186–90
        reptiles, 196–8
    humans, 177–84, 183*f*
social history, incentive stimuli, 409
social reward studies, Syrian hamsters
        (Mesocricetus auratus), 191
Sokoloff, Pierre, 315
Solomon, Richard, 147
somatosensation, neuroanatomy, 275–7
songbirds, 12–13
    song learning, 87–89
song–mating reward studies, 194–5
Søvik, Erik, 284–5
Spano, Philip Franco, 153
spatial learning
    eight-arm radial maze tests, 77–78
    hippocampal lesion effects, 82
Spealman, Roger, 295
Spea multiplicata (Mexican spadefoot toad), 198
species-typical responses, 39–40
Spence, Kenneth, 2, 109
Sperry, Roger, 330–1
Spindler, Joan, 32–35
Squire, Larry, 225
state of readiness, 292
STEP *see* striatal-enriched phosphatase (STEP)
stimulus–response learning, 23–28
    brain lesion effects, 82
stimulus–stimulus associative learning, 82
St Onge, Jennifer, 174
Strange, Bryan, 86–87
Strausfeld, Nicholas, 200, 284
stress system, 257–8
striatal circuits, novel stimuli, 323
striatal-enriched phosphatase (STEP), 300, 301*f*
    activation, 306
striatal output nuclei, motor systems, 281–2
striatonigrostriatal circuits, 290
striatum
    development, dopamine role, 165–6
    DOPAC:dopamine ratio, fed *vs.* starved rats,
        93–94
    dopamine hypothesis of schizophrenia, 207
    medium spiny neurons, 295
    motor systems, 283
    in vivo electrochemistry, 108–9
Stricker, Edward, 106
Sturnus vulgaris (European starling), 193, 194
substance P, 288

substantia nigra
  electrophysiology in humans, 103
  intense stimuli, 126
  maternal love, 180
superior olive, audition, 271
Surmeier, D James, 323
Sutherland, Earl, 149–50
synaptic plasticity, 143–4
Syrian hamsters (*Mesocricetus auratus*)
  pair bonds, 12
  social cooperation, 191–2
  social reward studies, 191
systematic desensitization, 38

Taeniopygia guttata (zebra finches), 193, 194
taste receptors, 273
tectospinal tracts, motor systems, 282
Ter-Pogossian, Michel, 113
terminal boutons, 286
terminology, problems with, 349–50
Δ^9-tetrahydrocannabinol (THC), 247–8
  conditioned place preference, SL327,
    blocking by, 250
  marijuana, 431
  reward properties, 54
  self-administered drug studies, 246
  see also marijuana
thalamostriatal projections, 440
thalamus, motor systems, 283
THC *see* Δ^9-tetrahydrocannabinol (THC)
theophylline, 321
thermoreception, 275–6
Thorazine *see* chlorpromazine
thioridazine, 226
Thorndike, Edward, 1–2, 27
threat conditioning, 358
  see also aversive conditioning
Tinbergen, Nikolaas, 26–27
Tolman, Edward C, 45–46, 77, 83–84
tone–shock association, conditioned
    avoidance responding, 64–66
tone signals, impending electrical shocks, 358
tonic activity, electrophysiology in *Macaca
    fascicularis* monkeys, 101
Trabucci, Michelle, 153
training
  effects of, 376
  electrophysiology of water-restricted rats, 104
Trainspotting (Welsh), 258–9
treadmill running, 95
trifluoperazine, 226
Tulving, Endel, 75
turnip mutant, 310
two-choice task, sequence of events, 72
two-factor theory, avoidance conditioning,
    36–38
two-way avoidance training in rats, 39–40

typical antipsychotic drugs, 229
  brain regions affected, 232–3
tyrosine hydroxylase, 196–7

unconditioned incentive stimuli, 409
Ungerstedt, Urbam, 96
Ungless, Mark, 131
Unterwald, Ellen, 318
Upon Further Reflection (Skinner), 49
uterine contractions, oxytocin, 185

Valenstein, Elliot, 333
Valium (diazepam), 387
van Rossum, Jacques, 151
vasopressin
  animal social cooperation, 184–6
  incentive learning, 186
  kidney fluid retention, 185
  monogamy-associated behavior, 185
ventral midbrain, 285
  information processing, 80
ventral striatum, incentive learning, 16, 290
ventral tegmental area
  feeding dopamine levels, 97
  glutamatergic synapses, 326–7
  reward learning mechanisms, 327
ventrolateral occipital cortex, 331
Verbal Learning (Skinner), 196
Vietnam war (1955-1975), drugs of abuse,
    260–1, 262
vision
  mental experience, 332
  neuroanatomy, 267–70
visual fields, 268
  testing of, 331
vocalization, rat social cooperation, 188–9
Voermans, Nicol, 86
Volkow, Nora, 239, 257, 335
von Economo, Constantin, 238
von Humboldt, Alexander, 99
Voruganti, Lakshmi, 247–8

Wang, Zuoxin, 190
Watson, John B, 2
wax-moth larvae, 75
WC44, 170
weather prediction task, fMRI, 84–85
weight gain, 228–9
Welsh, Irving, 258–9
what–when–where events, 75
White, Francis, 257
Wickens, Jeffrey, 104, 297
Wickens, Rebekah, 318
Wiegert, Simon, 306
Wiesel, Torston, 267–9
Wightman, Mark, 107–8
Wikler, Abraham, 262–3

WIN 55, 212–2, 250
winner effect, 191–2
Wise, Roy, 32–35, 98, 103, 125, 146, 251, 347–8
Wnt signaling pathway, 319
Woodbury, J Walter, 99

X-rays, discovery of, 111
Xu, Kathleen, 141, 142*f*, 319
Xylocopa appendiculata (carpenter bee), 201

Yalow, Rosalyn, 92
Yamamoto, Takashi, 274–5
Yao, Wei-Dong, 295
Yokel, Robert, 251

Zahm, Daniel S, 266
Zald, David, 115–16
Zarevics, Peter, 30–31
zebra finches *(Taeniopygia guttata)*, 193, 194
zebrafish *(Danio rerio)*, 13
    social cooperation, 199
    in vivo electrochemistry, 108
Zhang, Jongping, 295
Zigmond, Michael, 106
ziprasidone, 228
Zweifel, Larry, 166